D0026305

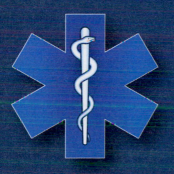

PREHOSPITAL EMERGENCY PHARMACOLOGY

SEVENTH EDITION

BRYAN E. BLEDSOE, DO, FACEP, FAAEM, EMT-P
Professor of Emergency Medicine
Director, Prehospital and Disaster Medicine Fellowship
University of Nevada School of Medicine
Attending Emergency Physician
University Medical Center of Southern Nevada
Las Vegas, Nevada

DWAYNE E. CLAYDEN, MEM, BHSC, PARAMEDIC
Academic Chair
Prehospital Care Programs
School of Health and Public Safety
SAIT Polytechnic
Calgary, Alberta Canada

PEARSON

Boston   Columbus   Indianapolis   New York   San Francisco   Upper Saddle River
Amsterdam   Cape Town   Dubai   London   Madrid   Milan   Munich   Paris   Montreal   Toronto
Delhi   Mexico City   São Paulo   Sydney   Hong Kong   Seoul   Singapore   Taipei   Tokyo

Publisher: Julie Levin Alexander
Publisher's Assistant: Regina Bruno
Editor-in-Chief: Marlene McHugh Pratt
Senior Managing Editor for Development: Lois Berlowitz
Assistant Editor: Jonathan Cheung
Director of Marketing: David Gesell
Executive Marketing Manager: Katrin Beacom
Marketing Manager: Brian Hoehl
Marketing Specialist: Michael Sirinides
Managing Editor for Production: Patrick Walsh
Production Liaison: Faye Gemmellaro

Production Editor: Emily Bush, S4Carlisle Publishing Services
Manufacturing Manager: Ilene Sanford
Manufacturing Buyer: Lisa McDowell
Art Director: Christopher Weigand
Cover Design: Jill Little
Interior Design: S4Carlisle Publishing Services
Editorial Media Manager: Amy Peltier
Media Project Manager: Lorena Cerisano
Composition: S4Carlisle Publishing Services
Printer/Binder: QuadGraphics/Dubuque
Cover Printer: Lehigh-Phoenix Color/Hagerstown

Copyright © 2012, 2005, 2001, 1996, 1992 by Pearson Education, Inc. All rights reserved. Manufactured in the United States of America. This publication is protected by Copyright and permission should be obtained from the publisher prior to any prohibited reproduction, storage in a retrieval system, or transmission in any form or by any means, electronic, mechanical, photocopying, recording, or likewise. To obtain permission(s) to use material from this work, please submit a written request to Pearson Education, Inc., Permissions Department, One Lake Street, Upper Saddle River, New Jersey 07458 or you may fax your request to 201-236-3290.

Library of Congress Cataloging-in-Publication Data

Bledsoe, Bryan E., (Date)
  Prehospital emergency pharmacology/Bryan E. Bledsoe, Dwayne E. Clayden. — 7th ed.
    p. ; cm.
  Includes index.
  ISBN-13: 978-0-13-513822-9
  ISBN-10: 0-13-513822-1
  I. Clayden, Dwayne E. II. Title.
  [DNLM: 1. Emergency Treatment. 2. Drug Therapy. WB 105]
  LC classification not assigned
  616.02'5—dc23

                                                    2011033619

NOTICE

The author and the publisher of this book have taken care to make certain that the information given is correct and compatible with the standards generally accepted at the time of publication. Nevertheless, as new information becomes available, changes in treatment and in the use of equipment and procedures become necessary. The reader is advised to carefully consult the instruction and information material included in each piece of equipment or device before administration. Students are warned that the use of any techniques must be authorized by their medical advisor, where appropriate, in accordance with local laws and regulations. The publisher disclaims any liability, loss, injury, or damage incurred as a consequence, directly or indirectly, of the use and application of any of the contents of this book.

10 9 8 7 6 5 4 3 2 1

Brady
is an imprint of

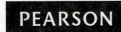

www.bradybooks.com

ISBN 10:   0-13-513822-1
ISBN 13: 978-0-13-513822-9

CONTENTS

PREFACE

Modern emergency medical service (EMS) is based on sound principles, practice, and research. The paramedic of today must be knowledgeable in all aspects of prehospital emergency medicine. Nowhere is this more important than when administering medications. *Prehospital Emergency Pharmacology* is a complete guide to the most common medications used in prehospital emergency care. This comprehensive text is designed with two purposes in mind: First, it is a complete pharmacology teaching text. Second, it is a handy reference to the most common medications and fluids used in prehospital care.

Welcome to the seventh edition of *Prehospital Emergency Pharmacology*. This text has been a cornerstone of EMS education for more than 25 years. The seventh edition has been extensively revised to reflect current trends in prehospital care. EMS is undergoing an essential evolutionary step in that modern prehospital practice must be based on sound scientific principles. We have been careful to ensure that the seventh edition reflects the trend toward evidenced-based practice. However, practices and formularies are different among regions and among countries. We have attempted to make the text as comprehensive as possible. We hope that *Prehospital Emergency Pharmacology* will prove a valuable aid to both the practicing paramedic and paramedic student.

It is the intent of the authors and publishers that this textbook be used as part of a formal paramedic education program taught by a qualified instructor and supervised by a licensed physician. The knowledge and skills outlined in this textbook are best learned in the classroom, skills laboratory, and then the clinical field setting. It is important to point out that this or any other text cannot teach skills. Care skills are learned only under the watchful eye of a paramedic instructor and perfected during clinical and field internships.

The care procedures presented here represent accepted practices in the United States and Canada. They are not offered as a standard of care. Paramedic-level care is to be performed only under the authority and guidance of a licensed physician. It is the reader's responsibility to know and follow local care protocols and standing orders as provided by medical advisers directing the system to which he or she belongs. Also, it is the reader's responsibility to stay informed of emergency care procedures and changes.

Bryan E. Bledsoe, DO, FACEP, FAAEM, EMT-P

Dwayne E. Clayden, MEM, BHSC, PARAMEDIC

ACKNOWLEDGMENTS

We wish to acknowledge the talents and efforts of the following people who contributed to *Prehospital Emergency Pharmacology*.

CHAPTER AUTHORS

We would like to thank Matthew S. Zavarella, MS, CRNA, NREMT-P, CFRN, CCRN, CEN for his work on the Chapter 4 Practice Problems. He has written example problems that are essential and vital to learning all aspects of pharmacology.

REVISED TEXT REVIEWERS

We appreciate the dedication of the text reviewers to this profession and especially appreciate their efforts in reviewing the revision of this text. The quality of the reviewers' comments and suggestions were invaluable as we revised this text. The assistance provided by these EMS experts is deeply appreciated.

Harvey Conner, AS, NREMT-P
Professor of EMS
Oklahoma City Community College EMS Program
Oklahoma City, OK

Jim Fox, EMT-PS, EMS-I
EMS Assistant Coordinator/ Instructor
Des Moines Fire Department
Des Moines, IA

Peter S. Golenia, PharmD, BCPS
Clinical Pharmacy Specialist, Emergency Medicine
Boston Medical Center
Boston, MA

Darren P. Lacroix, AAS, EMT-P
Educational Service Specialist
Gulf Coast Area Health Education Council, Del Mar College, Lacrdal Medical
Corpus Christi, TX

Richelle Laipply, PhD
Professor Allied Health
University of Akron
Akron, OH

Dean C. Meenach, AAS, RN, BSN, CEN, CCRN, EMT-P
Director of EMS Education
Mineral Area College
Park Hills, MO

Christopher T. Owens, PharmD, BCPS
Associate Professor & Chair
Department of Pharmacy Practice & Administrative Sciences
Idaho State University College of Pharmacy
Pocatello, ID

Valerie D. Simonds, MS, RN, NREMT-P
Professor (retired EMT Department Chair, Anne Arundel Community College,
Arnold, MD)
Adjunct faculty, University of Maryland, Maryland Fire and Rescue Institute (MFRI)
College Park, MD

Matthew S. Zavarella, MS, CRNA, NREMT-P, CFRN, CCRN, CEN
EMS Instructor
Westmoreland Community College
Pittsburgh, PA

DEVELOPMENT AND PRODUCTION

We would like to acknowledge the efforts and support of many talented individuals who assisted with the seventh edition.

First, we would like to thank Julie Alexander, publisher at Brady, and Marlene Pratt, editor-in-chief, for their ongoing support of this text and our other EMS projects. We would also like to thank Jonathan Cheung, Lois Berlowitz, and Faye Gemmellaro for their hard work in bringing this project to completion.

ABOUT THE AUTHORS

BRYAN E. BLEDSOE, DO, FACEP, FAAEM, EMT-P

Dr. Bryan Bledsoe is an emergency physician, researcher, and EMS author. Presently he is Professor of Emergency Medicine and Director of the EMS Fellowship program at the University of Nevada School of Medicine and an Attending Emergency Physician at the University Medical Center of Southern Nevada in Las Vegas. He is board-certified in emergency medicine.

Prior to attending medical school, Dr. Bledsoe worked as an EMT, a paramedic, and a paramedic instructor. He completed EMT training in 1974 and paramedic training in 1976 and worked for 6 years as a field paramedic in Fort Worth, Texas. In 1979, he joined the faculty of the University of North Texas Health Sciences Center and served as coordinator of EMT and paramedic education programs at the university. Dr. Bledsoe is active in emergency medicine and EMS research. He is a popular speaker at state, national, and international seminars and writes regularly for numerous EMS journals. He is active in educational endeavors with the United States Special Operations Command (USSOCOM) and the University of Nevada at Las Vegas.

Dr. Bledsoe is the author of numerous EMS textbooks and has in excess of 1 million books in print. Dr. Bledsoe was named a "Hero of Emergency Medicine" in 2008 by the American College of Emergency Physicians as a part of their 40th Anniversary celebration and was named a "Hero of Health and Fitness" by *Men's Health* magazine as part of their 20th anniversary edition in November of 2008. He is frequently interviewed in the national media. Dr. Bledsoe is married and divides his time between his residences in Midlothian, TX and Las Vegas, NV.

DWAYNE E. CLAYDEN, MEM, BHSC, PARAMEDIC

Dwayne Clayden is the Academic Chair, Prehospital Care Programs in the School of Health and Public Safety at SAIT Polytechnic, Calgary, Alberta Canada. He was previously Manager, Learning and Development for Alberta Health Services—Emergency Medical Services; Assistant Deputy Chief, Staff Development and Assistant to the Medical Director for the City of Calgary Emergency Medical Services in Calgary, Alberta, Canada. He was responsible for clinical competency assessment, field training, prehospital research, quality care, the in-house paramedic program, and the tactical EMS team.

In 2000 the Governor General of Canada presented Mr. Clayden with the Exemplary Service Medal for his contributions to EMS in Canada. In 1998 the Alberta Prehospital Professions Association presented him with the Award of Excellence for his contributions to Emergency Medical Services in Alberta.

Mr. Clayden began his career in 1978 as a police officer in Calgary. In 1980 he joined the Calgary Fire Department, Ambulance Division, as an emergency medical technician (EMT). Following his paramedic education at the Southern Alberta Institute of Technology (SAIT), he became a member of the Staff Development Division of the City of Calgary Emergency Medical Services. In 1987 he began his teaching career at SAIT, first in the EMT program and then in 1988 in the paramedic program. In August 2011 he returned to SAIT Polytechnic as the Academic Chair, Prehospital Care Programs.

From 1991 to 1996, Mr. Clayden was the publisher and editor-in-chief of *ON SCENE,* an EMS periodical for Canadian EMS. He has co-authored two texts with Dr. Bryan Bledsoe for Brady Publishing, *Prehospital Emergency Pharmacology* and *Pocket Reference for EMTs and Paramedics* and co-authored *Essentials of Paramedic Care, Canadian Edition.*

Mr. Clayden is very proud of his four children, Meagan, Lauren, Matthew, and Kaitlyn.

NOTICES

NOTICE ON DRUGS AND DRUG DOSAGES

Every effort has been made to ensure that the drug dosages presented in the textbook are in accordance with nationally accepted standards. When applicable, the dosages and routes are taken from the American Heart Association's Advanced Cardiac Life Support Guidelines. The American Medical Association's publication *Drug Evaluations,* the *Physicians' Desk Reference,* and Appleton & Lange's *Health Professions Drug Guide 2004* are followed with regard to drug dosages not covered by the American Heart Association's guidelines. It is the responsibility of the reader to be familiar with the drugs used in his or her system, as well as the dosages specified by the medical director. The drugs presented in this text should be administered only by direct order, whether verbally or through accepted standing orders, by a licensed physician.

NOTICE ON GENDER USAGE

The English language has historically given preference to the male gender. Among many words, the pronouns "he" and "his" are commonly used to describe both genders. Society evolves faster than language and the male pronouns still predominate in our speech. The authors have made great effort to treat the two genders equally, recognizing that a significant percentage of paramedics and patients are female. However, in some instances, male pronouns may be used to describe both male and female paramedics and patients solely for the purpose of brevity. This is not intended to offend any readers.

PRECAUTIONS ON BLOODBORNE PATHOGENS AND INFECTIOUS DISEASES

Prehospital emergency personnel, like all health care workers, are at risk for exposure to bloodborne pathogens and infectious diseases. In emergency situations it is often difficult to take or enforce proper infection control measures. However, paramedics must recognize their high-risk status. Readers should study the following information on infection control before turning to the main portion of this book.

Infection control is designed to protect emergency personnel, their families, and their patients from unnecessary exposure to communicable diseases.

Laws, regulations, and standards regarding infection control include the following:

- *Centers for Disease Control and Prevention (CDC).* The CDC has published extensive guidelines regarding infection control. Proper equipment and techniques that should be used by emergency response personnel to prevent or minimize risk of exposure are defined.

- *The Ryan White Act.* The Ryan White Act of 1990 allows emergency personnel to find out if they were exposed to an infectious disease while rendering patient care. Employers are required to name a "designated officer" to coordinate communications with the treating hospital.

- *Americans with Disabilities Act.* This act prohibits discrimination against individuals with disabilities, including those with contagious diseases. It guarantees equal employment opportunities and job protection if the infected individual can perform essential job functions and does not pose a threat to the safety and health of patients and coworkers.

- *Health Insurance Portability and Accountability Act of 1996 (HIPAA).* HIPAA significantly increased patient confidentiality and restricted access to medical records. Despite this, provisions were made in the act that allow for access to information related to possible exposure to infectious diseases. Thus, HIPAA does not prohibit infectious disease exposure notification, testing, and follow-up for EMS personnel.

- *Occupational Safety and Health Administration (OSHA) Regulations.* OSHA enacted a regulation entitled Occupational Exposure to Bloodborne Pathogens that classifies emergency response personnel as being at the greatest risk of occupational exposure to communicable diseases. This regulation requires employers to provide hepatitis B (HBV) vaccinations free of charge, maintain a written exposure control plan, and provide personal protective equipment. These requirements apply primarily to private employers. Applicability to local and state governmental employees varies by locality. Many states have developed their own OSHA plans.

- *National Fire Protection Association (NFPA) Guidelines.* This is a national organization that has established specific guidelines and requirements regarding infection control for emergency response agencies, particularly fire departments and emergency medical service agencies.

STANDARD PRECAUTIONS AND PERSONAL PROTECTIVE EQUIPMENT

Standard Precautions

Standard Precautions is a strategy that is based on the assumption that all blood and body fluids are infectious. It dictates that all EMS personnel use Standard Precautions with every patient. To achieve this, appropriate personal protective equipment (PPE) should be available in every emergency vehicle. The minimum recommended PPE includes the following:

- *Protective gloves.* Wear disposable protective gloves before initiating any emergency care. When an emergency involves more than one patient, change gloves between patients. When gloves have been contaminated, remove and dispose of them properly as soon as possible.
- *Masks and protective eyewear.* These should be worn together whenever blood spatter is likely to occur, such as with arterial bleeding, childbirth, endotracheal intubation and other invasive procedures, oral suctioning, and cleanup of equipment that requires heavy scrubbing or brushing. Both you and your patient should wear masks whenever the potential for airborne transmission of disease exists.
- *HEPA and N-95 respirators.* Due to the resurgence of tuberculosis (TB), you must protect yourself from infection through the use of a high-efficiency particulate air (HEPA) or N-95 respirator. Wear one whenever you care for a patient with confirmed or suspected TB, especially during procedures that involve the airway, such as the administration of nebulized medications, endotracheal intubation, or suctioning.
- *Gowns.* Disposable gowns protect your clothing from splashes. If large splashes of blood are expected, such as with childbirth, wear an impervious gown.
- *Resuscitation equipment.* Use disposable resuscitation equipment as your primary means of artificial ventilation in emergency care.

HANDLING CONTAMINATED MATERIAL

Many of the materials associated with the emergency response become contaminated with possibly infectious body fluids and substances. These include soiled linen, patient clothing and dressings, and used care equipment, including intravenous needles. It is important that prehospital personnel collect these materials at the scene and dispose of them appropriately to ensure their safety as well as that of their patients, their family members, bystanders, and fellow caregivers. Contaminated materials should be disposed of according to the following recommendations:

- Handle contaminated materials only while wearing the appropriate PPE.
- Place all blood- or body-fluid-contaminated clothing, linen, dressings, and patient care equipment and supplies in properly marked biological hazard bags and ensure that they are disposed of properly.
- Ensure that all used needles, scalpels, and other contaminated objects that have the potential to puncture the skin are properly secured in a puncture-resistant and clearly marked sharps container.
- Do not recap a needle after use; stick it into a seat cushion or other object, or leave it lying on the ground. These practices increase the risk of an accidental needlestick.

- Always scan the scene before leaving to ensure that all equipment has been retrieved and all potentially infectious material has been bagged and removed.

- If prehospital personnel are exposed to an infectious disease, have contact with body fluid with a route for system entry (such as an open wound on a hand when a glove tears while moving a soiled patient), or receive a needlestick with a used needle, the receiving hospital should be alerted and the service's infection control officer contacted immediately.

Following these recommendations will help protect paramedics and the people they care for from the dangers of disease transmission.

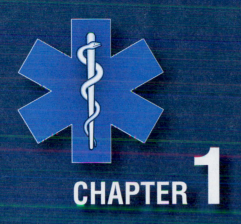

CHAPTER 1   GENERAL INFORMATION

OBJECTIVES

After completing this chapter, the reader should be able to:

- Define the terms *pharmacology, pharmacologists,* and *pharmacognosy.*
- List four medication sources and give examples of each source.
- Understand common pharmacological terminology and abbreviations.
- List four references for medication information and demonstrate how to find a medication in one of these references.
- Describe the four phases of medication development.
- Explain the legal regulations that apply to medications, including the schedule of controlled medications.
- Identify medications by their chemical name, generic name, trade name, and official name.
- List several examples of both liquid and solid medications.

INTRODUCTION

Drugs are chemical agents used in the diagnosis, treatment, or prevention of disease. When used in a medical setting, drugs, are commonly referred to as **medications**. The study of drugs and their actions on the body is called **pharmacology**. Scientists who study the effects of drugs on the body are called **pharmacologists**. It is through experimental pharmacology that medicine has made many of its most profound advances.

Historical Considerations

The use of herbs and minerals to treat various medical disorders is as old as the practice of medicine itself. Written records of drug use date back to early Egyptian times. Ancient Egyptians, Arabs, and Greeks probably passed formulations down through generations by word of mouth for centuries until they were recorded in pharmacopeias. Hippocrates, generally considered the father of modern medicine, wrote extensively on the use of drugs, although he rarely used them in the care of his patients. After the Renaissance, healers began to take a somewhat more scientific approach to disease and found that certain drugs were useful in treating some disorders but not others. Drug therapy was based largely on observation, and physicians were frequently unsure which body systems the drugs affected. Pharmacology had now become a distinct and growing discipline, separate from medicine.

One common additive to early medications was the purple foxglove plant. A common flowering plant, the purple foxglove was first described in A.D. 1250 by Welsh physicians. It was long thought to be a diuretic because of its role in the treatment of dropsy, an old term used to describe the generalized body edema associated with congestive heart failure. In 1785 William Withering described the use of the purple foxglove plant in the treatment of dropsy and other disorders. Although he did not associate the improvement seen in the treatment of dropsy with the foxglove's effect on the heart, he did note its effectiveness. He wrote, "It has a power over the motion of the heart to a degree yet unobserved in any other medicine." It was not until 1800 that the effect of foxglove specifically on the heart was actually described and its suspected action as a diuretic finally discarded.

Digitalis glycosides are the active agents in foxglove. Digitalis glycosides tend to increase myocardial contractile force. It is this increase in cardiac performance, with subsequently improved renal perfusion and filtration, that causes a reduction in the body swelling and not its diuretic effect as earlier thought. Even today digitalis glycosides remain one of the most commonly prescribed medications in the treatment of congestive heart failure and other cardiovascular disorders.

During the seventeenth and eighteenth centuries, tinctures of opium, coca, and digitalis were available. The related concept of vaccination from biologic extracts began in 1796 with Edward Jenner's smallpox inoculations. By the nineteenth century, atropine, chloroform, codeine, ether, and morphine were in use. The discoveries of animal insulin and penicillin in the early twentieth century dramatically changed the treatment of endocrine/metabolic and infectious diseases. Now, at the start of the twenty-first century, **recombinant DNA technology** has produced human insulin and recombinant tissue plasminogen activator (r-tPA). These medications have markedly changed the treatment of diabetes and cardiovascular disease.

Medicine changed dramatically in the early part of the twentieth century with the discovery of antibiotics. Prior to the introduction of the sulfa-class antibiotics in 1935, physicians had virtually no effective therapy for infections. Penicillin became widely available in the early 1940s, thus providing physicians a versatile yet inexpensive antibiotic. Additional antibiotics were subsequently developed. The introduction of antibiotic therapy resulted in a significant decrease in mortality and a resultant increase in life expectancy in the United States and other developed countries.

Pharmacognosy

Traditionally, **pharmacognosy** refers to the study of natural drug sources, such as plants, animals, or minerals and their products. Today, however, chemicals developed and used in the laboratory allow researchers to increase the number of medication sources. For example, oral contraceptives, which are synthetic analogues of human sex hormones, are manufactured via chemical methods (synthetically).

Researchers and drug developers also can now manipulate the molecular structure of substances, such as antibiotics, so that a slight change in chemical structure makes the drug effective against different organisms.

The hormone insulin, used to treat diabetes mellitus, was customarily obtained from the pancreas of slaughtered animals, mainly cattle and pigs. Although animal insulin is not chemically identical to human insulin, it is physiologically active in humans. Porcine insulin (insulin derived from pigs) most nearly resembles human insulin. The chemical alteration of three amino acids in porcine insulin makes it identical to human endogenous insulin. The chemically altered porcine insulin is marketed and usually referred to as "human insulin." Medication developers also can manufacture true human insulin from bacteria through recombinant deoxyribonucleic acid (DNA) technology.

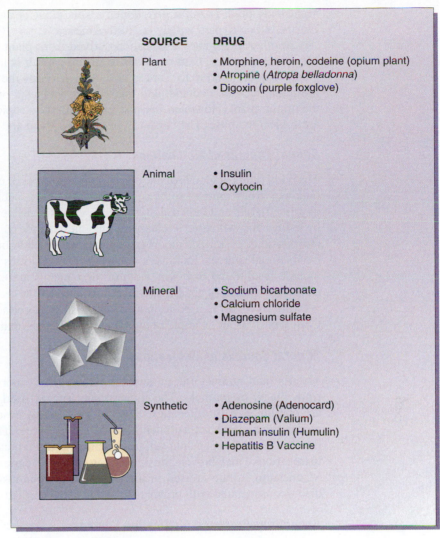

SOURCE	DRUG
Plant	• Morphine, heroin, codeine (opium plant) • Atropine (*Atropa belladonna*) • Digoxin (purple foxglove)
Animal	• Insulin • Oxytocin
Mineral	• Sodium bicarbonate • Calcium chloride • Magnesium sulfate
Synthetic	• Adenosine (Adenocard) • Diazepam (Valium) • Human insulin (Humulin) • Hepatitis B Vaccine

● **FIGURE 1–1**   Medication sources.

The four main sources of medications are plants, animals, minerals, and the laboratory (synthetic) (see Figure 1–1).

Plant Sources of Medications

Plants may be the oldest source of medications. The earliest concoctions using plants as medication sources consisted of the entire plant, including leaves, roots, bulb, stem, seeds, buds, and blossoms. Some of the extra material was harmful to human tissues. As the understanding of plants as a medication source became more sophisticated, researchers sought to isolate the active components (the components that caused the medication's effect) and avoid the harmful material.

The active components consist of several types and vary in character and effect. The most important are alkaloids (one of the largest groups of active components), which act as alkali. The organic alkaloids react with acids to form a salt. This salt, a neutralized or partially neutralized form, is more readily soluble in body fluids. The names of alkaloids and their salts usually end in -ine; examples include atropine, caffeine, and nicotine. Atropine sulfate is used in the treatment of slow heart rates and in certain types of toxicological emergencies. Atropine is derived from the deadly nightshade plant (*Atropa belladonna*). This plant is native to central and southern Europe but cultivated widely in North America.

Another emergency medication derived from plant sources is morphine sulfate. Morphine is used to treat moderate to severe pain. It is made from parts of the opium plant, which is native to Turkey and other parts of the Middle East. In addition to morphine, heroin, codeine, and many other analgesic preparations are derived from the opium plant. However, because of their psychotropic effects, narcotic analgesics are subject to abuse. They also can result in physical and psychological dependence.

Animal Sources of Medications

The body fluids or glands of animals can act as sources of medications. The medications obtained from animal sources include hormones, such as insulin (as previously discussed); oils and fats (usually mixed), such as cod-liver oil; and enzymes, produced by living cells, which act as catalysts. Enzymes include pancreatin and pepsin. Vaccines (suspensions of killed, modified, or attenuated microorganisms) also are obtained from animal sources. Examples of hormone medications derived from animal sources include insulin and oxytocin. Both of these agents are extracted from the desiccated endocrine glands of mammals. Insulin is used in the treatment of diabetes mellitus, whereas oxytocin is used to induce labor and treat certain types of vaginal bleeding. Cod-liver oil is an example of an oil derived from animals.

Mineral Sources of Medications

Metallic and nonmetallic minerals provide various inorganic material not available from plants or animals. The mineral sources are used as they occur in nature or are combined with other ingredients to yield acids, bases, or salts. Two emergency medications come from mineral (inorganic) sources. They are sodium bicarbonate ($NaHCO_3$) and magnesium sulfate ($MgSO_4$). Sodium bicarbonate is occasionally used to treat severe metabolic acidosis and is an adjunct in certain toxicological emergencies. Magnesium sulfate is used in the treatment of eclampsia, a life-threatening seizure disorder associated with pregnancy, and in some cardiac emergencies.

Laboratory-Produced Medication Sources

Researchers today produce an ever-increasing number of medications in the laboratory. The new medications may be natural (from animal or plant sources), **synthetic**, or a combination of the two. Examples of medications produced in the laboratory include thyroid hormone (natural), cimetidine (synthetic), and anistreplase (combination of natural and synthetic). Recombinant DNA research has led to another chemical source of organic compounds: The reordering of genetic information enables scientists to develop bacteria that produce insulin for humans. This technology is used to manufacture insulin, hepatitis B vaccine, glucagon, and several other products. Insulin is manufactured by taking the genetic code for human insulin and placing it into the cells of selected bacteria. These bacteria can then be grown in large quantities, thus producing a large amount of insulin at relatively low cost.

Many medications on the market today are synthetically derived. Common examples of emergency medications that are synthetically manufactured include fentanyl (Sublimaze), adenosine (Adenocard), and diazepam (Valium). Fentanyl is used for pain control and adenosine is used to treat cardiac arrhythmias. Diazepam is used to treat seizures, anxiety, and other neuropsychiatric disorders.

Sources of Medication Information

Obtaining information on medications can be difficult. Using multiple sources of information about medications is usually a good idea. Every book about medications, including this one, has a disclaimer regarding doses and current uses, referring the reader to local medical direction for the final word. Using multiple sources and comparing the author's statements about a medication may lead you to the best available information. EMS providers generally like small, short guides that they can carry in a shirt pocket. The widespread availability of the Internet now allows immediate access to numerous pharmacology databases. In addition, there are specific applications for smart phones specifically designed for medications and pharmacology (see Figure 1–2). These usually include important details about medications that the prehospital providers administer along with a long list of commonly prescribed medications and their classes. These EMS guides will be useful if you clearly understand the medications used in your system and have a working knowledge of commonly prescribed medication classes.

Many sources of medication information are available to the prehospital provider (see Table 1–1).

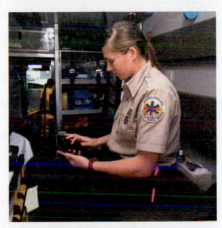

● **FIGURE 1–2** Smart phone pharmacology/ medication application. © Bryan E. Bledsoe

TABLE 1–1
Sources of Medication Information

Pharmacopeia: Official

- *United States Pharmacopeia (USP)* and *National Formulary (NF)*
- *British Pharmacopeia (BP)*
- *British National Formulary (BF)*
- *Compendium of Pharmaceuticals and Specialties (CPS)*, Canada

Compendia: Nonofficial

- *Drug Information/Hospital Formulary, American Hospital Formulary Service,* published by authority of the American Society of Hospital Pharmacists
- *Facts and Comparisons*
- *USP* dispensing information
- *Physician's Drug Reference*

Internet

- Drugs.com
- RxList.com
- WebMD
- *eMedicine*
- *micromedex*

Smart Phones

- *Epocrates*
- *Skyscape/DrDrugs®*
- *MediMath*
- *lexicomp*

MEDICATION RESEARCH AND BRINGING A MEDICATION TO MARKET

The pharmaceutical industry is highly motivated to bring profitable new medications to market. Proving the safety and reliability of these new medications, however, requires extensive research. While better understanding of biology is shortening the time needed to bring a new medication to market, the process still takes many years. To ensure the safety of new medications, the U.S. **Food and Drug Administration (FDA)** has developed a process for evaluating their safety and efficacy. The process, illustrated in Chart 1–1, adds even more time to the development cycle. Initial medication testing begins with the study of both male and female mammals. After testing a medication's toxicity, researchers evaluate its pharmacokinetics—it is absorbed, distributed, metabolized (biotransformed), and excreted—in animals. These animal studies also help determine the medication's therapeutic index (the ratio of its lethal dose to its effective dose). If the results of the animal testing are satisfactory, the FDA designates the medication as an Investigational New Drug (IND) and researchers can then test it in humans. Human studies take place in four phases.

Common Pharmacological Terminology and Abbreviations

It is common to use abbreviations in pharmacology. Abbreviations serve to expedite paperwork and promote efficiency. However, abbreviations should be used with caution as they can lead to confusion. Most hospitals and EMS systems will prepare a list

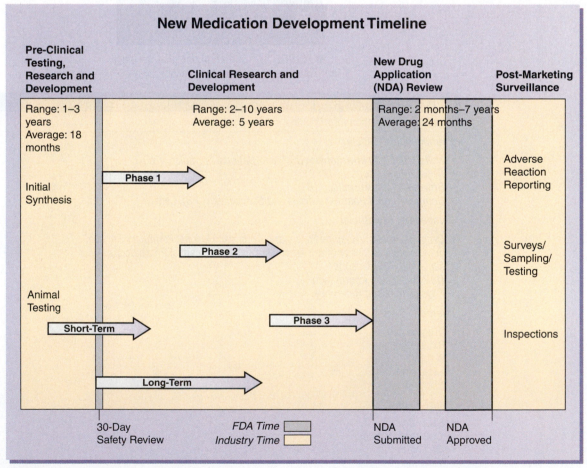

● **CHART 1–1** New medication development timeline.

of accepted abbreviations. Fortunately, the abbreviations used in pharmacology are fairly standard. It is important to be familiar with these abbreviations and with some of the common terminology applicable to the field of emergency pharmacology (see Table 1–2).

TABLE 1–2

Common Abbreviations

Abbreviation	Meaning	Abbreviation	Meaning
a.c.	Before meals	HPI	History of present illness
ACh	Acetylcholine	hr	Hour
ACLS	Advanced cardiac life support	IM	Intramuscular
ACS	Acute coronary syndrome	IO	Intraosseous
AMA	Against medical advice	IV	Intravenous
AMI	Acute myocardial infarction	IVP	Intravenous push
Amp	Ampule	IVPB	Intravenous piggyback
APAP	Acetaminophen	K^+	Potassium ion
ASA	Aspirin	kg	Kilogram
BP	Blood pressure	KVO	Keep vein open
c/o	Complains of	L	Liter
Ca^{++}	Calcium ion	Ⓛ	Left
CaCl	Calcium chloride	lb	Pound
CC	Chief complaint	LMA	Laryngeal mask airway
CHF	Congestive heart failure	LMP	Las menstrual period
cm	Centimeter	LOC	Loss of consciousness
cm^2	Cubic centimeter	LR	Lactated Ringer's
CO	Carbon monoxide	mcg	Microgram
CO_2	Carbon dioxide	MDI	Metered-dose inhaler
COPD	Chronic obstructive pulmonary disease	mEq	Milliequivalent
CP	Chest pain	mg	Milligram
CPAP	Continuous positive airway pressure	min	Minute
D/C	Discontinue	mL, ml	Milliliter
D_5W	5% dextrose in water solution	mm	Millimeter
Dig	Digitalis	N_2O	Nitrous oxide
DNR	Do not resuscitate	Na^+	Sodium ion
Dx	Diagnosis	$NaHCO_3$	Sodium bicarbonate
ED	Emergency department	NKA	No known allergies
ET	Endotracheal	NKDA	No known drug allergies
$EtCO_2$	End-tidal carbon dioxide	NPA	Nasopharyngeal airway
ETOH	Ethyl alcohol	NPO	Nothing by mouth
g	Gram	NS	Normal saline
GCS	Glasgow Coma Score	NSTEMI	Non-ST-segment elevation myocardial infarction
gr	Grain		
gtt(s)	Drop(s)	NTG	Nitroglycerin
HHN	Handheld nebulizer	O_2	Oxygen

(continued)

TABLE 1–2 (*continued*)

Common Abbreviations

Abbreviation	Meaning	Abbreviation	Meaning
OD	Overdose	SVN	Small volume nebulizer
OPA	Oropharyngeal airway	Tbsp	Tablespoon
oz	Ounce	t.i.d.	*ter in die* (three times a day)
p.c.	After meals	TKO	To keep open
PALS	Pediatric advanced life support	tPA	Tissue plasminogen activator
Pedi	Pediatrics	tsp	teaspoon
PMHx	Past medical history	Tx	Treatment or transport
p.o.	*per os* (by mouth)	UA	Unstable angina
p.r.	*per rectus* (per rectum)	y/o	Years old
p.r.n.	*pro re nada* (when necessary)	α	Alpha
PSHx	Past surgical history	β	Beta
q.h.	*quisque hora* (every hour)	Δ	Change (delta)
q.i.d.	*quarter in die* (four times a day)	$\downarrow$	Decrease or decreased
®	Right	°	Degree
r-tPA	Recombinant tissue plasminogen activator	°C	Degree Celsius (centigrade)
RL	Ringer's lactate	°F	Degree Fahrenheit
Rx	Treatment	=	Equal to
Sub-Q	Subcutaneous	♀	female
SL	Sublingual	>	Greater than
SpCO	Carboxyhemoglobin (CO-oximetry)	↑	Increase or increased
SpO$_2$	Oxygen saturation (oximetry)	<	Less than
Stat	*statin* (now or immediately)	♂	Male
STEMI	ST-segment elevation myocardial infarction	Ø	None (null)
SUX	Succinylcholine	≠	Not equal to

FDA CLASSIFICATION OF NEWLY APPROVED MEDICATIONS

The FDA has developed a method for immediately classifying new medications. This method of medication classification utilizes a number and a letter for each new medication in the IND phase or upon New Drug Application (NDA) review by the FDA. The manufacturer has a right to contest this classification and have it changed before the final classification is established.

Numerical Classification (Chemical)

1. A new molecular drug
2. A new salt of a marketed drug
3. A new formulation or dosage form not previously marketed
4. A new combination not previously marketed
5. A drug that is already on the market, a generic duplication

6. A product already marketed by the same company (This designation is used for new indications for a marketed drug.)

7. A drug product on the market without NDA approval (drug was marketed prior to 1938)

Letter Classification (Treatment or Therapeutic Potential)

A. Drug offers an important therapeutic gain (P-priority)

B. Drug that is similar to drugs already on the market (S-similar)

Other Classifications

A. Drugs indicated for AIDS and HIV-related disease

B. Drugs developed to treat life-threatening or severely debilitating illness

I. An orphan drug

NEW MEDICATION DEVELOPMENT

In the past, medications were found by trial and error. Now they are developed primarily by systematic research. Scientists still search for new organic and inorganic sources; however, they now focus most of their attention on the laboratory to discover needed medications.

The FDA carefully monitors new medication development, which can take many years to complete. Testing of new medications begins with animals to evaluate a medication's pharmacological use, dosage ranges, and possible toxic effects. Only after reviewing extensive animal studies and data on the safety and effectiveness of the proposed medication will the FDA approve the application for an investigational new medication.

Four phases of clinical evaluation involving human subjects follow approval of the IND. The clinical studies are intended to provide information on purity, bioavailability, potency, efficacy, safety, and toxicity. Depending on the results of testing, the studies can be stopped at any phase.

Phase I

The primary purposes of phase I testing are to determine the medication's pharmacokinetics, toxicity, and safe dose in humans.

In phase I, a clinical pharmacologist supervises studies involving a small number of healthy volunteers. All effects of the medication on the volunteers are recorded. The recorded clinical data determine the need for further testing.

Phase II

The primary purpose of phase II testing is to find the therapeutic medication level and watch carefully for toxic and side effects.

A small number of individuals who have the disease for which the medication is purported to be diagnostic or therapeutic are then given the medication. Supervisors carefully document toxic effects and adverse reactions to determine the medication's proper dosage. Researchers then review and compare data from the animal studies and human studies, closely monitoring effects on animal and human fertility and reproduction.

Phase III

The main purpose of phase III testing is to refine the usual therapeutic dose and to collect relevant data on side effects.

In phase III, large numbers of patients in medical research centers receive the medication. This larger sampling provides information about infrequent or rare adverse effects. Information collected during this phase helps determine risks associated with the new medication. Researchers also must perform various tests that take into account those patients who are so emotionally involved that they experience relief of symptoms based on suggestion. The administration of a placebo, a medically inert substance, to some patients provides control for such psychological responses. In one frequently used procedure, one-half of the patients receive the medication and one-half receive the placebo. To remove all bias, neither the patient nor the physician knows who has received the medication and who has received the placebo until completion of the study; this type of study is known as a double-blind study. In another type of study (crossover study) patients receive the medication for part of the time and a placebo for the rest of the time.

After the three phases, the FDA evaluates the results. If the FDA announces a favorable evaluation, the company developing the medication then completes a New Drug Application. FDA approval of the company's NDA means that the new medication has been accepted and can be marketed exclusively by its sponsoring company.

Phase IV

Phase IV testing involves post-marketing analysis during conditional approval. Once the medication is being used in the general population, the FDA requires the medication's maker to monitor its performance.

Phase IV is voluntary. After the NDA is approved, the medication company begins surveillance or post-market surveillance. It receives reports about the therapeutic results of the medication from physicians. The company must communicate adequately with the FDA and with the public during the medication's use. Some medications, such as benoxaprofen (Oraflex), have been found to be toxic and have been removed from the market after their initial release. At times, manufacturers have contended that a medication's benefits for a certain segment of the population outweigh its risks. Such was the manufacturer's response when the antidepressant tranylcypromine was withdrawn from the market. Eventually, but with certain restrictions, the FDA reinstated tranylcypromine in the market for use by patients with severe depression.

Expedited Medication Approval

Although most INDs undergo all four phases of clinical evaluation, a few can receive expedited approval. For example, because of the public health threat posed by acquired immunodeficiency syndrome (AIDS), the FDA and drug companies have agreed to shorten the IND approval process, allowing physicians to give qualified AIDS patients so-called Treatment INDs not yet approved by the FDA. Sponsors of medications that reach phase II or III clinical trials can apply for FDA approval of Treatment IND status. When the IND is approved, the sponsor supplies the medication to physicians whose patients meet appropriate criteria.

Orphan Drugs

Orphan drugs are drugs that are used to treat what are referred to as orphan diseases—relatively rare diseases that affect fewer than 200,000 people. Although these drugs are not widely marketed, they play an important role in modern health care. While some orphan drugs are useful for rare diseases, others produce high-risk adverse reactions that make liability insurance costs prohibitive. Many useful medications remain orphans because manufacturers cannot hope to recover the huge amounts of money spent in developing a new medication.

In 1983, Congress signed the Orphan Drug Act, which offers substantial tax credits to companies that develop orphan drugs. Small companies may receive federal financial grants to help them research and develop orphan drugs. As a result, thousands of patients may now use medications that until recently were unavailable. Despite legislation, many orphan drugs remain without developers.

Black Box Warnings

When a special problem arises with a medication that may lead to death or serious injury, the FDA may require the manufacturer to post those warnings in a prominently displayed "black box" in the labeling material. The FDA reserves boxed warnings for risks that can be minimized by conveying the information to health care personnel in this highlighted manner. **Black box warnings** must be considered when determining whether a medication should be a part of an emergency medical service (EMS) formulary.

UNLABELED USES OF MEDICATIONS

When approving a new medication, the FDA accepts it only for the indications for which phase II and phase III clinical studies have shown it to be safe and effective. These indications are approved (labeled); all others are not approved (unlabeled).

For example, the FDA may approve a new medication to treat hypertension if phase II and phase III studies showed that it was safe and effective for use in patients with hypertension. If the medication also works as an antianginal agent, the FDA cannot approve it for this indication unless formal studies in patients with angina pectoris are completed successfully. Such a medication is unapproved for treatment of angina pectoris, yet it may be used for this unlabeled indication, based on **empirical** evidence.

After prescribing a new medication approved to treat hypertension, a physician may discover that it also decreases the patient's angina. Then the physician may share this finding with colleagues in medical journals or at meetings, and they, too, may prescribe it for unlabeled uses.

The FDA recognizes that a medication's labeling does not always contain the most current information about its usage. Therefore, after the FDA approves a medication for one indication, a physician legally may prescribe it, a pharmacist may dispense it, and a nurse or paramedic may administer it for any labeled—or unlabeled—indication.

Although clinicians are not prohibited from prescribing, dispensing, or administering a medication for an unlabeled use, the FDA forbids the manufacturer from promoting a medication for any unlabeled indications. That is why medication package inserts and the *Physicians' Desk Reference* (a collection of drug manufacturers' product labeling) contain no information about unlabeled uses, and pharmaceutical sales representatives cannot discuss such uses. Nevertheless, many medications commonly are prescribed for unlabeled uses.

MEDICAL OVERSIGHT

Prehospital care has evolved as an extension of health care provided within the hospital setting. As such, all aspects of prehospital care have traditionally fallen under the supervision of physicians. This role is referred to as medical oversight and is currently enforced by legislation throughout Canada and the United States. Although the specifics of this legislation vary from province to province and state to state, it is based on a common theme involving all prehospital care providers acting under the direction and control of a physician. The prehospital care provider is acting as a delegate for the physician and is, in essence, working under the medical license of the physician providing medical control.

The Medical Director

The individual physician who assumes the medical oversight role described in the previous section is designated the **medical director**. The medical director is typically a licensed physician active in emergency medicine with an understanding of, and experience in, prehospital care. The specific duties of the medical director include development and implementation of medical control guidelines, education, quality assurance, equipment, and medication review, and assessment of competency. The role of the medical director has also evolved in recent years to include some scene response and field triage at mass casualty incidents. The medical director is responsible for the actions of care providers working under his or her medical control and, as such, is the ultimate authority with respect to all medical control and competency issues. Because prehospital care providers work under the license of the medical director, the medical director can be found medicolegally liable in cases of litigation involving prehospital care. In some systems, the medical director receives input from a medical control or medical advisory board, which generally has physician representation from the various institutions served by the EMS system. The roles and authority of these types of committees are system specific. Although the level of involvement of the medical director within an EMS system varies, ideally that individual should have ongoing exposure to activities in the field as a means of staying abreast of medical and operational issues. Care providers should view the medical director as a resource who can provide constructive feedback and answer questions as they arise. At the same time, the medical director must serve as a patient advocate, ensuring that patient care is the foremost priority.

Medical Control

Medical control constitutes one of the components of medical oversight and can be further subdivided into on-line and off-line medical control.

On-Line Medical Control

On-line medical control refers to orders given directly to prehospital care providers by a physician, generally via radio or telephone. Typically the prehospital care provider speaks to a physician in the emergency department to which the patient is being transported. Also known as a "base" physician, this individual is generally well acquainted with local medical control guidelines and the overall capabilities of the local EMS system and personnel.

Off-Line Medical Control

Off-line medical control essentially includes all aspects of medical oversight that do not involve direct medical control, including system design, protocol development, education, and quality improvement. To be effective, medical control must have the authority to discipline or limit the activities of those who deviate from an established standard of care. As an advancing field, prehospital care demands a commitment to lifelong learning, and it is the responsibility of both the care provider and the medical director to ensure that this process is ongoing. The education component of prehospital care is becoming increasingly important as the complexity of care, including medications and equipment, increases. The importance of training and education can be demonstrated by the ever-increasing number of medications and interventions provided in the field that have lethal potential if used inappropriately.

Medical Control Protocols and Guidelines

All treatments and interventions in the prehospital field are provided under the direct or indirect orders of a physician. Many of these orders are provided in the form of medical protocols that provide guidelines for treating patients in the field. Many systems provide **standing orders** or standing protocols that allow the care provider to treat patients without speaking to a physician. These **treatment protocols** are designed to facilitate management of specific presenting signs and symptoms rather than a specific diagnosis. Certain treatments and presenting problems may require base physician contact prior to implementation. Recently some EMS systems have implemented treat-and-release protocols that allow staff to release patients who respond to treatment and meet certain preestablished criteria. This is an example of the ever-increasing responsibility that prehospital care providers face, and it emphasizes the importance of education, judgment, and critical-thinking skills.

Legal Regulations, Standards, and Legislation

As a society develops and uses medications, it needs to establish controls regulating the manufacture, distribution, and use of those medications. In many cases a society's attitude and values, rather than formal controls, determine the acceptable limits of medication use. Formal drug controls range from individual institutional policies to governmental legislation.

International Controls

The United Nations, through its World Health Organization, attempts to influence international health by providing technical assistance and encouraging research for drug use. One committee has been established to cope with the problems associated with habit-forming drugs. Drug enforcement agencies in various nations cooperate, but no administrative or judicial structures enforce controls. As a result, control of international drug trade depends largely on the voluntary cooperation of nations.

Controls in the United States

Before a drug can be marketed, it must undergo extensive testing. This testing generally involves two phases, animal studies and clinical patient studies. Only after these extensive tests, and with governmental approval, can drugs be placed on the market. Even after clinical usage, the effectiveness of the drugs must be closely monitored. The FDA is the federal agency responsible for approval of drugs before they are made available to the general public.

Legislative control in the United States began in 1906, when Congress enacted the Pure Food and Drug Act. In addition to establishing the FDA, this act prohibited the sale of medicinal preparations that had little or no use and restricted the sale of drugs with a potential for abuse. The Pure Food and Drug Act named the **United States Pharmacopeia (USP)** and the **National Formulary (NF)** as official drug standards. Any drug bearing the official title *USP* or *NF* must conform to rigid standards regarding purity, preparation, and dosage.

The Pure Food and Drug Act was not as all-encompassing as its planners had envisioned it to be. For several years stronger drug laws were debated in both Congress and state legislatures. In the 1930s more than 100 people died from ingesting sulfanilamide, an antibacterial drug. Researchers discovered that the sulfanilamide had been prepared with a previously uninvestigated toxic substance called diethylene glycol. Finally in 1938, Congress enacted the Federal Food, Drug, and Cosmetic Act. Among the most important features of this act was the truth-in-labeling clause. The act required the following:

1. A statement accurately describing the package's contents
2. The usual names of the drugs, for official drugs (preparations listed in the pharmacopeia and adopted by the government as meeting pharmaceutical standards) and nonofficial drugs (drugs not listed in the pharmacopeia)

3. Indication of the presence, quantity, and proportion of certain drugs (such as alcohol, atropine, and bromides)
4. Warning of habit-forming drugs in the product and of their effects
5. The names of the manufacturer, packager, and distributor
6. Directions for use and warnings against unsafe use, including recommendations for dosage levels and frequency

The Kefauver Harris Amendment was an amendment to the Federal Food, Drug and Cosmetic Act, added in 1962, that required pharmaceutical manufacturers to provide proof of the safety and effectiveness of their drugs before being granted approval to produce and market the products. This also stopped the process of remarking inexpensive generic drugs under new "trade names."

Narcotics

A problem almost as old as medicine itself is abuse and addiction to certain drugs. Narcotics are among the drugs most frequently abused. Recognizing the need to control the sale of narcotics, the federal government enacted the Harrison Narcotic Act in 1914. This act served to control the importation, manufacture, and sale of the opium plant and its derivatives. It also controlled the derivatives of the coca plant. The primary drug derived from the coca plant is cocaine. As a result of this act, these drugs, as well as other drugs added to the list later, could be obtained only with special prescriptions. Only physicians who qualified and attained a special narcotic license could prescribe this class of drugs.

In 1970 major revisions were made in the use and control of narcotics and other drugs. This law, the Comprehensive Drug Abuse Prevention and Control Act of 1970 (commonly called the Controlled Substances Act of 1970), classifies the drugs used in medicine into five different schedules. A summary of the five schedules is found in Table 1–3.

The Controlled Substances Act

The Controlled Substances Act mandates that prescriptions for Schedule II medications cannot be refilled. Moreover, it requires that prescriptions for Schedule II medications be filled within 72 hours. Prescriptions for medications in this class cannot be called into the pharmacy over the telephone (except in special situations). Prescriptions for medications in Schedules III and IV may be refilled up to five times within six months. Prescriptions for Schedule V medications may be refilled at the discretion of the physician.

Responsibility for enforcing the Controlled Substances Act rests with the U.S. **Drug Enforcement Administration (DEA)**. Only physicians approved by the DEA may write prescriptions for scheduled drugs. The physician must indicate his or her DEA number on the prescription. Many states have enacted laws further regulating controlled substances.

Canadian Drug Legislation

Drug control in Canada falls under the direct supervision of the Department of National Health and Welfare. The Food and Drug Act, passed in 1941, empowers the governor-in-council to prescribe drug standards and limit variation in any food or drug. The 1953 Canadian Food and Drug Act (amended yearly) provides regulations for drug manufacture and sale. A comparison of the drug schedules in the United States and Canada is found in Table 1–3.

Canadian Narcotic Control Act and Regulations

In 1965, the Canadian Narcotic Control Act restricted the sale, possession, and use of narcotics. It further restricted narcotics to authorized personnel. This act defines who may prescribe a narcotic drug, such as physicians, dentists, research personnel, and their agents, and places conditions on the recipient of a narcotic prescription, requiring disclosure of all previous narcotics received within the past 30 days. In addition, the

TABLE 1-3

Schedule of Controlled Drugs

United States

Category	Examples
Schedule I	**Opiates**
No recognized medical use	Heroin
High abuse potential	
Research use only	**Hallucinogens**
	LSD
	Mescaline
	Ecstasy
	Depressants
	Methaqualone
Schedule II	**Opiates**
Written prescriptions required	Hydromorphone
No telephone renewals	Oxycodone
In an emergency, a prescription may be renewed by telephone	Morphine
	Fentanyl
	Stimulants
	Amphetamines
	Methylphenidate
	Depressants
	Secobarbital
Schedule III	**Opiates**
Prescriptions required to be rewritten after 6 months or five refills	Codeine of less than 1.8 g/dL
Prescriptions may be ordered by telephone	Hydrocodone with aspirin or acetaminophen
	Stimulants
	Benzphetamine
	Mazindol
	Depressants
	Butabarbital
	Ketamine
	Anabolic Steroids
	Ethylestrenol
	Fluoxymesterone
	Methyltestosterone
Schedule IV	**Opiates**
Prescriptions required to be rewritten after 6 months or five refills	Pentazocine
	Stimulants
	Fenfluramine
	Phentermine
	Depressants
	Benzodiazepines
	Chloral hydrate
Schedule V	Primarily small amounts of opiates, such as opium, dihydrocodeine, and diphenoxylate, when used as antitussives or antidiarrheals in combination products
Dispenses as any (nonnarcotic) prescription	
Some may be dispensed without prescription unless additional state regulations apply	

Canada

Category	Examples
Schedule H	**Hallucinogens**
Restricted drugs	Peyote
No recognized medicinal properties	LSD
	Mescaline
Narcotics Schedule	**Coca Leaf Derivatives**
Stringently restricted drugs	Cocaine
The letter *N* must appear on all labels and professional advertisements	**Opiates and Opiate Derivatives**
	Morphine
	Codeine
	Methadone
	Hydromorphone
	Meperidine
	Other Drugs
	Phencyclidine
	Cannabis
Schedule G	**Narcotic Analgesics**
Controlled drugs	Nalbuphine
Prescriptions are controlled because of the abuse potential of these drugs	Butorphanol
	Stimulants
	Amphetamines
	Barbiturates
	Phenobarbital
	Amobarbital
	Secobarbital
Schedule F	**Anxiolytics**
Prescription drugs	Benzodiazepines
Although not controlled drugs, agents in this category include some with a relatively low abuse potential	
The symbol *Pr* must appear on their labels	
Nonprescription Drug Schedule (group 3)	**Analgesics**
Drugs available only in the pharmacy and used only on a physician's recommendation	Low-dose codeine preparations
Limited public access	**Other Drugs**
	Insulin
	Nitroglycerin
	Muscle relaxants

act describes procedures for record keeping and dispensing by pharmacists. Hospital regulations are also outlined.

Methadone is covered individually in this act, which sets requirements for authorized practitioners who prescribe and dispense this drug.

Medication Storage

The proper storage and accounting of EMS system medications are important considerations. Several medications commonly used in EMS have very limited tolerance for extremes in temperature. When these medications are exposed to temperatures outside of the range of their tolerance they can lose effectiveness or become unsafe. EMS systems must have in place safeguards and policies and procedures to assure that medications are stored at the proper temperature.

Controlled substances are subject to abuse. Because of this, various precautions and safeguards must be in place to avoid **diversion** or **adulteration** of these medications. Federal and state laws require that controlled substances be stored in a securely locked and substantially built safe or cabinet. Those stored for immediate use (e.g., jump bags) must be tagged with a tamperproof tag or seal. Access to controlled substances is limited to those who will be administering or stocking the controlled substances. In most systems, there is a perpetual log that is kept to document the usage and wastage of controlled substances. This log generally reflects the following:

1. Date of medication administration
2. Patient name
3. Medication name
4. Medication strength
5. Dosage form
6. Quantity administered
7. Quantity wasted
8. Name of person administering/wasting the medication
9. Name of person witnessing any wastage

Controlled substances are usually counted daily or with personnel changes. Any discrepancies must me immediately reported. Routine and random audits of controlled substance stocks are common to assure compliance with federal and state laws (see Figure 1–3).

Drug Standards

The federal government establishes and enforces drug standards to ensure the uniform quality of drugs. Because some generic drugs affect patients differently than their brand name counterparts, standardization of drugs is necessary. Despite FDA standards, drugs sold or distributed by various manufacturers may have biological or therapeutic differences. An **assay** determines the amount of purity of a given chemical in a preparation in the laboratory (*in vitro*). While two generically equivalent preparations may contain the same amount of a given chemical (drug), they may have different therapeutic effects. This relative therapeutic effectiveness is determined by a **bioassay**, which attempts to ascertain their **bioequivalence**. The *United States Pharmacopeia* is the official standard for the United States. These standards pertain to the following drug properties:

> *Purity* refers to the uncontaminated state of a drug containing only one active component. In reality, a drug consisting of only one active compound rarely exists because manufacturers usually must add other ingredients to facilitate

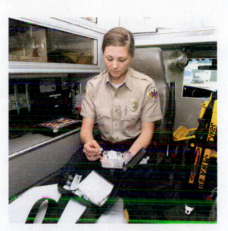

● **FIGURE 1–3** Narcotic counting and storage. © Bryan E. Bledsoe

drug formation and to determine absorption rate. As a result, standards of purity do not demand 100 percent pure active ingredients but specify the type and acceptable amount of extraneous material.

Bioavailability describes the degree to which a drug becomes absorbed and reaches general circulation. Factors affecting bioavailability include the particle size, crystalline structure, solubility, and polarity of the compound. The blood or tissue concentration of a drug is used to estimate bioavailability.

Potency of a drug refers to its strength or its power to produce the desired effect. Potency standards are set by testing laboratory animals to determine the definite measurable effect of an administered drug.

Efficacy refers to the how well the drug works in terms of treatment effect. Objective clinical trials attempt to determine efficacy, but absolute measurement remains difficult.

Safety and toxicity are determined by the incidence and severity of reported adverse reactions to the use of a drug. Some harmful effects may not appear for a considerable time. Safety and toxicity standards are being refined constantly as past experiences illuminate deficiencies in the standards.

Drug Names

Drugs are identified by four different names: chemical, generic, trade, and official. A drug's chemical name precisely describes its atomic and molecular structure. Because drugs are usually chemically complex in nature, so too are the chemical names. When a manufacturer decides to market a new drug, the United States Adopted Names (USAN) Council selects a generic name. The generic name, usually an abbreviated version of the chemical name, is frequently used. Manufacturers of pharmaceuticals rarely refer to drugs by their generic names. Instead, they select a name for a drug that is based on its chemical name or on the type of problem it is used to treat. This is referred to as the *trade name*. Trade names are always capitalized, whereas generic names are not. Trade names are protected by copyright. The symbol ® after the trade name means it is registered by and restricted to the drug manufacturer. The fourth method of naming a drug is the official name. The official name is followed by the initials *USP* or *NF,* which are official publications that list drugs conforming to standards set forth by the publication. The official name is usually the same as the generic name. Following is an example of the four names of a specific drug:

Chemical name:	*Ethyl 1-methyl-4-phenylisonipecotate hydrochloride*
Generic name:	Meperidine hydrochloride
Trade name:	Demerol Hydrochloride
Official name:	Meperidine hydrochloride, *USP*

Proprietary (Trade) Names

In recent years, controversy has developed regarding generic and nongeneric medications. When writing a prescription, a physician can order the medication by either the trade name or the generic name. Until recently, the pharmacist had to fill the prescription as written. Now, in many states, the pharmacist may substitute a less expensive generic medication for the prescription. As a rule, generic medications are not inferior in quality. They are usually cheaper because lesser known companies with minimal advertising and production costs manufacture them.

Most pharmaceutical manufacturers market their medications primarily under trade names rather than under generic names. Today a single medication may be sold under a number of trade names. For example, the asthma medication albuterol is sold under the names Proventil and Ventolin. The practice of using these trade names can be confusing to the medical provider and sometimes even to the physician, to say nothing of the inconvenience to the pharmacist, who must stock four or five different brands of the same medication.

Medications that share similar characteristics are grouped together as a pharmacological class (family), such as beta-blockers. A second grouping is the therapeutic classification, which groups medications by therapeutic use, such as antihypertensives. Thiazides and beta-blockers are both antihypertensives, but they share few characteristics.

COMPONENTS OF A MEDICATION PROFILE

A medication's profile describes its various properties. As a paramedic or paramedic student, you will become familiar with medication profiles as you study specific medications. A typical medication profile will contain the following information:

Names. These most frequently include the generic and trade names, although the occasional reference will include chemical names.

Classification. This is the broad group to which the medication belongs. Knowing classifications is essential to understanding the properties of medications.

Mechanism of action. The way in which a medication causes its effects; its pharmacodynamics.

Indications. Conditions that made administration of the medication appropriate (as approved by the Food and Drug Administration).

Pharmacokinetics. How the medication is absorbed, distributed, and eliminated; typically includes onset and duration of action.

Side effects/adverse reactions. The medication's untoward or undesired effects.

Routes of administration. How the medication is given.

Contraindications. Conditions that make it inappropriate to give the medication. Unlike when the medication is simply not indicated, a contraindication means that a predictable harmful event will occur if the medication is given in this situation.

Dosage. The amount of the medication that should be given.

How supplied. This typically includes the common concentrations of the available preparations; many medications come in different concentrations.

Special considerations. How the medication may affect pediatric, geriatric, or pregnant patients.

Medication profiles may also include other components, such as its interactions with other medications or with foods, when appropriate.

Medication Forms

Medications come in many forms and are packaged in numerous styles. Each form and each style has advantages and disadvantages. For example, medications taken by mouth tend to have a slow and unpredictable rate of absorption and thus a slower rate of onset of effect. Medications given intravenously, although rapidly acting, are much more difficult to administer. Medications may be packaged in unit–dose form, in which one dose of a medication comes in a labeled container or wrapper. They may also be packaged in bulk form, in which multiple doses of a medication are packaged in a container, bottle, or wrapper.

Medications are manufactured in many different forms including liquids, solids, suppositories, inhalants, sprays, creams, lotions, patches, and lozenges. To administer medications safely, you must be knowledgeable about the different effects of the many medication forms. For example, nitroglycerin administered sublingually (allowing it to dissolve under the tongue) can relieve anginal pain in less than 1 minute. The same medication administered as an ointment applied to the chest wall may not relieve acute pain at all; however, it may be used prophylactically for anginal pain. Common medication preparations are described in the following sections.

Liquid Medications

Liquid medications usually consist of a powder dissolved in a liquid. The medication is referred to as the **solute**. The liquid into which it is dissolved is called the **solvent**. In liquid medication preparations, the primary difference between one preparation and another is the solvent.

Solutions. Solutions are preparations that contain the medication dissolved in a solvent, usually water (for example, 5 percent dextrose in water).

Tinctures. Tinctures are medication preparations whereby the medication was extracted chemically with alcohol. They usually contain some dilute alcohol (for example, tincture of iodine).

Suspensions. Suspensions are medications that do not remain dissolved. After sitting for even short periods, these medications tend to separate. They must always be shaken well before use (for example, penicillin preparations).

Spirits. Spirit solutions contain volatile chemicals dissolved in alcohol (for example, spirit of ammonia).

Emulsions. Emulsions are preparations in which an oily substance is mixed with a solvent into which it does not dissolve. When mixed, it forms globules of fat floating in the solvent. An example of a common emulsion outside of medicine is oil and vinegar salad dressing.

Elixirs. Elixirs are preparations that contain the medication in an alcohol solvent. Flavoring, often cherry, is added to improve the taste (for example, Tylenol Elixir).

Syrups. Often medications are suspended in sugar and water to improve the taste. These are referred to as syrups (for example, cough syrup).

Liquid medications administered into the body through intramuscular, subcutaneous, or intravenous routes are called **parenteral medications**. Most medications used in emergency medicine are parenteral. Because they are introduced into the body, they must be sterile.

Liquid medications given parenterally are available in four packaging styles: vials, ampules, self-contained systems or syringes, and nebules. Sterile parenteral containers designed to carry a single patient dose are called **ampules** (see Figure 1–4). An ampule is a glass container with a thin neck, which usually is scored so it can be snapped off. After the tops are broken, the medication is drawn into a syringe for administration.

In emergency medicine many medications given parenterally are in self-contained systems or **prefilled syringes** (see Figures 1–5 and 1–6). These preparations save time by avoiding the problems inherent with ampules. Self-contained systems or prefilled syringes contain a single dose of a medication in a plastic bag or in a prefilled syringe with an attached needle. Prefilled syringes are often used during cardiopulmonary resuscitation and other advanced life support activities.

Vials are another type of container for parenteral medications (see Figures 1–7 and 1–8). Vials are bottles sealed with a rubber diaphragm and may contain a single

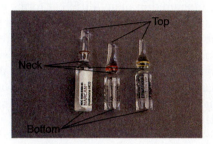

● **FIGURE 1–4** Ampules.

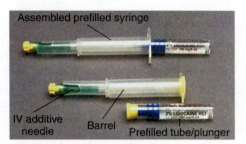

● **FIGURE 1–5** Prefilled syringes.

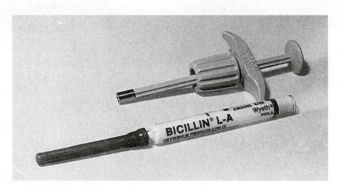

● **FIGURE 1–6** Tubex syringes.

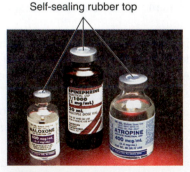

● **FIGURE 1–7** Multidose vials.

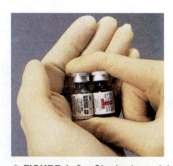

● **FIGURE 1–8** Single-dose vials.

or multiple doses. Multidose vials contain preservatives that enable them to be used for more than one dose, whereas single-dose vials do not contain such agents. Many medications used in emergency medicine are supplied in vials.

Nebules are used for medications that are premixed. For example, salbutamol (Ventolin) and ipratropium bromide (Atrovent) are both administered to the patient by nebulizer. Each nebule is filled with the amount of medication generally administered to an adult patient.

Solid Medications

Solid medications are usually administered orally, although many can be administered rectally. They include the following:

Powders. Powders are medications in powdered form. They are not as popular as pills, but some are still in use (for example, B.C. powder).

Capsules. Capsules consist of gelatin containers into which a powder is placed. The gelatin dissolves, liberating the powder (for example, amoxicillin capsules) into the gastrointestinal tract.

Tablets. Tablets are similar to pills. They are composed of a powder that has been compressed into an easily swallowed form and are often covered with a sugar coating to improve taste.

Suppositories

Administered rectally and vaginally, suppositories carry medications in a solid base that melts at body temperature. Suppositories produce local (analgesic, laxative, and anti-infective) and systemic (antiemetic, antipyretic, and analgesic) effects. Usually bullet shaped, most suppositories are about 1 inch (2.5 cm) long and require lubrication for insertion. Because they melt at body temperature, suppositories require refrigeration until administration. When placed into the body, either rectally or vaginally, they dissolve and are then absorbed into the surrounding tissue.

Inhalants

Inhalants are powered or liquid forms of a medication that are given using the respiratory route and are absorbed rapidly by the rich supply of capillaries in the lungs. Several frequently used methods of inhalation are nebulizers, metered-dose aerosol, or turbo inhalers or vaporizers.

IMPORTANT PHARMACOLOGICAL TERMINOLOGY

Important pharmacological terminology includes the following:

Adverse effect. An untoward effect is a side effect that proves harmful to the patient.

Antagonism. Antagonism signifies the opposition between two or more medications (for example, between naloxone and morphine).

Bolus. A bolus is a single, oftentimes large dose of medication (for example, diltiazem bolus, which is often followed by a diltiazem infusion).

Contraindications. Contraindications are the medical or physiological conditions present in a patient that would make it harmful to administer a medication of otherwise known therapeutic value.

Cumulative action. A cumulative action occurs when a medication is administered in several doses, causing an increased effect. This increased effect is usually due to a quantitative buildup of the medication in the blood.

Depressant. A depressant is a medication that decreases or lessens a body function or activity.

Habituation. Habituation is physical or psychological dependence on a drug.

Hypersensitivity. Hypersensitivity is a reaction to a substance that is normally more profound than seen in a population not sensitive to the substance (for example, an allergic reaction to penicillin).

Idiosyncrasy. An idiosyncrasy is an individual reaction to a medication that is unusually different from that seen in the rest of the population.

Indication. An indication refers to the medical condition or conditions in which the medication has proven to be of therapeutic value.

Potentiation. Potentiation is the enhancement of one medication's effects by another (for example, barbiturates and alcohol).

Refractory. Patients or conditions that do not respond to a medication are said to be refractory to the medication (for example, a patient with supraventricular tachycardia contractions who does not respond to adenosine).

Side effects. Side effects are the unavoidable, undesired effects frequently seen even in therapeutic medication dosages.

Stimulant. A stimulant is a medication that enhances or increases a bodily function (for example, caffeine in coffee).

Synergism. Synergism is the combined action of two medications. The action is much stronger than the effects of either medication administered separately.

Therapeutic action. A therapeutic action is the desired, intended action of a medication given in the appropriate medical condition.

Tolerance. When patients are receiving medications on a long-term basis, they may require larger and larger dosages of the medication to achieve a therapeutic effect. This increased requirement is termed tolerance.

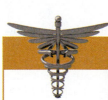

CASE STUDY

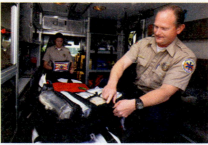

© Bryan E. Bledsoe

Rachel Lewis reports for her first shift with her Field Training Officer (FTO). Although she has been a volunteer paramedic for many years, this was her first full-time EMS job. Her first shift was designed to orient her to the EMS system and the ambulances. As a part of her orientation she had to complete a two-hour course on the Health Insurance Portability and Accountability Act (HIPAA). Next, she was introduced to the guidelines for use and storage of controlled substances. First, the FTO and Rachel carefully counted the controlled substances on the ambulance. He showed her how to access the controlled substances in the locked storage cabinet. Then, each vial of medication was removed and inspected for purity, expiration date, and signs of tampering. They carefully went through the supplies of morphine, fentanyl, diazepam, and lorazepam and then replaced them in the appropriate place. The FTO then detailed the daily sign-in and sign-out log mandated by the EMS system. He also explained the required procedures for administration, wastage, and documentation of controlled substances. By happenstance, Rachel's orientation day was the same day that a random check of controlled substances was conducted by EMS system management and the medical director. Through this audit she learned more about the safeguards in place to protect controlled substances from diversion and adulteration. Next, Rachel and her FTO began an inventory of the medical supplies on the ambulance. Although she understands the need for the paperwork, she was ready for her first call as a paid paramedic.

Questions

1. Why is it necessary to account for medications, including controlled substances, on a regular basis?
2. What controlled substances are used in your system and how are they accounted for?

CHAPTER REVIEW

Summary

Drugs are chemical agents used in the diagnosis, treatment, or prevention of disease. They are necessary for successful emergency care. It is important to be familiar with the commonly used emergency medications and with the terminology and abbreviations used in medicine so that communication with other medical personnel will be efficient and professional. Overall, it is essential to appreciate the inherent danger of any and all drugs and to use them properly. The rule to remember is, *When in doubt, do no harm.*

Key Words

adulteration   To make impure by adding extraneous, improper, or inferior ingredients.

ampules   a glass sterile parenteral container with a thin neck, which usually is scored so it can be snapped off and is designed to carry a single patient dose.

assay   A test that determines the amount and purity of a given chemical in a preparation in the laboratory.

bioassay   Test to ascertain a drug's availability in a biological model.

bioequivalence   Relative therapeutic effectiveness of chemically equivalent medications.

black box warning   Special warning placed on a medication label listing any special problems that may lead to death or serious injury.

controlled drug   Federal, state, and local laws control the use of a drug that may lead to drug abuse or drug dependence.

diversion   The use of prescription medications for recreational or nontherapeutic purposes.

drug   Any substance introduced into the body that changes a body function.

Drug Enforcement Administration (DEA)   Federal agency with responsibility for enforcing the Controlled Substances Act.

empirical Skill or knowledge based entirely on experience.

Food and Drug Administration (FDA) The federal agency responsible for approval of medications before they are made available to the general public.

medical director A licensed physician who serves as the chief medical officer of an EMS or educational program system. Each paramedic functions under the license of the system medical director.

medications Term typically used to describe use of drugs or similar agents in a therapeutic medical setting.

National Formulary The Pure Food and Drug Act named the *National Formulary (NF)* and the *United States Pharmacopeia (USP)* as official medication standards. Any medication bearing the official title *NF* or *USP* must conform to a rigid set of standards regarding purity, preparation, and dosage.

off-line medical control Also known as *indirect medical control;* the establishment of system policies and procedures, such as training, chart review, protocol development, audit, and quality improvement.

on-line medical control Also known as *direct medical control;* communication between field personnel and a medical control physician, with the medical control physician providing immediate direction for on-scene care.

parenteral medications Routes of administering medications into the body without going through the digestive tract.

pharmacognosy The study of natural drug sources.

pharmacologist Scientist who studies the effects of medications on the body.

pharmacology The study of drugs and their actions on the body.

prefilled syringes Self-contained systems where many medications are parenterally given.

recombinant DNA technology Also called genetic engineering; involves taking genetic material (DNA) from one organism and placing it into another.

solute A powder (medication) that is dissolved in a liquid (solvent).

solvent The liquid into which a medication (solute) is dissolved.

standing orders Written directives that may be carried out without, or prior to, contacting medical control.

synthetic Substance made by combining two or more simpler compounds.

treatment protocols Treatment guidelines for prehospital care. They may incorporate standing orders or may require contact with medical control prior to initiating advanced life support therapy.

United States Pharmacopeia The Pure Food and Drug Act named the *United States Pharmacopeia (USP)* and the *National Formulary (NF)* as official drug standards. Any medication bearing the official title *USP* or *NF* must conform to a rigid set of standards regarding purity, preparation, and dosage.

vials Bottles sealed with a rubber diaphragm and may contain a single or multiple doses for parenteral medications.

CHAPTER 2

PHARMACOKINETICS AND PHARMACODYNAMICS

OBJECTIVES

After completing this chapter, the reader should be able to:

- Define pharmacokinetics and pharmacodynamics.
- Define medication absorption and explain the factors involved in medication absorption.
- Explain the factors that can affect medication distribution.
- Explain biotransformation.
- Explain how a medication is eliminated from the body and list factors that affect elimination.
- Understand the mechanisms of action of medications.
- Explain the special considerations in medication therapy.

INTRODUCTION

To exert its desired biochemical and physiological effects on the body, a medication must reach its targeted tissues in a suitable form and in a sufficient concentration. The study of how medications enter the body, reach their site of action, and eventually become eliminated is termed **pharmacokinetics**. Once medications reach their targeted tissues, they begin a chain of biochemical events that ultimately leads to the physiological changes desired. These biochemical and physiological events are called the medication's **mechanism of action**.

After describing pharmacokinetics this chapter describes **pharmacodynamics**, or the mechanisms by which medications produce biochemical or physiological changes in the body. It describes the interaction between medications and receptors as well as medication action and medication effect. Pharmacotherapeutics addresses the different types of therapy and identifies factors that influence the choice of medication therapy and the patient's response to medications during therapy.

This chapter addresses the fundamentals of pharmacokinetics, pharmacodynamics, and pharmacotherapeutics as they apply to prehospital emergency care.

PHARMACOLOGY

Pharmacology is the study of medications and their interaction with the body. Medications do not confer any new properties on cells or tissues; they only modify or exploit existing conditions. They may be given for their local action (in which case systemic absorption of the medication is discouraged) or for systemic action. Although generally given for a specific effect, medications tend to have multiple actions at multiple sites, so they must be thought of in terms of their systemic effects rather than in terms of an isolated single effect. Pharmacology's two major divisions are pharmacokinetics and pharmacodynamics. Pharmacokinetics addresses how medications are transported into and out of the body. Pharmacodynamics deals with their effects once they reach the target tissues.

PHARMACOKINETICS

Strictly defined, pharmacokinetics is the study of the basic processes that determine the duration and intensity of a medication's effect. These four processes are absorption, distribution, biotransformation, and elimination.

To produce its desired effects, a medication must be present in the appropriate concentration at its various sites of action. Adenosine, a medication commonly used in the treatment of life-threatening arrhythmias must reach its target—cardiac tissue—rapidly and in a sufficient concentration to suppress the dysrhythmia. Several factors influence the concentration of a medication at its site of action. These factors include **absorption** of the medication into the circulatory system; **distribution** of the medication throughout the body; **biotransformation** of the medication into its active form, if required; and, finally, **elimination** of the medication from the body. All of these factors do not play a role in every medication used in prehospital care, but a fundamental understanding of each of these factors is essential.

REVIEW OF PHYSIOLOGY OF TRANSPORT

Pharmacokinetics is dependent on the body's various physiological mechanisms that move substances across the body's compartments. These mechanisms can be broken down into two broad categories based on their energy requirements and then further classified. A mechanism is referred to as **active transport** if it requires the use of energy to move a substance. This energy is achieved by the breakdown of high-energy chemical bonds found in chemicals such as ATP (adenosine triphosphate). ATP is broken down into ADP (adenosine diphosphate) liberating a considerable amount of biochemical energy. A common example of an active transport mechanism is the sodium–potassium (Na^+–K^+) pump. This is a protein pump that actively moves sodium ions into the cell and potassium ions out of the cell. Because this movement goes against the ion's concentration gradients, it must use energy.

Large molecules, such as glucose and most of the amino acids, do not readily pass through the cell membrane because of their size. These molecules are moved across the cell membrane with the help of special "carrier" proteins found on the surface of the target cells. These large molecules are "carried" across the cell membrane in a special transport process called carrier-mediated diffusion. Carrier-mediated diffusion can be an active process (active transport) or a passive process (facilitated diffusion) (see Figure 2–1). Once the molecule to be transported binds with the carrier protein, the configuration of the cell membrane changes, allowing the large molecule to enter the target cell. Insulin, an important hormone secreted by the endocrine pancreas, can increase the rate of carrier-mediated glucose transport from 10- to 20-fold. This is the principal mechanism by which insulin controls glucose use in the body.

Most medications travel through the body by means of passive transport, the movement of a substance without the use of energy. This requires the presence of concentration gradients in a solution. Diffusion and osmosis are forms of **passive transport**. Diffusion involves the movement of solute in the solution, whereas osmosis involves the movement of the solvent (usually water). In diffusion, the solute's molecules or

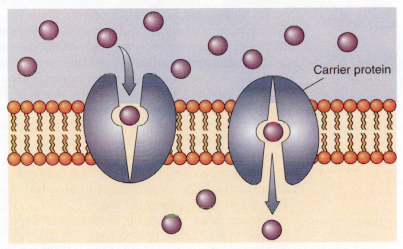

● FIGURE 2-1   Many large molecules require carrier proteins to move into the cell.

ions move down their concentration gradients from an area of higher concentration to an area of lower concentration. Conversely, in osmosis the solvent's molecules move up the concentration gradient to an area of higher concentration. Another way of looking at this is to think of osmosis as simply the diffusion of solvent from an area of high solvent concentration to an area of low solvent concentration. A final type of passive transport is filtration. This is simply the movement of molecules across a membrane down a pressure gradient, from an area of high pressure to an area of low pressure. This pressure typically results from the hydrostatic force of blood pressure.

Medication Absorption

Medication absorption encompasses a medication's progress from its pharmaceutical dosage form to a biologically available substance that can then pass through or across tissues. The transformation from dosage form to a biologically available substance must occur before the active medication ingredient reaches the systemic circulation. After a tablet or capsule disintegrates in the stomach or small intestine, enough liquid must be available for the active medication ingredients to dissolve before systemic absorption can occur. The body requires a solution of the medication's active ingredients to dissolve before systemic absorption can occur because tissues cannot absorb dry powders or dry crystals. Because syrups and suspensions occur in dosage form as solutions, their progress from medication administration to medication absorption is more rapid, leading to a quicker onset of medication action. However, some syrups are specifically designed to provide a delayed release of the medication.

Absorption is the process of movement of a medication from the site of application into the body and into the extracellular compartment. The duration and intensity of a medication's action is often related to the rate of absorption of the medication. Many factors affect medication absorption, including:

1. Solubility of the medication
2. Concentration of the medication
3. pH of the medication
4. Site of absorption
5. Absorbing surface area
6. Blood supply to the site of absorption
7. Bioavailability

The **solubility** is the tendency of a medication to dissolve. To facilitate medication absorption, the solubility of the administered medication must match the cellular constituents of the absorption site. Lipid-soluble (fat-soluble) medications can penetrate lipoid (fat-containing) cells; water-soluble medications cannot. For example, a water-soluble medication such as penicillin cannot penetrate the highly lipoid cells that act as barriers between the blood and brain. However a highly lipoid-soluble medication such as thiopental can penetrate the lipoid cells, cross into the brain, and induce an effect such as anesthesia. The human body is approximately 60 percent water. Thus, medications given in water solutions are more rapidly absorbed than those given in oil-based solutions, suspensions, or solid forms.

The concentration of a medication also affects the rate of absorption. Medications administered in high concentrations are absorbed much more rapidly than medications administered in low concentrations.

Another factor that affects medication absorption is the **pH** of a medication. The pH refers to how acidic or how basic (alkaline) the medication is. Most medications are either weak acids or weak bases. Acidic medications tend to be more rapidly absorbed when placed into an acidic environment (such as the stomach). Alkaline medications, on the other hand, are more rapidly absorbed when placed into an alkaline environment (such as the ileum).

The site of absorption directly affects the rate of medication absorption. Once administered, medications must pass through the various biological membranes until they reach the circulation. Medications placed on the skin (transdermal route) must pass through several cell layers before reaching the circulatory system. On the other hand, medications placed on mucous membranes (intranasal route) have many fewer cell layers through which to pass. Thus, medication absorption through mucous membranes is faster than medication absorption through the skin. It is sometimes useful to have slow absorption of a medication. A common emergency medication for which prolonged absorption is desired is nitroglycerin; nitroglycerin can be placed on the skin, where it is slowly absorbed over a prolonged period.

The surface area of the absorbing surface is an important determinant of the rate of medication absorption. Medications are absorbed quite rapidly from large surface areas. Inhaled medications are quickly distributed across the vast pulmonary epithelium. Medications administered by this route are rapidly absorbed into the circulation. In fact, some studies have shown that the rate of medication absorption through the inhaled route is nearly as rapid as administration by the intravenous route.

Finally, medication absorption is related to blood supply to the site of absorption. Some areas of the body have very rich blood supplies, whereas other areas do not. Medications placed in areas with rich blood supplies, such as the tissues under the tongue (sublingual), are absorbed rapidly. Medications placed in areas with poor blood supply, such as the fatty tissues (subcutaneous), are absorbed slowly. Muscle, as a rule, is more richly supplied with blood vessels than is subcutaneous tissue. Therefore, one would expect a medication to be absorbed more rapidly from muscle than from subcutaneous tissue (see Figure 2–2).

Knowledge of the various rates of medication absorption from each of the various routes is essential. (Routes of medication administration are discussed in detail in Chapter 3.) Epinephrine 1:1000, a medication commonly used in the management of acute allergic reactions, is generally given by the subcutaneous or intramuscular route. The reasons for choosing this site are many. First, epinephrine 1:1000 is a potent and concentrated medication. Rapid absorption of a large quantity of this medication into the circulation would certainly accentuate epinephrine's side effects such as tachycardia, trembling, and elevated blood pressure. Second, the therapeutic effects of epinephrine are fairly brief. The slower absorption obtained with subcutaneous injection allows prolonged release of the medication into the circulation, thus maintaining the desired effects for a longer period (see Table 2–1).

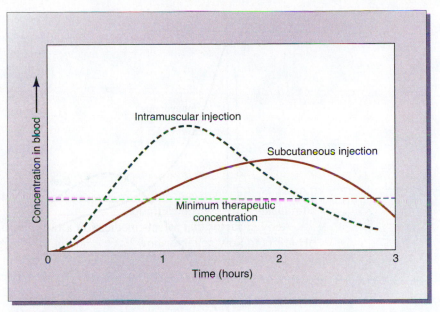

● **FIGURE 2–2** Comparision of medication levels following intramuscular and subcutaneous injections.

TABLE 2–1	
Comparison of Rates of Medication Absorption of Various Routes of Administration	
Route	**Rate of Absorption**
Oral	Slow
Subcutaneous	Slow
Topical	Moderate
Intramuscular	Moderate
Intranasal	Moderate
Intralingual	Rapid
Rectal	Rapid
Sublingual	Rapid
Endotracheal	Rapid
Inhalation	Rapid
Intraosseous	Immediate
Intravenous	Immediate

Systemic blood flow can also affect medication absorption. Factors that may *delay* absorption from parenteral sites include shock, acidosis, and peripheral vasoconstriction secondary to such things as hypothermia. Factors such as peripheral vasodilation, which can occur in hyperthermia and fever, may *increase* the rate of medication absorption.

Medication absorption time may be minimized by injecting the medication directly into the circulatory system by the intravenous (IV) route. The desired effects are seen much sooner, and the eventual blood levels of the medication are much more predictable. Consequently, most critical-care medications are given intravenously (see Figure 2–3).

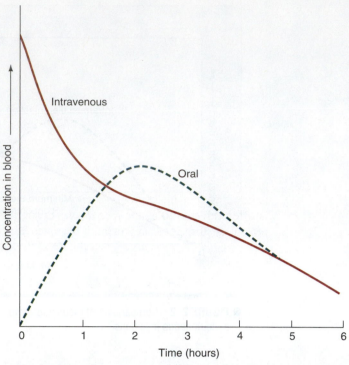

FIGURE 2–3 Comparison of medication levels following IV and oral medication administration.

Bioavailability is the measure of the amount of a medication that is still active after it reaches its target tissue. This is the bottom line as far as absorption is concerned. The goal of administering a medication is to assure sufficient bioavailability of the medication at the target tissue in order to produce the desired effect, after considering all of the absorption factors.

Distribution

Once a medication has entered the bloodstream, it must be distributed throughout the body. Most medications will pass easily from the bloodstream, through the interstitial spaces, into the target cells. Distribution is the process whereby a medication is transported from the site of absorption to the site of action.

Several factors can affect medication distribution:

1. Cardiovascular function
2. Regional blood flow
3. Medication storage reservoirs
4. Physiological barriers

As with medication absorption, medication distribution depends on cardiovascular function. Following administration and absorption, the medication is initially distributed to highly perfused body areas such as the brain, heart, kidneys, and liver. Delivery of the medication to the gastrointestinal system, skin, muscles, and fat is generally much slower. In certain conditions, such as shock and congestive heart failure, cardiac output will fall. When it does, medication distribution becomes much slower and much more unpredictable. When cardiac output is markedly diminished, some body areas are minimally perfused, and medication delivery to these areas is negligible.

Variances in *regional blood flow* can also affect medication distribution. For example, in cardiogenic shock, blood flow to the kidneys is often diminished. Medications that act specifically on the kidneys, such as diuretics, may not reach the kidneys in an adequate concentration to be effective.

In the body, a medication may be stored in various sites known as *medication reservoirs*. These reservoirs store medications by binding the medications to proteins present within the tissue in question. This action tends to delay the medication's **onset of action** and prolongs its duration of effect. There are two types of storage reservoirs: *plasma reservoirs* and *tissue reservoirs*.

During medication distribution through the vascular or lymphatic system, the medication comes in contact with proteins and remains free or binds to plasma carrier protein, storage tissue protein, or receptor protein. The portion of the medication that is bound to plasma proteins is called the *bound medication,* and the unbound portion is often referred to as the *free drug*. As soon as a medication binds to plasma carrier protein or storage tissue protein, it becomes inactive, rendering it unavailable for binding to a receptor protein and incapable of exerting therapeutic activity. However, a bound medication can free itself rapidly to maintain a balance between the amounts of free and bound medication. Only the free, or unbound, percentage of the medication remains active.

The percentage of medication that remains free and available for activity depends on the amount of plasma protein available for binding. The most common plasma protein involved in medication binding is **albumin**. However, other plasma proteins, such as **hemoglobin** and **globulins**, are utilized as well. This binding of medication to protein is usually reversible. The extent of binding depends on the physical properties of the medication itself. Some medications are highly bound, whereas others have limited binding. The degree to which a medication is bound is referred to as the **binding capacity**. Binding of a medication to plasma proteins tends to limit its concentration in the tissues.

Medications can also accumulate in the various tissues of the body. Common tissue reservoirs include fat, bone, and muscle tissue. Once in these compartments, the medication binds to proteins and similar substances. As with plasma protein binding, tissue binding is usually reversible. Some body compartments, such as the muscle tissue, can represent a sizable medication reservoir. Many medications are lipid soluble (fat soluble). These medications concentrate in the fatty tissues of the body, resulting in a prolonged medication effect.

Physiological barriers also affect medication distribution. Physiological barriers inhibit the movement of certain substances while permitting the passage of others. One of the most important physiological barriers is the **blood–brain barrier**. The blood–brain barrier refers to a network of capillary endothelial cells in the brain. These cells have no pores and are surrounded by a sheath of glial connective tissue that makes them impermeable to water-soluble medications. The network excludes most ionized medication molecules, such as dopamine, from the brain. However, it allows nonionized, unbound medication molecules, such as barbiturates, to pass readily and enter the brain. The blood–brain barrier is an effective boundary between the central nervous system and the peripheral nervous system. Delivery of medications and other substances to the brain is limited by the blood–brain barrier. It allows entry of certain medications and is considered a protective mechanism of the brain.

The so-called *placental barrier* can likewise prevent medications from reaching a fetus, although it is not the solid barrier that its name implies. The fetus is exposed to almost every medication that the mother takes. But because any medication must traverse the maternal blood supply and cross the capillary membranes into the placenta (fetal) circulation, delivering medications to a fetus requires them to be lipid soluble, nonionized, and non-protein-bound. This may slow some medications or reduce their placental transfer to benign levels.

Biotransformation

Like other chemicals that enter the body, medications are metabolized, or broken down into different chemicals (metabolites). The special name given to the **metabolism** of medications is biotransformation. Biotransformation can metabolize a drug into an active or inactive form. Generally speaking, it has one of two effects on most medications: (1) it can transform the medication into a more or less active metabolite, or (2) it can make the medication more water soluble (or less lipid soluble) to facilitate elimination. Some medications, such as lidocaine, are totally metabolized before elimination, others only partially, and still others not at all. The body will transform some molecules of most medications and eliminate others without transformation. Protein-bound medications are not available for biotransformation. Some so-called prodrugs (or parent medications) are not active when administered, but biotransformation converts them into active metabolites.

Many biotransformation processes occur in the liver. The endoplasmic reticula of hepatocytes (liver cells) contain microsomal enzymes that perform much of the metabolizing. (Smaller quantities of the enzymes are also found in the kidney, lung, and GI tract.) Because the blood supply from the GI tract passes through the liver via the portal vein, all medications absorbed in the GI tract pass through the liver before moving on through the systemic circulation. The first pass through the liver may partially or completely inactivate many medications. This first-pass effect is why some medications cannot be given orally but instead must be given intravenously to bypass the GI tract and prevent first-pass hepatic metabolism. It is also why medications that can be given either orally or intravenously may require a much higher oral dose than IV dose. Because we can observe the extent of first-pass metabolism, we can predict how much to increase a dose of an oral medication to deliver an effective amount of the medication into the general circulation.

Through biotransformation, the body detoxifies and disposes of foreign substances. Because medications are unnatural to the body, they are disposed of, as are other toxins. In most cases, the enzyme system increases the water solubility of a medication so that the renal system can excrete it. The lipid solubility of some medications may be altered enzymatically so that the end products enter into and are excreted through the biliary system. Using the renal or the biliary pathway for disposal, the body usually transforms the medication into a readily eliminated, pharmacologically inactive product.

Biotransformation begins immediately following introduction of the medication into the body. Certain medications are rapidly biotransformed, and others are not. For example, the emergency medication epinephrine is active as administered. However, it is very rapidly metabolized to inactive forms before elimination. Because of this rapid biotransformation, epinephrine must be readministered approximately every 3 to 5 minutes if still required.

Some medications are inactive when administered. Once they have been absorbed, they must be converted to an active form, either in the blood or by the target tissue. The inactive precursor is referred to as a prodrug. Several medications used in prehospital care must be converted into an active form before they can exert their desired effects. Diazepam (Valium), a medication used in the treatment of seizures, is relatively inactive as administered. Once in the body it is converted to its active metabolite, desmethyldiazepam, which then induces the desired effects (see Figure 2–4).

Elimination

Medications are eventually eliminated from the body in either their original form or as metabolites. Medication **excretion** refers to movement of a medication or its metabolites from the tissues back into the circulation and from the circulation into the organs of excretion. Medications may be excreted by the kidneys into the urine, by the liver into the

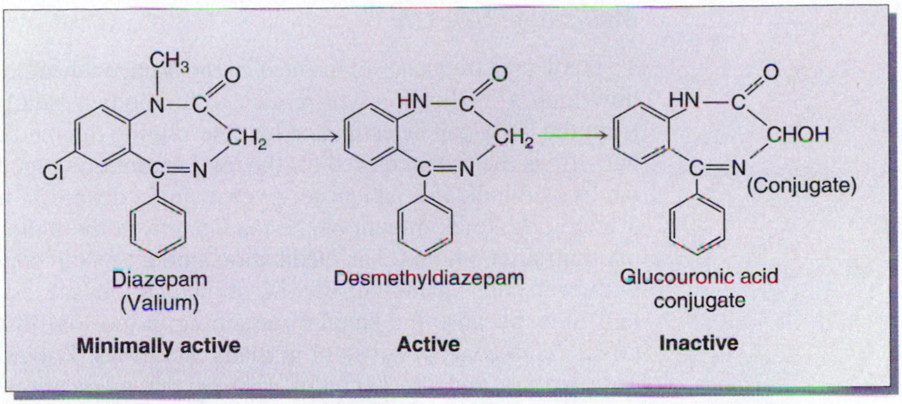

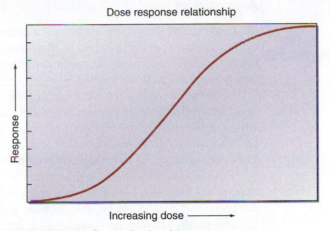

● **FIGURE 2–4** Metabolites of diazepam.

Dose response relationship

● **FIGURE 2–5** The medication dose–response curve.

bile, by the intestines into the feces, or by the lungs with the expired air. Additionally, medications may be excreted through sweat, saliva, and breast milk. Excretion through sweat glands is rarely a significant mechanism for elimination. Excretion through mammary glands becomes a concern when nursing mothers take medications. Medications may also be removed artificially by direct interventions, such as peritoneal dialysis or hemodialysis. The rate of elimination varies with the medication and the state of the body. During shock states, the kidneys are poorly perfused. In such cases, medications that are primarily eliminated by the kidneys remain present in the body for longer periods. The slower the rate of elimination, the longer the medication stays in the body.

Medication Dosing

The amount of medication administered in any giving setting is referred to as the **dose**. The dosage of a medication includes the amount of the medication administered, the frequency of medication administration, and the number of doses administered. For example, the antibiotic azithromycin (Zithromax) has the following dosage for treatment of common infections. A loading dose of 500 milligrams is administered on day 1. This is followed by subsequent 250 milligrams doses each day for the next four days. The dosage of a medication is important in determining the subsequent amount of medication in the body. Generally speaking, the effects (beneficial and toxic) tend to increase as the dosage of medication increases and can be reflected in the medication dose–response curve (see Figure 2–5). The most desirable dosage is one that gives enough medication effect to treat the condition in question without causing toxic effects.

Medication Half-Life

To predict the frequency of the medication dosage schedule, the physician must determine how long a medication will remain in the body. Usually the rate of medication loss from the body can be estimated by determining the medication's **half-life**. Medication half-life is the time required for the total amount of a medication in the body to diminish by one-half. If a patient receives a single dose of a medication with a half-life of 5 hours, the total amount of the medication in the patient's body would diminish by one-half after 5 hours. The medication amount would continue to decrease accordingly with each subsequent half-life. Most medications are essentially eliminated after five half-lives because the amount remaining is too low to exert a beneficial or adverse effect. This concept is useful in many situations. For example, if a medication overdose occurs and the excretion rate of the medication is not compromised, about 97 percent of the original dose will be eliminated after five half-lives.

Accumulation

Medication half-life is also useful when assessing medication accumulation. A medication that is not readministered is eliminated almost completely after five half-lives, but a regularly administered medication reaches a constant total body amount, or steady state, after about five half-lives.

Although a medication was once at a steady state, the medication's concentration in the blood fluctuates above and below the average concentration. Stated another way, although the medication was once at steady state, its concentration does not remain uniform; rather, it increases, peaks, and declines, although within a constant range. These changes can be minimized by continuous infusions of a drug at a constant rate.

For some medications, the time required to reach therapeutic blood concentration may be too long. For example, when using digoxin, with a half-life of about 1.6 days, the physician would not be able to wait 8 days (1.6 days times five half-lives) to achieve steady-state blood concentration levels to control a life-threatening arrhythmia, such as atrial fibrillation. Therefore, an initial large dose, called a **loading dose**, would be administered to reach the desired therapeutic blood concentration level. Consequently, smaller **maintenance doses** would be given daily to replace the amount of medication eliminated since the last dose. These dosages maintain a therapeutic blood concentration in the body at all times.

Clearance

Medication clearance refers to the removal of a medication from the body. A medication with a slow clearance rate is removed from the body slowly; one with a high clearance rate is removed rapidly. A medication with a high clearance rate may require more frequent administration and higher doses than a comparable medication with a low clearance rate. A medication with a low clearance rate can accumulate to a toxic concentration in the body unless it is administered less frequently or at lower doses.

Onset, Peak, and Duration

Besides absorption, distribution, metabolism, and excretion, three other factors play an important role in a medication's pharmacokinetics:

1. Onset of action
2. Peak concentration
3. Duration of action

The onset of action refers to the time it takes to observe the desired effect. In many situations, the onset of action is related to the time when the medication is sufficiently absorbed to reach an effective blood level and is sufficiently distributed to its site of action to elicit a therapeutic response.

As the body absorbs more of the medication, the medication concentration in the blood rises, more medication reaches the site of action, and the therapeutic response often increases. These occurrences characterize the peak concentration level for the medication dose administered.

As soon as the medication begins to circulate in the blood, it also begins to be eliminated. Eventually medication elimination exceeds its absorption rate because less of the medication dose remains to be absorbed. At this point, the medication concentration in the blood and the medication's effect begin to decline. When the blood concentration falls below the minimum needed to produce an effect, medication action ceases, although some medication remains in the blood. Therefore, the duration of action is the length of time that medication concentration is sufficient in the blood to produce a therapeutic response.

A medication's onset, peak, and duration are determined by several factors. These include its bioavailability (the extent to which a medication's active ingredient is absorbed and transported to its site of action) and medication concentration in the blood. The rate of clearance and elimination are major factors in a medication's concentration in the blood. However, some medications may have a duration of effect that extends well beyond their half-life.

PHARMACODYNAMICS

Pharmacodynamics is the study of the mechanisms by which specific medication dosages act to produce biochemical or physiological changes in the body.

Mechanisms of Action of Medications

Medications can act in four different ways. They may bind to a receptor site, change the physical properties of cells, chemically combine with other chemicals, or alter a normal metabolic pathway. Each of these actions involves a physiochemical interaction between the medication and a functionally important molecule in the body.

Medications That Act by Binding to a Receptor Site

Most medications operate by binding to a receptor. Almost all medication receptors are protein molecules on the surfaces of cells. They are part of the body's normal regulatory stimulation/inhibition function, and can be stimulated or inhibited by chemicals. Each different receptor's name generally corresponds to the medication that stimulates it. For example, if an opiate stimulates the receptor, then the receptor is an opioid receptor. When multiple medications stimulate the same receptor, standard practice is to use the generic name.

The force of attraction between a medication and a receptor is called their **affinity**. The greater the affinity, the stronger the bond. Different medications may bind to the same type of receptor site, but the strength of their bonds may vary. The binding site's shape determines its receptivity to other chemicals, whether they are medications or endogenous substances. These binding sites are relatively specific—a nonopiate medication generally will not affect an opiate binding site, although occasionally a medication with a similar receptor binding site will unexpectedly cross-react. Receptors can also have subtypes. At least five subtypes of adrenergic receptors, for example, are important to prehospital practice.

A medication's pharmacodynamics also involves its ability to cause the expected response, called its efficacy. Just as different medications may have different affinities for a site, they may also have different efficacies; that is, medication A may cause a stronger response than medication B. Affinity and efficacy are not directly related.

Medication A may cause a stronger response than medication B, even though medication B binds to the receptor site more strongly than medication A.

When a medication binds with its specific type of receptor, a chemical change occurs that ultimately leads to the medication having its desired effect on the body. In most cases, medications will either stimulate or inhibit the cell's normal biochemical actions. In fact, a medication cannot impart a new function to a cell. Some medications may interact with a receptor and directly result in the desired effect. Other medications, however, may interact with a receptor and cause the release or production of a second compound. This secondary compound, or second messenger, includes such compounds as calcium or cyclic adenosine monophosphate (cAMP). Cyclic AMP is the most common second messenger. It has a multitude of effects inside the cell. These secondary messengers are particularly important in the endocrine system, because they principally occur in endocrine glands. Once cAMP is formed inside the cell, it activates still other enzymes, usually in a cascading action. That is, the first enzyme activates another enzyme, which activates a third enzyme, and so forth. This is important in that it amplifies the action so that even a small amount of a medication (or hormone) acting on the cell surface can initiate a powerful, cascading, activating force for the entire cell.

The number of receptors on a target cell usually does not remain constant on a daily basis or even from minute to minute. This is because the receptor proteins are often destroyed during the course of their function. At other times, they are either reactivated or remanufactured by the protein-manufacturing mechanism of the cell. Binding of a medication (or hormone) to a target cell receptor causes the number of receptors to decrease. This process is termed downregulation of the receptors. It results in a decreased responsiveness of the target cell to the medication or hormone as the number of available active receptors decreases. In other cases, but less commonly, a medication (or hormone) can cause the formation of more receptors than normal. This process, upregulation, increases the target tissue's sensitivity to the particular medication or hormone.

Chemicals that stimulate a receptor site generally fall into two broad categories, **agonists** and **antagonists**. Agonists bind to the receptor and cause it to initiate the expected response. Antagonists bind to a site but do not cause the receptor to initiate the expected response. Some medications, agonist–antagonists (also called partial agonists), may do both. Nalbuphine (Nubain), for instance, stimulates some of the opioid agonists' analgesic properties, but partially blocks others such as respiratory depression.

Receptor-mediated medication actions work like a lock (the receptor) and key (the agonist). If you put the key in the lock and turn it, the lock will open. An antagonist is like a key that fits into the lock, but will not turn and cannot open the lock. Target tissues generally have many receptors, so to take the analogy another step, imagine that to get maximal effect a single key (agonist) must move around and open many doors (trigger many biochemical responses). An agonist–antagonist would be a key that unlocks and opens a door but gets stuck in the lock. That is, the medication will cause the expected effect, but that medication will also block another medication from triggering the same receptor. This competitive antagonism is considered surmountable because a sufficiently large dose of the agonist can overcome the antagonism.

Noncompetitive antagonism can also occur. Continuing the lock, key, and door analogy, imagine the door is barred. This antagonism would be insurmountable; no amount of agonist could overcome it. Noncompetitive antagonism occurs because the binding of the antagonist at a different site causes a deformity of the binding site that actually prevents the agonist from fitting and binding. Irreversible antagonism may also occur when a competitive antagonist permanently binds with a receptor site. When this occurs, no amount of agonist will stimulate the receptor. For the effects of such an antagonist to wear off, the body must create new receptors.

Two medications may appear to be antagonists while actually acting independently. This physiological antagonism can occur when one medication's effects counteract another's. Although neither agent chemically affects the other, their net effect is antagonistic. An example of a receptor, agonist, antagonist, and agonist–antagonist can be described using an opiate receptor. These receptors occur naturally in the brain and respond to natural endorphins. Morphine sulfate acts as an agonist. It binds to the opiate receptor and causes the expected response of pain relief. Naloxone (Narcan) acts as an antagonist. It will bind to the opiate receptor, but will not initiate the pain relief. It will prevent morphine sulfate from binding to the site and thus effectively blocks the morphine and its response. If the patient is given nalbuphine (Nubain), an agonist–antagonist, it will bind to the opiate receptor and relieve pain, but it is less efficacious than morphine. The nalbuphine blocks morphine from the receptor like an antagonist, but stimulates the receptor on its own like an agonist, although to a lesser extent.

Medications That Act by Changing Physical Properties

Some medications change the physical properties of a part of the body. Medications that change the osmotic balance across membranes are good examples of this type of medication action. The osmotic diuretic mannitol (Osmotrol), for instance, increases urine output by increasing the blood's osmolarity, or osmotic "pull." This increased osmolarity triggers the normal regulatory systems to decrease water reabsorption in the renal tubules, thereby reducing the total amount of water in the body.

Medications That Act by Chemically Combining with Other Substances

Medications that participate in chemical reactions that change the chemical nature of their substrates (the chemical or substance on which a medication acts) play a large role in prehospital practice. For example, isopropyl alcohol, which is often used to disinfect skin before percutaneous needle insertion for phlebotomy or IV cannulation, denatures the proteins on the surface of bacterial cells. This ruptures the cells, destroying the bacteria. The antacids are another example. They act by chemically neutralizing the hydrochloric acid in the stomach. Sodium bicarbonate given intravenously chemically neutralizes some of the acids in the bloodstream, effectively making the blood more alkalotic.

Medications That Act by Altering a Normal Metabolic Pathway

Some anticancer and antiviral medications are chemical analogs of normal metabolic substrates. In a process that has been dubbed a counterfeit incorporation mechanism, these medications can be incorporated into the products of metabolism of cancer cells. Because these medications are not really the expected substrate, the anticipated product either will not form or, if formed, will be substantially or completely inactive.

Medication Potency and Efficacy

Medication potency refers to the relative amount of a medication required to produce the desired response. Comparing the medication potency of one medication with that of another medication can reveal which is the more potent medication. The power of a medication to produce a therapeutic effect is called the medication's efficacy. Medications that are agonists have both affinity and efficacy. Medications that are antagonists have affinity but not efficacy, because they do not produce a physiological response. Classic illustrations of this principle are the medications epinephrine and propranolol (Inderal). Epinephrine, once administered, is transported to its various target tissues—namely, the heart, the lungs, and the peripheral blood vessels. Once at these target tissues, it finds and binds to its receptors, which are called beta-receptors. If the medication is able to bind to these beta-receptors, then the desired physiological

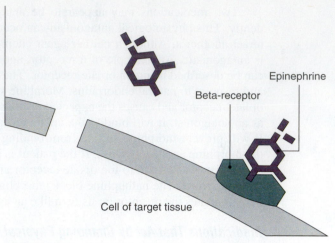

● **FIGURE 2–6** Epinephrine interacting with beta-receptor.

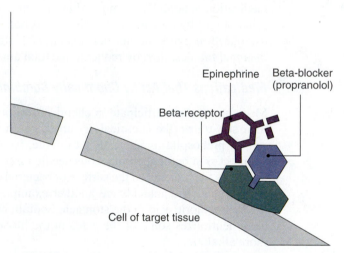

● **FIGURE 2–7** Beta-receptor blocked by propranolol.

response will be seen. Several medications themselves are inactive but can bind to beta-receptors in much the same manner as epinephrine. These medications are referred to as beta-blockers, and the prototype medication of this group is propranolol. If a beta-blocker has already bound to the receptor, then epinephrine cannot bind, and the desired effect is effectively blocked (see Figures 2–6 and 2–7). A more detailed discussion of beta-receptors and beta-blockers can be found in Chapter 6.

Therapeutic Index

Once again, for a medication to be effective it must reach a certain concentration at the target tissue. The minimal concentration of a medication necessary to cause the desired response is referred to as the **therapeutic threshold**, or **minimum effective concentration**. A concentration below this therapeutic threshold will not induce a clinical response. There is also a point at which the medication concentration can get high enough to be toxic or even fatal. The general goal of medication therapy is to give the minimum concentration of a medication necessary to obtain the desired response (see Figure 2–8).

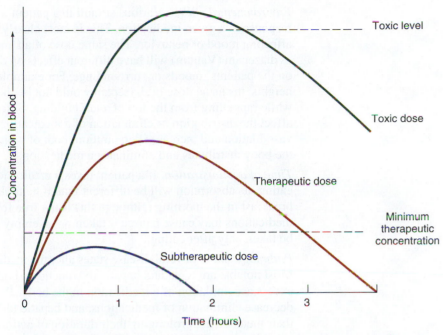

● **FIGURE 2–8** Comparison of blood levels following subtherapeutic, therapeutic, and toxic doses of the same medication.

The difference between the minimum effective concentration and the **toxic level** varies significantly from medication to medication. The difference between these two concentrations is referred to as the **therapeutic index** and is usually obtained in the laboratory. Certain medications, such as digoxin, have very little difference between the effective dose and the toxic dose. Such medications are said to have a low therapeutic index. Medications such as naloxone (Narcan), the narcotic antagonist, have a significant margin between the effective dose and the toxic dose and are said to have a high therapeutic index. Prehospital care providers should be familiar with the therapeutic indexes of the medications they use.

Factors Altering Medication Response

Different individuals may have different responses to the same medication. Factors that alter the standard medication–response relationship include the following:

- *Age.* The liver and kidney functions of infants are not yet fully developed, so their response to medications may be altered. Likewise, as we age, the function of these organs begins to deteriorate. As a result, infants and the elderly are most susceptible to having an altered response to a medication.

- *Body mass.* The more body mass a person has, the more fluid that is potentially available to dilute a medication. A given amount of medication will have a higher concentration in a person with little body mass than in a much larger person. Thus, most medication dosages are stated in terms of body mass. For example, the standard dose of lidocaine for a patient in cardiac arrest is a 0.5 mg/kg. A 100-kg patient will receive 150 mg of lidocaine, whereas a 50-kg patient will receive only 75 mg.

- *Gender.* Most differences in medication response due to gender result from the relative body masses of men and women. The different distribution and amounts of body fat also affect the amounts of medication available at any given time.

- *Environmental milieu.* Various stimuli in a patient's environment affect his response to a given medication. This is most clearly seen with medications affecting mood or behavior. The same dose of an antianxiety medication such as diazepam (Valium) will have different effects on different patients, depending on the patients' moods or surroundings. For example, if a patient is afraid of heights, his usual dose of diazepam would not be likely to help him remain calm while rappelling from the top of a tall building. Surrounding conditions may also affect the distribution or elimination of a medication. Heat, for example, causes vasodilation and increases perspiration, both of which may alter the rate at which the body distributes and eliminates a medication.

- *Time of administration.* If a patient takes a medication immediately after eating, its absorption will be different than if he took the same medication before breakfast in the morning (although this is not true for all medications). Some medications may cause nausea if taken on an empty stomach and must therefore be taken only after eating.

- *Pathologic state.* Several disease states alter the medication–response relationship. Most notable are renal and hepatic dysfunctions, both of which may lead to excess accumulation of a medication in the body. Renal failure is likely to decrease elimination of medications, and hepatic failure may decrease or inhibit their metabolism, prolonging their duration of action. Acid–base disturbances may alter a medication's solubility or the extent to which it ionizes, thus changing its absorption rate.

- *Genetic factors.* Genetic traits such as a lack of specific enzymes or a lowered basal metabolic rate alter medication absorption or biotransformation and thus modify the patient's response.

- *Psychological factors.* A patient's mental state can also affect his response to a medication. The best known example of this is the placebo effect. Essentially, if a patient believes that a medication will have a given effect, then he is much more likely to perceive that the effect has occurred.

Special Considerations in Medication Therapy

Age, pregnancy, and lactation are important considerations in medication therapy. Both children and the elderly are particularly susceptible to the adverse effects of medications. Consequently, medication dosages often must be modified for persons in these age groups. Likewise, special precautions must be taken when administering medications to a pregnant patient, because many medications will also affect the fetus. Certain medications are excreted into the breast milk, which becomes a particular concern in mothers who are breast-feeding their infants. The following sections discuss these special considerations in medication therapy.

Pediatric Patients

Children are typically smaller than adults, and medication dosages must be reduced accordingly. Pediatric medication dosages are typically based on the child's body weight or body surface area (BSA). Thus, it is essential that prehospital personnel determine or approximate a child's weight before administering a medication. Often, the parents can provide an approximate weight from a recent doctor's visit. In emergencies the child's body weight can be estimated by determining the child's age and finding the average body weight for that age on a reference table.

Neonates (infants from birth to 4 weeks) are a special concern. Common sites of medication metabolism and elimination, such as the liver and kidneys, are not well developed in neonates. Thus both medication metabolism and excretion may be impaired. Medication dosages for neonates must often be modified to reflect these factors.

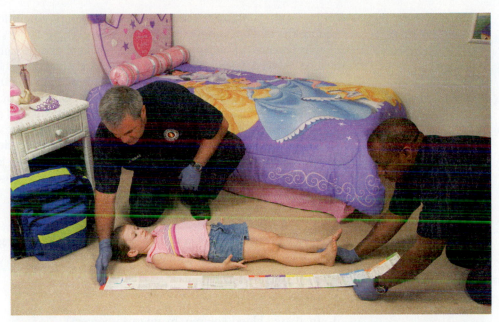

● **FIGURE 2–9**   A Broselow tape is useful for calculating medication dosages for pediatric patients.

The American Heart Association (AHA) and the American Academy of Pediatrics (AAP) publish recommended medication dosages for most emergency medications. Often, the doses of common emergency medications are listed on easy-to-use reference cards. To use these, prehospital care providers simply look up the child's age or weight. Below the age or weight are the recommended dosages for common emergency medications.

Another popular device for determining pediatric medication dosages is the Broselow tape (see Figure 2–9). The Broselow tape is simply unfolded and placed alongside the supine child to measure the child from the top of the head to the bottom of the feet. The tape is divided into various color-coded medication dosage charts based on the child's length (which is directly related to the child's weight and body surface area). Prehospital care providers simply use the dosage chart that corresponds to the child's length. In addition to medication dosages, the Broselow tape contains recommended endotracheal tube sizes, defibrillator settings, and other important emergency information.

Geriatric Patients

The elderly age group is the fastest growing segment of the U.S. population, and older adults are frequent users of the emergency medical services (EMS) system. The aging process begins at the cellular level and affects virtually every body system. Common physiological effects of aging include the following:

1. Decreased cardiac output
2. Decreased renal function
3. Decreased brain mass
4. Decreased total body water
5. Decreased body fat
6. Decreased serum albumin
7. Decreased respiratory capacity

These changes can lead to altered pharmacodynamics and pharmacokinetics for many medications. With aging, the rate of metabolism and the excretion of medications can be significantly decreased. In addition, there is often decreased protein binding because the level of serum albumin decreases. These factors combine to increase the relative potency of a medication. Consequently, the dosages of many medications must be reduced when administered to an elderly patient.

The elderly are more apt to suffer from more than one disease process at a time. In addition, they may be on chronic medications, which may affect the emergency medications paramedics need to administer in the prehospital setting. Multiple medical problems make medication dosing much more difficult. For example, treating a patient with congestive heart failure may be more difficult if the patient also has renal failure. In this case, the dosage of furosemide (Lasix) may need to be increased, and the dosage of morphine may need to be decreased. All factors must be considered before administering medications to the elderly.

Pregnancy and Lactation

Pregnancy presents two pharmacological problems. First, pregnancy causes a number of anatomical and physiological changes in the mother, including:

1. Increased cardiac output
2. Increased heart rate
3. Increased blood volume (by up to 45 percent)
4. Decreased protein binding
5. Decreased hepatic metabolism
6. Decreased blood pressure

These anatomical and physiological changes must be considered prior to administering medications or fluids to a pregnant patient.

The second consideration associated with pregnancy is that any medication administered to the mother has the potential to cross the placenta and affect the fetus. Some medications cross the placenta rapidly, but others do not. Thus, medications should be administered in pregnancy only when the potential benefits outweigh the risks. The U.S. Food and Drug Administration (FDA) categorizes most medications based on their safety in pregnancy (see Table 2–2).

TABLE 2–2	
FDA Pregnancy Categories	
Category	**Description**
A	**Controlled studies show no risk:** Well-controlled studies in pregnant women have failed to demonstrate risk to the fetus.
B	**No evidence of risk in humans:** Animal studies have not demonstrated a risk to the fetus, but there are no adequate studies in pregnant women.
	OR
	Adequate studies in pregnant women have not demonstrated a risk to the fetus in the first trimester and there is no risk in the last trimester, but animal studies have demonstrated adverse effects.
C	**Risk cannot be ruled out:** Animal studies have demonstrated adverse effects, but there are no adequate studies in pregnant women; however, benefits may be acceptable despite the potential risk.
	OR
	No adequate animal studies or adequate studies of pregnant women have been done.
D	**Positive evidence of risk:** Fetal risk has been demonstrated. In certain circumstances, benefits could outweigh the risks.
X	**Contraindicated in pregnancy:** Fetal risk has been demonstrated. This risk outweighs any possible benefit to the mother. Avoid using in pregnant or potentially pregnant patients.

As with pregnancy, medication therapy can affect a breast-feeding infant. Many medications are excreted readily into the breast milk. If the mother continues to breast-feed while receiving these medications, the medications can be excreted into the breast milk and be ingested by the baby. If a breast-feeding mother is to receive medications, she should be instructed to stop breast-feeding and pump her breasts. She should dispose of the expressed milk until she is certain that the medication has been cleared from her system. During the time she is pumping her breasts, she should switch the infant to a commercial formula.

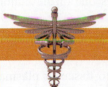

CASE STUDY

It's another Sunday morning and the crew of Rescue 1 are responding to an unconscious person at a known "shooting gallery" not far from downtown. "Shooting galleries" are areas where IV drug abusers often congregate and inject their drugs. Paramedics have been to this location numerous times. It is a popular area for heroin addicts to inject their drugs. Upon arrival, paramedics enter the rundown house and find an unconscious male on an old mattress. Other people on scene report that the patient recently "mainlined" an unknown quantity of heroin. Paramedics utilize Standard Precautions and assess the patient. His pupils are pinpoint and his breathing is about 10 times per minute. Paramedics quickly place a saline lock and administer a dose of the narcotic antagonist naloxone. Following this, the patient slowly arouses and becomes oriented. As usually occurs at this location, the patient refuses subsequent care and completes a refusal of transport form.

Robert Samuels, an EMT student riding with Rescue 1, questions the paramedics about the call. The paramedics describe how narcotics such as heroin bind to receptors in the brain that cause respiratory and central nervous system depression. Heroin acts as a "key" on the receptors that are much like "locks." The administration of naloxone, a narcotic antagonist, actually displaced some of the heroin molecules from the receptors. When this occurred, the naloxone molecules bound to the receptors in place of the heroin thus reversing the respiratory depression and similar untoward effects. Because of this, the patient aroused and refused further care.

Questions

1. Why can naloxone be also used for other medications such as hydromorphone and morphine?
2. Give another example of an antidote that is occasionally used in the prehospital setting.

CHAPTER REVIEW

Summary

A basic understanding of pharmacokinetics and pharmacodynamics is essential for prehospital personnel to anticipate the desired therapeutic effects as well as any possible side effects of the medications they administer. Such factors as rate of absorption, elimination, minimum therapeutic concentration, and toxic levels should be considered in all medications.

Key Words

absorption   The process whereby a medication is moved from the site of application into the body and into the extracellular fluid compartment.

active transport   A mechanism of transport that requires the use of energy to move a substance.

affinity   The tendency of a medication to combine with a specific medication receptor.

agonist   A medication or other substance that binds with a specific medication receptor and causes a physiological response.

albumin   Protein found in almost all animal tissue. It constitutes one of the major proteins in human blood.

antagonist   A medication or other substance that blocks a physiological response or that blocks the action of another medication or substance.

binding capacity   The degree to which a medication is bound to tissue or plasma proteins.

biotransformation   Biotransformation, also called metabolism, is the process of changing a medication into a different form, either active or inactive, by the body.

blood–brain barrier   Protective mechanism that selectively allows the entry of specific compounds into the brain. It is an effective boundary between the central nervous system and the peripheral nervous system.

distribution   The process whereby a medication is transported from the site of absorption to the site of action.

dose   A measured portion of a medication taken at one time.

dosage   The amount of a medicine or other agent administered for a given case or condition.

efficacy   The power of a medication to produce a therapeutic effect.

elimination   The process whereby a medication is removed from the body by excretion into the urine, feces, bile, saliva, sweat, breast milk, or expired air.

excretion   The elimination of waste products from the body. *Excretion* is often used interchangeably with the term *elimination*.

globulin   One of a broad category of simple proteins found in the body.

half-life   The time required for a level of a medication in the blood to be reduced by 50 percent of its beginning level.

hemoglobin   An iron-containing compound found within the blood cell that is responsible for the transport and delivery of oxygen to the body cells.

loading dose   The initial dose of a medication given in a sufficient amount to achieve a therapeutic plasma level.

maintenance dose   The dose of a medication necessary to maintain a constant therapeutic plasma level.

mechanism of action   Biochemical and physiological events when medications reach their targeted tissues.

metabolism   The sum total of all physical and chemical changes that occur within the body. In pharmacology it is often used interchangeably with the term *biotransformation*.

minimum effective concentration   The minimum amount of medication needed in the bloodstream to cause the desired therapeutic effect.

onset of action   The time interval between the administration of a medication and the first sign of its onset; onset of action is influenced by the physical and chemical properties of a medication as well as by its route of administration.

passive transport   A mechanism of transport that does not require the use of energy to move a substance.

pH   A scientific method of expressing the acidity or alkalinity of a solution, which is the logarithm of the hydrogen ion concentration divided by 1. The higher the pH, the more alkaline the solution; the lower the pH, the more acidic the solution.

pharmacodynamics   The study of a medication's action on the body.

pharmacokinetics   The study of how medications enter the body, reach their site of action, and eventually are eliminated.

solubility   The tendency of a medication to dissolve.

therapeutic index   An index of the medication's safety profile, which is determined by calculating the difference between the medication's therapeutic threshold and toxic level. It is typically determined in the laboratory.

therapeutic threshold   The minimum amount of medication needed in the bloodstream to cause a desired therapeutic effect.

toxic level   The plasma level at which severe adverse reactions are expected or likely.

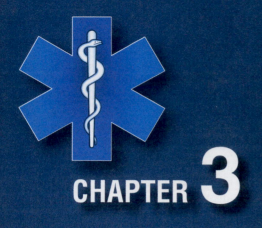

CHAPTER 3

ADMINISTRATION OF MEDICATIONS

OBJECTIVES

After completing this chapter, the reader should be able to:

- State the necessary components of a verbal or standing medication order.
- Explain the six rights of medication administration.
- Explain the advantages and disadvantages of enteral versus parenteral administration.
- List and explain four enteral tract routes.
- List and explain 12 parenteral routes.
- Briefly explain the following routes of medication administration:
  a. Transdermal
  b. Sublingual
  c. Subcutaneous route
  d. Intramuscular route
  e. Intravenous bolus
  f. Intravenous piggyback
  g. Via the endotracheal tube
  h. Via an intraosseous infusion
  i. Intranasal
- Describe the different methods of administering medications through inhalation therapy.
- Describe the special considerations in administering medications to a pediatric patient.
- Briefly explain the following pediatric routes of medication administration:
  a. Intramuscular route
  b. Subcutaneous route
  c. Intravenous route
  d. Rectal
  e. Introsseous

INTRODUCTION

In emergency medicine, medications must be administered promptly, in the correct dose, and by the correct route. Many medications, when given by the appropriate route and dose, can be beneficial. However, those same medications, when given by an inappropriate route or dose, can be fatal. Norepinephrine, for example, is a potent medication used to treat severe hypotension. It is designed to be given by slow, intravenous infusion. If given in an intravenous bolus, however, it may be fatal. This admonition applies to most medications used in emergency medicine.

The emergency scene is often hectic. Paramedics often prepare and administer medications in the worst of environments. Consequently, it is essential that all prehospital personnel develop safe habits regarding medication preparation and medication administration. These safe habits serve to protect both the patient and the paramedic.

This chapter presents the procedures for medication preparation and administration of medications used in emergency medical practice.

PATIENT CARE USING MEDICATIONS

Paramedics are responsible for the standard of care for patients in their charge. The ability to administer prehospital medications can benefit many patients; however, this responsibility cannot be taken lightly. You are, therefore, personally responsible—legally, morally, and ethically—for the safe and effective administration of medications. The following guidelines will help you to meet that responsibility:

- Know the precautions and contraindications for all medications you administer.
- Practice proper medication administration technique.
- Observe and document medication effects.
- Maintain a current knowledge in pharmacology.
- Establish and maintain professional relationships with other health care providers.
- Understand the pharmacokinetics and pharmacodynamics.
- Have a current medication reference available.
- Take careful medication histories including:
  - Name, strength, and daily dose of prescribed medications
  - Over-the-counter medications
  - Vitamins
  - Herbal medications
  - Folk medicine or folk remedies
  - Allergies
- Evaluate the compliance, dosage, and adverse reactions.
- Consult with medical direction when appropriate.

THE MEDICATION ORDER

Prehospital personnel are responsible for preparing and administering many emergency medications and fluids. The selection and administration of a particular medication depends on an accurate and complete patient assessment. The results of this assessment must be relayed to medical control or applied to prehospital treatment protocols or standing orders. An inaccurate or incomplete patient assessment may lead to administration of the wrong medication.

Medical oversight was discussed in Chapter 1. A review of the information regarding medical oversight, medical control, and medical control protocols is suggested.

The first step in medication administration is the medication order. The order may be in the form of a direct verbal order or through written standing treatment orders. The order generally specifies the following:

1. Medication desired
2. Dose desired

3. Administration route
4. Administration rate

If possible, verbal medication orders should be written down when they are received. After receiving the order, the paramedic should repeat the entire order back to the medical control physician. Doing so ensures that there is no misunderstanding related to the medication order. A typical medication order interchange is as follows:

Medical Control: Start an IV of normal saline at 125 mL per hour and administer 5 mg of diazepam intravenously over 1 minute.

Medic 1: Confirming an IV of normal saline at 125 mL per hour and 5 mg of diazepam intravenously over 1 minute.

Medical Control: Affirmative Medic 1.

In systems that utilize protocols, paramedics first review the appropriate protocols. They then confirm the ordered medication, dosage, route, and rate of medication administration and, if possible, have another crew member review and double-check the protocol. Finally, paramedics prepare and administer the medication as detailed in the protocol.

It is essential to use good judgment regarding medication administration. Paramedics should always carefully evaluate the orders they receive. Occasionally, orders will be received that differ from accepted local prehospital protocols. In these cases, paramedics must contact the medical control physician and advise him or her of the discrepancy. If, after discussion of the discrepancy, the medical control physician does not change the order, paramedics should follow the order. The exceptions to this rule, of course, are orders that paramedics believe will harm the patient. If paramedics believe a particular medication or dose will harm the patient, they should notify the medical control physician that they are withholding the medication and give the reason for doing so. Paramedics must document well the circumstances surrounding the controversy and submit documentation to the system medical director for resolution. Although prehospital care providers are responsible to the medical control physician, they have a higher duty to protect the health and well-being of their patients.

SIX RIGHTS OF MEDICATION ADMINISTRATION

After paramedics have received the medication or fluid order, they should then administer the medication in question. In performing medication administration, prehospital care providers adhere to the six rights of medication administration:

1. Right patient
2. Right medication
3. Right dose
4. Right route
5. Right time
6. Right documentation

Right Patient

Ensuring that the right patient receives the right medication is usually not a problem in prehospital care because typically only one patient is being treated. However, in some circumstances more than one patient may be undergoing treatment, especially in multiple casualty incidents. In cases with multiple patients, it is prudent to use some label to distinguish patients. Some systems prefer to use the patient's last name. However, it is not uncommon for several members of one family to be involved in an emergency. Each family member usually has the same last name, and some have the same first name (e.g., William and William Jr.). In these cases, it is best to assign numbers (e.g., Patient 1 and Patient 2) or letters of the alphabet (e.g., Patient A and Patient B) to each patient to avoid confusion.

Confusion regarding multiple patients is more of a problem for medical control than for individual paramedics. A multiple casualty incident may utilize several ambulances, with similar call signs. Personnel in each ambulance will contact medical control regarding the patient or patients they are transporting. Care should be taken to distinguish the patients and units to avoid confusion and possible medication error. Errors can be minimized by using effective scene management techniques such as the incident command system. In this system, each patient is designated with a number or letter at the time of triage. Radio communications, both initial and subsequent, should refer to the patient by this designation to help avoid confusion both in the field and at medical control.

Right Medication

A common error in prehospital medication administration is the selection of the wrong medication. Most emergency medications are supplied in ampules, vials, or prefilled syringes. Many look very similar. To ensure that the right medication is selected, paramedics should carefully read the label. If the medication is supplied in a box, they should check the label on the box and compare it with the label on the vial or ampule itself after removing it from the box. Paramedics can never assume that a medication is correct simply because it is in the correct place in the medication box. They must always read and check the label three times.

Medication preparations and concentrations can vary. In addition to checking the medication name, paramedics should always check to ensure that the medication concentration is the one desired. This check is especially important for medications that are carried in differing concentrations (e.g., epinephrine 1:1000 and epinephrine 1:10 000 or lidocaine 100 mg for intravenous bolus and lidocaine 1 g for intravenous infusion).

When following a physician's verbal order, repeat the order back to confirm that you both intend the same thing for the patient. Inspect the label on the medication at least three times before giving the medication to the patient: first as you remove the medication from the medication box or cabinet; second, as you draw the medication into the syringe; and third, immediately before you administer the medication. The expiration date of a medication should always be checked prior to administration. The medication should be held up to the light and inspected for discoloration or particles in the solution. Expired and discolored medications should be discarded. Routine (preferably daily) medication box inspections should detect any expired medications. However, paramedics should always double-check the medication prior to administration.

One of the most common medication administration errors is failure to confirm the medication name. If you have any question about a medication, do not administer it without confirmation. Showing the medication container to your partner and asking for confirmation is an easy way to further ensure that you are giving the right medication.

Right Dose

Administration of the correct medication dose is crucial. Errors in dosage occur in either calculating the correct dose or preparing the correct dose. Most medication orders are fairly straightforward, and many medications are supplied in unit–dose forms. In these cases, medication dosage calculation and medication preparation are easy. However, some medications, especially those administered by intravenous infusion, are much more difficult to calculate. For these medications, paramedics should refer to standardized dosage charts to assist with preparation and administration of the desired dose.

Right Route

Most medications used in prehospital care are designed to be given by the intravenous route. However, certain medications can be given by other routes depending on the physician's orders. It is the paramedic's responsibility to know the various routes by which a particular medication can be administered. For example, the injectable forms of the medications hydroxyzine (Vistaril) and promethazine (Phenergan) are occasionally used in the treatment of nausea. Promethazine can be administered both intravenously and intramuscularly. Hydroxyzine, in comparison, can be administered only by the intramuscular route.

Right Time

Most medication orders for prehospital care call for immediate (**stat**) administration of the medication. These orders are generally one-time orders. However, certain medications may be administered repeatedly, especially in cardiac arrest situations, in which medications are administered at specific time intervals.

An important consideration is the rate at which a medication should be administered. The rate is usually expressed as the period of time over which the medication in question should be administered. Many medications can be administered rapidly as an intravenous bolus. Others must be administered at a specific rate. Diazepam, for example, should never be administered faster than 1 mL/min (5 mg/min). The rate of medication administration is particularly crucial for intravenous infusion medications (e.g., lidocaine, dopamine, nitroglycerin, and norepinephrine).

Right Documentation

The medications you administer in the field do not stop affecting your patient when he enters the hospital. As a result, you must completely document all of your care, especially any medications you have administered, so that long after you have gone on to your next call, other providers will know what medications your patient has been given.

GENERAL ADMINISTRATION ROUTES

The two primary channels for getting medications into the body are enteral (through the **alimentary canal**, or gastrointestinal [GI] tract) and parenteral routes. The GI tract provides a fairly safe but relatively slow-acting site for medication absorption. Oral, sublingual, and rectal preparations are given via the GI tract. Administration by the parenteral route can involve all routes other than the GI tract. This chapter deals primarily with medications given by injection. Paramedics use the parenteral route to provide a rapid onset of action of the medication. The parenteral route also is used when the GI route would inactivate the medication, in unconscious patients, and in unstable or seriously ill patients who require precise administration and monitoring. In acute care medicine, administration is almost always parenteral because the onset of action is much quicker and usually more predictable.

TABLE 3–1

Comparison of Enteral vs Parenteral Routes

Advantages	Disadvantages
Enteral Route	
Simple	Slow rate of onset
Safe	Cannot be given to unconscious or nauseated patients
Generally less expensive	
Low potential for infection	Absorbed dosage may vary significantly because of actions of digestive enzymes and the condition of the intestinal tract
Parenteral Route	
Rapid onset	Administration often difficult and painful
Can be given to unconscious and nauseated patients	Usually more expensive
Absorbed dosage and action are more predictable	Side effects usually more severe
	Potential for infection

Table 3–1 compares the relative advantages and disadvantages of enteral versus parenteral administration.

Enteral Tract Routes

The common enteral routes of administration used in general medical practice are as follows:

Oral (PO). The best and most convenient way of administering medications is by mouth. Most medications are available in oral preparations. The effects of oral administration are often not seen until 30 to 45 minutes after administration and therefore not generally considered a medication administration route in prehospital care.

Orogastric/nasogastric tube (OG/NG). Via tube is generally considered another option for oral administration of medications. This route is generally used for oral medications when the patient already has the tube in place for other reasons.

Sublingual (SL). Some medications can be administered sublingually (i.e., under the tongue). When administered in this fashion, the medication is placed under the tongue, where it quickly dissolves. The medication is then absorbed into the vast capillary network present in the mucous membranes. Nitroglycerin, a medication frequently used in the management of angina pectoris, is administered by this route.

Buccal. The buccal area is the mucous membrane on the side of the cheek. Absorption through this route between the cheek and gum is similar to sublingual absorption. Glucose gel can be administered through the buccal route when an IV cannot be established. This route should be used only for conscious patients with an intact gag reflex.

Rectal (PR). Rectal administration may have both **local** and **systemic** effects. It may be necessary to administer some medications rectally, especially if the patient is nauseated. The rectal route is frequently used in infants and children, who may not be able to swallow oral medications. Absorption of rectally administered medications is highly variable but generally somewhat slower than by the oral route.

Parenteral Routes

Any method of administration that does not involve passage through the digestive tract is termed parenteral. Parenteral routes include the following:

Topical. Certain medications can be placed on the skin, where they are slowly absorbed into the capillary network underneath the skin. The rate of onset varies, but the duration of action is prolonged. This route is often used to administer nitroglycerin in the emergency setting.

Intradermal. Medications can be injected into the dermal layer of the skin. The amount of medication that can be given via this route is limited, and systemic absorption (into the bloodstream) is very slow. Generally, this route is reserved for diagnostic skin tests, such as allergy testing.

Intranasal. Intranasal administration of selected medications has become a popular route of prehospital medication administration. The medication is aerosolized and instilled in the nose, whereby the medication is rapidly absorbed through the massive vascular network in the nasal tissues. This route is often considerably more comfortable for the patient than other routes.

Subcutaneous. With subcutaneous administration, medications are injected into fatty, subcutaneous tissue under the skin and overlying the muscle. The rate of absorption is slower than that seen with intramuscular and intravenous administration. Epinephrine 1:1000, which is used in the treatment of acute asthma and other respiratory emergencies, is almost always administered subcutaneously. A maximum of 2 mL of a medication can be given subcutaneously.

Intramuscular. The most commonly used route of parenteral medication administration is the intramuscular route. The medication is injected into muscle tissue, from which it is absorbed into the bloodstream. This method of administration has a predictable rate of absorption but is considerably slower than intravenous administration.

Intravenous. Most medications used in emergency medicine are designed to be administered intravenously. These can be in the form of an intravenous (IV) **bolus** or as a slow **intravenous infusion**, sometimes referred to as a **piggyback** infusion. The rate of absorption is rapid and predictable. Of all the routes frequently employed, however, IV administration of medications has the most potential for causing adverse reactions.

Endotracheal. When an IV or IO line cannot be started, it is sometimes possible to administer emergency medications down an endotracheal tube, which permits absorption into the capillaries of the lungs. It has been shown that this route has a rate of absorption as fast as the IV route. Medications that can be administered endotracheally include epinephrine, lidocaine, naloxone, and atropine.

Sublingual injection. In the rare instance in which neither an IV line can be started nor an endotracheal tube inserted, certain medications can be injected into the vast capillary network immediately under the tongue.

Intraosseous. When an IV line cannot be started, many emergency medications and fluids can be administered intraosseously. A needle can be placed in the anterior aspect of the proximal tibia (adult and child) or in the proximal humerus (adult), through which medications and fluids can be administered. The onset of action is similar to that for IV administration.

Inhalational. Medications can be administered directly into the respiratory tract in cases of respiratory distress resulting from reversible airway disease including asthma and certain types of chronic obstructive pulmonary disease. These medications are usually nebulized into a water vapor and breathed with normal respiration.

Umbilical. Both the umbilical vein and umbilical artery can provide an alternative to IV administration in newborns.

Vaginal. Medications can be placed into the vagina, where they are absorbed into surrounding tissues. Most vaginal medications are supplied in creams or vaginal suppositories. The onset of action is slow, and the effects are generally limited to the lower female genital tract.

MEDICATION ADMINISTRATION AND PREPARATION

Preparation

Medications can be injected into several body spaces, and the type of injection depends on the body space that is used. The techniques and equipment used for each injection type vary. All injections require a liquid form of the prescribed medication and some type of syringe and needle. The paramedic must know and use the correct type of needle and syringe for the different kinds of injections. For example, an intramuscular (IM) injection requires a long IM needle. A short subcutaneous needle would not reach the muscle, and pain or tissue damage could result.

Dead Space

Manufacturers calibrate syringes so that dead space compensation (amount of medication left behind when syringe is emptied) is not necessary.

Reconstitution and Withdrawal from a Vial

Liquid and powdered medications for parenteral administration are packaged in **sterile** vials. The paramedic can withdraw liquid medication into the syringe, but powdered forms must be reconstituted first. The paramedic must use sterile technique during all medication preparation and injection procedures to decrease the risk of infection. Ideally, a filter needle is used.

Small air bubbles may adhere to the interior surface of the syringe when medication is withdrawn from a vial. This small amount of air would not harm the patient if injected, but it could change the dose of medication actually administered. Therefore, the paramedic should remove the air bubbles. To do so, he holds the syringe with the needle pointed upward, taps the side of the syringe until the bubbles accumulate at the hub, then slowly pushes the plunger until the air is expelled. If the amount of medication is not accurate after this procedure, the paramedic withdraws more of the medication to complete the prescribed dose.

Withdrawal from an Ampule

Liquid medications for parenteral administration also can be packaged in sterile ampules. Powdered ones rarely are packaged in ampules. Before administering medication from an ampule, the paramedic must withdraw it carefully.

Skin Preparation

After filling the syringe, the paramedic must prepare the patient's skin for injection. If the skin is soiled, it should be washed and dried thoroughly if possible. Then an alcohol swab is used to clean the skin. A 2% chlorhexidine gluconate 70% isopropyl alcohol (Chloraprep) swab may be used as well.

Care should be taken not to touch the patient's skin with anything except the sterile swab. When using a disinfectant, the paramedic should always begin at the point where the needle will be inserted and wipe in a spiral pattern from the center outward. Cleaning from the puncture site outward carries bacteria away from the site.

Before injecting the medication, the disinfected area should be allowed to dry for about 1 minute, if possible. Blowing on or fanning the area to hasten the drying process is discouraged because these activities increase the risk of contamination. Injecting while the skin is still moist can introduce cleansing agents into the tissues and causes irritation. Allowing the skin to dry before injection in many cases reduces injection pain.

MEDICAL DIRECTION

Paramedics do not practice autonomously. You will operate under the license of a medical director who is responsible for all of your actions; this responsibility extends to the administration of medication.

The medical director determines which medications you will use and the routes by which you will deliver them. Some states have a "state medication list" whereby the medications a service may carry are dictated by law or legislation or a regulatory agency. While some medications can be administered via off-line medical direction (written protocols), you will need specific authorization for others after consulting on-line or direct medical direction. You must strictly abide by all of your medical director's guidelines.

Knowing all medication administration protocols is essential, especially which medications to administer under protocols and which to deliver only after authorization from medical direction. You cannot afford wasting valuable time looking up procedures and directives for the critical patient who requires immediate medication therapy. Furthermore, because inappropriate medication delivery can have serious consequences, you may face severe legal ramifications even if your patient suffers no harm.

Standard Precautions

Establishing routes for medication delivery presents the constant potential for exposure to blood and other body fluids. Always take appropriate Standard Precautions to decrease your risk of exposure. The type of Standard Precautions you use will vary according to the delivery route and your patient's condition. At a minimum, you should wear gloves and goggles. Optimally you will also wear a mask. Remarkably, the simplest form of Standard Precautions is often the most neglected: hand washing. Washing your hands before and after patient contact is one of the most effective ways to decrease your exposure to infectious material.

MEDICAL ASEPSIS

Medical **asepsis** describes a medical environment free of pathogens. Many paramedical procedures, especially those related to medication administration, place the patient at increased risk for infection. The external environment is full of microorganisms, many of them pathogenic. Techniques such as intravenous access or endotracheal intubation can allow pathogens to enter the patient's body, where they may cause local or systemic complications.

Sterilization

The most aseptic environment is a sterile one. A sterile environment is free of all forms of life. Generally, environments are sterilized with extensive heat or chemicals.

A sterile environment is difficult to attain in the prehospital setting. Consequently, you must practice **medically clean techniques** to minimize your patient's risk of infection. Medically clean techniques involve the careful handling of sterile equipment to prevent contamination. For example, much of the equipment used for medication administration is in sterile packaging. Once you open the package, you must use a medically clean technique to keep the equipment clean and uncontaminated until you use it. If you drop a piece of equipment on a dirty surface, you must discard it and obtain a new piece. Other medically clean techniques, including hand washing, glove changing, and discarding equipment in opened packages, help to prevent equipment and patient contamination. Remember, too, that many patients have lowered immunity levels or carry infectious diseases. Thus, keeping the ambulance and equipment clean is another essential medically clean procedure.

Disinfectants and Antiseptics

When administering medications you must use disinfectants and antiseptics to ensure local cleanliness. Do not confuse disinfectants and antiseptics; the distinction is important. **Disinfectants** are toxic to living tissue. You will therefore use them only on nonliving surfaces or objects such as the inside of an ambulance or laryngoscope blades after use. Never use disinfectants on living tissue.

Antiseptics are not toxic to living tissue. They destroy or inhibit pathogenic micro-organisms already living on surfaces and are generally used to cleanse the local area before needle puncture. Common antiseptics include alcohol and other preparations used either alone or together. Frequently, antiseptics are diluted disinfectants.

DISPOSAL OF CONTAMINATED EQUIPMENT AND SHARPS

Blood and body fluid can harbor infectious material that endangers the health care provider, family, bystanders, or the patient himself. Many times the patient is infected with pathogenic organisms long before signs and symptoms appear. Therefore, you must treat all blood and body fluids as potentially infectious.

Medication administration commonly involves needles in direct contact with the patient's blood and body fluid. Once used, a needle represents a significant risk. Inadvertent needle sticks, the most common accident in health care as a whole, can transmit diseases between the patient and paramedic. Properly handling needles and other sharps before and after patient use can prevent many of these accidental needle sticks. To minimize the risk of an accidental needle stick, take these precautions:

- *Minimize the tasks you perform in a moving ambulance.* Use needles as sparingly as possible in the back of a moving ambulance. When appropriate, perform all interventions involving needles on scene. If en route, it may be occasionally necessary to have the driver pull the ambulance over to the side of the road and stop briefly if you have to use a needle.

- *Immediately dispose of used sharps in a sharps container.* You should dispose of all sharps, including needles and prefilled syringes, directly into the sharps container without removing or bending a needle. You should also dispose of items such as used ampules in the sharps container. Avoid dropping sharps onto the floor for later disposal. In the heat of the moment, you may forget the sharp or misplace it.

- *Never recap a needle.* The risks of a needlestick injury are too high. Never recap a needle.

MEDICATION ROUTES USED IN EMERGENCY MEDICINE

Emergency medications are administered parenterally by either the transdermal, sublingual, subcutaneous, intramuscular, intravenous, endotracheal, intraosseous, or **inhalational route.** Paramedics must always use universal precautions in patient care, particularly with medication administration. This section outlines the procedure for administration by each of these routes. Prior to the administration of any medication, the following steps should be completed:

Administration of Medication

1. Identify any patient allergies prior to base hospital contact.
2. Take and record vital signs.
3. Determine if the order is consistent with training and scope of practice.
4. Confirm order by repeating:
   a. Medication
   b. Dosage, volume, and concentration
   c. Route of administration
5. Write down the order and time of order.
6. Select proper medication and check the name of the medication:
   a. When the medication is first selected
   b. When drawing up the medication
   c. Prior to administering to patient
   d. When replacing medication in storage or disposing of ampule
7. Check for cloudiness, particles, discoloration, and expiration date.
8. Confirm order and medication with partner.
9. Prior to administration of any medication, check the six rights:
   a. Right patient
   b. Right medication
   c. Right dose or amount
   d. Right route
   e. Right time
   f. Right documentation
10. Record medication, dose and volume, route, and time and check and record patient vital signs.
11. Properly dispose of needles in an approved sharps container.

All medication administration skill checklists are given in Appendix E.

Transdermal Administration

Medications given by the transdermal route promote slow, steady absorption. Nitroglycerin, hormones, and analgesics are commonly administered transdermally. Transdermal delivery can also produce localized effects, as with anti-inflammatories and other bacteriostatic and softening agents. Applying medication locally avoids passing larger quantities of the medication throughout the entire body, where it is not needed. Transdermal medications include lotions, ointments, creams, foams, wet dressings, adhesive-backed applications, and suppositories.

Sublingual

Sublingual medications are absorbed through the mucous membranes beneath the tongue. The sublingual region is extremely vascular and permits rapid absorption with systemic delivery. These medications are generally dissolvable tablets or sprays. Commonly administered sublingual medications are nitroglycerin and lorazepam.

Intranasal (IN)

Intranasal administration of medications is an effective way to achieve rapid medication delivery without intravenous access. This is particularly important in children. The mucosal tissues of the nose are very vascular and have a great blood supply (this serves to heat and humidify incoming air). The instillation of a water-based medication onto the nasal mucosa allows a fairly rapid and predictable absorption of the medication. Usually the medication is placed into a device, such as the mucosal atomization device (MAD) that aerosolizes the liquid medication and disperses it across the nasal mucosa where it is absorbed into the circulatory system. The analgesic fentanyl and the sedative/hypnotic midazolam are the most frequently administered via this route.

Subcutaneous Injection

Subcutaneous (SC) injections provide a slow, sustained release of medication and a longer duration of action and are used when the total volume injected is no more than 1 mL of liquid. Many medications, including insulin, heparin, and epinephrine, are given by the SC route.

SC injection sites, all areas relatively distant from bones and major blood vessels, include the area over the scapula, the lateral aspects of the upper arm and thigh, and the abdomen. At least a 1 inch (2.5 cm) pinched fold of skin and tissue is necessary for administering SC injections. Burned, edematous, or scarred skin should not be used as an SC injection site, nor should the area 2 inches (5 cm) in diameter around the umbilicus or belt line.

Aspiration is not necessary with SC injection because subcutaneous tissue usually contains only small blood vessels. Therefore, the danger of unintended IV injection is minimal.

Intramuscular Injection

Intramuscular injection is useful when medication action faster than that provided by SC injection is desired but rapid effects are not required. The onset of action usually occurs within 10 to 15 minutes after an IM injection. However, the blood flow to the injection site affects the absorption rate. The most common muscles into which medications are administered are the deltoid and the gluteus. In general, 5 mL of fluid can be administered with an IM injection, but a maximum of 1 mL of medication can be given into the deltoid, whereas 10 mL can be given into the gluteus. Accurate identification of injection sites is important because major blood vessels and nerves traverse the muscle groups used for IM injections. Therefore, using an inappropriate injection site could result in permanent damage to the patient. The technique for administering an IM injection is the same for both adult and pediatric patients.

Intravenous Administration

Medications are administered intravenously to obtain an immediate onset of action, to obtain the highest possible blood concentration of a medication, and to treat conditions that require the constant titration of medication. In many cases, life-threatening situations such as shock require such constant titration.

Sites used for IV administration include the veins on the hand and wrist, the forearm veins that traverse the antecubital fossa, and the external jugular veins. The veins on the scalp and umbilical vessels (for infants), and the superficial veins of the leg and foot can be utilized when other sites cannot be used.

As mentioned previously, there are two distinct methods of IV medication administration: (1) the IV bolus and (2) slow IV infusion (sometimes called "piggyback"). Emergency medications administered by the IV bolus technique are usually administered with prefilled syringes. Many medications, however, are still available only in ampule or vial form.

In all but a few cases, it is essential that an IV be established before administering medications intravenously. Establishing an IV line makes the repeated administration of medications less traumatic for the patient.

Endotracheal Administration

The endotracheal route is no longer considered a primary route for medication administration in the emergency setting. If an IV cannot be established, then the intraosseous route is the next preferred route. When administering a medication via the endotracheal tube, the dose should be increased to 2 to 2.5 times the intravenous dose.

Intraosseous Injection

In instances where an IV cannot be established and the patient needs emergency medications or fluids, an intraosseous line can be established. When the paramedic is unable to establish an IV after two attempts in a critical patient, the intraosseous (IO) line should be attempted. The IO was primarily used in pediatric patients but is now widely used in both children and adults.

A needle is placed into the anterior proximal tibia (approximately 1 to 3 cm below the tibial tuberosity) or in the proximal humerus. The needle is advanced through the cortex of the bone into the bone marrow cavity. Entry into the marrow cavity is evidenced by a lack of resistance after penetrating the bony cortex, the needle standing upright without support, the ability to aspirate bone marrow into a syringe connected to the needle, or the free flow of the infusion without significant subcutaneous infiltration. Fluids and medications administered into the marrow cavity quickly enter the circulatory system. The onset of action of medications administered by this route is similar to that found with IV injection. Virtually all emergency medications can be administered through this route.

Inhalational Administration

Many medications used in the treatment of respiratory emergencies are administered by inhalation. The most common example is oxygen. In addition, some medications are designed to be administered into the respiratory tree. The most common of these are the bronchodilators, including metaproterenol (Alupent), racemic epinephrine, isoetharine (Bronkosol), ipratropium (Atrovent), and salbutamol (Ventolin). If these medications are administered directly into the respiratory tree, they can quickly reach their site of action with minimal absorption delays. Following are three common methods for administering these medications:

> *Metered-dose inhalers*. Metered-dose inhalers are aerosolized forms of the medication in a small canister. Most bronchodilators are supplied in this form. Many patients have inhalers at home and use them routinely. The canister is attached to a mouthpiece. The patient places his or her lips around the mouthpiece, begins to inhale, and presses the canister. When the canister is pressed, a metered amount of the medication is delivered in aerosol form. The amount of medication delivered is accurate and limited. Metered-dose inhalers are designed for single-patient use. Some metered-dose inhalers come equipped with a spacer. The spacer is a cylindrical canister between the inhaler and the mouthpiece. Prior to administration, the patient will depress the inhaler sending a measured dose of

medication into the spacer. The patient will then breathe in and out of the spacer through the mouthpiece, thus inhaling the medication into the lungs. The system is particularly useful for patients who have a hard time operating and inhaling the metered-dose inhaler. This is common in the elderly and in young children. The spacer, when used in conjunction with a metered-dose inhaler, is very effective.

Dry powder inhalers. Several manufacturers provide respiratory medications in specialized delivery devices that deliver the drug as a dry powder without a propellant. Among these are the Advair Diskus and the Spiriva HandiHaler. Generally speaking, these medications are used for maintenance therapy and not for emergent care.

Small-volume nebulizer. Small-volume nebulizers, also called updraft or handheld nebulizers, are the most commonly used method of administering inhaled medications in the emergency setting. The nebulizer has a chamber into which a solution of the medication, usually diluted with 2 to 3 mL of sterile saline, is placed. Oxygen or compressed air is blown past the chamber, causing the medication to be aerosolized. The patient inhales the aerosolized medication with each breath. This method of bronchodilator administration is advantageous because it delivers supplemental oxygen, delivers the medication over a 5- to 10-minute interval, and is supplied in single-dose ampules.

PEDIATRIC ADMINISTRATION TECHNIQUES

Administering medications safely to a child requires special attention to the six rights because any medication error can have a much greater impact on a child than on an adult. For each route of administration, the paramedic must modify adult administration techniques for a pediatric patient. No matter which route is used, the paramedic should attempt to elicit the child's cooperation to make medication administration as easy as possible. If the child is unable to cooperate, the paramedic may need to ask a parent to assist and hold the child during administration.

Although absorption from the GI tract is less predictable than from other routes, oral administration may be used. In prehospital care, the administration of Tylenol may be required in febrile patients. Administering medications to a child may be a challenge.

If an infant or small child must be restrained for medication administration, the paramedic should use a syringe without a needle to administer small, controlled doses. To minimize the risk of choking or aspirating, the paramedic should hold the child's head upright or to the side.

The paramedic then slides the syringe into the child's mouth about halfway back between the gums and cheeks and squirts a small amount of medication. This administration technique offers several advantages. Placing the medication deep in the side of the mouth makes it difficult for the child to lose the medication by spitting or drooling. Although medication administration may take longer because the medication is given in small amounts, this technique reduces the risk of choking, coughing, and vomiting because it does not stimulate the gag reflex.

Intramuscular Injection

For an IM injection the paramedic should use the smallest gauge needle appropriate for the medication, usually a needle that is 25 to 22 gauge. The needle length should not exceed 1 inch (2.5 cm), except in the adult-sized adolescent, who may require a 1.5-inch (3.8-cm) needle. Draw up only the exact quantity of the medication to be administered—no more, no less.

The recommended injection sites vary with age. The *vastus lateralis* and *rectus femoris* muscles are the recommended sites for an infant or toddler. For a child who has been walking for about 1 year, the paramedic can give the injection in the ventro-gluteal or dorsogluteal area. Walking develops muscles and thus reduces the risk of sciatic nerve damage during an IM injection. For an older child, an injection site such as the deltoid, gluteus maximus, ventrogluteus, vastus lateralis, or rectus femoris may be used. The same injection technique used in an adult is used in a child. If necessary, the child's parent or the paramedic's partner may be asked to hold the child still during injection.

Subcutaneous Administration

Subcutaneous administration is the same in a child as in an adult. Injection sites include the abdomen and the middle third of the upper arm or thigh. The needle should be 27 to 23 gauge and 3/8 to 5/8 inch (1 to 1.5 cm) long.

Intravenous Administration

Pediatric IV administration is the same as for an adult, with the caution that any medication error can have a much greater impact on a child than on an adult.

Rectal Administration

Medication absorption from the rectum may be unpredictable. Nevertheless, medications may be administered rectally when oral administration or other routes are not available. For example, in a febrile patient having a seizure, administration of medications by other routes would be difficult. In this situation, the rectal administration of diazepam (Valium) or lorazepam (Ativan) may be indicated.

CHAPTER REVIEW

Summary

It is essential that acute-care personnel be competent with all of the medication routes used in emergency medicine. These skills can be developed only after repeated practice in the classroom and the clinical setting. It is important for paramedics to be familiar with all of the medications used in routine prehospital care in their system and the routes by which the medications are administered. If there is any doubt concerning an order or an administration route, the medical control physician or a medication reference source should be consulted. Each time a medication is administered, the paramedic should ensure he or she has met each of the six rights of medication administration: right patient, right medication, right dose, right route, right time, and right documentation.

This book is not a substitute for a rigorous classroom instruction session on medication administration. It is designed purely as a teaching aid for the student and as a reference source for others.

Key Words

alimentary canal   The digestive tract.

antiseptic   Cleaning agent that is not toxic to living tissue.

asepsis   A condition free of pathogens.

bolus A method of intravenous medication administration by which a medication is rapidly administered rather than infused over a period of time.

disinfectant Cleansing agent that is toxic to living tissue.

dry powder inhaler Proprietary respiratory medication delivery system that allows a patient to inhale the drug as a dry powder with the aid of a propellant.

endotracheal A route of medication administration by which medications are administered down an endotracheal tube.

inhalational route Route via which a medication is introduced into the body through the respiratory tract.

intradermal A parenteral route of medication administration by which a medication is injected into the dermal layer of the skin.

intramuscular A common parenteral route of medication administration by which a medication is injected into the skeletal muscle.

intranasal Adminstration of medication through the nasal passage via use of an atomizer.

intraosseous A route of fluid and medication administration in which select medications or fluids are injected into the bone marrow. This route is considered an alternative to venous access in children under the age of 6 years.

intravenous A commonly used parenteral route of medication administration by which a medication is injected directly into venous circulation.

intravenous infusion A method of medication administration by which a medication or fluid is given over time.

local Limited to one area of the body.

medically clean technique Careful handling to prevent contamination.

metered-dose inhaler A device for administering medication by inhalation; it consists of a canister containing a liquid that, when activated, delivers the medication via a fine mist.

piggyback infusion A method of administering a medication by slow IV infusion.

rectal An enteral route of medication administration by which a medication is instilled in the rectum.

stat Latin abbreviation meaning "immediately."

sterile Free of all forms of life.

subcutaneous A common parenteral route of medication administration by which a medication is injected into the loose connective tissue between the dermis and the muscle.

sublingual A route of medication administration by which a medication is absorbed across the rich blood supply of the tongue.

systemic Throughout the body.

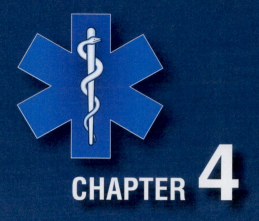

CHAPTER 4

MEDICATION DOSAGE CALCULATIONS

OBJECTIVES

After completing this chapter, the reader should be able to:

- Define the metric system.
- Identify and utilize the common metric prefixes, multiples, and submultiples.
- Convert between units of the metric system.
- Convert between units of the metric system and the customary or apothecary system.
- Utilize the rules of the metric system.
- Solve a basic order word problem using either the ratio and proportion, cross multiplication, or formula method.
- Recognize an order based on patient's weight.
- Solve an order problem based on patient weight using the simple three-step method.
- Recognize the two basic types of concentration problems.
- Define and recognize a weight/volume percentage solution.
- Find the amount of solute in a weight/volume percentage solution using either the formula method or the ratio and proportion method.
- Find the concentration of a solution using either the formula method or the ratio and proportion method.
- Recognize an intravenous drip problem.
- Organize the information from an intravenous drip problem.
- Recognize and be familiar with the dimensional analysis method of solving intravenous drip problems.
- Recognize and be familiar with the rule of fours method of solving intravenous drip problems.
- Solve an intravenous drip problem using either the dimensional analysis or the intravenous rule of fours method.
- Recognize an intravenous drip problem based on patient weight.
- Organize the information from an intravenous drip problem that is based on patient weight.
- Solve an intravenous drip problem based on patient weight using either the dimensional analysis or rule of fours method.
- Recognize an intravenous order of milliliters per hour that needs to be converted to drops per minute.
- Utilize the formula method to solve a conversion from milliliters per hour to drops per minute.

INTRODUCTION

Administration of the correct medication dosage is essential to proper prehospital medical care. This skill will be tested in written exams, practical skill stations, and on a daily basis in the prehospital environment. Medications used in emergency medicine are available from many different manufacturers. They also vary in concentration, volume, and packaging. The importance of being familiar with the common emergency medication preparations and calculating correct dosages cannot be overemphasized. All prehospital personnel should be able to prepare the correct medication dose quickly and accurately from available ampules, vials, pills, tablets, or other prepackaged medications regardless of medication concentration, volume, or packaging. This responsibility requires knowledge, skill, and practice. This chapter will help paramedics prepare to meet that responsibility.

Familiarity with the systems of measurement frequently used in medicine, especially the metric system, is essential to meet this responsibility. Conversion from one system to another is often required.

It is important to point out that there are several smart phone applications that perform medication dosage calculations. These programs vary in their level of sophistication but are quite useful. However, phones fail and cellular signals are lost. Because of this, EMS personnel must always be able to rapidly and accurately perform medical dosage calculations the old-fashioned way—with pencil and paper.

In this chapter a review of the metric system, common mathematical operations, and dosage calculations are presented. The practice problems at the end of this chapter provide an opportunity to hone the skills learned.

SECTION 1: THE METRIC SYSTEM

The International System of Units (SI), or the metric system, is an international system of measurement that originated in France during the period of the French Revolution. It has been internationally developed and is approved for use in the United States with some minor modifications. The metric system is the standard system of weights and measures used worldwide in the sciences, including medicine and pharmacology. However, tradition has caused some apothecary and household weights and measures, known as the customary system, to endure in the United States.

The metric system is a decimal system based on multiples or submultiples of the number 10. All units are either 10 times larger or 1/10 as large as the next unit. Because the metric system is based on 10, the conversion from one unit to another is simple. To change from one multiple or submultiple to another requires moving only a decimal point. Greek prefixes are used to express these multiples and submultiples. Different prefixes produce units that are of an appropriate size for the application that is needed.

Units of the Metric System

There are many units in the metric system. The following units of the metric system are approved for use in the United States and are the units most commonly used in the prehospital environment:

- Meter (m) for length
- Degrees Celsius (°C) for temperature
- Gram (g) for mass
- Liter (L) for volume

The liter (L) is not an SI unit. That is why the abbreviation, or symbol, is capitalized. The SI unit for volume is the cubic meter (m^3). However, the liter (L) is an approved and preferred unit of volume in Europe, Canada, and the United States. Other nonmetric units that are acceptable to use in the United States include the minute, the hour, and the nautical mile.

Multiples, Submultiples, and Prefixes of the Metric System

Units are used like home bases. Very large numbers or very small numbers can be difficult to manage. The metric system answers this problem with an easy solution: Multiples or submultiples are used in a decimal system and each is given a prefix to attach to the base unit. Although Table 4–1 does not list all of them, it lists some of the common multiples, submultiples, and prefixes of the metric system. Symbols over 1 million are capitalized; all others are lowercase.

Instead of using a large number of zeros, a person making metric conversions can simply change the prefix. A quantity of 1000 g of something is much easier to work with mathematically if it is converted to 1 kg.

Metric Conversions

Converting within the metric system is logical and simple. The most common multiples or prefixes used in the prehospital setting are the *kilo-,* the *milli-,* and the *micro-.* One can convert between these multiples by a factor of 1000 by either multiplying or dividing by 1000 depending on the need. Examples of common metric conversions follow:

$$1 \text{ kg} = 1000 \text{ g}$$
$$1 \text{ g} = 1000 \text{ mg}$$
$$1 \text{ mg} = 1000 \text{ mcg}$$
$$1 \text{ L} = 1000 \text{ mL}$$

Let us say we have 1 mg of a medication and we need to divide it up to work with it more effectively. Rather than deal with fractions, we can simply convert it to 1000 mcg. Now, it will be easier to divide and work with.

TABLE 4–1

Common Multiples, Submultiples, and Prefixes of the Metric System

Multiples and Submultiples	Prefix Name	Prefix Symbol
$1\,000\,000\,000 = 10^9$	*giga-*	G
$1\,000\,000 = 10^6$	*mega-*	M
$1\,000 = 10^3$	*kilo-*	k
$100 = 10^2$	*hecto-*	h
$10 = 10^1$	*deka-*	da
	Base Unit	
$0.1 = 10^{-1}$	*deci-*	d
$0.01 = 10^{-2}$	*centi-*	c
$0.001 = 10^{-3}$	*milli-*	m
$0.000\,001 = 10^{-6}$	*micro-*	μ or mc
$0.000\,000\,001 = 10^{-9}$	*nano-*	n

TABLE 4–2

Common Conversion Factors between the Metric and Customary Systems

Metric		Customary
5 mL	=	1 tsp
15 mL	=	1 T (tablespoon)
30 mL	=	1 fl oz
950 mL	=	1 qt
3.8 L	=	1 gal
2.54 cm	=	1 inch
65 mg	=	1 gr
0.45 kg	=	1 lb
1 kg	=	2.2 lb

Some conversions between the customary and the metric systems may still be necessary. Just ask anyone in the United States how much he weighs. What unit will he respond? Pounds. Because prehospital medicine uses the metric system, common conversion factors between the two systems are provided in Table 4–2.

The following temperature conversion formulas may also prove helpful:

$$°C = (°F - 32) \times \frac{5}{9}$$

$$°F = \left(°C \times \frac{9}{5}\right) + 32$$

Rules of the Metric System

Units

The written names of all metric units start with lowercase letters unless they begin a sentence. The units meter, gram, liter, and so on begin with lowercase letters. The one exception, however, is degrees Celsius. The unit *degrees* is lowercase, but the word *Celsius* is capitalized. Normal body temperature would be written as

37 degrees Celsius

Symbols (Abbreviations)

Generally, the metric symbols or the abbreviations are written in lowercase letters. For example:

km for kilometer

mg for milligram

Just as *L* for *liter* is capitalized because it is not an SI unit, unit abbreviations derived from a person's name are also capitalized:

L for liter

Pa for pascal

mL for milliliter

Plurals

The full written names of units (e.g., meter, gram, and liter) are made plural only when the numerical value that precedes them is more than 1. One exception to this rule is 0 degrees Celsius.

> 0 degrees Celsius
>
> 2 liters
>
> 0.25 liter, *not* 0.25 liters

Symbols for units are not made plural:

> 50 mL = 50 milliliters
>
> 50 mL, *not* 50 mLs

Spacing

A space is used between the number and the symbol (abbreviation) to which it refers:

> 5 km
>
> 10 mg
>
> 40° C

Hyphens

Hyphens between a number and a metric unit are not necessary when used as a one-thought modifier. If a hyphen is used, the name of the metric value should be written out. Hyphens should not be used with symbols (abbreviations).

> 1-liter bag, *not* 1-L bag
>
> 5-kilometer run, *not* 5-km run

Spaces

Spaces are used in place of commas when writing metric values that contain five or more digits. For values with four digits, either a space or no space is acceptable. The spaces are added on either side of the decimal point.

> 1 234 567 km, *not* 1,234,567 km
>
> 2000 mL or 2 000 mL
>
> 0.123 456 kg

Period

A period is not used with metric unit names and symbols (abbreviations) except at the end of a sentence.

> 50 cm, *not* 50 cm.

Decimal Point

A period is used as a decimal point within numbers to designate decimal fractions. When the number is less than 1 (a decimal fraction), a 0 is written before the decimal point. This leading 0 is especially important in medication calculations because it draws attention to the decimal point and prevents medication dosage errors. Common fractions are not used in the metric system.

0.5 mg, *not* .5 mg

SECTION 2: FIND THE ORDERED DOSE

The ordered dose is the most simple dosage calculation for the prehospital care provider. In this type of problem, the paramedic is given an order to administer a medication to a patient. There are three components to locate in this type of problem: the doctor's order, the concentration of the medication on hand, and what unit to administer.

The Doctor's Order

The order from the physician includes the amount of the medication and should also include the route of administration. The routes of administration include subcutaneous, intramuscular, intravenous (IV), endotracheal, sublingual, intraosseous, intralingual, transdermal, oral, and rectal. Orders can be verbal or written as a standing order or protocol. The order in the example that follows is known as a *basic order*.

Concentration

The second item to identify is the concentration or "what's on hand," as referred to by some texts. The paramedic is given the concentration of either a vial, an ampule, a prefilled syringe, or a tablet. Concentrations can be listed as common fractions, ratio percentages, percentage solutions, or by mass (e.g., grams and milligrams).

Unit to Administer

It is essential to look at the doctor's order and identify the unit of measurement that will be administered to the patient. Some texts refer to the unit to administer as "what you are looking for."

All three components can be identified in the following example.

EXAMPLE PROBLEM

A physician orders 2.5 mg of morphine to be administered IV to a patient with substernal chest pain. You have a 1 mL vial that contains 10 mg of morphine (10 mg/mL). How many milliliters are you going to have to draw into a syringe and push IV into your patient?

Note: Some problems may not ask, "How many milliliters?" They may simply ask, "How much are you going to administer?" You will have to deduce "milliliters" from the context of the problem.

To solve dosage calculation problems consistently and accurately you must be organized. Developing the habit of organization early will make medication dosage problems seem easier. So, before starting any calculations, write down all of the components to the problem.

Doctor's order:	2.5 mg of morphine IV
Concentration:	10 mg/mL or 10 mg per 1 mL
Unit to administer:	mL

(continued)

Example Problem (continued)

Now that you have identified the three components, you will need to solve the problem. There are three methods that can be used. The first two methods are basic algebraic equations and the third is a formula.

Ratio and Proportion Method

1. On the left side of the proportion, put the ratio that is known:

$$10 \text{ mg} : 1 \text{ mL} ::$$

2. On the right side of the proportion, put the ratio that is unknown (usually the ratio composed of the order). It is essential that you put the *units* on both sides of the equation in the same sequence:

$$10 \text{ mg} : 1 \text{ mL} :: 2.5 \text{ mg} : x \text{ mL}$$

3. Now put the proportion in the form of a basic algebraic equation. The extremes can be placed to the left of an equal sign and the means to the right:

$$10x = 2.5 \times 1$$

4. Multiply the right side:

$$10x = 2.5$$

5. Divide both sides by the number in front of x and check to see if the answer's unit matches what you are looking for:

$$x = 0.25 \text{ mL}$$

Cross Multiplication Method

The cross multiplication method is very similar to the ratio and proportion method. It simply sets up the problem using common fractions. The first fraction can be the concentration. The second fraction is the doctor's order over what is to be administered.

$$\frac{10 \text{ mg}}{1 \text{ mL}} = \frac{2.5 \text{ mg}}{x \text{ mL}}$$

Cross multiply the fractions by multiplying the numerators by the opposite denominators. The resulting algebraic equation is exactly the same as from the preceding equation:

$$10x = 2.5 \times 1$$
$$10x = 2.5$$
$$x = 0.25 \text{ mL}$$

In both methods, remember to place the unit to administer, or "what you are looking for," into the answer.

Formula Method

Some people prefer to memorize a formula to solve this type of problem. The following formula will be helpful if you prefer this method:

$$\text{Volume to be administered } (x) = \frac{\text{Volume on hand} \times \text{Ordered dose}}{\text{Concentration on hand}}$$

Using the preceding example (on page 67), place each of the components in their proper places in the formula, as illustrated in the following example.

1. Fill in the formula:

$$x = \frac{(1 \text{ mL})(2.5 \text{ mg})}{10 \text{ mg}}$$

2. Cancel any like units (mg):

$$x = \frac{(1 \text{ mL})(2.5 \text{ mg})}{10 \text{ mg}}$$

3. Work the algebra:

$$x = \frac{2.5}{10} \text{ mL}$$

$$x = 0.25 \text{ mL}$$

SECTION 3: FIND THE UNITS PER KILOGRAM

Finding the units per kilogram adds a new dimension to the problems in the previous section. Instead of a basic order, the doctor will order a certain number of units (e.g., grams and milligrams) of a medication to be administered based on the patient's weight, almost always in kilograms. This is referred to as an order based on patient's weight. Look at the following example.

EXAMPLE PROBLEM

The doctor orders 5 mg/kg of bretylium IV to be administered to your patient. You have premixed syringes with 500 mg/10 mL. Your patient weights 220 lb. How many milliliters will you administer?

You can see that the order of 5 mg/kg of bretylium is a little different than a basic order. Start by writing down all of the key information. In this type of problem, add a patient weight category. Always begin with organizing the information:

Doctor's order:	5 mg/kg bretylium IV
Concentration:	500 mg/mL
Unit to administer:	mL
Patient's weight:	220 lb

Look at the order. It is directly tied to the patient's weight. Put another way, the order is saying, "For every kilogram of patient, give 5 mg of bretylium."

In the following three-step method, only step 2 is new. The other steps have been covered in previous sections.

(continued)

Example Problem (continued)

Three-Step Method
1. Convert the patient's weight from pounds to kilograms.
2. Convert the ordered dose based on patient's weight to a basic order.
3. Find the ordered dose.

Step 1: Convert pounds to kilograms.

$$220 \text{ lb} \div 2.2 = 100 \text{ kg}$$

or

$$220 \text{ lb} \times 0.45 = 99 \text{ kg}$$

Note: For ease of computation, 99 kg could then be approximated to 100 kg without compromising patient care.

Step 2: Convert the order by weight to a basic order.
This step can be calculated by using a formula or by using the ratio and proportion method.

Formula Method

$$x = \frac{\text{Ordered dose} \times \text{Weight (kg)}}{1 \text{ kg}}$$

Set up the formula.

$$x = \frac{5 \text{ mg} \times 100 \text{ kg}}{1 \text{ kg}}$$

The unit of kilogram in the numerator cancels out the unit of kilogram in the denominator, leaving milligrams. Now, work the math:

$$x = 500 \text{ mg}$$

This is the basic ordered dose. You can now proceed to step 3 or look at the ratio and proportion method.

Ratio and Proportion Method

$$5 \text{ mg} : 1 \text{ kg} :: x \text{ mg} : 100 \text{ kg}$$
$$x = 5 \times 100$$
$$x = 500 \text{ mg}$$

Either way, this is now a basic order that can be worked with. Draw a line through the order based on patient weight and write in the new basic order of 500 mg over it. This habit will help keep information organized. Now, the ordered dose must be calculated.

Step 3: Find the ordered dose.
Because you now have a basic order, find the ordered dose using the method that you prefer from Section 2.

Answer: 10 mL

SECTION 4: CONCENTRATION PROBLEMS

Prehospital care providers encounter two types of concentration problems. The first type of concentration problem, amount of solute problems, tests knowledge of the solutions that paramedics work with. The second type not only helps in finding the concentration in an IV bag but is also a major step used when solving IV drip problems (Sections 5 and 6).

Amount of Solute

Concentration problems dealing with amount of solute are seen more often on tests than in practical applications. They involve searching for the amount of solute in a weight/volume percentage solution. Weight/volume percentage is a commonly used percentage concentration with prehospital solutions. It always expresses the number of grams of solute in a total of 100 mL of solution.

For example, 50 percent dextrose in water, or $D_{50}W$, is a common prehospital medication. This expression means that there are 50 g of dextrose in every 100 mL of solution. The fraction expression of the weight/volume percentage solution is as follows:

$$\frac{50 \text{ g}}{100 \text{ mL}} \text{ of dextrose in water}$$

Knowing this, it is obvious that when there are 50 mL of this solution, there are 25 g of dextrose. Following are a couple of examples of how this type of problem could be worded.

EXAMPLE PROBLEM

You have a 250 mL bag of D_5W. How many grams of dextrose are in the bag?

Formula Method

$$\text{Number of grams } (x) = \text{Percentage of solution} \times \text{Volume of solution}$$

Filling in the formula and working the problem solves the preceding example:

$$x = \frac{5 \text{ g}}{100 \text{ mL}} \times 250 \text{ mL}$$

$$x = \frac{1250}{100} \text{ g}$$

$$x = 12.5 \text{ g}$$

Hint: If the problem had asked for answers in milligrams, the grams would need to be converted to milligrams to find the correct answer.

(continued)

Example Problem (continued)

Ratio and Proportion or Cross Multiplication Method

This problem could also be worked using either the ratio and proportion or cross multiplication methods:

$$5 \text{ g} : 100 \text{ mL} :: x \text{ g} : 250 \text{ mL} \quad or \quad \frac{5 \text{ g}}{100 \text{ mL}} = \frac{x \text{ g}}{250 \text{ mL}}$$

$$100x = 5 \times 250$$

$$100x = 1250$$

$$x = 12.5 \text{ g}$$

These same types of problems can be twisted around. What if the number of grams to be administered and the percentage were given and the amount to be infused was the unknown? Look at the following example.

EXAMPLE PROBLEM

The doctor orders 12.5 g of 5 percent dextrose to be infused. How many milliliters will be infused?

A formula, the ratio and proportion method, or cross multiplication may be used to solve this type of problem.

Formula Method

$$\text{Volume } (x) = \frac{\text{Amount ordered (g)}}{\text{Percentage}}$$

$$x = \frac{12.5 \text{ g}}{5 \text{ percent}}$$

or mathematically the same:

$$x = 12.5 \text{ g} \times \frac{5 \text{ g}}{100 \text{ mL}}$$

$$x = 12.5 \text{ g} \times \frac{100 \text{ mL}}{5 \text{ g}}$$

$$x = \frac{1250}{5} \text{ mL}$$

$$x = 250 \text{ mL}$$

Ratio and Proportion Method

Still using the preceding example, we can use the ratio and proportion method to find the answer:

$$5 \text{ g} : 100 \text{ mL} :: 12.5 \text{ g} : x \text{ mL}$$

$$5x = 1250$$

$$x = 250 \text{ mL}$$

Find the Concentration of a Solution

In most facilities and EMS systems, the pharmacy or medication manufacturer prepares solutions for IV use. However, in small hospitals, rural EMS systems, and other settings (such as testing sites), paramedics are required to measure, prepare, and administer these solutions.

The second type of concentration problem is used to find the concentration of a particular premixed IV solution (or syringe, vial, or the like). It is also used as a major step in solving IV drip problems. It is important to know the answer to the question "What do they mean by concentration?" The usual answer is how many milligrams or micrograms of a medication are contained per 1 mL of a given solution. There are other ways to express concentration, but when prehospital care workers are referring to an IV solution's concentration they usually mean a per milliliter concentration.

EXAMPLE PROBLEM

One gram of lidocaine has been added to a 250 mL bag of D_5W. What is the concentration?

Formula Method

A standard formula is used to express concentration. Once it is set up, it is simply a matter of reducing the fraction to a denominator of 1.

$$x = \frac{\text{Solute (grams or milligrams of drug)}}{\text{Solvent (liters or milliliters of volume)}}$$

Set up the formula:

$$x = \frac{1 \text{ g lidocaine}}{250 \text{ mL } D_5W}$$

Convert grams to milligrams (lidocaine is ordered in milligrams):

$$x = \frac{1000 \text{ mg lidocaine}}{250 \text{ mL } D_5W}$$

Reduce the fraction to a denominator of 1:

$$x = \frac{1000 \text{ mg lidocaine}}{250 \text{ mL } D_5W} \div \frac{250}{250}$$

$$x = \frac{4 \text{ mg lidocaine}}{1 \text{ mL } D_5W}$$

This result can be expressed verbally as "The concentration is 4 milligrams per milliliter" or "4 to 1." This is the per milliliter concentration.

Ratio and Proportion Method

$$1000 \text{ mg} : 250 \text{ mL} :: x \text{ mg} : 1 \text{ mL}$$

$$250x = 1000$$

$$x = 4 \text{ mg/mL}$$

Both of these methods can be used to find the per milliliter concentration of any solution.

Calculating IV drips has been a quandary for many prehospital care providers for a long time. Asking any paramedic, nurse, or doctor to set up an IV drip without a calculator, reference, electric pump, or computerized device is likely to produce all kinds of moans and excuses. But that is exactly what paramedics are expected to do at test stations and in the prehospital environment. There is an easy way to solve drip problems. This section will examine both the dimensional analysis and the rule of fours methods. Paramedics may choose the method that works best for them.

IV Drip

In some cases, patients require medication to be infused on a continual basis. Paramedics will receive orders to administer a certain number of units (usually milligrams or micrograms) of a medication per minute to a patient through an IV. Known as an infusion, it is also referred to as an IV drip because it involves calculating the number of drops that "drip" and are delivered intravenously each minute to deliver the amount of medication the doctor is ordering.

Even though most of these IV infusions are commercially available already premixed, paramedics will be tested on mixing the medication and starting the infusion correctly. If an occasion occurs in which paramedics do not have a premixed bag, they will know what to do. This process involves drawing medication from a vial or ampule into a syringe and mixing it into an IV bag. Then, paramedics will be required to set a drip rate based on the doctor's order and the administration set that is available. The solution is the number of drops that fall each minute (gtt/min).

Formula Method (Dimensional Analysis)

If paramedics have a chemistry or algebra background, they will understand the formula method and probably prefer it. It very systematically and mathematically calculates the IV drip rate. If they do not like math or chemistry, they may not like this method. They do need to understand it, however. This method shows how a drip rate is calculated and answers a lot of questions that may arise later. Organization of the material is still the key to success.

EXAMPLE PROBLEM

A doctor orders 2 mg/min of lidocaine to be administered to a patient who was experiencing an arrhythmia. You have a vial that contains 1 g of lidocaine in 5 mL. Your ambulance carries only 250 mL bags of D_5W. Your administration set is a microdrip set (60 gtt/mL). At how many drops per minute will you adjust your administration set to drip?

Before starting any calculations, organize the information just as you were doing in Section 2. There are a couple of new categories in this type of problem.

Order:	2 mg lidocaine IV
On hand:	1 g lidocaine/5 mL
Bag:	250 mL D_5W
Administration set:	60 gtt/mL
Unit to administer:	gtt/min

Example Problem (continued)

Formula (Dimensional Analysis) Method

$$x = \frac{\text{IV bag volume (mL)}}{\text{Amount of drug in bag}} \times \frac{\text{Unit ordered}}{1 \text{ min}} \times \frac{\text{Administration set (gtt)}}{1 \text{ mL}}$$

1. Fill in the formula:

$$x = \frac{250 \text{ mL}}{1 \text{ g}} \times \frac{2 \text{ mg}}{1 \text{ min}} \times \frac{60 \text{ gtt}}{1 \text{ mL}}$$

Note: The 5 mL in the vial on hand is not figured into the equation.

2. Convert the grams in the bag to match the milligrams in the doctor's order:

$$x = \frac{250 \text{ mL}}{1000 \text{ mg}} \times \frac{2 \text{ mg}}{1 \text{ min}} \times \frac{60 \text{ gtt}}{1 \text{ mL}}$$

3. Cancel out like units and zeros. Confirm that the remaining units are what you are looking for:

$$x = \frac{25}{10} \times \frac{2}{1 \text{ min}} \times \frac{6 \text{ gtt}}{1}$$

4. Multiply and reduce the fraction:

$$x = \frac{300 \text{ gtt}}{10 \text{ min}}$$

$$x = \frac{30 \text{ gtt}}{1 \text{ min}} \quad \text{or} \quad 30 \text{ gtt/min}$$

You can now set your drip rate on the IV administration set. Remember, in most ambulances and test centers, an electric or computerized IV pump will not be available and you will have to set the rate by hand.

Rule of Fours Method

This method is called the rule of fours because it is based on multiples of the number 4. This is also known as the "easy" way. Many people find it far simpler than the formula method or dimensional analysis. It requires the memorization of a process, not a formula, and requires only simple logic and very little math. Look at the same example problem from earlier:

EXAMPLE PROBLEM

A doctor orders 2 mg/min of lidocaine to be administered to a patient who was experiencing an arrhythmia. You have a vial that contains 1 g of lidocaine in 5 mL. Your ambulance carries only 250 mL bags of D₅W. Your administration set is a microdrip set (60 gtt/mL). At how many drops per minute will you adjust your administration set to drip?

We begin by organizing the information from the problem similarly to how it was done in the previous example. However, this time we add a new category: the concentration of the IV solution (1 g into 250 mL).

(continued)

Example Problem (continued)

Note: Finding the concentration in the bag is the *key* to solving IV drip problems when using this method. Refer to Section 4 to review this process.

Order:	2 mg/min lidocaine IV
On hand:	1 g lidocaine/5 mL
Bag:	250 mL D_5W
Concentration:	4 mg/mL
Administration set:	60 gtt/mL
Unit to administer:	gtt/min

1. *Compare.* Now that the information is organized, a logical comparison can be made between the concentration and the administration set. Looking at the concentration we could say that in every 1 mL there are 4 mg of lidocaine. We could also say that there are 60 drops in each milliliter. Therefore, in every 60 drops there are 4 mg or 60 gtt/4 mL.

2. *Set up.* Set up the rule of fours "clock" based on step 1. Drops go on the inside of the clock, and milligrams go on the outside. The relationship between the 4 mg and the 60 gtt becomes the 12 o'clock position. Halfway around the clock is the logical half of that relationship. So, 30 gtt equals 2 mg and so on around the clock.

4 mg/mL CLOCK

1 gram into 250 mL yields 4 mg/mL

3. *Look.* Find the doctor's order on the outside of the "clock" and compare it with the drops per minute on the inside. This is the rate at which the administration set is to drip.

$$x = 30 \text{ gtt/min}$$

It is that easy. Different "clocks" can be set up depending on the concentration in the IV bag and/or the administration set available. These parameters can change. The process of setting up the "clock" will be the same and work every time. You will find that there are just a few "clocks" that you will use regularly.

SECTION 6: CALCULATE AN IV DRIP BASED ON PATIENT WEIGHT

This section takes the calculation in the previous section just one step further. It adds the dimension of patient weight. IV drip medication orders can be based on patient weight just as basic orders can.

EXAMPLE PROBLEM

An order is received to administer 10 mcg/kg/min of dopamine IV. You have a vial that contains 200 mg of dopamine in 10 mL (200 mg/10 mL). You also have 250 mL bags of D_5W with a microdrip administration set. Your patient weighs 176 pounds. At how many drops per minute will you adjust your administration set to drip?

Example Problem (continued)

Organize the material as before. This time the category of patient weight is added. Remember that finding the concentration in the bag is still the key to solving drip problems.

Order:	10 mcg/kg/min
On hand:	200 mg dopamine/10 mL
Bag:	250 mL D_5W
Administration set:	60 gtt/mL
Concentration:	800 mcg/mL
Patient's weight:	176 lb
Unit to administer:	gtt/min

1. Convert the patient's weight to kilograms. 176 lb ÷ 2.2 = 80 kg
2. Convert the doctor's order from micrograms per kilogram per minute to micrograms per minute. 10 µg × 80 kg = 800 mcg/min
3. You now have the ordered dose. Find the concentration in the bag and use the "clock" or use the dimensional analysis method to solve.

200 milligrams into 250 mL yields 800 mcg/mL

Answer: 60 gtt/min

The dimensional analysis method may also be used to solve this type of problem. After converting the patient's weight and the doctor's order, use the formula from Section 5.

SECTION 7: MILLILITERS PER HOUR TO DROPS PER MINUTE

Sometimes, doctors order IVs to be infused in milliliters per hour or over a specific period of time. To set an IV's administration set, the order must be converted to drops per minute. This section shows how to convert that type of order. A simple conversion formula is all that is needed.

EXAMPLE PROBLEM

The doctor orders you to start an IV of normal saline to run at 100 mL/hr. You have a macrodrip set of 15 gtt/mL. At how many drips per minute will you set your administration set to drip?

Note: Macrodrip administration sets can vary in size.

Formula Method

$$x = \frac{\text{Ordered amount (mL)}}{\text{Order time (min)}} \times \frac{\text{Administration set (gtt)}}{1\ \text{mL}}$$

1. Fill in the formula. Convert the doctor's order in hours to minutes when you enter the ordered time:

$$x = \frac{100\ \text{mL}}{60\ \text{min}} \times \frac{15\ \text{gtt}}{1\ \text{mL}}$$

(continued)

Example Problem (continued)

2. Cancel units, zeros, and multiply:

$$x = \frac{150 \text{ mL}}{6 \text{ min}}$$

3. Simplify the fraction:

$$x = \frac{25 \text{ gtt}}{1 \text{ min}} \quad \text{or} \quad 25 \text{ gtt/min}$$

PRACTICE PROBLEMS

Section 1

Solve the following conversion problems. Answers may be found in the Answer Key at the back of the book.

1. 1 g	= _____ mg			**9.** 37°C	= _____ °F		
2. 1 mg	= _____ μg			**10.** 104°F	= _____ °C		
3. 1 mg	= _____ g			**11.** 1/4 gr	= _____ mg		
4. 0.8 mg	= _____ μg			**12.** 2 Tbsp	= _____ mL		
5. 1.5 L	= _____ mL			**13.** 180 lb	= _____ kg		
6. 400 000 mg	= _____ g			**14.** 7 lb	= _____ kg		
7. 800 mg	= _____ g			**15.** 25 kg	= _____ lb		
8. 500 mL	= _____ L						

Section 2

Solve the following dosage calculation problems. Answers may be found in the Answer Key at the back of the book.

1. You arrive at the physician's office and find the staff performing CPR on a 45-year-old male who came to the clinic complaining of chest pain. After appropriate measures were initiated the first medication to administer in this cardiac arrest per protocol is epinephrine 1mg IVP. Epinephrine 1:10 000 comes prepackaged in a prefilled syringe 0.1 mg/mL. The patient weighs 180 lbs. How many milliliters would you administer?

2. Your patient is actively seizing. Your benzodiazepine of choice is midazolam which comes in a multidose vial of 20 mLs. The concentration of the vial is 5 mg/mL. The first dose of versed is unsuccessful in terminating the patient's seizure and you need to administer 10 mg of midazolam. How many milliliters would you administer?

3. Your patient meets the criteria for treating symptomatic bradycardia. Following current AHA recommendations, you administer of 0.5 mg of atropine IV. The atropine is supplied in your ambulance in a syringe as 1 mg/10 mL. How many milliliters will you give?

4. A 14-year-old male patient fell from his skateboard and suffered an apparent isolated closed radial/ulnar fracture. The analgesic of choice available in your county's jurisdiction is fentanyl. It is packaged in a 2 mL ampule with a concentration of 25 mcg/mL. You want to administer 50 mcgs. How many milliliters would you administer?

5. After determining that your patient meets your chest pain activation criteria and alerting the receiving facility cardiac catheterization team you continue to appropriately manage the patient's chest discomfort. Your next action is to

administer 2.5 mgs of morphine sulfate every 3–5 minutes until the patient has a significant reduction in their chest discomfort. The morphine is prepackaged in a 1 mg/mL syringe. How many milliliters would you administer?

6. A patient is suffering from uncontrolled hypertension with apparent end organ damage. After consulting with medical command you are directed to administer 20 mg of labetalol over 1–2 minutes. The vial of labetalol reads 5 mg/mL. How many milliliters would you administer?

7. Your patient is suffering mild shortness of breath after being stung by a bee. He also has several large red blotches and complains of severe pruritis. The medication of choice is subcutaneous epinephrine 1:1000 0.3–0.5 mg. You decide to initially start with a 0.3 mg dose. The epinephrine is prepackaged in an ampule that reads 1 mg/mL. How many milliliters will you administer?

8. Your patient is exhibiting paroxysmal supraventricular tachycardia (PSVT). Vagal maneuvers are ineffective and medical control orders 12 mg of adenosine rapid IV push. The vial reads 3 mg/mL. How many milliliters will you administer?

9. Your patient is experiencing sustained hemodynamically stable ventricular tachycardia. Protocol directs you to first attempt a 150 mg bolus of amiodarone over 3–5 minutes. The patient is 45 years old and weighs 75 kg. The amiodarone syringe reads 15 mg/mL. How many milliliters will you administer?

10. After performing a thorough assessment of an unknown unresponsive patient your glucometer reading reveals the patient's blood glucose level to be 40 mg/dL. With no apparent contraindications and a patent free flowing IV you decide to administer 25 g of dextrose IV bolus. The prefilled syringe reads 0.5 g/mL. How many milliliters will you administer?

Section 3

Solve the following dosage calculation problems. Answers may be found in the Answer Key at the back of the book.

1. While assisting the flight team, you are asked to draw up the succinylcholine for the rapid sequence intubation of your patient. The nurse asks you to draw up 2 mg/kg of succinylcholine. Your patients weight is estimated at approximately 150 lb. The succinylcholine concentration is 20 mg/mL. How many milliliters will you administer?

2. After successfully intubating the patient and confirming ETT placement, the flight team prepares a vecuronium infusion for continued paralysis to facilitate mechanical ventilation. The dosing of the vecuronium is 0.1 mg/kg based on the weight of the patient in question #1. Norcuron when reconstituted is 10 mg/2mL. How many milliliters will you administer?

3. After assessing the ABCs and performing CPR, an 8-month-old's heart rate is approximately 30 bpm. Your partner establishes an IO and your next intervention is to administer 0.01 mL/kg of 1:10 000 epinephrine. The epinephrine syringe label reads epinephrine 1:10 000 0.1 mg/mL. Your patient weighs approximately 16 lb. How many milliliters will you administer?

4. After consulting with poison control and verifying your suspicions that your patient overdosed on amitriptyline—a tricyclic antidepressant, you are ordered to administer 1 mEq/kg of sodium bicarbonate at 1 mEq/kg to a patient who weighs 160 lb. It comes prepackaged in a syringe with the label reading 50 mEq/50 mL. How many milliliters will you administer?

5. A severely bradycardic 44 lb pediatric patient does not respond to your initial treatments. Standing orders tell you to administer 0.01 mg/kg epinephrine IV. Your ampule reads 10 mg/10 mLs. How many milliliters will you administer?

Section 4

Solve the following concentration problems. Answers may be found in the Answer Key at the back of the book.

1. You are mixing your standard concentration of dopamine for an interfacility transport. However the physician asks you to double the amount of dopamine you normally add to your drip so you can decrease the flow rate and still achieve the same dosage. This is because the patient is in acute renal failure already. The ED physician requests you mix 800 mg of dopamine in a 250 mL bag of D_5W. What is the per milliliter concentration?

2. How many grams of sodium chloride are in a 1000 mL bag of 0.9 percent normal saline?

3. You are transporting a dialysis patient to the emergency department after receiving dialysis. She has a magnesium infusion running. The clinic had mixed 1g of magnesium in a 100 mL bag of D_5W for infusion over 120 minutes. What is the per milliliter concentration?

4. There is a prefilled syringe of 1 percent lidocaine in your ambulance. It contains 5 mL. How many milligrams does it contain?

5. While taking your annual pharmacology competencies a question reads "a bag of norepinephrine is mixed by placing 4 mg of norepinephrine in 250 mL of D_5W. What is the final concentration in mcg/mL?" What is your answer?

6. After converting a patient in atrial flutter to sinus rhythm in the emergency department, the patient is placed on a procainamide infusion. The infusion is prepared by placing 2 grams of procainamide in 250 mLs of 0.9% saline. What is the per milliliter concentration?

7. You are transporting a patient from the ED to the cardiac catheterization laboratory. The patient has dopamine currently infusing to maintain his or her blood pressure. The label on the dopamine bag reads 400 mg of dopamine in 250 mLs of 0.9% saline. The bag now has 150 mL left in it. What is the per milliliter concentration in the bag now?

8. Just before leaving the ED, the pharmacist hands you a bag of epinephrine that you are to begin infusing on your septic hypotensive patient. The pharmacist mixed the infusion by adding 15 mg of epinephrine in 250 mL of 0.9% saline. You are to begin the infusion at 2 mcg/mL. What is the current concentration in mcg/mL?

9. During clinical rotations in the ICU you are caring for a renal patient on a furosemide infusion. The infusion was prepared by mixing 500 mg of furosemide in a 50 mL bag of 0.9% saline. What is the current concentration in mg/mL?

10. After treating your patient with labetalol prehospitally for a hypertensive emergency, the ED physician decides to continue with a maintenance infusion at 1.5 mg/min titrated to keep the patients MAP BP below 100 mmHg. The pharmacist mixes the infusion by placing 400 mgs of labetalol in 80 mLs of 0.9% saline. What is the current concentration in mg/mL ?

Section 5

Solve the following IV drip problems. Answers may be found in the Answer Key at the back of the book.

1. You are preparing a dopamine drip for a hypotensive patient. You have to prepare the dopamine infusion first. On hand you have a vial that contains 400 mg of dopamine in 10 mL (400 mg/10 mL). To decrease the overall fluid volume infused you chose a 250 mL bag of D_5W and a micro drip administration set (60 gtt/mL). Based on your calculations the patient should receive 400 mcg/min to adequately support his or her blood pressure. How many drops per minute will you adjust your administration set to drip?

2. After administering IV epinephrine to a severe anaphylaxis patient, you elect to support his or her blood pressure with an epinephrine infusion. Your protocol directs you to start the infusion at 1 mcg/kg/min and titrate to a systolic BP of 80 mmHg. You are ordered to place 1 mg into a 250 mL bag of D_5W. At what rate will you set your micro drip (60 gtt/mL) administration set?

3. After successful conversion of a patient in atrial flutter to sinus rhythm in the emergency department the patient is placed on an IV antiarrhythmic drip. The cardiologist chooses procainamide and writes an order for a continued infusion at 2 mg/min. The pharmacist places 1 gram of procainamide in a 250 mL bag of D_5W. At what rate will you set your micro drip (60 gtt/mL) administration set?

4. In an attempt to raise a bradyacardic patient's heart rate and blood pressure, you choose to start an epinephrine infusion. Your partner opens 2 (two), 1 mg 1:1000 ampules of epinephrine and injects them into a 250 mL bag of normal saline. Utilizing a solution set with a modified micro drip administration set (45 gtt/mL), what would you set the rate at to achieve 4 mcg/kg/min?

5. You are ordered to administer a lidocaine drip at 2 mg/min. You have 2 g of lidocaine added to a 500 mL bag. What is the drip rate with a microdrip administration set (60 gtt/mL)?

6. Solve problem 5 using a macro drip administration set (10 gtt/mL).

7. After converting a patient from a supraventricular tachycardia with a diltiazem bolus you want to prevent the rhythm from spontaneously reoccurring. You mix 125 mg of diltiazem in a 125 mL bag of D_5W. Utilizing a standard micro drip (60 gtt/mL) solution set what would you set the rate at to obtain a rate of 10 mg/hour ? What is the drip rate?

8. You are transporting a patient who had an acute inferior wall MI to a tertiary care hospital for coronary revascularization. You consult with your medical director before you leave and decide to supplement the patient's BP by using dobutamine 500 mcg/kg/min. You place 800 mg of dobutamine into a 500 mL bag of 0.9% normal saline. What is the drip rate with a micro drip administration set (60 gtt/mL)?

9. Solve problem 5 using a macro drip administration set (15 gtt/mL).

10. You have an order to administer lidocaine at 4 mg/min. The 1 L bag of normal saline has had 4 g of lidocaine added. What is the drip rate with a micro drip administration set (60 gtt/mL)?

Section 6

Solve the following IV drip problems based on patient weight. Answers may be found in the Answer Key at the back of the book.

1. When preparing to hang a your dopamine drip you realize that the pharmacy had not supplied you with your normal concentration/strength when you last switched medication boxes at the hospital. The dopamine that you currently have is mixed 800 mg in 250 mL of D_5W. Your patient weighs 176 lb and your starting dosage is 5 mcg/kg/min. What is the drip rate with a micro drip administration set (60 gtt/mL)?

2. A 22 lb pediatric patient requires an epinephrine drip at 0.1 mcg/kg/min. You place 1 mg of epinephrine in a 250 mL bag of D_5W. What is the drip rate with a micro drip administration set (60 gtt/mL)?

3. Your patient in problem 2 does not significantly improve and the doctor doubles the order to 0.2 mcg/kg/min. What is the drip rate?

4. The patient in the emergency department that you just brought in was diagnosed with a dissecting thoracic aortic aneurysm. In order to lower his blood pressure and to prevent further dissection the patient is placed on a sodium

nitroprusside drip. The patient weighs 95 kg. The sodium nitroprusside drip is prepared by placing 100 mg of sodium nitroprusside in 250 of D_5W. The physician orders the drip to be started at 2 mcg/kg/min. Utilizing a standard micro drip 60 gtt administration set what would you drip rate be?

5. You are transporting a 176 lb trauma patient with a suspected transected spinal cord in severe spinal shock. He is hypotensive and was started on a neosynephrine drip to maintain his systemic vascular resistance and blood pressure prior to leaving the rural ED. The drip was mixed by adding 60 mg of phenylephrine to 250 mL of 0.9% normal saline. The patient's blood pressure continues to drop and you are instructed to increase the dose to 0.5 mcg/kg/min. Utilizing a standard micro drip 60 gtt administration set what would your drip rate be?

6. You are transporting a patient to a burn center after sustaining full thickness burns over 60% BSA. He is currently intubated, chemically sedated, and paralyzed. In addition he is on a fentanyl drip for acute pain management. The drip was prepared by mixing 2000 mcg of fentanyl in 40 mL of D_5W. The patient's weight is 176 lbs. You want to increase the drip to 0.1 mcg/kg/min, utilizing a micro drip set. What should the new rate be set at?

7. Your cardiac patient is exhibiting the signs and symptoms of cardiogenic shock. Among other procedures, protocol calls for a dopamine drip at 10 mcg/kg/min. The patient's wife states that her husband weighs 150 lb. The premixed dopamine bag label reads 800 mg in 250 mL bag of D_5W and you are utilizing a micro drip set. What should the drip rate to be?

8. A patient in the ED was unresponsive to both IV atropine and an epinephrine infusion, and the transcutaneous pacer was unable to maintain capture. The patient was placed on an isoproterenol infusion in a final attempt to increase the patient's heart rate. The infusion was mixed by placing 4 mgs of isoproterenol in 250 mL of D_5W. The cardiologist wants the drip started at 0.1 mcg/kg/min, the patient's weight is 220 lb. Using a micro drip (60 gtt administration set) what would you calculate the drip rate at?

9. You are completing your report after delivering a patient to the emergency center, and you notice that the dopamine dose ordered by medical control is missing from your notes. To avoid any problems, you decide to determine the ordered dose based on the information available. The patient weighs 176 lb and the IV infusion is flowing through a micro drip administration set at 30 gtt/min. The label you put on the 500 mL bag of normal saline reads "800 mg dopamine added." What was the doctor's original dose per kilogram per minute order?

10. You are in the same situation as you were in problem 9. The patient weighs 220 lb. The infusion set is a micro drip set and is flowing at 30 gtt/min. The label on the 250 mL bag of D_5W reads "200 mg dopamine added." What was the doctor's original dose per kilogram per minute order?

Section 7

Solve the following problems of converting milliliters per hour to drops per minute. Answers may be found in the Answer Key at the back of the book.

1. Protocol calls for suspected right ventricular infarct chest pain patients to receive a 500 mL fluid bolus then the IV to be run at 300 mL per hour. You are using a 15 gtt/mL macro drip administration set. What will your drip rate be set at?

2. You are transporting a patient between an urgent care facility and the hospital. The physician wants a total of 200 mL infused in the 60 minute transport. An IV of 0.9% NaCL is already running with a 15 gtt/mL administration set. What will you set your drip rate at?

3. After assessing your acute abdominal pain patient, you follow your protocol and establish a large bore IV. Your goal is to run your IV fluid at 120 mL/hr. You are using a macro drip administration set (10 gtt/mL.) What is the drip rate?

4. A 6-week-old pediatric patient is admitted to the emergency center severely dehydrated. The order reads to infuse 100 mL of 0.45 percent sodium chloride in 2.5 percent D_5W over 1 hour. This is to be followed with 200 mL/hr of the same fluid over 8 hours. What are the two drip rates using a micro drip set?

5. Using the Parkland Formula you determine that your burn patient should receive 600 mL over the first hour (60 minutes) Your partner sets up your IV fluid using a macrodrip administration set of 10 gtts/mL. What is the drip rate?

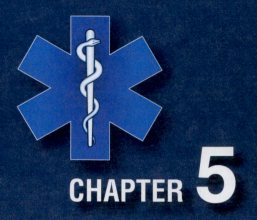

CHAPTER 5

FLUIDS, ELECTROLYTES, AND INTRAVENOUS THERAPY

OBJECTIVES

After completing this chapter, the reader should be able to:

- Identify the body's major fluid compartments and the proportion of total body water they contain.
- List the major electrolytes and discuss the role they play in maintaining a fluid balance within the human body.
- Define the following cell physiology terms and explain the role each process plays in human fluid dynamics:
  - Diffusion
  - Osmosis
  - Active transport
  - Facilitated diffusion
- Identify the major elements of blood and describe their purposes.
- Define hypotonic, hypertonic, and isotonic solutions.
- List the various fluid replacement products and describe the advantages and disadvantages of field use.
- State the size and type of intravenous catheter to be used for particular applications.
- Explain the different types of intravenous fluids that can be used.
- State which intravenous administration sets should be used and in what circumstances.
- List the possible sites an intravenous tube can be inserted and the rationale for each.
- Demonstrate the procedure for inserting an intravenous tube.
- Describe the procedure for collecting blood samples from an intravenous tube.

INTRODUCTION

One of the most important aspects of prehospital care is the administration of intravenous (IV) fluids and electrolytes. There are two major reasons for administering intravenous fluids during the prehospital phase of emergency medical care. The first is to immediately replace intravascular blood volume, and the second is to provide an easily accessible route for the administration of lifesaving emergency medications.

FLUIDS

Water is the most abundant substance in the human body. Approximately 60 percent of the total body weight is water, which is located within two fluid compartments, or spaces. The largest of these fluid compartments is the **intracellular** fluid (ICF) compartment, which includes all fluids found within the cells. Three-fourths of all body water is within the intracellular compartment. The remaining water can be found outside of the cell membrane in the **extracellular** fluid (ECF) compartment. There are two major components of the ECF: **intravascular fluid**, which is found within the blood vessels and outside of the cell membranes; and the **interstitial fluid**, that fluid found outside the cell membrane yet not within any defined blood vessels. The relationship of the various fluid compartments is illustrated as follows:

Extracellular Fluid	15 percent of total body weight
(Interstitial Fluid	10.5 percent of total body weight)
(Intravascular Fluid	4.5 percent of total body weight)
Intracellular Fluid	45 percent of total body weight
Total Body Water	60 percent of total body weight

Internal Environment

The internal environment is the extracellular fluid, which bathes each body cell. An important balance must be maintained regarding the internal environment. Whenever one aspect of the internal environment deviates from normal, as frequently occurs in injury and illness, the body immediately responds and attempts to return to normal. The body's tendency to maintain all of its physiological activities in proper balance, including the internal environment, is called **homeostasis**.

ELECTROLYTES

In addition to the body fluids, some important chemicals are also required for life. These chemicals are divided into two main classes: **electrolytes** and nonelectrolytes. Chemicals that take on an electrical charge when placed in water are called electrolytes; chemicals that do not take on an electrical charge are called nonelectrolytes. All electrolytes are measured in quantities called milliequivalents (mEq). Sodium bicarbonate, a common emergency medication, is an electrolyte. When placed in water, it quickly divides into charged particles, or ions. All dosages of sodium bicarbonate are calculated in milliequivalents. Certain electrolytes, when dissolved in water, take on a positive charge. These are called **cations**. The major cations—sodium (Na^+), calcium (Ca^{2+}), potassium (K^+), and magnesium (Mg^{2+})—have a special significance. Sodium (Na^+) and calcium (Ca^{2+}) have their greatest concentration in the extracellular fluid, and potassium (K^+) and magnesium (Mg^{2+}) are more concentrated in intracellular space. Imbalances in any one of these electrolytes can result in major problems.

Sodium (Na^+)

Sodium is the most abundant extracellular cation and is especially important in the regulation of body water. Sodium is also important in nerve impulse transmission and in the transfer of calcium into the cell. The most common source of sodium is sodium chloride, or table salt. Sodium is often found in conjunction with chloride (Cl^-) or bicarbonate (HCO_3^-).

Regulation of sodium occurs in the kidney, primarily through reabsorption in the tubules. Aldosterone is the hormonal regulator. Secreted by the adrenal cortex aldosterone increases renal absorption of sodium. Because of sodium's high attraction for water, alterations in sodium and water balance are closely related. An imbalance in one leads to an imbalance in the other. Hypernatremia, or too much sodium, may be due to either an acute gain in sodium or a loss of water without corresponding loss of sodium.

Calcium (Ca^{2+})

Calcium is necessary for the structure of bone and teeth. It also functions as an enzyme cofactor for blood clotting and is required for hormone secretion, membrane stability and permeability, and muscle contraction. One common source of calcium is dairy products.

Most calcium in the body is located in bone tissue, with the remainder found in the plasma and body cells. Inside the cells, calcium is necessary for energy used by muscle fibers to contract. The strength of the contraction is directly related to the concentration of calcium. Calcium is often found in conjunction with phosphate (HPO_4^-).

Blood levels of calcium are closely regulated by parathyroid hormone (PTH), vitamin D, and calcitonin (from the thyroid gland). Renal regulation of calcium requires PTH, which is secreted in response to low plasma levels.

Potassium (K$^+$)

Potassium is necessary in the transmission and conduction of nerve impulses, maintenance of normal cardiac rhythms, and skeletal smooth muscle contraction. It is also required for glycogen deposits in the liver and skeletal muscles. In this capacity, potassium works closely with sodium, momentarily trading places with sodium across the cellular membranes to maintain electrical neutrality. This action conducts nerve impulses from one end of the cell to the other. It becomes extremely important in the conduction of cardiac rhythms and the movement of calcium into the cell for muscle contraction.

Magnesium (Mg^{2+})

Approximately 40 to 60 percent of magnesium is stored in muscle and bone. Most of the remainder is stored intracellularly and appears to be related to potassium and calcium. Magnesium activates the enzyme (ATPase) that is essential for normal cell membrane function and is the energy source for the sodium-potassium pump. Physiological effects include relaxing smooth muscle and increasing the stability of cardiac cells, thus reducing the potential for arrhythmias.

Electrolytes that take on a negative charge are called anions. Examples of anions found within the body include chlorine (Cl^-), bicarbonate (HCO_3^-), phosphate (HPO_4^-), and most of the organic (carbon-based) molecules. In addition to the fluid balance mentioned earlier, electrical neutrality must be carefully maintained between cations and anions.

CELL PHYSIOLOGY

To maintain physiological homeostasis, there must be an exchange of electrolytes and water materials across the membrane of the cell. The cell membrane is very complex. It is said to be semipermeable, meaning that it allows certain compounds to pass readily across it while restricting the passage of others. Many materials must pass across the cell membrane including oxygen, carbon dioxide, nutrients, fluids, and electrolytes. There are three major ways to move substances across the cell membrane: **diffusion,** facilitated diffusion, and active transport. Diffusion and facilitated diffusion are passive processes, whereas active transport requires energy expenditure by the cell (see Figure 5–1).

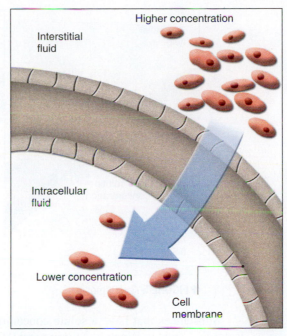

● FIGURE 5–1 Diffusion.

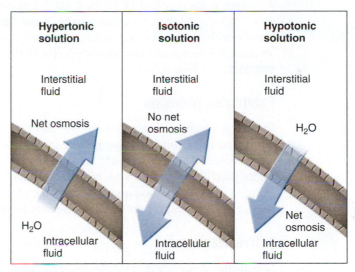

● FIGURE 5–2 Relationships and effects of hypertonic, isotonic, and hypotonic.

Diffusion

Diffusion occurs when concentrations of various substances become higher on one side of the semipermeable cell membrane. When this difference occurs, an osmotic gradient is created. The side of the cell membrane with the higher concentration is said to be **hypertonic** with respect to the other side. Conversely, the side of the membrane with the lower concentration is said to be **hypotonic** in relation to the other (see Figure 5–2). When both sides of the cell membrane have an equal concentration of the substance in question, the system is said to be **isotonic**. These concepts underpin the rationale for IV therapy. IV fluids with a solute concentration less than that of blood are said to be hypotonic solutions. An example of a hypotonic solution is 0.45 percent sodium chloride (one-half normal saline).

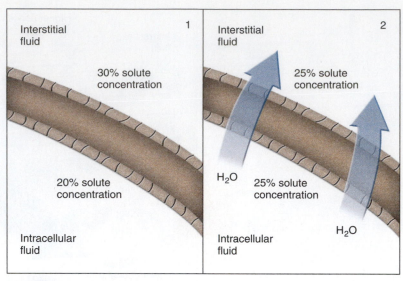

● **FIGURE 5–3** Osmosis.

Substances that have a solute concentration equal to that of blood are said to be isotonic. Lactated Ringer's solution and 0.9 percent sodium chloride are examples of isotonic fluids. An example of a hypertonic solution is 50 percent dextrose in water. Although not a classical IV fluid, it plays a major role in prehospital care. One of the most important substances that passes across the cell membrane is water. Water diffuses readily across the cell membrane from an area of higher water concentration to an area of lesser water concentration. The diffusion of water in this manner is called **osmosis** (see Figure 5–3).

Facilitated Diffusion

Certain molecules can move across the cell membrane by a process known as facilitated diffusion. Glucose is an example of such a molecule. Facilitated diffusion requires the assistance of "helper proteins" on the surface of the cell membrane. These proteins, once activated, bind to the glucose molecule. After binding, the protein changes its configuration and transports the glucose molecule into the cell, where it is released. The transport protein is then ready for another glucose molecule.

Active Transport

Sometimes it is desirable for the body to maintain a gradient along a cell membrane. This is especially true regarding the ions sodium (Na^+) and potassium (K^+). To sustain life, the concentration of sodium outside the cell membrane must be significantly higher than that inside the cell. Also, the concentration of potassium must be maintained at a much higher level within the cell. To maintain the gradient, the sodium must be pumped out of the cell and potassium must be pumped into the cell. Both of these processes require energy. This is an example of active transport.

BLOOD

One of the most important aspects of the extracellular fluid, and thus the internal environment, is blood. Blood is the main element involved in the oxygenation of body cells, transport of nutrients, transport of control maintenance factors (hormones), waste removal, and temperature regulation. Blood is a complex substance divided into two basic components: plasma and formed elements.

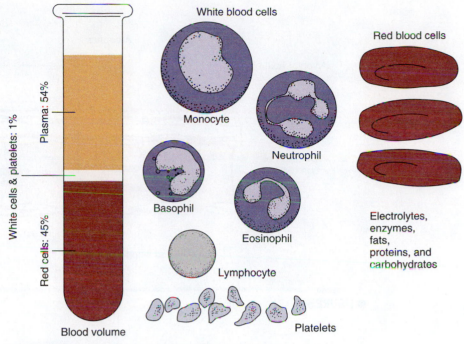

White blood cells

Red blood cells

Plasma: 54%

White cells & platelets: 1%

Red cells: 45%

Monocyte

Neutrophil

Basophil

Eosinophil

Lymphocyte

Platelets

Electrolytes,
enzymes,
fats,
proteins, and
carbohydrates

Blood volume

● **FIGURE 5–4**   Various components of blood.

Plasma

Plasma is the complex fluid portion of blood. Plasma communicates continually through pores in the capillaries with the fluid that is circulating between the cells (interstitial fluid). Plasma is approximately 92 percent water and contains a number of formed elements (see Figure 5–4).

Formed Elements

Formed elements consist of plasma proteins, plasma lipids, electrolytes, nutrients, and cellular elements such as red blood cells, white blood cells, and platelets. The formed elements make up approximately 45 to 50 percent of blood volume. The continuous movement of blood keeps the formed elements dispersed throughout the plasma, where they are available to carry out the following functions:

1. *Respiratory:* delivery of oxygen to the cells and exchange of carbon dioxide
2. *Nutritional:* delivery of other substances needed for cellular metabolism (glucose and other carbohydrates, amino acids, fatty acids, vitamins, minerals, and trace elements)
3. *Regulatory:* delivery of substances such as electrolytes and hormones
4. *Excretory:* removal of cellular debris and waste products such as those of cellular metabolism (carbon dioxide, water, and acids)
5. *Protective:* defense against injury and invading microorganisms

There are three major classes of blood cells. The first are the red blood cells, or **erythrocytes** (see Figure 5–5). Erythrocytes have an important iron-containing protein called **hemoglobin**. Hemoglobin is responsible for the transport of oxygen and carbon dioxide. A significant percentage of blood, approximately 45 percent, is red blood cells. The percentage of red blood cells present is referred to as the **hematocrit**.

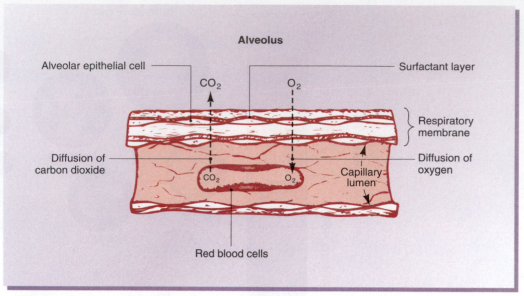

Alveolus

Alveolar epithelial cell

Surfactant layer

CO_2 O_2

Respiratory membrane

Diffusion of carbon dioxide

CO_2 O_2

Capillary lumen

Diffusion of oxygen

Red blood cells

● **FIGURE 5–5**   The red blood cell.

White blood cells, or **leukocytes**, are the second type of cells found in the blood. The leukocytes, such as neutrophils, play a role in combating infection by phagocytizing bacteria. Other leukocytes, such as lymphocytes, produce antibodies to help fight infection. The last type of blood component present is platelets, or **thrombocytes**, which are responsible for blood clotting.

Blood Types

An antigen is the protein identifier in most cells. The presence or absence of a particular antigen identifies that cell as either "self" or "foreign." Once a cell is identified as foreign, specific antibodies to that cell are formed. Subsequently, all antigens (cells with that specific foreign identifier) are attacked and destroyed. This is termed an antigen–antibody reaction. When the reaction occurs because two types of blood are mixed, it is called a **transfusion reaction**. At least two commonly occurring antigens, each of which can trigger antigen–antibody reaction, have been found in human blood cells, especially on the cell membrane surfaces. There are two types of antigens in the blood that are more likely than others to cause reactions: the ABO system of antigens and the Rh system.

ABO Types

The ABO group consists of two major antigens, labeled A and B, that are found on the surfaces of red blood cells (RBCs). These antigens can appear by themselves or together or be entirely absent. The result of their presence or absence is one of the four blood types:

Type A. Individuals with blood type A carry the A antigen on the RBCs.

Type B. Individuals with blood type B carry the B antigen on the RBCs.

Type AB. Individuals with blood type AB carry the A and B antigens on the RBCs.

Type O. Individuals with blood type O carry neither antigen on the RBCs.

In the ABO system, the body spontaneously develops antibodies to the other blood types. This system determines which blood type or types each person can receive without triggering a transfusion reaction (see Table 5–1).

TABLE 5–1			
ABO Blood Types			
Blood Types	**Antibodies**	**Can Receive**	**Can Donate to**
Type A	B antibodies	Type A or O	Type A, AB
Type B	A antibodies	Type B or O	Type B, AB
Type AB	No antibodies	Type AB, A, B, O	Type A, B, AB
Type O	A and B antibodies	Type O	Type A, B, AB, O

Rh Factor

The second important system in blood transfusion is the Rh system. The Rh antigen, type D, is widely prevalent. People with this type of antigen are said to be Rh positive; those without the type D antigen are said to be Rh negative. Approximately 85 to 95 percent of Americans are Rh positive.

Antibodies to the Rh factor do not occur naturally and must be acquired through exposure to Rh-positive blood. This process is most evident in Rh-positive babies born to Rh-negative mothers. The mother must be given a vaccine after each birth to prevent the formation of antibodies to any subsequent Rh-positive fetuses. In adult Rh-negative patients, a similar but delayed reaction can occur if Rh-positive blood is received. On receiving the second Rh-positive transfusion, a severe and potentially life-threatening reaction may occur in the patient.

IV THERAPY

As mentioned earlier, there are two major indications for IV therapy. The first is to replace fluid losses, which may occur as a result of hemorrhage caused by trauma or from severe diarrhea, vomiting, heat exhaustion, or burns. It is best to replace the fluid losses with intravenous fluids of similar isotonicity. The second is to provide a route for the administration of medications.

There are two major classes of IV fluids: colloids and crystalloids. **Colloids** contain compounds of high molecular weight, usually proteins, which do not readily diffuse across the cell membrane. In addition, they exert colloid osmotic pressure, which means they tend to attract water into the intravascular space. Thus, a small amount of a colloid can be administered to a patient with a greater than expected increase in intravascular volume. This is because the colloid will draw water from the interstitial space and the intracellular compartment to increase the intravascular volume. Common examples of colloids include the following:

Plasma protein fraction (Plasmanate). Plasmanate is a protein-containing colloid. The principal protein present is albumin, which is suspended, along with other proteins, in a saline solvent.

Albumin. Albumin infusions contain only human albumin. Each gram of albumin holds approximately 18 mL of water in the bloodstream.

Dextran. Dextran is not a protein but a large sugar molecule with osmotic properties similar to those of albumin. It comes in two molecular weights (40 000 and 70 000 Da). Dextran 40 has 2 to 2.5 times the colloid osmotic pressure of albumin.

Hetastarch (Hespan). Hetastarch, like dextran, is a sugar molecule with osmotic properties similar to those of protein. It does not appear to share many of dextran's side effects.

Polygeline (Haemaccel). Haemaccel is a gelatinous colloid with osmotic properties similar to albumin. It is relatively free of side effects and is temperature stable with an excellent shelf life.

Colloid replacement therapy, at present, does not have a role in prehospital care except under rare circumstances. Colloid products are expensive and most of them have a short shelf life.

Crystalloids contain only water and electrolytes. These substances all readily diffuse across the cell membrane. Crystalloids are the primary solutions used in prehospital intravenous fluid therapy. Because there are multiple fluid preparations, it is often helpful to classify them according to the tonicity related to plasma:

Isotonic solutions. Isotonic solutions have an electrolyte composition similar to that of blood plasma. When placed into a normally hydrated patient, they do not cause a significant fluid or electrolyte shift.

Hypertonic solutions. Hypertonic solutions have a higher solute concentration than does plasma. These fluids tend to cause a fluid shift out of the intracellular compartment into the extracellular compartment when administered to a normally hydrated patient. Later, there is a diffusion of solutes in the opposite direction.

Hypotonic solutions. Hypotonic solutions have less of a solute concentration than does plasma. When administered to a normally hydrated patient, they cause a movement of fluid from the extracellular compartment into the intracellular compartment. Later, solutes move in an opposite direction.

Paramedics choose replacement fluids based on patient needs and the patient's underlying problem. As a rule, hemorrhage occurs so fast that there is not time for a significant fluid shift between the extracellular and intracellular space. Consequently, replacement fluids are most commonly isotonic; lactated Ringer's solution and Normal Saline are used most often. If the patient is dehydrated because of fluid loss from diarrhea or fever, then there is a greater deficit of water than sodium. In this case, the paramedic may be asked to use hypotonic fluids such as one-half Normal Saline.

Some replacement fluids contain a single element, such as sodium chloride or dextrose, whereas others contain multiple elements. Solutions such as lactated Ringer's are designed so that the concentration of electrolytes is very similar to that of the plasma; they are thus referred to as balanced salt solutions.

Three of the most commonly used solutions in prehospital care are lactated Ringer's solution, 0.9 percent sodium chloride (Normal Saline), and 5 percent dextrose in water (D_5W).

Lactated Ringer's solution. Lactated Ringer's solution is an isotonic electrolyte solution. It contains sodium chloride, potassium chloride, calcium chloride, and sodium lactate in water.

Normal saline. Normal saline is an electrolyte solution containing sodium chloride in water that is isotonic with extracellular fluid.

5 percent dextrose in water. D_5W is a hypotonic glucose solution used to keep a vein open and to supply the calories necessary for cell metabolism. Although it has an initial effect of increasing the circulatory volume, glucose molecules rapidly move across the vascular membrane. The resultant free water follows almost immediately, leaving little effect on circulating blood volume.

Both lactated Ringer's solution and Normal Saline are used to replace fluid volume because their administration causes an immediate expansion of the circulatory volume. However, as was noted earlier, due to the movement of the electrolytes and water, two-thirds of either of these solutions is lost to the interstitial space within

TABLE 5–2

Approximate Ionic Concentrations (mEq/L) and Calories per Liter

	Ionic Concentrations (mEq/L)							
	Sodium	Potassium	Calcium	Chloride	Lactate	Calories per Liter	Osmolarity[a] (mOsm/L)	pH Range[b]
5% Dextrose Injection, USP						170	252	3.5–6.5
10% Dextrose Injection, USP						340	505	3.5–6.5
0.9% Sodium Chloride Injection, USP	154			154			308	4.5–7.0
Sodium Lactate Injection, USP (M/6 Sodium Lactate)	167				167	54	334	6.0–7.3
2.5% Dextrose & 0.45% Sodium Chloride Injection, USP	77			77		85	280	3.5–6.0
5% Dextrose & 0.2% Sodium Chloride Injection, USP	34			34		170	321	3.5–6.0
5% Dextrose & 0.33% Sodium Chloride Injection, USP	56			56		170	365	3.5–6.0
5% Dextrose & 0.45% Sodium Chloride Injection, USP	77			77		170	406	3.5–6.0
5% Dextrose & 0.9% Sodium Chloride Injection, USP	154			154		170	560	3.5–6.0
10% Dextrose & 0.9% Sodium Chloride Injection, USP	154			154		340	813	3.5–6.0
Ringer's Injection, USP	147.5	4	4.5	156			309	5.0–7.5
Lactated Ringer's Injection	130	4	3	109	28	9	273	6.0–7.5
5% Dextrose in Ringer's Injection	147.5	4	4.5	156		170	561	3.5–6.5
Lactated Ringer's with 5% Dextrose	130	4	3	109	28	180	525	4.0–6.5

[a]Normal physiological isotonicity range is approximately 280–310 mOsm/L. Administration of substantially hypotonic solutions may cause hemolysis, and administration of substantially hypertonic solutions may cause vein damage.
[b]pH ranges are USP for applicable solution; corporate specification for non-USP solutions.

1 hour. The second reason for initiating an IV infusion in the field is to provide a route for the administration of medications. The following IV fluids are most frequently used in prehospital emergency care (see Table 5–2).

℞ Plasma Protein Fraction (Plasmanate)

Class: Natural colloid

Description

Plasma protein fraction is a protein-containing colloid that is suspended in a saline solvent. The principal protein in plasma protein fraction is serum human albumin.

Other proteins present include globulin and gamma globulin. Plasma protein fraction is prepared from large pools of human plasma. It is quite expensive and has a very short shelf life. Although rarely used in the prehospital phase of emergency medical care, plasma protein fraction is preferred by some emergency specialists in the management of hypovolemic states, especially burn shock. After a patient sustains a severe burn, fluid is lost from the blood into the surrounding tissue. Plasma protein fraction, because it remains in the circulating blood volume, is effective in maintaining adequate blood volume and blood pressure. It is usually used in combination with lactated Ringer's solution or Normal Saline.

Mechanism of Action

Plasmanate is a protein-containing colloid that remains in the intravascular compartment. It increases intravascular volume by attracting water from other fluid compartments by virtue of its colloid osmotic pressure.

Indications

Hypovolemic shock, especially burn shock
Hypoproteinemia (low protein states)

Contraindications

There are no major contraindications to plasma protein fraction when used in the treatment of life-threatening hypovolemic states.

Precautions

It is important to monitor constantly the response of the patient and adjust the rate of infusion accordingly. The patient should be monitored for elevated blood pressure and pulmonary edema during and following plasmanate administration.

Side Effects

Chills, fever, urticaria (hives), nausea, and vomiting have all been reported with plasma protein fraction use.

Interactions

Solutions should not be mixed with or administered through the same administration sets as other intravenous fluids.

Dosage

The plasma protein fraction infusion rate should be titrated according to the patient's hemodynamic response. In the management of shock secondary to burns, the physician's orders regarding the rate of administration must be closely followed. Standard formulas for IV fluid administration have been developed. The medical control physician will use these formulas in judging the correct rate of intravenous administration.

Route

Intravenous infusion

How Supplied

Plasma protein fraction is supplied in 250 mL and 500 mL bottles of a 5 percent solution. An administration set is usually attached.

Class: Artificial colloid

Description

Dextran is a colloid that differs significantly from plasma protein fraction. Instead of proteins, dextran contains chains of sugars that are approximately the same molecular weight as serum albumin. Thus, because of their large molecular size, they remain within the circulating blood volume for an extended period. Although not as effective as plasma protein fraction, dextran has proved effective as an adjunctive aid in the management of hypovolemic shock. Dextran is supplied in two molecular weights. Dextran 40 has an average molecular weight of approximately 40,000 Da. Dextran 40 is secreted by the kidneys much more readily than the higher molecular weight form, dextran 70 (molecular weight of 70,000 Da). The higher molecular weight form tends to be broken down into glucose instead of being secreted in the dextran form, as occurs with dextran 40. The decision on which type of dextran to use in prehospital care rests with the system medical director. Because dextran is excreted through the urine, urine output is usually maintained with the administration of dextran.

Mechanism of Action

Dextran is a sugar-containing colloid used as an intravascular volume expander. It remains in the intravascular compartment for approximately 12 hours. It increases intravascular volume by attracting water from other fluid compartments by virtue of its colloid osmotic pressure.

Indication

Hypovolemic shock

Contraindications

Dextran should not be administered to patients who have a known hypersensitivity to the medication. It should not be administered to patients with congestive heart failure, renal failure, or known bleeding disorders.

Precautions

A major drawback to the use of dextran is that it coats the red blood cells, thus preventing accurate blood typing and possibly hindering administration of whole blood if required. A tube of blood should be drawn before administering dextran for blood typing at the hospital.

Allergic reactions, ranging from mild to severe anaphylaxis, have been known to occur following the administration of dextran. If these occur, therapy should be immediately discontinued. In the case of mild reactions, the patient should be closely monitored, and emergency resuscitative medications should be readily available. Severe allergic reactions may require the administration of epinephrine, diphenhydramine (Benadryl), and possibly corticosteroids. It is usually preferable to use crystalloid solutions, such as lactated Ringer's solution, rather than dextran, in the management of profound hypovolemic shock.

Side Effects

Rash, itching, dyspnea, chest tightness, and mild hypotension have all been reported with dextran use. The incidence of these side effects is very low, however, and reactions are generally mild.

Increased bleeding time has also been reported with dextran use due to its interference with platelet function.

Interactions

Dextran should not be administered to patients who are receiving anticoagulants because it significantly retards blood clotting.

Dosage

The dosage of dextran is titrated according to the patient's physiological response. In the management of burn shock, it is especially important to follow standard fluid resuscitation regimens to prevent possible circulatory overload.

Route

Intravenous infusion

How Supplied

Dextran 40 and dextran 70 are supplied in 250 and 500 mL bottles.

℞ Hetastarch (Hespan)

Class: Artificial colloid

Description

Hetastarch is an artificial colloid differing from both plasma protein fraction and dextran. Hetastarch is derived from amylopectin and chemically resembles glycogen. The average molecular weight is approximately 450,000 Da, which gives it colloidal properties similar to those of human albumin. Intravenous infusion of hetastarch results in plasma volume expansion slightly greater than the amount infused.

Because the colloidal properties of hetastarch are quite similar to those of human albumin, it has proved effective in the management of hypovolemic shock, especially burn shock. It does not appear to share the blood-typing problems seen with dextran.

Mechanism of Action

Hetastarch is a starch-containing colloid used as an intravascular volume expander. Following administration, the plasma volume is expanded slightly in excess of the volume of hetastarch administered. This effect has been observed for up to 24 to 36 hours. Hetastarch increases intravascular volume by virtue of its colloid osmotic pressure.

Indications

Hypovolemic shock, especially burn shock
Septic shock

Contraindications

There are no major contraindications to hetastarch when used in the management of life-threatening hypovolemic states.

Precautions

It is important to constantly monitor the response of the patient and adjust the rate of infusion accordingly. The patient should be monitored for signs of pulmonary edema and elevated blood pressure during and following hetastarch administration.

Large volumes of hetastarch may alter the body's coagulation mechanism. Hetastarch should be used with caution in patients who are receiving anticoagulants.

Side Effects

Nausea, vomiting, mild febrile reactions, chills, itching, and urticaria (hives) have been reported with hetastarch administration. Severe anaphylactic reactions have been rarely reported.

Interactions

Hetastarch should not be administered to patients who are receiving anticoagulants.

Dosage

The hetastarch infusion rate should be titrated according to the patient's hemodynamic response. In the management of burn shock, the physician's orders regarding the rate of administration must be closely followed. Standard formulas for colloid administration to burn patients have been developed. It is important to remember that a fall in blood pressure in burn shock occurs much later than with hemorrhagic causes.

Route

Intravenous infusion

How Supplied

Sterile 6 percent hetastarch in 0.9 percent sodium chloride is supplied in 500 mL bottles.

℞ Polygeline (Haemaccel)*

Class: Artificial colloid

Description

Haemaccel, although not used in North America, is utilized by EMS systems throughout the rest of the world. Haemaccel is a manufactured protein derived

*Not currently used in North America.

from gelatin obtained from cattle in the United States. It is sterile, pyrogen free, and contains no preservatives. Furthermore, studies have shown that it remains effective after freezing and thawing. The molecular weight of Haemaccel is approximately 35 000 Da. In addition to polygeline, Haemaccel contains Na^+ (145 mEq), K^+ (5.1 mEq), Ca^{2+} (6.25 mEq), and Cl^- (145 mEq). The pH is approximately 7.3. Following administration of 1 L, the colloidal osmotic pressure of Haemaccel draws an additional 500 mL or so of fluid into the intravascular space.

Mechanism of Action

Haemaccel is a gelatinous colloid used as an intravascular volume expander. The half-life of Haemaccel is approximately 8 hours. It increases intravascular fluid volume by attracting water from other fluid compartments by virtue of its colloid osmotic pressure.

Indication

Hypovolemic shock

Contraindications

Haemaccel is contraindicated in patients with known hypersensitivity to any of its components. It should be used with caution in patients with a history of anaphylaxis.

Precautions

Although rare, be alert for allergic reactions and possible anaphylaxis.

Side Effects

Transient skin reactions (wheals, urticaria), tachycardia, bradycardia, nausea, vomiting, dyspnea, hypotension, fall in temperature, and shivering have been reported with Haemaccel administration. If these occur, the infusion should be stopped.

Interactions

None reported

Dosage

The dosage of Haemaccel is titrated according to the patient's physiological response. In the management of burn shock, it is especially important to follow standard fluid resuscitation regimens to prevent possible circulatory overload.

Route

Intravenous infusion

How Supplied

Haemaccel, 3.5 percent, is supplied in 500 mL plastic infusion bottles.

℞ Lactated Ringer's Solution (Hartmann's Solution)

Class: Isotonic crystalloid solution

Description

Lactated Ringer's solution is one of the most frequently used IV fluids in the management of hypovolemic shock. It is an isotonic crystalloid solution containing electrolytes in the following concentrations:

Sodium (Na^+) 130 mEq/L
Potassium (K^+) 4 mEq/L
Calcium (Ca^{2+}) 3 mEq/L
Chloride (Cl^-) 109 mEq/L

In addition to the electrolytes mentioned earlier, lactated Ringer's solution contains 28 mEq of lactate (lactic acid), which acts as a buffer.

Mechanism of Action

Lactated Ringer's solution replaces water and electrolytes.

Indications

Hypovolemic shock
Keep open IV

Contraindications

Lactated Ringer's solution should not be used in patients with congestive heart failure or renal failure.

Precautions

Patients receiving lactated Ringer's solution should be monitored to prevent circulatory overload.

Side Effects

Rare in therapeutic dosages

Interactions

Few in the emergency setting

Dosage

Crystalloids, such as lactated Ringer's solution, diffuse out of the intravascular space and into the surrounding tissues in less than an hour. Thus, it is often necessary to replace 1 L of lost blood with 3 to 4 L of lactated Ringer's solution.

In severe hypovolemic shock, lactated Ringer's solution should be infused through large-bore (14- or 16-gauge) IV cannulas. These infusions should be administered "wide open" until a systolic blood pressure of approximately 100 mmHg is achieved. When this blood pressure is attained, the infusion should be reduced to about 100 mL/hr. If the blood pressure falls again, then the infusion rate should be increased and adjusted accordingly. Adjunctive devices, such as the pneumatic anti-shock garment (PASG) and extremity elevation, may be used in the management of severe hypovolemic shock.

Route

Intravenous infusion

How Supplied

Lactated Ringer's solution is supplied in 250, 500, and 1000 mL bags and bottles.

℞ 5 Percent Dextrose in Water (D₅W)

Class: Hypotonic dextrose-containing solution

Description

When vigorous fluid replacement is not indicated, 5 percent dextrose in water (D_5W) may be used. D_5W can be used for the administration of intravenous medications. D_5W is hypotonic, which prevents circulatory overload in patients with congestive heart failure.

Mechanism of Action

D_5W provides nutrients in the form of dextrose as well as free water.

Indications

IV access for emergency medications
For dilution of concentrated medications for intravenous infusion

Contraindications

D_5W should not be used as a fluid replacement for hypovolemic states. Dextrose-containing solutions should be avoided in patients with head injury or stroke.

Precautions

Dextrose-containing solutions are acidic and may produce local venous irritation. Subcutaneous administration from extravasation may result in tissue necrosis.

As with any IV fluid, it is important to watch for signs of circulatory overload when administering D_5W.

When treating hypoglycemia, it is imperative that a tube of blood be drawn before administering D_5W or 50 percent dextrose ($D_{50}W$).

Side Effects

Rare in therapeutic dosages

Interactions

D_5W should not be used with phenytoin (Dilantin) or inamrinone (Inocor).

Dosage

D_5W is usually administered through a minidrip (60 drops/mL) set at a rate of "to keep open" (TKO).

Route

Intravenous infusion

How Supplied

D_5W is supplied in bags and bottles of 50, 100, 150, 250, 500, and 1000 mL.

℞ 10 Percent Dextrose in Water ($D_{10}W$)

Class: Hypertonic dextrose-containing solution

Description

Ten percent dextrose in water ($D_{10}W$) is a hypertonic solution. Like D_5W, $D_{10}W$ is used only when vigorous fluid replacement is not indicated. $D_{10}W$ has twice as much carbohydrate as does D_5W, which makes it of use in the management of hypoglycemia.

Mechanism of Action

$D_{10}W$ provides nutrients in the form of dextrose as well as free water.

Indications

Neonatal resuscitation
Hypoglycemia

Contraindications

$D_{10}W$ should not be used as a fluid replacement for hypovolemic states. Dextrose-containing solutions should be avoided in patients with head injury or stroke.

Precautions

Dextrose-containing solutions are acidic and may produce local venous irritation. Subcutaneous administration from extravasation may result in tissue necrosis.

As with any IV fluid, it is important to be alert for signs of circulatory overload.

When treating hypoglycemia, it is imperative that a tube of blood be drawn before administering $D_{10}W$ or 50 percent dextrose ($D_{50}W$).

Side Effects

Rare in therapeutic dosages

Interactions

$D_{10}W$ should not be used with phenytoin (Dilantin) or inamrinone (Inocor).

Dosage

The administration rate of $D_{10}W$ usually depends on the patient's condition.

Route

Intravenous infusion

How Supplied

$D_{10}W$ is supplied in bottles and bags of 50, 100, 150, 250, 500, and 1000 mL.

℞ 0.9 Percent Sodium Chloride (Normal Saline)

Class: Isotonic crystalloid solution

Description

The use of 0.9 percent sodium chloride, or Normal Saline (as it is often called), has several applications in emergency medicine. Normal saline contains 154 mEq/L of sodium ions (Na^+) and approximately 154 mEq/L of chloride (Cl^-) ions. Because the concentration of sodium is near that of blood, the solution is considered isotonic. Normal saline is especially useful in heat stroke, heat exhaustion, and diabetic ketoacidosis.

Mechanism of Action

Normal saline replaces water and electrolytes.

Indications

Heat-related problems (heat exhaustion, heat stroke)
Freshwater drowning
Hypovolemia
Diabetic ketoacidosis
Keep open IV

Contraindication

The use of 0.9 percent sodium chloride should not be considered in patients with congestive heart failure because circulatory overload can be easily induced.

Precautions

Normal saline contains only sodium and chloride. When large amounts of Normal Saline are administered, it is quite possible for other important physiological electrolytes to become depleted. In cases in which large amounts of fluids may have to be administered, it might be prudent to use lactated Ringer's solution.

Side Effects

Rare in therapeutic dosages

Interactions

Few in the emergency setting

Dosage

The specific situation being treated dictates the rate at which Normal Saline is administered. In severe heat stroke, diabetic ketoacidosis, and freshwater drowning, it is quite likely that paramedics will be called on to administer the fluid quite rapidly. In other cases, it is advisable to administer the fluid at a moderate rate (e.g., 100 mL/hr).

Route

Intravenous infusion

How Supplied

Normal saline is supplied in 250, 500, and 1000 mL bags and bottles. Sterile Normal Saline for irrigation should not be confused with that designed for intravenous administration.

℞ 0.45 Percent Sodium Chloride (One-Half Normal Saline)

Class: Hypotonic crystalloid solution

Description

One-half Normal Saline (0.45 percent sodium chloride) solution is a hypotonic crystalloid solution containing approximately one-half the concentration of sodium and chloride as does blood plasma.

Mechanism of Action

One-half Normal Saline replaces free water and electrolytes.

Indication

Patients with diminished renal or cardiovascular function for whom rapid rehydration is not indicated

Contraindication

Cases in which rapid rehydration is indicated

Precautions

One-half Normal Saline contains only sodium and chloride. When large amounts of one-half Normal Saline are administered, it is possible for other important physiological electrolytes to become depleted. In cases in which large amounts of fluids must be administered, it might be prudent to use lactated Ringer's solution.

Side Effects

Rare in therapeutic dosages

Interactions

Few in the emergency setting

Dosage

The specific situation and patient condition dictate the rate at which one-half Normal Saline is administered.

Route

Intravenous infusion

How Supplied

One-half Normal Saline is supplied in 250, 500, and 1000 mL bags and bottles.

℞ 5 Percent Dextrose in 0.45 Percent Sodium Chloride (D₅1/2NS)

Class: Hypertonic dextrose-containing crystalloid solution

Description

Five percent dextrose in 0.45 percent sodium chloride ($D_5$1/2NS) is a versatile fluid. It contains the same amount of sodium and chloride as does one-half Normal Saline. Dextrose has been added for its nutrient properties, providing 80 calories per liter.

Mechanism of Action

$D_5$1/2NS replaces free water and electrolytes and provides nutrients in the form of dextrose.

Indications

Heat exhaustion
Diabetic disorders
For use as a To keep open (TKO) solution in patients with impaired renal or cardiovascular function

Contraindication

$D_5$1/2NS should not be used when rapid fluid resuscitation is indicated. Dextrose-containing solutions should be avoided in patients with head injury or stroke.

Precautions

Dextrose-containing solutions are acidic and may produce local venous irritation. Subcutaneous administration from extravasation may result in tissue necrosis.

As with any IV fluid, it is important to watch for signs of circulatory overload when administering $D_5$1/2NS.

When treating hypoglycemia, it is imperative that a tube of blood be drawn before administering $D_5$1/2NS or 50 percent dextrose (D_{50}W).

Side Effects

Rare in therapeutic dosages

Interactions

D$_5$1/2NS should not be used with phenytoin (Dilantin) or inamrinone (Inocor).

Dosage

The specific situation and patient condition dictate the rate at which D$_5$1/2NS should be administered.

Route

Intravenous infusion

How Supplied

D$_5$1/2NS is supplied in bottles and bags containing 250, 500, and 1000 mL of the fluid.

℞ 5 Percent Dextrose in 0.9 Percent Sodium Chloride (D$_5$NS)

Class: Hypertonic dextrose-containing crystalloid solution

Description

Five percent dextrose in 0.9 percent Normal Saline is a hypertonic crystalloid to which 5 g of dextrose per 100 mL of fluid has been added for its nutrient properties (80 calories per liter).

Mechanism of Action

D$_5$NS replaces free water and electrolytes and provides nutrients in the form of dextrose.

Indications

Heat-related disorders
Freshwater drowning
Hypovolemia
Peritonitis

Contraindications

D$_5$NS should not be administered to patients with impaired cardiac or renal function. Dextrose-containing solutions should be avoided in patients with head injury or stroke.

Precautions

Dextrose-containing solutions are acidic and may produce local venous irritation. Subcutaneous administration from extravasation may result in tissue necrosis.

D_5NS contains only the electrolytes sodium and chloride. When large amounts of fluids must be administered, it might be prudent to use lactated Ringer's solution to prevent depletion of the other physiological electrolytes.

When treating hypoglycemia, it is imperative that a tube of blood be drawn before administering D_5NS or 50 percent dextrose ($D_{50}W$).

Side Effects

Rare in therapeutic dosages

Interactions

D_5NS should not be used with phenytoin (Dilantin) or inamrinone (Inocor).

Dosage

The specific situation and patient condition dictate the rate at which D_5NS is given.

Route

Intravenous infusion

How Supplied

D_5NS is supplied in bags and bottles containing 250, 500, and 1000 mL of the solution.

℞ 5 Percent Dextrose in Lactated Ringer's Solution (D_5LR)

Class: Hypertonic dextrose-containing crystalloid solution

Description

Five percent dextrose in lactated Ringer's solution (D_5LR) contains the same concentration of electrolytes as does lactated Ringer's solution. In addition to the electrolytes, however, 5 g of dextrose per 100 mL of fluid has been added for nutrient properties. This added dextrose causes the solution to be hypertonic and adds 80 calories per liter.

Mechanism of Action

D_5LR replaces water and electrolytes and provides nutrients in the form of dextrose.

Indications

Hypovolemic shock
Hemorrhagic shock
Certain cases of acidosis

Contraindications

D_5LR should not be administered to patients with decreased renal or cardiovascular function. Dextrose-containing solutions should be avoided in patients with head injury or stroke.

Precautions

Patients receiving D$_5$LR should be constantly monitored for signs of circulatory overload. It is essential that a blood sample be drawn before administering D$_5$LR to patients with hypoglycemia.

Dextrose-containing solutions are acidic and may produce local venous irritation. Subcutaneous administration from extravasation may result in tissue necrosis.

Side Effects

Rare in therapeutic dosages

Interactions

D$_5$LR should not be used with phenytoin (Dilantin) or inamrinone (Inocor).

Dosage

In severe hypovolemic shock, D$_5$LR should be infused through a large-bore catheter (14 or 16 gauge). This infusion should be administered "wide open" until a blood pressure of 100 mmHg is achieved. When the blood pressure is attained, the infusions should be reduced to 100 mL/hr. In other cases, the specific situation and patient condition dictate the rate of administration.

Route

Intravenous infusion

How Supplied

D$_5$LR is supplied in bags and bottles containing 250, 500, and 1000 mL of the fluid.

INSERTION OF INDWELLING IV CATHETER

One of the earliest stages in the management of an acutely ill or injured patient is the placement of an IV catheter. In trauma cases an IV catheter provides access for fluid resuscitation, whereas in medical disorders it provides a route for medications that must be given intravenously.

Before inserting an IV catheter, several decisions must be made to ensure the best possible care for the patient. They are as follows:

What Size Catheter Should Be Inserted?

When managing patients with trauma who require rapid fluid administration, it is imperative that a large catheter, 16 gauge, be inserted. It is important to remember that patients who are likely to need whole blood on arrival at the hospital require a large-bore catheter (18 gauge or larger). Medical patients may receive an 18- or 20-gauge catheter.

What Type of IV Catheter Should Be Inserted?

As a rule, an over-the-needle catheter is all that should be used in the prehospital setting. Butterfly catheters are usually too small to administer large amounts of fluids rapidly. Butterfly catheters should be carried for use in children, however. Occasionally, an adult with exceptionally small veins may be encountered, and, in this case, a butterfly catheter may be inserted if one of the other types of catheters cannot be placed.

What Type of IV Fluid Should Be Used?

Usually, the decision of what type of IV fluid to use is left up to the base station physician or written in the protocols. It is important to be familiar with the types of fluids that have been discussed in this chapter.

What Type of Administration Set Should Be Used?

There are two general types of IV administration sets. The macrodrip, or standard, set delivers in the neighborhood of 10 to 20 gtt/mL, depending on the manufacturer. Minidrip, or microdrip, sets deliver anywhere from 50 to 60 gtt/mL, depending on the manufacturer. If a large quantity of fluids will be administered, then a macrodrip set should be used. Whenever a paramedic is going to administer a medication, he or she should use a minidrip set. This is especially true for piggyback medication infusions. Many systems also use Buretrol or Volutrol sets for administering aminophylline and similar medications. If these sets are used, paramedics should remember them when preparing to administer medications such as aminophylline.

Where Should the IV Be Inserted?

Routinely, IV infusions should be started in the larger veins of the forearm. These are usually the most accessible and the least painful for the patient. When these veins are not available, as often occurs in shock and trauma, then any of the other peripheral sites should be attempted.

The veins of the leg and the external jugular in the neck are considered peripheral veins. When treating medical or traumatic emergencies, the rule of thumb for starting an intravenous infusion is "any port in a storm." In a cardiac/traumatic arrest, the antecubital vein is a preferred site.

Procedure for Intravenous Cannulation

Once the preceding five decisions have been made, then the actual procedure of inserting the IV can begin. The procedure is as follows:

1. Observe Standard Precautions.
2. Receive the order.
3. Confirm the order and write it down.
4. Prepare the equipment and don gloves and protective eyewear:
   a. Appropriate IV fluid
   b. Appropriate administration set
   c. Appropriate indwelling catheter
   d. Extension IV tubing
   e. Tourniquet
   f. Antibiotic swab
   g. 2 × 2 gauze pad
   h. 1-inch tape
   i. Short arm board
5. Remove the envelope from the IV fluid.
6. Inspect the fluid, making sure that it is not discolored and does not contain any particulate matter; check that it contains the amount of fluid it should have. Do not administer if discolored, if particles are present, or if less than the indicated quantity of fluid is present.
7. Open and inspect the IV tubing.
8. Attach the extension tubing.

9. Close the clamp on the tubing.

10. Remove the sterile cover from the IV fluid and the administration set.

11. Insert the administration set into the IV fluid.

12. Squeeze the drip chamber to fill it with fluid.

13. Bleed all of the air out of the IV tubing.

14. Hang the bag on an IV pole (or have a bystander hold it) at the appropriate height.

15. Place the tourniquet on the patient to occlude venous flow only.

16. Select a suitable vein and palpate it (see Figures 5–6 and 5–7).

17. Prepare the site by cleansing it with an antibiotic swab.

18. Make the puncture using appropriate sterile technique, enter the vein, observe flashback, and advance the catheter (see Figures 5–8 through 5–10).

19. Connect the IV tubing and remove tourniquet.

20. Slowly open the valve.

21. Confirm that the fluid is flowing appropriately without any evidence of infiltration.

22. Cover with a sterile 2 × 2 gauze pad or adhesive bandage.

23. Securely tape the IV catheter and tubing down.

24. Adjust the flow rate.

25. Apply a short arm board.

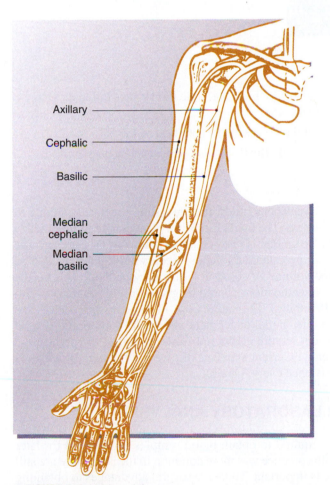

● **FIGURE 5–6** Veins of the arm.

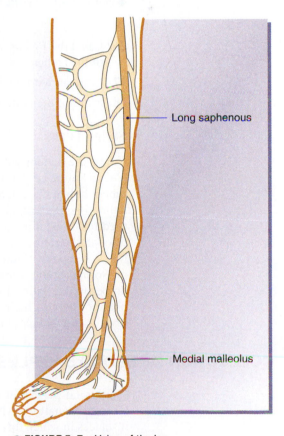

● **FIGURE 5–7** Veins of the leg.

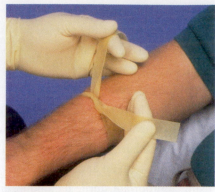

● **FIGURE 5–8**   Apply the tourniquet.

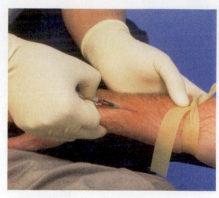

● **FIGURE 5–9**   Puncture the skin.

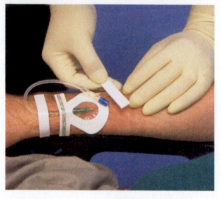

● **FIGURE 5–10**   Secure the catheter.

26. Label the IV bag with the patient's name, date, time the IV was initiated, gauge of the catheter, and your initials.

27. Confirm with medical control the successful completion of the IV.

28. Monitor the patient for the desired effects and any undesired ones as well.

Saline Locks

Unless the patient will receive intravenous fluids, the prevailing practice is simply to place a Saline Lock for venous access. The Saline Lock is a plastic male adapter with a rubber hub at the end and a plastic tip that is inserted directly into an IV catheter. The Saline Lock is primarily used for precautionary venous access only, but may also be used for blood draw and limited volume IV solution infusion by puncture of a needle through the rubber hub. IV push medications should be given only through an IV infusion setup (IV solution and IV tubing). The Saline Lock must be flushed with 2 cc's of Normal Saline for injection after initial attachment and each blood draw. If used properly, the Saline Lock will not require additional flushing during the prehospital phase of care to maintain patency. Current standard of care for flushing of a Saline Lock to prevent clot blockage is once every 8 hours.

COLLECTION OF BLOOD SAMPLES FOR LABORATORY ANALYSIS

Prehospital personnel may be required to obtain blood samples in the field for later laboratory analysis. Although this practice was more common in the past, there are still instances in which this practice is important. There are several advantages to obtaining blood samples in the field.

First, it provides the emergency physician with information about the patient before medical intervention. This information is especially important in cases of suspected hypoglycemia when 50 percent dextrose is administered (although electronic glucometers are very accurate and thus the need for blood samples prior to glucose administration is diminishing). In situations in which a patient may be trapped or transport to the hospital is otherwise delayed, blood samples can be taken to the hospital before the patient so that blood can be typed, cross-matched, and ready when the patient eventually arrives in the emergency department. Whenever a prehospital intervention might affect the subsequent care of the patient (e.g., administering dextran, which may inhibit blood typing), the paramedic should always draw a blood sample according to local protocol.

Most commonly, blood samples are taken when an IV is started. The paramedic should always follow Standard Precautions when caring for a patient and especially when handling a blood sample. Standard Precautions should be taken. After placing the IV catheter and before connecting the IV line, a 10 mL syringe can be attached to the catheter and blood gently withdrawn from the vein. The syringe can be removed and the IV line connected. It is important to withdraw the blood from the syringe slowly. Withdrawing it rapidly can damage the blood cells, causing them to rupture and leak their contents, which in turn can erroneously alter the blood chemistries and render the sample useless.

Once blood is withdrawn from a patient, it is usually placed into evacuated blood collection tubes (Vacutainer). These tubes have a vacuum that allows the tube to fill with a predetermined amount of blood. Most tubes contain a chemical to keep the blood from clotting. Each tube has a different colored rubber top, depending on its use and contents. The type of tube a paramedic may be asked to draw may vary from region to region. After withdrawing the blood as described earlier, an 18-gauge needle is placed on the syringe. The needle is inserted into the rubber top and the tube is allowed to fill with blood. The paramedic should not attempt to overfill the tube or press on the plunger of the syringe, but allow the vacuum to fill the vial.

After the vials are filled, they should be inverted several times to mix the blood and the anticoagulant. The types and color of tubes, and the order in which they are drawn, can vary from system to system. The patient's name, date, time drawn, paramedic's name, and incident number (if any) are immediately written on the vial. The tubes are given to the appropriate emergency department personnel on arrival. The paramedic documents on the patient report form the time the blood was drawn and to whom it was given. At critical scenes, labeling tubes may be difficult. As an alternative until tubes can be labeled, tape the tubes to the IV bag.

BLOOD TRANSFUSIONS

When mismatched blood is transfused, the donor's antibodies can bind to antigens on the recipient's red blood cells (RBCs). This reaction, known as a transfusion reaction, causes clumping of RBCs in the blood (agglutination) and subsequent hemolysis (RBCs breaking apart). Transfusion reaction can be prevented only by complete and careful type matching between donor and recipient.

Paramedics occasionally transport a patient receiving blood. These patients need careful monitoring for signs and symptoms of transfusion reaction. The severity of the reaction depends on the degree of incompatibility, the amount of blood given, and the rate of administration. Onset is usually rapid, either during or immediately after a transfusion. More rarely, it occurs later. Signs and symptoms include anxiety; facial flushing; pain in the neck, chest, and lumbar area; tachycardia; cold, clammy skin; hypotension; nausea or vomiting; dizziness; hives; headaches; and fever.

When signs and symptoms of transfusion reaction appear, the transfusion should be discontinued immediately. A physician should be consulted as soon as possible and a crystalloid infusion for medication administrations maintained. Typically, a fluid bolus is administered to assure adequate urine output. A diuretic such as mannitol (Osmitrol) and an antihistamine such as diphenhydramine (Benadryl) may be indicated. One of the most lethal effects of transfusion reaction is renal failure, which can begin within a few minutes to a few hours and may progress to death.

CASE STUDY

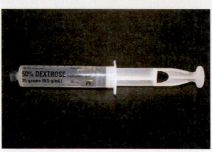

© Bryan E. Bledsoe

In the old NBC television series *Emergency!* paramedics Johnny Gage and Roy Desoto would often call Rampart General and receive orders for "D_5W and transport." For many years D_5W was often used in EMS as a free-water replacement solution. However, more recent studies have shown that administering dextrose (glucose) containing solutions to victims of stroke or brain trauma actually worsened outcomes. The brain and other central nervous system tissues depend almost exclusively on glucose as an energy source. In addition, the brain is the only tissue type that does not require insulin to facilitate glucose entry into the cells. During periods of ischemia (e.g., stroke, brain trauma) the oxygen level in the affected brain cells and tissues is decreased. Thus, when supplemental glucose is administered, glucose entry into the brain cells and tissues is increased. However, without adequate oxygen supplies to break down the glucose totally, much of the excess glucose is converted to lactic acid—a strong acid. As lactic acid levels increase, the pH of the cells and tissues subsequently decreases, ultimately leading to damage or even death of the cells and tissues. Because of this, it is no longer considered safe to administer glucose-containing solutions to these patients (unless bona fide hypoglycemia is documented).

CHAPTER REVIEW

Summary

As with the skills of medication administration, the insertion of an IV requires vigorous mannequin, classroom, and clinical training under the supervision of a qualified instructor.

Key Words

cations   A positive charge that certain electrolytes take when dissolved in water.

colloid   A substance of high molecular weight, such as plasma proteins. Colloids tend to remain in the intravascular space, as opposed to crystalloids, which tend to diffuse out.

crystalloid   A solution containing crystalline substances, such as Normal Saline.

diffusion   The movement of solute (substances dissolved in a solution) from an area of greater concentration to an area of lesser concentration.

electrolytes A chemical substance that dissociates into charged particles when placed in water.

erythrocytes Red blood cells; responsible for transport of oxygen.

extracellular The space outside the cell membrane.

hematocrit A measure of the number of red blood cells found in the blood, stated as a percentage of the total blood volume.

hemoglobin An important iron-containing protein that erythrocytes have.

homeostasis The body's natural tendency to keep the natural environment constant.

hypertonic A state in which a solution has a higher solute concentration on one side of a semipermeable membrane than on the other side.

hypotonic A state in which a solution has a lower solute concentration on one side of a semipermeable membrane than on the other side.

intracellular The space and materials within the cell membrane.

intravascular The space within the blood vessels.

interstitial fluid Fluid outside the cell membrane yet not within any defined blood vessel.

isotonic A state in which solutions on opposite sides of a semipermeable membrane are equal in concentration.

leukocytes White blood cells; responsible for fighting infection.

osmosis The movement of a solvent (water) across a semipermeable membrane from an area of lesser (solute) concentration to an area of greater (solute) concentration; osmosis is a form of diffusion.

plasma The complex fluid portion of blood.

semipermeable membrane A specialized biological membrane, such as that which encloses the body's cells, that allows passage of certain substances and restricts the passage of others.

thrombocytes Blood platelets which are responsible for blood clotting.

transfusion reaction The reaction when two types of blood are mixed.

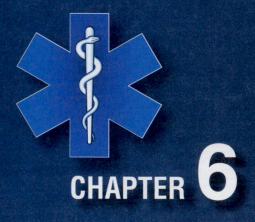

CHAPTER 6

THE AUTONOMIC NERVOUS SYSTEM

OBJECTIVES

After completing this chapter, the reader should be able to:

- Describe the anatomy and physiology of the autonomic nervous system.
- Compare sympathetic and parasympathetic actions.
- Explain the function of the sympathetic nervous system.
- List the five adrenergic receptors and explain the effect of each one on body organs.
- Explain the function of the parasympathetic nervous system.

INTRODUCTION

The autonomic nervous system is a part of the peripheral nervous system and is responsible for control of involuntary, or visceral, bodily functions. It controls crucial cardiovascular, respiratory, digestive, urinary, and reproductive functions. It also plays a key role in the body's response to stress.

Many of the medications used in emergency care act directly or indirectly on the autonomic nervous system. Thus, it is essential that prehospital personnel have a good understanding of the structure and function of the autonomic nervous system. This chapter discusses the anatomy and physiology of the autonomic nervous system as it applies to emergency pharmacological therapy.

THE AUTONOMIC NERVOUS SYSTEM

The nervous system is the body's principal control system. It regulates virtually all bodily functions via electrical impulses transmitted through nerves. Closely related to the nervous system is the endocrine system. Like the nervous system, the endocrine system is an important control system. However, unlike the nervous system, it exerts its effect on the body through the release of specialized chemical substances called **hormones**.

The nervous system is customarily divided into the central nervous system and the peripheral nervous system. The **central nervous system (CNS)** consists of the brain and spinal cord. In contrast, the **peripheral nervous system (PNS)** is composed

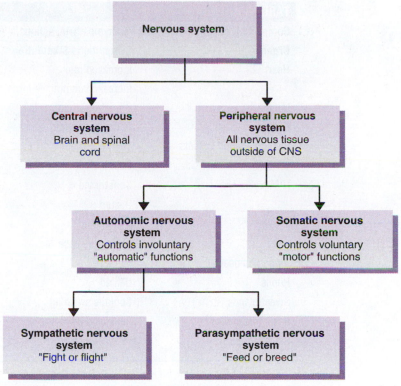

● **FIGURE 6–1** Functional organization of the nervous system.

of the cranial nerves and the spinal nerves. The peripheral nervous system can be further divided into the somatic nervous system and the autonomic nervous system. The **somatic nervous system (SNS)** controls voluntary motor functions such as movement. The **autonomic nervous system (ANS)** controls involuntary automatic functions (see Figure 6–1).

The two functional divisions of the autonomic nervous system are the sympathetic nervous system and the parasympathetic nervous system. The **sympathetic nervous system** allows the body to function under stress. It is often referred to as the *fight-or-flight* aspect of the nervous system. The parasympathetic nervous system, on the other hand, primarily controls vegetative functions such as digestion of food. It is often referred to as the *feed-or-breed* or *rest-and-repose* aspect of the autonomic nervous system. The parasympathetic nervous system is in constant opposition to the sympathetic nervous system (see Table 6–1).

Autonomic Nervous System Anatomy and Physiology

Although the autonomic nervous system is located primarily outside of the central nervous system, it arises from the central nervous system. The nerves of the autonomic nervous system exit the central nervous system and subsequently enter specialized structures called autonomic **ganglia**. In the autonomic ganglia, the nerve fibers from the central nervous system interact with nerve fibers that extend from the ganglia to the various target organs. Autonomic nerve fibers that exit the central nervous system and terminate in the autonomic ganglia are called *preganglionic nerves*. Autonomic nerve fibers that exit the ganglia and terminate in the various target tissues are called *postganglionic nerves*. The ganglia of the sympathetic nervous system are located

TABLE 6–1

Comparison of Sympathetic and Parasympathetic Actions

Organ	Sympathetic Stimulation	Parasympathetic Stimulation
Heart	Increased rate	Decreased rate
	Increased contractile force	Decreased contractile force
Lungs	Bronchodilation	Bronchoconstriction
Kidneys	Decreased output	No change
Systemic blood vessels		
Abdominal	Constricted	None
Muscle	Constricted α	None
	Dilated β	None
Skin	Constricted	None
Liver	Glucose release	Slight glycogen synthesis
Blood glucose	Increased	None
Pupils	Dilated	Constricted
Sweat glands	Copious sweating	None
Basal metabolism	Increased up to 100%	None
Skeletal muscle	Increased strength	None

close to the spinal cord, whereas the ganglia of the parasympathetic nervous system are located close to the target organs (see Figure 6–2).

No actual physical connection exists between two nerve cells or between a nerve cell and the organ it innervates. Instead, there is a space between nerve cells called a synapse. The space between a nerve cell and the target organ is called a neuroeffector junction. Specialized chemicals called **neurotransmitters** are used to conduct the nervous signal between nerve cells or between a nerve cell and its target organ. Neurotransmitters are released from presynaptic neurons and subsequently act on postsynaptic neurons or on the designated target organ. When released by the nerve ending, the neurotransmitter travels across the synapse and activates membrane receptors on the adjoining nerve or target tissue. The neurotransmitter is then either deactivated or taken back up into the presynaptic neuron. The primary neurotransmitters of the autonomic nervous system are **acetylcholine (ACh)** and **norepinephrine.** Acetylcholine is utilized in the preganglionic nerves of the sympathetic nervous system and in both the preganglionic and postganglionic nerves of the parasympathetic nervous system. Norepinephrine is the primary postganglionic neurotransmitter of the sympathetic nervous system. Synapses that use ACh as the neurotransmitter are called **cholinergic** synapses. Synapses that use norepinephrine as the neurotransmitter are called **adrenergic** synapses.

The Sympathetic Nervous System

The sympathetic nervous system arises from the thoracic and lumbar region of the spinal cord. Preganglionic nerves leave the spinal cord through the spinal nerves and end in the sympathetic ganglia. There are two types of sympathetic ganglia: sympathetic chain ganglia and collateral ganglia (see Figure 6–3). In addition, special preganglionic sympathetic nerve fibers innervate the adrenal medulla. Postganglionic nerves that exit the *sympathetic chain ganglia* extend to several peripheral target tissues of

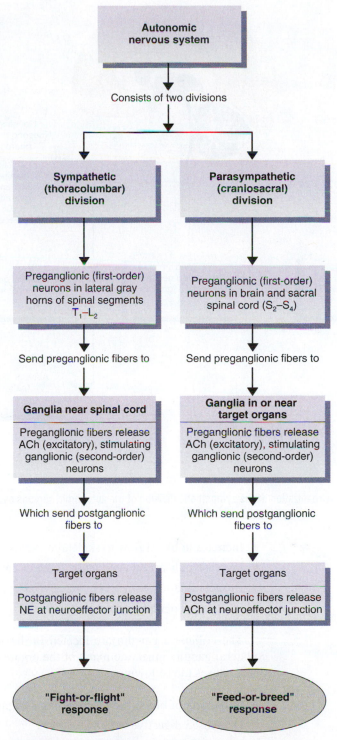

● FIGURE 6–2 Components of the autonomic nervous system.

the sympathetic nervous system. When stimulated, these fibers have several effects, including the following:

- Stimulation of secretion by sweat glands
- Constriction of blood vessels in the skin

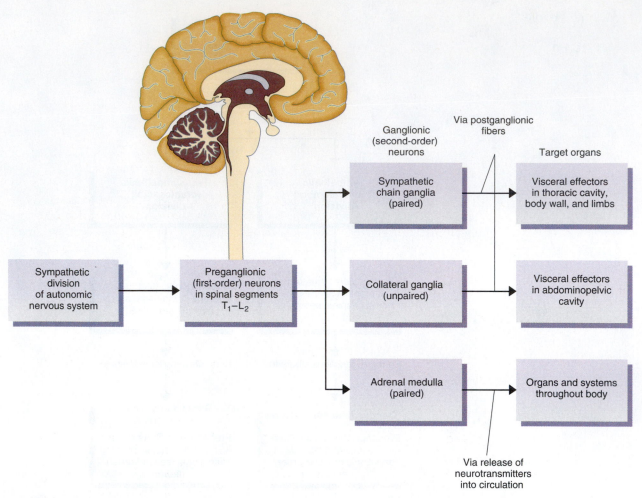

● **FIGURE 6–3** Organization of the sympathetic division of the autonomic nervous system.

- Increase in blood flow to skeletal muscles
- Increase in heart rate and in the force of cardiac contractions
- Bronchodilation
- Stimulation of energy production

The collateral ganglia are located in the abdominal cavity. Nerves leaving the collateral ganglia innervate many of the organs of the abdomen. Stimulation of these fibers causes the following:

- Reduction of blood flow to abdominal organs
- Decreased digestive activity
- Relaxation of smooth muscle in the wall of the urinary bladder
- Release of glucose stores from the liver

Sympathetic nervous system stimulation also results in direct stimulation of the **adrenal medulla**. The adrenal medulla in turn releases the hormones norepinephrine (noradrenalin) and **epinephrine** (adrenalin) into the circulatory system. Approximately 80 percent of the hormones released by the adrenal medulla are epinephrine, with norepinephrine constituting the remaining 20 percent. Once released, these hormones are carried throughout the body, where they cause their intended effects by acting on hormone receptors. The release of norepinephrine and epinephrine by the adrenal medulla stimulates tissues that are not innervated by sympathetic nerves. In addition, these substances prolong the effects of direct sympathetic stimulation. All of these effects serve to prepare the body to deal with stressful and potentially dangerous situations.

Adrenergic Receptors

Sympathetic stimulation ultimately results in the release of norepinephrine from postganglionic nerves. The nervous impulse subsequently crosses the synapse and interacts with adrenergic receptors. Shortly thereafter, the norepinephrine is taken up by the presynaptic neuron for reuse or is broken down by enzymes present within the synapse (see Figure 6–4). Sympathetic stimulation also results in the release of epinephrine and norepinephrine from the adrenal medulla. Both epinephrine and norepinephrine also interact with specialized receptors on the membranes of the target organs. These receptors, called *adrenergic receptors,* are located throughout the body. Once stimulated by the appropriate hormone, they cause a response in the organ or organs they control.

The two known types of sympathetic receptors are the adrenergic receptors and the dopaminergic receptors. The adrenergic receptors are generally divided into five types. These five receptors are designated *alpha$_1$* (α_1), *alpha$_2$* (α_2), *beta$_1$* (β_1), and *beta$_2$* (β_2), and beta$_3$ (β_3) The α_1-receptors cause peripheral vasoconstriction, mild bronchoconstriction, and stimulation of metabolism. The α_2-receptors are found on the *presynaptic* surfaces of sympathetic neuroeffector junctions. Stimulation of α_2-receptors is inhibitory. They serve to prevent overrelease of norepinephrine in the synapse. When the level of norepinephrine in the synapse gets high enough, the α_2-receptors are stimulated and norepinephrine release is inhibited. Stimulation of β_1-receptors causes an increase in heart rate, cardiac contractile force, and cardiac automaticity and conduction. Stimulation of β_2-receptors causes vasodilation and bronchodilation. Stimulation of β_3 adrenergic receptors, which are primarily located in adipose tissues, causes the breakdown of fat (lipolysis) and the generation of heat (thermogenesis) in skeletal muscle (see Table 6–2). *Dopaminergic receptors* located outside of the central nervous system, although not fully understood, are believed to cause dilation of the renal, coronary, and cerebral arteries. These have limited application in clinical practice.

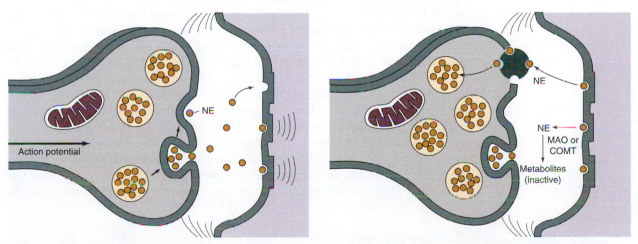

● **FIGURE 6–4** Physiology of an adrenergic synapse. Norepinephrine is released from the presynaptic nerve and stimulates receptors on the postsynaptic nerve. Subsequently, the norepinephrine is either taken up by the presynaptic nerve or deactivated by enzymes present in the synapse.

TABLE 6–2

Actions of the Adrenergic Receptors

Receptor	Actions
alpha$_1$ (α_1)	Peripheral vasoconstriction
	Increased contractile force (positive inotropic effect)
	Decreased heart rate (negative chronotropic effect)
alpha$_2$ (α_2)	Decreased catecholamines in circulation (vasodilation and decreased blood pressure)
beta$_1$ (β_1)	Increased heart rate (positive chronotropic effect)
	Increased contractile force (positive inotropic effect)
	Increased automaticity (positive dromotropic effect)
beta$_2$ (β_2)	Peripheral vasodilation
	Bronchodilation
	Uterine smooth muscle relaxation
	Gastrointestinal smooth muscle relaxation
Beta$_3$ (β_3)	Lipolysis
	Thermogenesis
Dopaminergic	Renal vasodilation
	Mesenteric vasodilation

Medications that stimulate the sympathetic nervous system are referred to as **sympathomimetics**. Medications that inhibit the sympathetic nervous system are called **sympatholytics**. Some medications are pure α-agonists, whereas others are pure α-antagonists. Some medications are pure β-agonists, whereas others are pure β-antagonists. Medications such as epinephrine stimulate both α- and β-receptors. Medications such as the **bronchodilators** are termed β selective, because they act more on β$_2$-receptors than on β$_1$-receptors.

The Parasympathetic Nervous System

The **parasympathetic nervous system** arises from the brain stem and the sacral segments of the spinal cord. The preganglionic neurons are typically much longer than those of the sympathetic nervous system because the ganglia are located close to the target tissues. Parasympathetic nerve fibers that leave the brain stem travel within four of the cranial nerves including the oculomotor nerve (III), the facial nerve (VII), the glossopharyngeal nerve (IX), and the vagus nerve (X). These fibers synapse in the parasympathetic ganglia with short postganglionic fibers, which then continue to their target tissues. Postsynaptic fibers innervate much of the body including the intrinsic eye muscles, the salivary glands, the heart, the lungs, and most of the organs of the abdominal cavity. The sacral segment of the parasympathetic nervous system forms distinct pelvic nerves that innervate ganglia in the kidneys, bladder, sex organs, and terminal portions of the large intestine (see Figure 6–5). Stimulation of the parasympathetic nervous system results in the following:

- Pupillary constriction
- Secretion by digestive glands
- Increased smooth muscle activity along the digestive tract

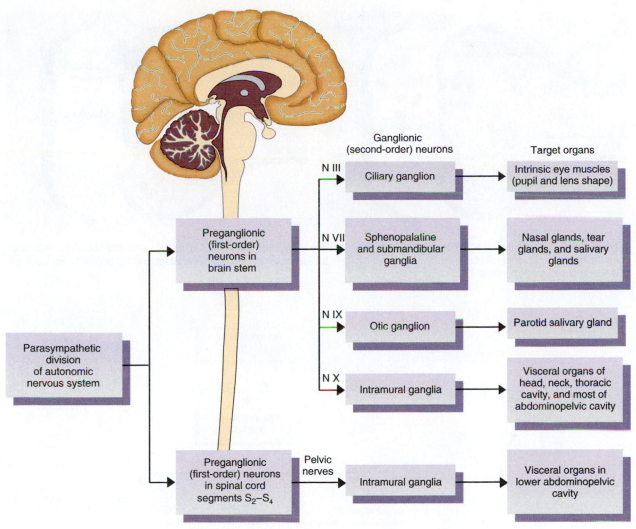

● **FIGURE 6–5**   Organization of the parasympathetic division of the autonomic nervous system.

- Bronchoconstriction
- Reduction in heart rate and cardiac contractile force

Through these and other functions, the processing of food, energy absorption, relaxation, and reproduction are facilitated.

All preganglionic and postganglionic parasympathetic nerve fibers use acetylcholine as a neurotransmitter. Acetylcholine, when released by presynaptic neurons, crosses the synaptic cleft and activates receptors on the postsynaptic neuron or on the neuroeffector junction. Acetylcholine is also the neurotransmitter for the somatic nervous system and is present in the neuromuscular junction. Acetylcholine is very short lived. Within a fraction of a second after its release, acetylcholine is deactivated by another chemical called acetylcholinesterase. Acetic acid and *choline,* which are produced when acetylcholine is deactivated, are taken back up by the presynaptic neuron (see Figure 6–6).

The parasympathetic system has two main types of ACh receptors, nicotinic and muscarinic (see Figures 6–7 and 6–8). Knowing these receptors' locations and functions will greatly simplify learning the functions of medications in this class. Nicotinic$_N$ (neuron) receptors are found in all autonomic ganglia, where

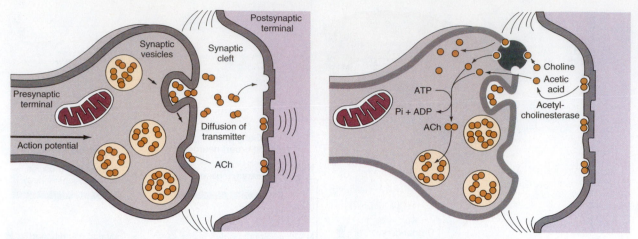

● **FIGURE 6–6** Physiology of a cholinergic synapse. Acetylcholine is released from the presynaptic nerve and stimulates receptors on the postsynaptic nerve. Subsequently, the acetylcholine is broken down by acetylcholinesterase and the products are taken up by the presynaptic nerve fiber.

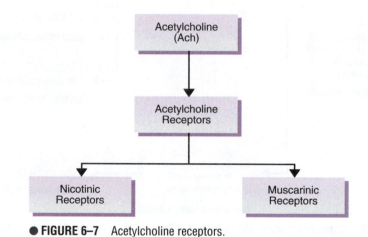

● **FIGURE 6–7** Acetylcholine receptors.

```
Acetylcholine
Receptors
    |
    +------------------+----------------------+
    |                  |                      |
Neuromuscular      Autonomic                 CNS
(Nicotinic)    (Muscarinic & Nicotinic)  (Muscarinic & Nicotinic)
```

● **FIGURE 6–8** Location and classes of acetylcholine receptors.

acetylcholine serves as the presynaptic neurotransmitter of both the parasympathetic and sympathetic nervous systems. Nicotinic$_M$ (muscle) receptors are found at the neuromuscular junction and initiate muscular contraction as part of the somatic nervous system (see Figure 6–9). Muscarinic receptors are found in many organs thoughout the body and are primarily responsible for promoting the parasympathetic

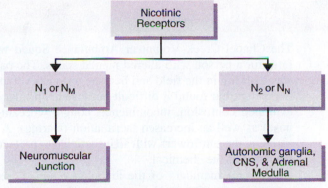

● **FIGURE 6–9** Location and classes of nicotinic receptors.

TABLE 6-3

Location and Effect of Muscarinic Receptors

Organ	Functions	Location
Heart	Decreased heart rate	Sinoatrial node
	Decreased conduction rate	Atrioventricular node
Arterioles	Dilation	Coronary
	Dilation	Skin and mucosa
	Dilation	Cerebral
GI tract	Relaxed	Sphincters
	Increased	Motility
	Increased salivation	Salivary glands
	Increased secretion	Exocrine glands
Lungs	Bronchoconstriction	Bronchiole smooth muscle
	Increased mucous production	Bronchial glands
Gallbladder	Contraction	
Urinary bladder	Relaxation	Urinary sphincter
	Contraction	Detrusor muscle
Liver	Glycogen synthesis	
Lacrimal glands	Secretion (increased tearing)	Eye
Eye	Contraction for near vision	Ciliary muscle
	Constriction	Pupil
Penis	Erection	

response. Table 6–3 summarizes the locations and actions of the muscarinic receptors.

The emergency medication atropine is an antagonist to the parasympathetic nervous system and is used to increase heart rate. Atropine binds with ACh receptors, thus preventing ACh from exerting its effect. Medications such as atropine, which block the actions of the parasympathetic nervous system, are referred to as parasympatholytics or anticholinergics. Medications that stimulate the parasympathetic nervous system are referred to as parasympathomimetics.

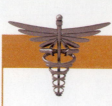

The Chapel Creek Volunteer Ambulance Squad was summoned to a local sunflower farm for a person with altered mental status. The patient, a 23-year-old migrant worker, was working in the field and became progressively more confused. Paramedics assessed the patient but found it difficult because his primary language was Spanish. The patient exhibited confusion, incontinence, cough, wheezing, headache, and rhinorrhea (runny nose) as well as increased lacrimation (tearing). A supervisor said that they had been spraying the sunflowers with an insecticide to protect the blooms. He could not remember the name of the chemical.

Several members of the ambulance squad are also farmers and suspect that the insecticide was from a class of chemicals known as organophosphates. Chemicals in this class stimulate cholinergic receptors (muscarinic, nicotinic, and central nervous system receptors) and cause the classic signs and symptoms of cholinergic poisoning. Based upon the symptoms, paramedics administered a small, test dose of 1 milligram of atropine sulfate—a potent anticholinergic medication. The patient exhibited no change following the test dose, thus indicating moderate to severe cholinergic poisoning. Based upon this, repeated doses of atropine were administered and the patient's symptoms started to improve. The patient was transported to the hospital and made an uneventful recovery.

CHAPTER REVIEW

Summary

The autonomic nervous system is a part of the peripheral nervous system and is responsible for control of involuntary, or visceral, bodily functions. It maintains the body's internal environment by controlling crucial cardiovascular, respiratory, digestive, urinary, and reproductive functions. It also plays a key role in the body's response to stress.

Because many of the medications used in prehospital care act directly or indirectly on the autonomic nervous system, it is essential that prehospital personnel have a good understanding of the structure and function of the autonomic nervous system.

Key Words

acetylcholine (ACh)   Chemical neurotransmitter found in all autonomic preganglionic synapses and in parasympathetic postganglionic synapses.

adrenal medulla   An endocrine gland, located atop the kidney, that manufactures and secretes epinephrine and norepinephrine.

adrenergic   Related to or pertaining to the sympathetic nervous system.

autonomic nervous system (ANS)   Part of the peripheral nervous system responsible for control of involuntary, or visceral, bodily functions.

bronchodilator   A medication that helps to improve breathing by relaxing the smooth muscle of the bronchioles, causing bronchodilation.

central nervous system (CNS)   The central portion of the nervous system, consisting of the brain and spinal cord.

cholinergic   Related to or pertaining to the parasympathetic nervous system.

epinephrine   A naturally occurring hormone that stimulates the adrenal glands, increases cardiac output, and causes bronchodilation.

hormones   Specialized chemical substances released by an effect of the endocrine system.

neurotransmitter   A substance that is released from the axon terminal of a presynaptic neuron. On excitation it travels across the synaptic cleft to either excite or inhibit the target cell. Examples include acetylcholine, norepinephrine, and dopamine.

norepinephrine   A naturally occurring hormone that also serves as a sympathetic neurotransmitter. It is found in most postganglionic synapses.

parasympathetic nervous system (PNS)   The division of the autonomic nervous system that is responsible for controlling vegetative functions.

peripheral nervous system   The portion of the nervous system outside the brain and spinal cord. It is composed of the cranial nerves and peripheral nerves.

somatic nervous system (SNS)   The portion of the nervous system that controls voluntary motor functions such as movement.

sympathetic nervous system   The division of the autonomic nervous system that prepares the body for stressful situations.

sympatholytic (or antiadrenergic)   Medications that block beta adrenergic receptors and slow the heart rate.

sympathomimetic   A medication or other substance that causes effects such as those of the sympathetic nervous system (also called adrenergic).

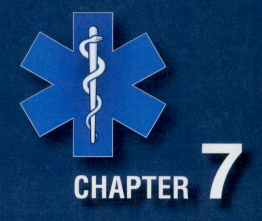

OBJECTIVES

After completing this chapter, the reader should be able to:

- Describe and list the pharmacokinetics, indications, contraindications, and dosages for the sympathomimetics epinephrine, norepinephrine, phenylephrine, isoproterenol, dopamine, dobutamine, inamrinone, milrinone and vasopressin.
- Discuss the pharmacology of vasopressin and its role in cardiac arrest management.
- Explain the class of medications known as adrenergic antagonists.
- Describe and list the pharmacokinetics, indications, contraindications, and dosages for the adrenergic antagonists propranolol, sotalol, metoprolol, labetalol, atenolol, and esmolol.
- Discuss the use of antiarrhythmic medications in modern prehospital practice.
- Describe and list the pharmacokinetics indications, contraindications, and dosages for the antiarrhythmics lidocaine, procainamide, adenosine, verapamil, diltiazem, amiodarone, phenytoin, edrophonium chloride, and magnesium sulfate.
- Explain the role of the parasympatholytic atropine and list the pharmacokinetics, indications, contraindications, and dosages for its use.
- Describe digitalis and list the pharmacokinetics, indications, contraindications, and dosages for its use.
- Describe the indications for anticoagulant therapy in emergency care.
- Discuss the use of fibrinolytics and platelet aggregation inhibitors in the treatment of acute coronary syndrome (ACS).
- Describe and list the pharmacokinetics, indications, contraindications, and dosages for aspirin and the fibrinolytic agents streptokinase, anistreplase, alteplase, tenecteplase, and retaplase recombinant.
- List the pharmacokinetics, indications, contraindications, and dosages for sodium bicarbonate.
- Explain the pharmacokinetics, indications, contraindications, and dosages for morphine and nitrous oxide in the treatment of cardiac chest pain.
- Discuss the use of diuretics in the management of congestive heart failure.
- List the pharmacokinetics, indications, contraindications, and dosages for the diuretics furosemide and bumetanide.
- Discuss the use of the natriuretic peptide nesiritide for the management of congestive heart failure.

- Describe the action of nitroglycerin in cardiac chest pain and congestive heart failure.
- List the pharmacokinetics, indications, contraindications, and dosages for the antianginal agents nitroglycerin, nitroglycerin spray, and nitroglycerin paste.
- Define and explain a hypertensive emergency and contrast it with a hypertensive urgency.
- List the pharmacokinetics, indications, contraindications, and dosages for the antihypertensives nicardipine, clevidipine, nifedipine, enalaprilat, captopril, sodium nitroprusside, and hydralazine.
- Detail the renin-angiotensin-aldosterone system (RAAS) and detail the effect of common antihypertensive medications on this system.
- List the pharmacokinetics, indications, contraindications, and dosages for calcium chloride.

INTRODUCTION

Most prehospital emergency medications are used in the treatment of cardiac emergencies. These medications, because of the nature of their actions, may be accompanied by many side effects. Some general classifications follow for our discussion of the emergency cardiovascular medications:

Gases

Oxygen

Sympathomimetics (Sympathetic agonists)

Epinephrine
Norepinephrine (Levophed)
Phenylephrine (Neo-Synephrine)
Isoproterenol (Isuprel)
Dopamine HCl (Intropin)
Dobutamine (Dobutrex)
Inamrinone (Inocor)
Milrinone (Primacor)
Vasopressin (Pitressin)

Adrenergic Antagonists (Sympathetic antagonists)

Propranolol (Inderal)
Sotalol HCl (Sotacor, Betapace)
Metoprolol (Lopressor)
Labetalol (Trandate, Normodyne)
Atenolol (Tenormin)
Esmolol (Brevibloc)

Antiarrhythmics

Lidocaine (Xylocaine)
Procainamide (Pronestyl)
Adenosine (Adenocard)
Verapamil (Isoptin, Calan)
Diltiazem (Cardizem)
Amiodarone HCl (Cordarone)
Phenytoin (Dilantin)
Edrophonium chloride (Tensilon)
Magnesium sulfate

Parasympatholytics (Parasympathetic antagonists)

Atropine sulfate

Cardiac Glycosides

Digoxin (Lanoxin)

Anticoagulants

Heparin (UFH)
Enoxaparin (Lovenox)

Platelet-Aggregation Inhibitors

Aspirin
Clopidogrel (Plavix)
Abciximab (ReoPro)
Eptifibatide (Integrilin)
Tirofiban (Aggrastat)

Fibrinolytics

Streptokinase (Streptase)
Anistreplase (Eminase, Apsac)
Alteplase, tissue plasminogen activator (r-tPA) (Activase)
Tenectplase (TNKase)
Reteplase Recombinant (Retavase)

Alkalinizing Agents

Sodium bicarbonate

Analgesics

Morphine sulfate
Nitrous oxide (Nitronox, Entonox)

Diuretics

Furosemide (Lasix)
Bumetanide (Bumex)

Natriuretic Agents

Nesiritide (Natrecor)

Antianginal Agents

Nitroglycerin (Nitrostat)
Nitroglycerin paste (Nitroglycerin Ointment)
Nitroglycerin spray (Nitroglycerin Spray)
Nitroglycerin infusion (Tridil)

Antihypertensives

Nicardipine (Cardene)
Clevidipine (Cleviprex)
Nifedipine (Procardia, Adalat)
Enalaprilat (Vasotec)
Captopril (Capoten)
Sodium nitroprusside (Nitropress, Nipride)
Hydralazine (Apresoline)

Other Cardiovascular Medications

Calcium chloride

OXYGEN

Oxygen is an important medications used in prehospital care. It is required by the body's cells to facilitate the breakdown of glucose into usable energy forms. Without oxygen, the breakdown of glucose is ineffective and incomplete. This breakdown without oxygen is termed **anaerobic metabolism**. Anaerobic metabolism yields **lactic acid**, a strong acid, as its end product. This acid, in conjunction with an increased carbon dioxide level, leads to systemic acidosis.

Oxygen is an odorless, tasteless, colorless gas that vigorously supports combustion. It is present in room air at a concentration of approximately 21 percent. This concentration is adequate for our daily activities. In injury and illness, however, the body needs increased levels of oxygen to maintain homeostasis.

Recent studies have demonstrated that increased concentrations of oxygen can be toxic. Excessive amounts of oxygen can cause the formation of toxic chemicals called *oxygen free radicals* or *reactive oxygen species*. The oxygen free radicals can damage and even destroy body tissues in a process called *oxidative stress*. Oxidative stress has now been linked to numerous disease processes including atherosclerosis, Alzheimer's disease, Parkinson's disease, and others. Highly oxygen-dependent tissues, such as the brain and heart, are particularly vulnerable to the effects of oxidative stress. Neonates, as they transition to extrauterine life, are also susceptible to the effects of oxidative stress. It has been determined that oxidative stress plays a major role in cardiac arrest and reperfusion injury. The current recommendations are to administer oxygen only to those patients who are **hypoxic** based upon physical exam findings and **pulse oximetry**. Even then, oxygen administration should be judicious. Oxygen therapy should only correct hypoxia.

 Oxygen

Class Gas

Description

Oxygen is an odorless, tasteless, colorless gas necessary for life.

Mechanism of Action

Oxygen enters the body through the respiratory system and is transported to the cells by hemoglobin, found in the red blood cells. Oxygen is required for the efficient breakdown of glucose into a usable energy form. Its onset of action following administration is immediate. The administration of enriched oxygen increases the oxygen concentration in the alveoli, which subsequently increases the oxygen saturation of available hemoglobin.

Pharmacokinetics

Onset: Immediate
Peak Effects: < 1 minute
Duration: < 2 minutes
Half-Life: N/A

Indication

Hypoxia. Oxygen is indicated whenever hypoxia is suspected or present as documented by physical examination findings and/or pulse oximetry.

Contraindications

Non-hypoxic patients. There is no advantage to administering oxygen to the normoxic (non-hypoxic) patient. Elevated oxygen levels (hyperoxia) should be avoided.

Precautions

Oxygen should only be administered in a concentration that will correct hypoxia. It should be titrated to avoid hyperoxia. The administration of high concentrations of oxygen to neonates for a prolonged period of time can damage the infant's eyes (*retinopathy of prematurity*). Although this is rarely a problem in prehospital care, it is a consideration in long-distance and prolonged transport. Oxygen delivered at a flow rate of 6 lpm or greater should be humidified to prevent drying of the mucous membranes of the upper respiratory system. When possible, oxygen administration should be monitored by use of pulse oximetry. *Pulse oximetry* is a noninvasive method for accurately measuring the oxygen saturation of hemoglobin. It is relatively inexpensive, easy to use, and quite accurate in detecting oxygen delivery problems.

Side Effects

There are few, if any, acute side effects associated with oxygen administration. Hyperoxia has been associated with free-radical induction and oxidative stress. Prolonged administration of high-flow, nonhumidified oxygen may cause drying of the mucous membranes, resulting in irritation and possibly nosebleeds.

Interactions/Incompatibilities

There are no interactions associated with oxygen administration. However, oxygen may increase the toxicity of certain herbicides (e.g., paraquat and diaquat) in patients who have ingested these poisons. These chemicals are sometimes sprayed on illicit agricultural products such as marijuana. Poisoning by these agents is uncommon.

Dosage

The dosage of oxygen is based on the patient's underlying problems. In the prehospital setting oxygen should be administered at the least concentration that will correct the patient's hypoxia. Oxygen delivery rates vary based upon the delivery device utilized (see Table 7–1). Pulse oximetry should be used to guide care.
General guidelines follow:

- Cardiac arrest and other critical patients—Provide only enough oxygen to correct hypoxia. In non-hypoxic patients, room air (21% oxygen) is usually adequate.
- Chronic obstructive pulmonary disease—35 percent oxygen concentration (increase as needed).

How Supplied

Oxygen is supplied in pressurized cylinders of varying size (see Table 7–2). Liquid oxygen is becoming more common in prehospital care. The sizes and types of liquid oxygen containers vary.

TABLE 7–1

Oxygen Delivery by Device

Oxygen Delivery Device	Flow Rate (lpm)	Percentage Delivered
Nasal cannula	1–6	24–44
Simple face mask	8–10	40–60
Venturi mask	4–12	24–50
Partial rebreathing mask	6–10	35–60
Nonrebreathing mask	6–10	60–95
Bag, valve, and mask with reservoir	10–15	40–90
Demand valve	10–15	100

TABLE 7–2

Capacity of Common Oxygen Cylinders

Cylinder Name	Volume (L)
D	400
E	660
M	3000

SYMPATHOMIMETICS

The term **sympathomimetic** means to mimic the actions of the sympathetic nervous system. Medications in this group do exactly that. They either act directly on receptors of the sympathetic nervous system or act indirectly by stimulating the release of **endogenous** catecholamines. **Catecholamine** is the name used to describe several medications that are chemically similar. These medications are epinephrine, norepinephrine (Levophed), isoproterenol (Isuprel), dopamine (Intropin), and dobutamine (Dobutrex). All of these agents, except isoproterenol and dobutamine, can be found naturally in the body. Isoproterenol and dobutamine are synthetic catecholamines. All sympathomimetics, monoamine oxidase inhibitors (MAOIs), and tricyclic antidepressants (TCAs) may increase blood pressure. To understand and appreciate the actions and roles of the sympathomimetics fully, it is essential to first review the sympathetic nervous system.

Sympathetic Nervous System

The sympathetic nervous system is sometimes called the fight-or-flight system. It is this part of the nervous system that prepares the body to deal with various stresses, whether real or imagined. Sometimes it is referred to as the **adrenergic system**. Both it and the other aspect of the autonomic nervous system, the parasympathetic nervous system, functionally oppose each other to maintain **homeostasis**. The parasympathetic system is sometimes called the **cholinergic system**.

As indicated by Table 7–3, the sympathetic nervous system tends to stimulate those organs needed to deal with stressful situations. It also tends to inhibit the use of organs not needed, such as the digestive tract.

The sympathetic nervous system uses the hormone **norepinephrine** to transmit impulses from the nerve to the effector cell. Chemicals that propagate the nervous impulse, such as norepinephrine, are called **neurotransmitters**. In emergency situations

TABLE 7–3

Comparison of Sympathetic and Parasympathetic Actions

Organ	Sympathetic Stimulation	Parasympathetic Stimulation
Heart	Increased rate	Decreased rate
	Increased contractile force	Decreased contractile force
Lungs	Bronchodilation	Bronchoconstriction
Kidneys	Decreased output	No change
Systemic blood vessels		
Abdominal	Constricted	None
Smooth muscle	Constricted (α)	None
	Dilated (β)	None
Skin	Constricted	None
Liver	Glucose release	Slight glycogen synthesis
Blood glucose	Increased	None
Pupils	Dilated	Constricted
Sweat glands	Copious sweating	None
Basal metabolism	Increased up to 100%	None
Skeletal muscle	Increased strength	None
	Heat generation	None
Adipose tissues	Fat breakdown	None

the norepinephrine released by the nerve endings may be augmented with epinephrine and norepinephrine secreted from the adrenal medulla. Like the adrenergic nerves, the adrenal medulla secretes norepinephrine. About 20 percent of the catecholamines secreted by the adrenals are in the form of norepinephrine. The remaining 80 percent are in the form of epinephrine (adrenalin).

When released, norepinephrine acts on specialized chemical receptors. These receptors are located at various points throughout the body. Once stimulated by the appropriate catecholamine, they cause a response in the organ or organs they control. There are two types of receptors, the **adrenergic receptors** and the **dopaminergic receptors**. The adrenergic receptors are further divided into five different types. These five types of receptors are designated *alpha₁* (α_1), *alpha₂* (α_2), *beta₁* (β_1), *beta₂* (β_2), and *beta₃* (β_3). The α_1-receptors cause peripheral vasoconstriction and occasionally mild bronchoconstriction. The α_2-receptors, when stimulated, inhibit the release of norepinephrine. This effect is antagonistic to the actions of α_1 receptors and over time can cause peripheral vasodilation. The β_1-receptors, once stimulated, cause an increase in cardiac rate, cardiac force, and cardiac automaticity and conduction. The β_2-receptors cause vasodilation and bronchodilation. The β_3-receptors stimulate the breakdown of fat (lipolysis) and the generation of heat (thermogenesis) in skeletal muscle. Dopaminergic receptors, though not totally understood, are believed to cause dilatation of the renal, coronary, and cerebral arteries. See Chapter 6 for a more detailed discussion of the autonomic nervous system.

Catecholamines

Certain medications stimulate certain receptors to one degree or another. Norepinephrine, for example, has an effect on both α- and β-receptors. However, its effects are considerably stronger on α-receptors than on β-receptors. Consequently, norepinephrine

TABLE 7–4

Comparison of Effects of α- and β-Adrenergic Receptor Activity on Selected Organs

Organ	α-adrenergic Receptors	β-adrenergic Receptors
Heart	No cardiac effect	Increased heart rate (β_1)
		Increased contractile force (β_1)
		Increased automaticity (β_1)
Systemic blood vessels	Vasoconstriction	Vasodilation (β_2)
Lungs	Mild bronchoconstriction	Bronchodilation (β_2)

is primarily regarded as an α-receptor-stimulating agent. Epinephrine, like norepinephrine, acts on both α- and β-receptors. However, unlike norepinephrine, epinephrine has a much greater effect on β-receptors and is considered a β-receptor-stimulating agent. Isoproterenol, the synthetic catecholamine, although rarely used in emergency medicine, acts entirely on β-receptors with no α effects noted. Dopamine acts on both α- and β-receptors depending on the dosage. In addition, when used in certain doses, it acts on the dopaminergic receptors. This dopaminergic effect is quite useful because it tends to keep blood flowing to the renal arteries, even in emergency situations. One of the long-term major complications of severe medical emergencies such as cardiac arrest is renal failure.

Medications that cause an increase in the cardiac rate are called positive chronotropic agents. Medications that cause an increase in cardiac force are referred to as positive inotropic agents. Medications that cause an increase in the rate of cardiac impulse conduction through the AV node are referred to as positive in dromotropic agents.

The primary use of the sympathomimetics in emergency medicine is to increase the blood pressure in cardiogenic and septic shock. These medications raise the blood pressure by one of two different methods. Medications that stimulate α-receptors elevate blood pressure merely by peripheral vasoconstriction. Vasoconstriction reduces the size of the vascular pool, thus increasing the blood pressure. Medications that act on β-receptors elevate blood pressure by causing an increase in cardiac output. Cardiac output can be defined as follows:

$$\text{Cardiac output} = \text{Stroke volume} \times \text{Heart rate}$$

Thus,

$$\text{Blood pressure} = \text{Cardiac output} \times \text{Peripheral vascular resistance}$$

The β-receptor-stimulating medications, including epinephrine and dopamine, cause an increase in both heart rate (positive chronotropic) and **stroke volume** (positive inotropic). The different receptor effects are summarized in Table 7–4.

℞ Epinephrine

Class Sympathetic agonist

Description

Epinephrine is a naturally occurring catecholamine with both α- and β-adrenergic stimulant effects.

Mechanism of Action

Epinephrine acts directly on α- and β-adrenergic receptors. Its effect on β-receptors is much more profound than its effect on α-receptors. The effects of epinephrine include the following:

- Increased heart rate
- Increased cardiac contractile force
- Increased electrical activity in the myocardium
- Increased systemic vascular resistance
- Increased blood pressure
- Increased automaticity

Interestingly, it has been found that the beneficial effects of epinephrine in cardiac arrest are more due to its alpha adrenergic effects (vasoconstriction) than its beta adrenergic effects (as previously thought). Epinephrine has been the mainstay in the treatment of various forms of cardiac arrest and is still recommended primarily because of its vasopressor effects. Studies have shown that epinephrine increases a return of spontaneous circulation (ROSC) but has not been found to increase long-term survival.

Epinephrine's effects usually appear within 90 seconds of administration, and they are usually of short duration. Therefore, it must be administered every 3–5 minutes to maintain therapeutic levels. Epinephrine is still recommended in the treatment of cardiac arrest.

Pharmacokinetics

Onset: < 2 minutes [intravenous/endotracheal tube (IV/ET)]

Peak Effects: < 5 minutes (IV/ET)

Duration: 5–10 minutes (IV/ET)

Half-Life: 5 minutes

Indications

Epinephrine is used in cardiac arrest (asystole, ventricular fibrillation, pulseless ventricular tachycardia, pulseless electrical activity), severe anaphylaxis, and severe reactive airway disease. It is also used in symptomatic bradycardia refractory to atropine.

Contraindications

Epinephrine 1:10 000 is contraindicated in patients who do not require extensive cardiopulmonary resuscitative efforts. With simple allergic reactions and asthma, the 1:1000 dilution should be used and is administered intramuscularly.

Precautions

Epinephrine, like all catecholamines, should be protected from light. It can be deactivated by alkaline solutions such as sodium bicarbonate. Thus, it is essential that the IV line be adequately flushed between administrations of epinephrine and sodium bicarbonate.

Side Effects

Epinephrine can cause palpitations, anxiety, tremulousness, headache, dizziness, nausea, and vomiting. Because of its strong inotropic and chronotropic properties, epinephrine increases myocardial oxygen demand. Even in low doses it can cause myocardial ischemia. When administering epinephrine in the emergency setting, these effects should be kept in mind. Like most of the other medications used in emergency medicine, epinephrine is effective only when the myocardium is adequately oxygenated.

Interactions/Incompatibilities

Epinephrine is pH dependent and can be deactivated when administered with highly alkaline solutions such as sodium bicarbonate. The effects of epinephrine can be intensified in patients who are taking antidepressants.

Dosage

Epinephrine 1:10 000 can be administered intravenously, intraosseously, or endotracheally. Common doses include the following:

Cardiac arrest (adults). The dose of epinephrine in cardiac arrest is 1.0 mg of a 1:10 000 solution intravenously or via an intraosseous device. This can be repeated every 3–5 minutes as required. Higher dosages may be ordered by medical control and are potentially helpful in the cardiac arrest setting for patients who are on beta-blocker therapy. If an IV cannot be started, epinephrine can be administered endotracheally. The endotracheal dose should be increased to at least 2–2.5 times the intravenous dose but is generally ineffective.

Cardiac arrest (children). The initial dose of epinephrine in pediatric cardiac arrest is 0.01 mg/kg of a 1:10 000 solution intravenously (0.1 mL/kg). This should be repeated at the same dose every 3–5 minutes as needed.

Severe anaphylaxis or severe asthma (adults). Intravenous epinephrine should be used only for life threatening, severe anaphylaxis and severe asthma. Less severe cases (allergic reactions) should be treated with epinephrine 1:1000 intramuscularly or with an inhaled β-agonist. In severe anaphylaxis or asthma (non-cardiac arrest), the initial dose should be 0.05–0.01 mg intravenously (5–10% of cardiac arrest dose). The dose may be repeated every 5 to 15 minutes as required. An epinephrine drip may be required in severe cases.

Severe anaphylaxis or severe asthma (children). Intravenous epinephrine should be used only for life threatening, severe anaphylaxis and severe asthma. Less severe cases should be treated with epinephrine 1:1000 intramuscularly or with an inhaled β-agonist. In severe anaphylaxis or asthma the initial dose should be 0.01 mg/kg intravenously. The dose may be repeated every 5–15 minutes as required. An epinephrine drip may be required in severe cases.

℞ Norepinephrine (Levophed)

Class Sympathetic agonist

Description

Norepinephrine is a naturally occurring catecholamine. It acts on both α- and β-adrenergic receptors. However, its action on α-receptors is more profound.

Mechanism of Action

Because of its action on α-receptors, norepinephrine is a potent peripheral vaso-constrictor. This vasoconstriction serves to increase blood pressure in cardiogenic shock and other hypotensive emergencies.

Pharmacokinetics

Onset: Immediate
Peak Effects: < 1 minute
Duration: 1–2 minutes
Half-Life: 3 minutes

Indications

Norepinephrine is used in hypotension (systolic blood pressure < 70 mmHg) not related to hypovolemia (e.g., septic shock). It is now considered a first-line agent.

Contraindications

Norepinephrine should not be given to patients who are hypotensive from hypovolemia.

Precautions

Because of the powerful effects of norepinephrine, it is essential to measure the blood pressure every 5–10 minutes to prevent dangerously high blood pressures. Fluid replacement should be initiated prior to administration of norepinephrine. Norepinephrine should be given through the largest vein readily available because it may cause local tissue necrosis if it extravasates. Phentolamine (Regitine) can be diluted in saline and infiltrated into the area of extravasation to help minimize necrosis and sloughing. Like the other sympathomimetics, norepinephrine can increase myocar-dial oxygen demand. It should be used with caution in persons with cardiac ischemia. Norepinephrine typically induces renal and mesenteric vasoconstriction. However, in septic patients, norepinephrine improves renal blood flow and urine output.

Side Effects

Norepinephrine can cause anxiety, tremulousness, headache, dizziness, nausea, and vomiting. It can also cause bradycardia as a reflex response to increased peripheral vasoconstriction. Because of its inotropic and chronotropic properties, norepineph-rine increases myocardial oxygen demand. Even in low doses it can cause myocar-dial ischemia. When administering norepinephrine in the emergency setting, these effects should be kept in mind.

Interactions/Incompatibilities

Norepinephrine can be deactivated by alkaline solutions such as sodium bicarbon-ate. Concomitant administration with β-blockers can result in markedly elevated blood pressure.

Dosage

The current dosage recommended by the American Heart Association for norepinephrine is 0.1–0.5 mcg/minute (maximum of 30 mcg/minute). Higher doses

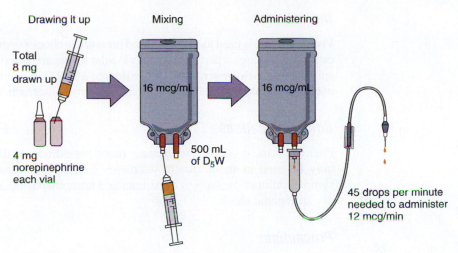

Drawing it up   Mixing   Administering

Total
8 mg
drawn up

4 mg
norepinephrine
each vial

16 mcg/mL

500 mL
of D₅W

16 mcg/mL

45 drops per minute
needed to administer
12 mcg/min

● **FIGURE 7–1**   Preparation of norepinephrine infusion.

may be required to maintain adequate blood pressure. An effective dilution can be obtained by placing 8 mg in 500 mL of D₅W. This will give a concentration of 16 mcg/mL. The same concentration can be attained by placing 4 mg in 250 mL of D₅W (see Figure 7–1).

Because of its potency, norepinephrine is given only in extremely diluted IV infusions. To control its administration, it should be piggybacked into an already established IV line and administered via a controlled pump.

℞ Phenylephrine (Neo-Synephrine)

Class Sympathetic agonist

Description

Phenylephrine is a synthetic catecholamine that acts primarily on α-adrenergic receptors.

Mechanism of Action

Phenylephrine is a potent, synthetic catecholamine that acts almost exclusively on α-receptors. Because it has no significant β-receptor-stimulating capabilities, its actions are primarily on the vascular smooth muscle heart and lungs thus increasing peripheral vascular resistance and blood pressure. When used topically on mucosal membranes, it reduces mucosal swelling and edema and makes it an excellent adjunct for nasal procedures such as nasotracheal intubation.

Pharmacokinetics

Onset: Immediate
Peak Effects: < 1 minute
Duration: 15–20 miutes
Half-Life: 2 minutes

Indications

Phenylephrine is used to support blood pressure in shock (systolic B P < 70 mmHg)—especially in cases where peripheral vascular resistance is reduced (e.g., septic shock, spinal shock). However, it is not considered a first-line agent. Phenylephrine is also useful in shrinking nasal mucosal tissues prior to nasotracheal intubation.

Contraindications

Phenylephrine is not used to increase blood pressure in cardiogenic shock. It should only be used in shock due to decreases in peripheral vascular resistance. Other sympathomimetics, such as dopamine and norepinephrine, should be used in cases of cardiogenic shock.

Precautions

It is important to be careful when administering phenylephrine. Extravasation can causes tissue sloughing at the injection site.

Side Effects

Phenylephrine can cause nervousness, headache, blurred vision, lacrimation, urinary retention, and rebound nasal congestion. It can also cause tremor, arrhythmias, hypertension, angina, nausea, and vomiting. Many of these side effects are dose related.

Interactions/Incompatibilities

Phenylephrine can be deactivated by alkaline solutions such as sodium bicarbonate. It should be used with caution in patients with digitalis toxicity because it may aggravate tachyarrhythmias.

Dosage

The usual dosage of phenylephrine is 100–180 mcg/min (approximately 0.5–2 mcg/kg/min). The maintenance dose is typically 46–60 mcg/min once blood pressure is stabilized. Because of its potency, phenylephrine should be given only by IV infusion. An established IV line, into which the phenylephrine is piggybacked, should be maintained.

℞ Isoproterenol (Isuprel)

Class Sympathetic agonist

Description

Isoproterenol is a synthetic catecholamine. It acts primarily on β-adrenergic receptors.

Mechanism of Action

Isoproterenol is a potent, synthetic catecholamine that acts almost exclusively on β-receptors. Because it has no significant α-receptor-stimulating capabilities, its actions are primarily on the heart and lungs. Isoproterenol is seldom used anymore.

Pharmacokinetics

Onset: Immediate
Peak Effects: < 1 minute
Duration: Varies
Half-Life: < 1.5 minutes

Indications

Isoproterenol is available for use in very selected patients such as denervated hearts (transplants) and beta-blocker overdoses. It is also useful in high-degree heart blocks (Mobitz II and third-degree blocks) when transcutaneous pacing is unavailable.

Contraindications

Isoproterenol is not used to increase blood pressure in cardiogenic shock. It should only be used in shock resulting from bradycardias. Other sympathomimetics, such as dopamine and norepinephrine, should be used in cases of cardiogenic shock.

Precautions

When administering isoproterenol, the patient must be monitored for signs of ventricular irritability. These signs may take the form of premature ventricular contractions, ventricular tachycardia, or even ventricular fibrillation. It is important to be careful when administering isoproterenol. Like epinephrine, it significantly increases myocardial oxygen demand. The increase in myocardial oxygen uptake may increase myocardial infarction size. In patients who have not suffered a myocardial infarction, isoproterenol may cause myocardial ischemia. External pacing, if available, should be used instead of isoproterenol.

Side Effects

Isoproterenol can cause nervousness, headache, tremor, arrhythmias, hypertension, angina, nausea, and vomiting. Many of these side effects are dose related.

Interactions/Incompatibilities

Isoproterenol can be deactivated by alkaline solutions such as sodium bicarbonate. It should be used with caution in patients with digitalis toxicity because it may aggravate tachyarrhythmias.

Dosage

The usual dosage of isoproterenol is 1 mg diluted in 500 mL of D_5W; this will give a concentration of 2 mcg/mL. It should be titrated until the desired heart rate is attained or until signs of ventricular irritability, such as premature ventricular contractions, occur. The usual infusion rate is 2–10 mcg/min. Isoproterenol should be given only by IV infusion. An established IV line, into which the isoproterenol is piggybacked, should be maintained. Isoproterenol is best administered via a controlled pump.

Class Sympathetic agonist

Description

Dopamine is a naturally occurring catecholamine. It is a chemical precursor of nor-epinephrine. It acts on α, β_1, and dopaminergic adrenergic receptors. Its effect on adrenergic receptors is dose dependent.

Mechanism of Action

Dopamine is used in the treatment of hypotension associated with cardiogenic shock. It is chemically related to both epinephrine and norepinephrine and increases blood pressure by acting on both α- and β_1-adrenergic receptors. Dopamine's effect on β_1-receptors causes a positive inotropic effect on the heart. It does not increase myocardial oxygen demand as much as isoproterenol and epinephrine do and does not have the same powerful chronotropic effects. Dopamine also acts on α-adrenergic receptors, causing peripheral vasoconstriction. Dopamine increases both the systolic blood pressure and the pulse pressure (the difference between the systolic and diastolic blood pressures), but, as a rule, there is usually less effect on the diastolic pressure.

Pharmacokinetics

Onset: < 5 minutes

Peak Effects: 5–8 minutes

Duration: < 10 minutes

Half-Life: 2 minutes

Indications

Dopamine is used in hemodynamically significant hypotension (systolic blood pressure of 70–100 mmHg) not resulting from hypovolemia, and in cardiogenic shock. It is also used in symptomatic bradycardia refractory to atropine.

Contraindications

Dopamine should not be used as the sole agent in the management of hypovolemic shock unless fluid resuscitation is well under way. Dopamine should be used in patients with known **pheochromocytoma** (a tumor of the adrenal gland).

Precautions

Dopamine increases the heart rate and can induce or worsen supraventricular and ventricular arrhythmias. Whenever the dosage of dopamine surpasses 20 mcg/kg/min, its α effects predominate and it functions very much like norepinephrine. Dopamine, like the other catecholamines, should not be administered in the presence of tachyarrhythmias or ventricular fibrillation.

Side Effects

Dopamine can cause nervousness, headache, arrhythmias, palpitations, chest pain, dyspnea, nausea, and vomiting. Many of these side effects are dose related.

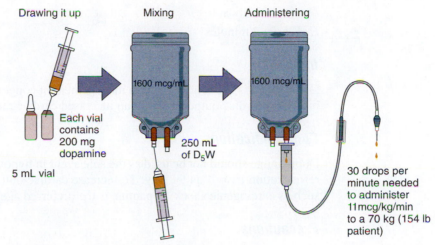

Drawing it up   Mixing   Administering

Each vial contains 200 mg dopamine

5 mL vial

1600 mcg/mL

250 mL of D_5W

1600 mcg/mL

30 drops per minute needed to administer 11mcg/kg/min to a 70 kg (154 lb patient)

● **FIGURE 7–2**   Preparation of dopamine infusion.

Interactions/Incompatibilities

Like all of the catecholamines, dopamine can be deactivated by alkaline solutions such as sodium bicarbonate. If the patient is taking MAOIs (a type of antidepressant), the dose should be reduced. Dopamine may cause hypotension when used concomitantly with phenytoin (Dilantin).

Dosage

The standard method of preparing a dopamine infusion is to place 800 mg in 500 mL of D_5W or by adding 400 mg to 250 mL of D_5W; this gives a concentration of 1600 mcg/mL. The effects of dopamine are dose dependent.

    The initial infusion is from 2 to 10 mcg/kg/min. This rate may be increased until the blood pressure improves (see Figure 7–2) or until a maximum of 20 mcg/kg/min. Dopamine is administered only by IV drip, which should be piggybacked into an already established IV infusion. Dopamine is best administered via a controlled pump.

℞ Dobutamine (Dobutrex)

Class Sympathetic agonist

Description

Dobutamine is a synthetic catecholamine. It acts primarily on β_1-receptors but is a less potent β-agonist than is isoproterenol.

Mechanism of Action

Dobutamine increases the force of the systolic contraction (positive inotropic effect) with little chronotropic activity. For these reasons, it is useful in the management of congestive heart failure when an increase in heart rate is not desired.

Pharmacokinetics

Onset: 2–10 minutes
Peak Effects: 10–20 minutes

Duration: Varies

Half-Life: 2 minutes

Indication

Dobutamine is used for short-term management of congestive heart failure when an increased cardiac output, without an increased cardiac rate, is desired.

Contraindications

Dobutamine should not be used as the sole agent in hypovolemic shock unless fluid resuscitation is well under way. To increase cardiac output in severe emergencies, such as cardiogenic shock, dopamine is the preferred agent.

Precautions

Tachycardia and an increase in the systolic blood pressure are common following the administration of dobutamine. Increases in heart rate of more than 10 percent may induce or exacerbate myocardial ischemia. Premature ventricular contractions (PVCs) can occur in conjunction with dobutamine administration. As with any sympathomimetic, blood pressure should be monitored.

Side Effects

Dobutamine can cause nervousness, headache, hypertension, arrhythmias, palpitations, chest pain, dyspnea, nausea, and vomiting. Many of these side effects are dose related.

Interactions/Incompatibilities

Dobutamine may be ineffective when administered to patients taking beta-blockers because these medications can block the beta-receptors on which dobutamine acts. Patients taking TCAs are at increased risk of hypertension with dobutamine administration.

Dosage

The desired dosage range for dobutamine is between 2 and 20 mcg/kg/min. Doses of 5–10 mcg/kg/min are common. Dobutamine should be administered according to the patient's response (see Figure 7–3).

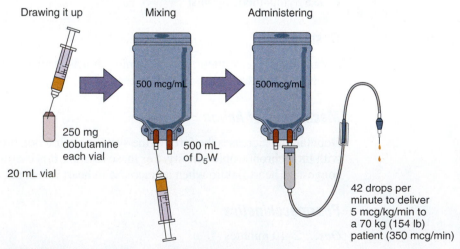

● **FIGURE 7–3**   Preparation of dobutamine infusion.

Dobutamine should be diluted in either 500 mL or 1 L of D_5W and administered via IV infusion. Dobutamine is best administered via a controlled pump.

℞ Inamrinone (Inocor)

Class Inotrope (phosphodiesterase inhibitor)

Description

Inamrinone is a rapidly acting inotropic agent. It is a *phosphodiesterase* inhibitor and does not act on adrenergic receptors.

Mechanism of Action

Inamrinone, like the other medications previously presented, increases cardiac output promptly following intravenous administration. It is a positive inotrope and has some vasodilatory properties. Unlike the other medications, however, it does not stimulate either α- or β-adrenergic receptors. The exact mechanism by which inamrinone increases blood pressure is not well understood. It does not increase cardiac output in the same manner as the digitalis preparations. Clinically, inamrinone resembles dobutamine in its effects. Because inamrinone does not stimulate β-adrenergic receptors, it may be effective in cases of congestive heart failure that do not respond to dobutamine or to one of the other inotropic agents.

Pharmacokinetics

Onset: 2–5 minutes
Peak Effects: 10 minutes
Duration: 0.5–2.0 hours
Half-Life: 4–6 hours

Indication

Inamrinone is used in short-term management of severe congestive heart failure refractory to diuretics, vasodilators, and conventional inotropic agents.

Contraindications

Inamrinone should not be administered to patients with a known hypersensitivity to the medication or to the bisulfite class of chemicals.

Precautions

Inamrinone should not be used in cases of congestive heart failure occurring immediately after myocardial infarction. Like dobutamine, inamrinone may increase myocardial ischemia. As with the other inotropic agents, the blood pressure, pulse, and electrocardiogram (ECG) should be constantly monitored. Inamrinone should not be diluted in solutions containing dextrose (e.g., D_5W). Inamrinone should be diluted with 0.9 percent sodium chloride (normal saline) or 0.45 percent sodium chloride (one-half normal saline).

Side Effects

Inamrinone can cause arrhythmias, hypotension, nausea, vomiting, abdominal pain, and decreased platelets (thrombocytopenia).

Interactions/Incompatibilities

Furosemide (Lasix) should not be administered into an intravenous line delivering inamrinone. A chemical reaction occurs between these two medications, resulting in the formation of a precipitate in the intravenous line. Inamrinone should not be diluted in solutions containing dextrose.

Dosage

For congestive heart failure (CHF) the dose should be 5–10 mcg/kg/min IV. Therapy should be initiated with an IV bolus of 0.75 mg/kg (one dose) given slowly during a 2- to 5-minute interval. This should be followed by a maintenance infusion of 5–15 mcg/kg/min. This infusion can be prepared by placing one ampule (100 mg) in 500 mL of normal saline solution. This will give a concentration of 0.2 mg/mL (200 mcg/mL).

An additional bolus of 0.75 mg/kg given slowly over 2 to 3 minutes can be given 30 minutes later if required.

The overall rate of inamrinone administration must be carefully adjusted and based on the patient's clinical response.

Inamrinone should be administered only by the IV route, either as a bolus or by infusion, as described earlier. Inamrinone is best administered via a controlled pump.

℞ Milrinone (Primacor)

Class Inotrope (phosphodiesterase inhibitor)

Description

Milrinone is a rapidly acting inotropic agent. It is a phosphodiesterase inhibitor and does not act on adrenergic receptors.

Mechanism of Action

Milrinone, like the other medications previously presented, increases cardiac output promptly following intravenous administration. It is a positive inotrope and has some vasodilatory properties. Unlike the other medications, however, it does not stimulate either α- or β-adrenergic receptors. The postulated mechanism is via increased cardiac output due to positive inotropy as a result of inhibition of cyclie guanosine monophosphate (cGMP)-dependent phosphodiasterase. It does not increase cardiac output in the same manner as the digitalis preparations. Clinically, milrinone resembles dobutamine in its effects but has less tachycardia. Because milrinone does not stimulate β-adrenergic receptors, it may be effective in cases of congestive heart failure that do not respond to dobutamine or to one of the other inotropic agents.

Pharmacokinetics

Onset: 5–15 minutes
Peak Effects: Not specified

Duration: 3–6 hours
Half-Life: 2-3 hours

Indication

Milrinone is used in short-term management of severe congestive heart failure refractory to diuretics, vasodilators, and conventional inotropic agents.

Contraindications

Milrinone should not be administered to patients with a known hypersensitivity to the medication or to the bisulfite class of chemicals.

Precautions

Milrinone should not be used in cases of congestive heart failure occurring immediately after myocardial infarction. Like dobutamine, milrinone may increase myocardial ischemia. As with the other inotropic agents, the blood pressure, pulse, and electrocardiogram (ECG) should be constantly monitored. Milrinone should be diluted with 0.9 percent sodium chloride (normal saline) or 5 percent dextrose in water (D_5W).

Side Effects

Milrinone can cause arrhythmias, hypotension, nausea, vomiting, abdominal pain, and decreased platelets (thrombocytopenia).

Interactions/Incompatibilities

Furosemide (Lasix) should not be administered into an intravenous line delivering milrinone. A chemical reaction occurs between these two medications, resulting in the formation of a precipitate in the intravenous line.

Dosage

For congestive heart failure (CHF) the dose should be 50 mcg/kg IV/IO given slowly over a 10-minute interval. This should be followed by a maintenance infusion of 0.375 mcg/kg/min.

The overall rate of milrinone administration must be carefully adjusted and based on the patient's clinical response.

Milrinone should only be administered by the IV/IO route, either as a bolus or by infusion, as described earlier. Milrinone is best administered via a controlled pump.

℞ Vasopressin (Pitressin)

Class Hormone; vasopressor

Description

Vasopressin is a polypeptide hormone extracted from the posterior pituitaries of animals. It possesses pressor and antidiuretic hormone (ADH) properties. Conclusive evidence supporting the use of vasopressin in cardiac arrest is lacking.

Mechanism of Action

Vasopressin, in higher doses, acts as a non-alpha-adrenergic vasoconstrictor through direct stimulation of smooth muscle receptors. It can be used as an alternative to epinephrine during CPR.

Pharmacokinetics

Onset: Variable
Peak Effects: Variable
Duration: 30–60 minutes
Half-Life: 10–20 minutes

Indications

Vasopressin is used to increase peripheral vascular resistance during CPR (as an alternative to epinephrine or after epinephrine has been used). Because the effects of vasopressin have not been shown to differ from those of epinephrine in cardiac arrest, 1 dose of vasopressin 40 units IV/IO may replace either the first or second dose of epinephrine in the treatment of cardiac arrest.

Contraindications

Vasopressin is contraindicated in patients with a chronic nephritis, ischemic heart disease, PVCs, or advanced arteriosclerosis. When used in CPR, these contraindications may not apply.

Precautions

Vasopressin should be used with caution in patients with epilepsy, migraine, asthma, heart failure, and angina.

Side Effects

Side effects include blanching of the skin, abdominal cramps, nausea, hypertension, bradycardia, and minor arrhythmias.

Interactions/Incompatibilities

None in advanced cardiac life support (ACLS) setting.

Dosage

Adult dose. 40 units IV/IO (single dose only). Can replace first or second dose of epinephrine in cardiac arrest.
Pediatric dose. Usage in cardiac arrest not detailed.

ADRENERGIC ANTAGONISTS

Adrenergic antagonists are a unique class of medications that antagonize adrenergic receptor sites. Certain medications block only α-receptors, whereas others block only β-receptors. Some of the β-blockers are so selective that they block only β_1- or β_2-receptors. The medications that block the β-receptors are receiving the most use.

They are useful in the treatment of hypertension, cardiac arrhythmias, and angina pectoris. The prototypical sympathetic blocker is propranolol (Inderal), a nonselective beta-blocker that is both a β_1- and β_2-antagonist. Although used selectively in emergency medicine, beta-blockers do play a role in the treatment of certain cardiac arrhythmias and hypertension.

It is thought that some ventricular arrhythmias, such as ventricular tachycardia and recurrent ventricular fibrillation, can be caused by excessive β-receptor stimulation. Administration of beta-blockers may inhibit these arrhythmias. Propranolol should not be used in combination with verapamil. The **concomitant** blocking of slow calcium channels by verapamil, and the β-receptor antagonism caused by propranolol, may result in asystole.

℞ Propranolol (Inderal)

Class Nonselective beta-blocker (Class II antiarrhythmic)

Description

Propranolol is a nonselective β-antagonist. It inhibits the effects of circulating catecholamines.

Mechanism of Action

Propranolol nonselectively blocks both β_1- and β_2-adrenergic receptors. It causes a reduction in heart rate (negative chronotropic effect), cardiac contractile force (negative inotropic effect), blood pressure, and myocardial oxygen demand. It is useful in treating recurrent ventricular tachycardia and recurrent ventricular fibrillation that does not respond to other antiarrhythmics. It may also be of value in the treatment of tachyarrhythmias resulting from digitalis toxicity and selected supraventricular tachycardias.

Pharmacokinetics

Onset: < 2 minutes (IV)
Peak Effects: 5 minutes (IV)
Duration: 1–2 hours (IV)
Half-Life: 2–3 hours (IV)

Indications

Propranolol can be considered in:

- Stable, narrow-complex tachycardias if rhythm remains uncontrolled or unconverted by adenosine or vagal maneuvers or if SVT is recurrent
- Control ventricular rate in patients with atrial fibrillation or atrial flutter
- Certain forms of polymorphic VT (associated with acute ischemia, familial Long QT Syndrome, catecholaminergic)

Contraindications

Propranolol is contraindicated in patients with bradycardia, a history of asthma, COPD, and congestive heart failure.

Precautions

Because propranolol may decrease heart rate, atropine should be readily available. In bradycardia refractory to atropine, transcutaneous pacing should be utilized. Propranolol should be used with caution in diabetics because it may mask the signs and symptoms of hypoglycemia. Glucagon can be used in the management of severe beta-blocker overdose. It helps to maintain the heart rate and blood pressure.

Side Effects

Propranolol may cause bradycardia, hypotension, lethargy, congestive heart failure, dyspnea, wheezing, and weakness.

Interactions/Incompatibilities

Propranolol should be used with caution in patients who have received intravenous calcium channel blockers. It should be used with caution in patients taking antihypertensive agents.

Dosage

Propranolol may produce significant, even life-threatening, side effects. When administered intravenously, care must be taken to dilute 1 mg in 10 mL of D_5W or saline. The standard dosage is 0.5–1.0 mg administered *slowly* (over 1 minute). Propranolol should not be administered faster than 1 mg/min. This can be repeated, if needed, up to a total dose of 0.1 mg/kg. Throughout administration, careful blood pressure monitoring is required. Like all medications acting on the heart, it should be administered only to patients who are on cardiac monitors. Propranolol should be administered intravenously in the treatment of life-threatening tachyarrhythmias.

Sotalol (Sotacor, Betapace)

Class Beta-blocker (Class II and Class III antiarrhythmic properties)

Description

Sotalol is a nonselective beta-adrenergic blocking agent.

Mechanism of Action

Sotalol blocks stimulation of β_1- (myocardial) and β_2- (pulmonary, vascular, and uterine) adrenergic receptor sites.

Pharmacokinetics

Onset: Variable
Peak Effects: 2–3 hours
Duration: 24 hours
Half-Life: 7–18 hours

Indications

Sotalol is indicated for the treatment of hemodynamically stable monomorphic ventricular tachycardia.

Contraindications

Sotalol is contraindicated in patients with bronchial asthma, allergic rhinitis, severe sinus node dysfunction, sinus bradycardia and second- and third-degree atrioventricular (AV) block (unless a functioning pacemaker is present), cardiogenic shock, severe or uncontrolled heart failure, and known hypersensitivity. It should be avoided in patients with a prolonged QT interval.

Precautions

Sotalol may cause new or worsen existing arrhythmias. Such proarrhythmic effects range from an increase in frequency of PVCs to the development of more severe ventricular tachycardia, ventricular fibrillation, and **torsade de pointes**.

Side Effects

Central nervous system effects include fatigue, weakness, anxiety, dizziness, drowsiness, insomnia, memory loss, mental status changes, nervousness, and nightmares. Respiratory effects include bronchospasm and wheezing. Cardiovascular effects include arrhythmias, bradycardia, congestive heart failure, pulmonary edema, orthostatic hypotension, and peripheral vasoconstriction.

Interactions/Incompatibilities

General anesthesia, IV phenytoin, and verapamil may cause additive myocardial depression. Additive bradycardia may occur with digitalis glycosides. Additive hypotension may occur with other antihypertensives, acute ingestion of alcohol, or nitrates. Sotalol should be used cautiously within 14 days of MAOI therapy (may result in hypotension). Sotalol may interact with class IA antiarrhythmic medications such as disopyramide, quinidine, and procainamide and class III medications such as amiodarone.

Dosage

In clinical studies 1.5 mg/kg was infused over 5 minutes; however, current U.S. package labeling recommends any dose of the drug should be infused slowly over a period of 5 hours.

℞ Metoprolol (Lopressor)

Class Selective beta-blocker (Class II antiarrhythmic)

Description

Metoprolol is a β-antagonist that blocks both β_1- and β_2-adrenergic receptors. Unlike propranolol, however, metoprolol is selective for β_1-adrenergic receptors. It has minimal, if any, effect on β_2-adrenergic receptors at doses less than 100 mg.

Mechanism of Action

Metoprolol causes a reduction in heart rate, systolic blood pressure, and cardiac output following administration because of its selective effects on β_1-adrenergic receptors. In addition, metoprolol appears to inhibit tachycardia, especially in the period following an acute myocardial infarction. Because of these effects, metoprolol is thought to be protective of the heart and is used to reduce potential complications in selected patients who have suffered an acute myocardial infarction. Metoprolol has proved effective in reducing the incidence of ventricular fibrillation and chest pain in these patients, thus reducing overall patient mortality in the post–myocardial infarction period.

Pharmacokinetics

Onset: Immediate (IV)
Peak Effects: 20 minutes (IV)
Duration: 5–8 hours
Half-Life: 3–4 hours

Indication

Metoprolol is used in patients with suspected or definite acute myocardial infarction who are hypertensive and do not have any contraindications. It can also be considered in the following conditions:

- Stable, narrow-complex tachycardias if rhythm remains uncontrolled or unconverted by adenosine or vagal maneuvers or if SVT is recurrent
- Control ventricular rate in patients with atrial fibrillation or atrial flutter
- Certain forms of polymorphic VT (associated with acute ischemia, familial Long QT Syndrome, catecholaminergic)

Contraindications

Metoprolol is contraindicated in any patient with a heart rate of less than 45 beats per minute, a systolic blood pressure less than 100 mmHg, or congestive heart failure. In addition, metoprolol is contraindicated in patients with first-degree heart block with a PR interval greater than 0.24 second (only in ACS patients), second-degree heart block (either Mobitz I or Mobitz II), or third-degree block. It is also contraindicated in any patient showing either early or late signs of shock. Metoprolol should not be administered to any patient with a history of asthma or bronchospastic disease in the prehospital setting.

Precautions

The blood pressure, pulse rate, ECG, and respiratory status should be continuously monitored during metoprolol therapy. Prehospital personnel should be alert for signs and symptoms of congestive heart failure, bradycardia, shock, heart block, or bronchospasm when administering metoprolol. The presence of any of these signs or symptoms is an indication for discontinuing the medication.

Side Effects

Metoprolol may cause bradycardia, hypotension, lethargy, congestive heart failure, dyspnea, wheezing, and weakness.

Interactions/Incompatibilities

Metoprolol should not be administered to patients who have received intravenous calcium channel blockers. It should be administered with caution to patients taking antihypertensive agents.

Dosage

An initial bolus of 5 mg metoprolol should be given by slow IV injection. If the vital signs remain stable, a second 5 mg bolus should be given 2 minutes after the first. Finally, if the first two boluses are well tolerated, a third 5 mg bolus should be administered 2 minutes after the second bolus. The total dose should not exceed 15 mg. As mentioned previously, the vital signs and ECG should be constantly monitored.

Metoprolol should be administered only by slow IV injection in the manner described earlier.

℞ Labetalol (Trandate, Normodyne)

Class Nonselective beta-blocker (Class II antiarrhythmic)

Description

Labetalol is a nonselective β-blocker and a selective α_1-blocker.

Mechanism of Action

Labetalol differs considerably in its action from the β-blockers previously presented. Like propranolol, labetalol is a nonselective β-adrenergic antagonist showing no preference for either β_1- or β_2-receptors. However, unlike the other β-blockers, labetalol also blocks α_1-adrenergic receptors. Blockage of α_1-receptors inhibits peripheral vasoconstriction, thus causing peripheral vasodilation. Because of these properties, labetalol is a potent agent for lowering blood pressure in cases of hypertensive crisis. It lowers blood pressure by decreasing cardiac output through its β_1-blocking properties (to a limited degree) and by causing peripheral vasodilation through its α_1-blocking properties.

Pharmacokinetics

Onset: 2–5 minutes (IV)

Peak Effects: 5–15 minutes (IV)

Duration: 2–4 hours (IV)

Half-Life: 3–8 hours

Indications

Labetalol is indicated for the acute management of hypertensive emergency. A hypertensive emergency is a markedly elevated blood pressure causing end-organ changes (e.g., altered mental status, chest pain, renal failure). Headache and anxiety associated with an elevated blood pressure are not indications for parenteral antihypertensive therapy.

Contraindications

Labetalol is contraindicated in patients with bronchial asthma, congestive heart failure, heart block, bradycardia, or cardiogenic shock.

Precautions

As with all β-blockers the blood pressure, pulse rate, ECG, and respiratory status should be continuously monitored. Prehospital personnel should be alert for signs and symptoms of decongestive heart failure, bradycardia, shock, heart block, or bronchospasm when administering labetalol. The appearance of any of these signs or symptoms is an indication for discontinuing the medication. Because of the effects of labetalol on β_1-receptors, postural hypotension might occur and should be anticipated. The patient should be supine at all times during medication administration.

Side Effects

Labetalol may cause bradycardia, hypotension, lethargy, congestive heart failure, dyspnea, wheezing, and weakness.

Interactions/Incompatibilities

Labetalol should not be administered to patients who have received intravenous calcium channel blockers. It should be administered with caution to patients taking antihypertensive agents.

Dosage

The following are two accepted methods of administering labetalol in the treatment of hypertensive crisis:

1. Twenty milligrams of labetalol can be administered by slow IV injection over 2 minutes. Immediately before the injection and at 5 and 10 minutes after the injection, the supine blood pressure should be recorded. Additional injections of 40 mg can be given every 10 minutes until a desired supine blood pressure is achieved or 300 mg of the medication has been given.
2. 500 mg of labetalol can be added to 250 mL of D_5W. This gives a concentration of 1.0 mg/mL. This solution should be administered at a rate of 2 mg/min to a maximum dose of 300 mg. The blood pressure should be continuously monitored.

Labetalol should be administered by slow IV/IO injection or infusion as described earlier.

℞ Atenolol (Tenormin)

Class Selective beta-blocker (Class II antiarrhythmic)

Description

Atenolol is a selective β-antagonist with a propensity for β_1-adrenergic receptors. It inhibits the effects of circulating catecholamines.

Mechanism of Action

Atenolol selectively blocks both β_1-adrenergic receptors. It causes a reduction in heart rate (negative chronotropic effect), cardiac contractile force (negative inotropic effect), blood pressure, and myocardial oxygen demand. It is useful in treating recurrent tachyarrhythmias.

Pharmacokinetics

Onset: < 2 minutes

Peak Effects: 5 minutes

Duration: 24 hours

Half-Life: 6–7 hours

Indications

Atenolol can be considered in:

- Stable, narrow-complex tachycardias if rhythm remains uncontrolled or unconverted by adenosine or vagal maneuvers or if SVT is recurrent.
- Control ventricular rate in patients with atrial fibrillation or atrial flutter.
- Certain forms of polymorphic VT (associated with acute ischemia, familial Long QT Syndrome, catecholaminergic).

Contraindications

Atenolol is contraindicated in patients with bradycardia, a history of asthma, COPD, and decompensated congestive heart failure.

Precautions

Because atenolol may decrease heart rate, atropine should be readily available. In bradycardia refractory to atropine, transcutaneous pacing should be utilized. It can precipitate congestive heart failure in patients who are predisposed to this condition and should thus be used with caution in these patients.

Side Effects

Atenolol may cause bradycardia, hypotension, lethargy, congestive heart failure, dyspnea, wheezing, and weakness.

Interactions/Incompatibilities

Atenolol should not be administered to patients who have received intravenous calcium channel blockers. It should be used with caution in patients taking antihypertensive agents.

Dosage

Atenolol should be administered at a dose of 5 mg IV/IO over 5 minutes. It can be repeated at 5 mg in 10 minutes if the arrhythmia persists or recurs.

Esmolol (Brevibloc)

Class Selective beta-blocker (Class II antiarrhythmic)

Description

Esmolol is a β_1 selective (cardioselective) β-blocker with a very short half-life.

Mechanism of Action

Esmolol is a selective β_1-blocker. It has a very rapid onset and a short duration of action (9 minutes). Esmolol is used to slow rapid heart rates in patients with supraventricular tachycardia including atrial flutter and atrial fibrillation. Patients with extremely rapid heart rates can develop congestive heart failure or angina because the rapid heart rate may prevent adequate filling of the ventricles. The duration of action of esmolol is so brief that it should be administered by intravenous infusion.

Pharmacokinetics

Onset: < 5 minutes

Peak Effects: 10–20 minutes

Duration: 10–30 minutes

Half-Life: 2–9 minutes

Indication

Esmolol may be considered for the following conditions:

- Stable, narrow-complex tachycardias if rhythm remains uncontrolled or unconverted by adenosine or vagal maneuvers or if SVT is recurrent.
- Control ventricular rate in patients with atrial fibrillation or atrial flutter.
- Certain forms of polymorphic VT (associated with acute ischemia, familial Long QT Syndrome, catecholaminergic).

Contraindications

Esmolol should not be used in patients with sinus bradycardia, heart block greater than first degree, cardiogenic shock, or overt congestive heart failure.

Precautions

A significant number of patients receiving esmolol may experience hypotension (systolic less than 90 mmHg). Hypotension can occur at any dose but primarily is dose related. If hypotension develops, the dosage should be reduced. Patients with congestive heart failure may have worsening of their symptoms with esmolol. Because esmolol may depress cardiac contractility, it should be used with extreme caution in patients prone to congestive heart failure. Patients with bronchospastic disease (e.g., asthma and COPD) should not receive β-blockers, including esmolol, unless the medical control physician deems that the benefits outweigh the risks.

Side Effects

Esmolol may cause bradycardia, dizziness, hypotension, lethargy, congestive heart failure, dyspnea, wheezing, and weakness.

Interactions/Incompatibilities

Esmolol should not be administered to patients who have received intravenous calcium channel blockers. It should be administered with caution to patients taking antihypertensive agents. Morphine can increase the blood levels of esmolol, requiring a reduction in dosage. Esmolol should not be used in cases of supraventricular tachycardia caused by epinephrine, dopamine, and norepinephrine.

Dosage

Esmolol therapy is started by administering a loading dose of 500 mcg/kg over 1 minute. After 1 minute the dose should be followed by a maintenance dose of 50 mcg/kg/min for 4 minutes. If an adequate therapeutic effect is not seen, the loading dose should be repeated for 1 minute and then the maintenance dose is increased to 100 mcg/kg/min. The dose can be titrated at 4-minute intervals by repeating the loading dose for 1 minute and increasing the maintenance dose by 50 mcg/kg/min at 4-minute intervals until the desired effect is obtained. The maintenance dose should not exceed 300 mcg/kg/min. In the event of an adverse reaction, the dose of esmolol can be reduced or discontinued immediately. Esmolol is supplied in a premixed solution containing 2500 mg in 250 mL and vials containing 10 mg/mL. Esmolol should be administered intravenously.

ANTIARRHYTHMICS

Many different medications are useful in the treatment and prevention of cardiac arrhythmias. Some medications are useful in the treatment of atrial arrhythmias, whereas others are useful in the treatment of ventricular arrhythmias. As a result, it is essential to distinguish between these two types of arrhythmias. The common antiarrhythmic medications are often classified in the Vaughan-Williams classification system based on their action (see Table 7–5 and Figure 7–4).

The most common antiarrhythmic medications used in emergency medicine include the following:

Lidocaine (Xylocaine). Lidocaine was once the most common medication used in the treatment of arrhythmias. It has largely been replaced by amiodarone.

Procainamide (Pronestyl). Procainamide is useful in the suppression of ventricular arrhythmias and treatment of atrial fibrillation. It is generally not a first-line medication.

TABLE 7–5

Antiarrhythmic Classifications and Examples

General Action	Class	Prototype	ECG Effects
Sodium channel blockers	IA	Quinidine, procainamide*, disopyramide	Widened QRS, prolonged QT
	IB	Lidocaine*, phenytoin, mexiletine	Widened QRS, prolonged QT
	IC	Flecainide*, propafenone Moricizine*	Prolonged PR, widened QRS
Beta-blockers	II	Propranolol*, acebutolol, esmolol, metoprolol	Prolonged PR, bradycardias
Potassium channel blockers	III	Bretylium*, amiodarone	Prolonged QT
Calcium channel blockers	IV	Verapamil*, diltiazem	Prolonged PR, bradycardias
Miscellaneous	V	Adenosine, digoxin	Prolonged PR, bradycardias

*Prototype.

Class I effect
Sodium channel blockade

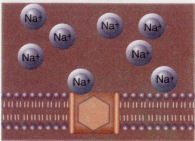

Class II effect
Noncompetitive alpha- and beta-blockade

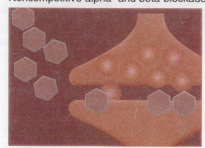

Class III effect
Potassium channel blockade

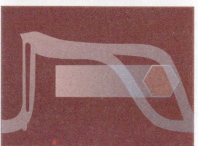

Class IV effect
Calcium channel blockade

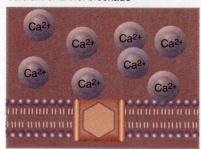

● **FIGURE 7–4**   Vaughan Williams classification of antiarrhythmic medications.

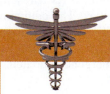

CASE PRESENTATION

EMS is dispatched to a residence to aid a man with chest pain. The patient is conscious and breathing and has a history of "heart attacks." On arrival paramedics are directed to a 63-year-old male (weight 80 kg) sitting on the couch in the living room. The patient is pale, cool, and diaphoretic.

Physical Examination

CNS: The patient is conscious, alert, and oriented × 4

Resp: Respirations are 24 and of normal depth; lung sounds clear bilaterally; trachea is midline; no signs of trauma

CVS: Carotid and radial pulses are strong and irregular; skin is pale, cool, and diaphoretic

ABD: Soft and nontender

Muscl/Skel: Patient able to move extremities on command; no weaknesses to hand grip

Vital Signs

Pulse: 72/min, irregular, strong

Resp: 24/min, shallow

BP: 122/72 mmHg

SpO₂: 95 percent

ECG:	Regular sinus rhythm with multifocal PVCs at 10/min
Hx:	**P** No provoking factors
	Q Crushing pain
	R Radiating to neck
	S 10/10, worst pain ever
	T Started suddenly 1/2 hour ago
Past Hx:	The patient's wife states that her husband has had several episodes of chest pain brought on by exertion over the past few weeks. He was diagnosed with angina 6 years ago and had a "heart attack" last year. He has nitroglycerin spray, which he has used twice, prior to arrival of the ambulance. The patient takes nitroglycerin spray and ASA.

Treatment

Oxygen was administered by a nasal cannula at 2 lpm. An IV was started with an 18-gauge catheter in the left arm and run TKO. The paramedics noticed a change on the ECG monitor to ventricular bigeminy. The patient was given nitroglycerin spray 0.4 mg with no relief; 2.5 mg of morphine was administered and provided slight relief of pain. ASA was not given because the patient already takes ASA daily. Transport to the hospital was initiated. The pain was rated at 8/10, and another nitroglycerin spray and 2.5 mg of morphine were given. A 12-lead ECG confirmed ST elevation in both the inferior and lateral leads. The destination hospital was informed of a potential candidate for fibrinolytic therapy and a second 18-gauge IV was initiated and run TKO. On arrival at the hospital the patient was treated with a fibrinolytic medication and then admitted to the CCU to recover.

Adenosine (Adenocard). Adenosine is a naturally occurring nucleoside useful in the treatment of supraventricular tachycardias and is considered a first-line medication in emergency care of tachyarrhythmias (narrow- and wide-complex).

Verapamil (Isoptin, Calan). Verapamil is a slow calcium channel blocker. It is occasionally used in the treatment of selective arrhythmias.

Diltiazem (Cardizem). Diltiazem is a calcium channel blocker and is used to slow the rapid ventricular rate that often accompanies atrial flutter and atrial fibrillation.

Amiodarone HCl (Cordarone). Amiodarone is a class III antiarrhythmic agent that decreases sinus automaticity, reduces the speed of conduction, and increases the refractory period of the AV node.

Phenytoin (Dilantin). Phenytoin is infrequently used in the emergency setting as an antiarrhythmic agent. It has proven effectiveness, however, in the management of life-threatening arrhythmias resulting from digitalis toxicity.

Edrophonium chloride (Tensilon). Edrophonium chloride is an anticholinesterase agent that has proven effectiveness in terminating paroxysmal supraventricular tachycardias that do not respond to vagal maneuvers. Its usage is rapidly declining, with verapamil and adenosine being preferred.

Magnesium sulfate. Magnesium is a cofactor in many of the chemical and enzyme reactions that occur in the body. Magnesium deficiency is associated with a high frequency of cardiac arrhythmias and sudden death. Pharmacologically, it functions like a physiological calcium channel blocker.

Propranolol (Inderal). Propranolol, discussed in the previous section, plays a role in the treatment of supraventricular arrhythmias. Students are encouraged to review the section on propranolol and integrate the information with that on the medications mentioned here.

Class Antiarrhythmic

Description

Lidocaine is an amide-type local anesthetic. It is used to treat life-threatening ventricular arrhythmias.

Mechanism of Action

Lidocaine was once the most frequently used antiarrhythmic agent in prehospital care. However, after several decades of scrutiny, lidocaine has now become secondary therapy to newer antiarrhythmic agents such as amiodarone. Lidocaine depresses depolarization and automaticity in the ventricles. It has very little effect on atrial tissues. In therapeutic doses it does not slow AV conduction and does not depress myocardial contractility. However, while prophylaxis with lidocaine reduces the incidence of ventricular fibrillation, recent research suggests that lidocaine actually increased all-cause mortality rates. Thus, the practice of prophylactic administration of lidocaine is not recommended.

Lidocaine is most apt to suppress ventricular arrhythmias when the level of the medication in the blood is between 1.5 and 6.0 mcg/mL of blood. A 75–100 mg bolus of lidocaine will maintain adequate blood levels for only 20 minutes (see Figure 7–5). Therefore, once an arrhythmia is suppressed, the lidocaine bolus should be followed by a 2 to 4 mg/min infusion to ensure therapeutic blood levels.

Pharmacokinetics

Onset: < 3 minutes

Peak Effects: 5–7 minutes

Duration: 10–20 minutes

Half-Life: 1.5–2.0 hours

Indications

Lidocaine is used in ventricular tachycardia and ventricular fibrillation refractory to amiodarone.

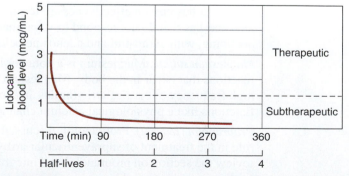

● **FIGURE 7–5** Blood levels of lidocaine following bolus without drip.

Contraindications

Lidocaine is usually contraindicated in second-degree Mobitz II and third-degree blocks. Lidocaine slows conduction of the electrical impulse from the atria to the ventricles. Decreased ventricular rates may accompany high-grade heart block, resulting in escape beats that are premature ventricular contractions. Whenever PVCs occur in conjunction with bradycardia (heart rate less than 60 beats per minute), the bradycardia should be treated first. The medication of choice is atropine sulfate, followed by transcutaneous pacing if atropine is not effective.

Precautions

Central nervous system depression may occur when the dosage exceeds 300 mg/hr. Symptoms of central nervous system depression include a decreased level of consciousness, irritability, confusion, muscle twitching, and eventually seizures. Exceedingly high doses can result in coma and death. Routine prophylactic lidocaine therapy in patients with acute myocardial infarction is no longer recommended.

Side Effects

Lidocaine may cause drowsiness, slurred speech, seizures, confusion, hypotension, bradycardia, heart blocks, nausea, vomiting, and respiratory and cardiac arrest.

Interactions/Incompatibilities

Lidocaine should be used with caution when administered concomitantly with procainamide, amiodarone, phenytoin, quinidine, and β-blockers because medication toxicity may result.

Dosage

Hemodyamically stable monomorphic ventricular tachycardia. The initial dose of lidocaine should be 1.0–1.5 mg/kg. Boluses of 0.5–0.75 mg/kg can be repeated every 5–10 minutes as required to a maximum dose of 3.0 mg/kg. Once the arrhythmia has been suppressed, a lidocaine drip should be initiated at 2–4 mg/min.

The dosage of lidocaine should be reduced 50 percent in patients over 70 years of age and in patients with liver disease, heart failure, bradycardias, or conduction disturbances. Lidocaine is generally given in an IV bolus followed by an infusion (see Figure 7–6). It can also be given endotracheally, however, when an IV/IO line

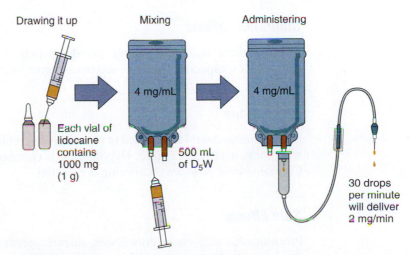

● **FIGURE 7–6** Preparation of lidocaine infusion.

cannot be established. The dose should be increased to 2–2.5 times the intravenous dose when administering it endotracheally.

Procainamide (Pronestyl)

Class Antiarrhythmic

Description

Procainamide is an ester-type local anesthetic. It is used to treat life-threatening ventricular arrhythmias refractory to other antiarrhythmics.

Mechanism of Action

Procainamide is effective in suppressing ventricular ectopy. It may be effective in cases in which lidocaine has not suppressed life-threatening ventricular arrhythmias. Procainamide reduces the automaticity of the various pacemaker sites in the heart. Procainamide slows intraventricular conduction to a much greater degree than does lidocaine.

Pharmacokinetics

Onset: 10–30 minutes
Peak Effects: 15–20 minutes
Duration: 3–6 hours
Half-Life: 3 hours

Indications

Procainamide can be used to treat ventricular tachycardia with a pulse. It can also be used in the treatment of pre-excited atrial fibrillation.

Contraindications

Procainamide should not be administered to patients with severe conduction system disturbances, especially second- and third-degree heart blocks.

Precautions

Procainamide should be avoided in patients with prolonged QT syndrome and those with congestive heart failure. Hypotension is common with intravenous infusion. Constant blood pressure monitoring is essential.

Side Effects

Procainamide may cause drowsiness, seizures, confusion, hypotension, bradycardia, heart blocks, nausea, vomiting, and respiratory and cardiac arrest.

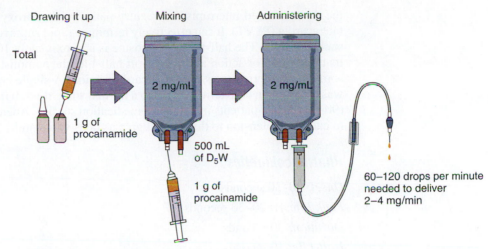

Drawing it up   Mixing   Administering

Total

1 g of procainamide

2 mg/mL   500 mL of D$_5$W

1 g of procainamide

2 mg/mL

60–120 drops per minute needed to deliver 2–4 mg/min

● **FIGURE 7–7**   Preparation of procainamide infusion.

Interactions/Incompatibilities

The hypotensive effects of procainamide may be increased if administered with antihypertensive medications. The chance of neurological toxicity by both lidocaine and procainamide increases when the medications are administered together.

Dosage

In treating ventricular tachycardia or atrial fibrillation, procainamide should be administered at 20–50 mg/min until the arrhythmia is suppressed. This should be discontinued if any of the following occur:

1. Arrhythmia is suppressed.
2. Hypotension ensues.
3. QRS complex is widened by 50 percent of its original width.
4. A total of 17 mg/kg of the medication has been administered.

The maintenance infusion of procainamide is 1–4 mg/min. The duration of procainamide's effect is shorter than that of lidocaine, requiring a more rigorous approach. Procainamide should be administered by slow IV/IO bolus (20 mg/min) followed by a maintenance infusion. Generally, 1 g of procainamide is placed in 500 mL of D$_5$W or NS. This gives a final concentration of 2 mg/mL (see Figure 7–7).

℞ Adenosine (Adenocard)

Class Antiarrhythmic (Class V antiarrhythmic)

Description

Adenosine is a naturally occurring nucleoside that slows AV conduction through the AV node. It has an exceptionally short half-life and a relatively good safety profile.

Mechanism of Action

Adenosine is a naturally occurring substance (purine nucleoside) that is present in all body cells. Adenosine decreases conduction of the electrical impulse through the AV node and interrupts AV reentry pathways in paroxysmal supraventricular tachycardia (PSVT). It can effectively terminate rapid supraventricular arrhythmias such as PSVT. The half-life of adenosine is approximately 10 seconds. Because of its rapid onset of action and very short half-life, the administration of adenosine is sometimes referred to as chemical cardioversion. A single bolus of the medication was effective in converting PSVT to a normal sinus rhythm in a significant number (90 percent) of patients in the initial medication studies. Adenosine does not appear to cause hypotension to the same degree as does verapamil.

Pharmacokinetics

Onset: 20–30 seconds
Peak Effects: 20–30 seconds
Duration: 30 seconds
Half-Life: 10 seconds

CASE PRESENTATION

At 1900 hours paramedics are dispatched to a residence to aid a 42-year-old female complaining of shortness of breath and chest pain. The patient is conscious and breathing. On arrival the paramedics are met by the patient's son, who directs the ambulance crew to the kitchen. They find the patient seated in a chair. The patient looks anxious, scared, and pale.

Physical Examination

CNS:	The patient is conscious, alert, and oriented × 4; appears anxious
Resp:	Respirations are 24 and shallow, with difficult, labored breathing; lung sounds clear bilaterally; trachea is midline; no signs of trauma
CVS:	Carotid and radial pulses are present and rapid, pulse weaker radially; skin is pale and cool
ABD:	Soft and nontender
Muscl/Skel:	Patient able to move extremities on command; no weaknesses to hand grip

Vital Signs

Pulse:	220/min, regular, weak	
Resp:	24/min, shallow, with difficulty breathing normally	
BP:	110/60 mmHg	
SpO$_2$:	97 percent	
ECG:	Supraventricular tachycardia	
Hx:	**P**	Was cooking at onset of symptoms
	Q	Palpitations, squeezing discomfort with a feeling of SOB
	R	Nonradiating
	S	3/10
	T	Started suddenly about 30 minutes ago

Past Hx: The patient states that this has never happened before. She was cooking dinner when it suddenly "hit" her. She thought it would go away if she sat down, but it seemed to just get worse. She states that her heart feels like it is going to "jump" out of her chest and that she is having a hard time catching her breath. She does not take any medication except vitamins and is not allergic to anything.

Treatment

Oxygen was administered by nasal cannula at 2 lpm and an 18-gauge IV was initiated in her left antecubital vein and run TKO. A 12-lead ECG confirmed the SVT, and paramedics had the patient attempt the Valsalva maneuver without successful conversion of the SVT.

They advised the patient about adenosine, explaining the potential side effects; 6 mg of adenosine was then administered by rapid IV push. Although the patient felt some of the side effects of the adenosine, the first dose did not convert the SVT. The paramedics then administered a second dose of adenosine, this time increasing the dose to 12 mg. After a 4-second interval of a second-degree heart block, the patient's rhythm converted to a regular sinus rhythm. The patient stated that she was free of symptoms. She was transported to the hospital for further assessment, and a 12-lead ECG done en route did not show any acute evidence of a myocardial infarction. The patient was released shortly after with no apparent lasting effects of the SVT.

Indication

Adenosine is the preferred agent in the treatment of tachyarrhythmias refractory to vagal maneuvers including supraventricular tachycardia (narrow-complex tachycardia) and stable ventricular tachycardia (wide-complex tachycardia). It can be used as a diagnostic agent to determine whether the condition is wide- or narrow-complex tachycardia.

Contraindications

Adenosine should not be administered in cases of irregular (atrial fibrillation) or polymorphic (*torsade de pointes*) tachycardia. It is contraindicated in patients with second- or third-degree heart block, sick sinus syndrome, or those with known hypersensitivity to the medication. It should not be given to patients with asthma.

Precautions

Adenosine typically causes arrhythmias at the time of cardioversion. These generally last a few seconds or less and may include PVCs, premature atrial contractions, sinus bradycardia, sinus tachycardia, and various degrees of AV block. In extreme cases, transient asystole may occur. If this occurs, appropriate therapy should be initiated. Adenosine should be used cautiously in patients with asthma.

Side Effects

Adenosine can cause facial flushing, headache, shortness of breath, dizziness, and nausea, among others. Because the half-life of adenosine is so brief, side effects are generally self-limited.

Interactions/Incompatibilities

Methylxanthines (e.g., aminophylline and theophylline) may decrease the effectiveness of adenosine, thus requiring larger doses. Dipyridamole (Persantine) can potentiate the effects of adenosine. The dosage of adenosine may need to be reduced in patients receiving dipyridamole.

Dosage

The initial dose of adenosine is 6 mg given as a rapid intravenous bolus over a 1- to 2-second period. To be certain that the medication rapidly reaches the central circulation, it should be given directly into a vein or into a proximal medication port of a functioning IV/IO line. It should be followed immediately by a rapid saline flush. If the initial dose does not result in conversion of the PSVT within 1 to 2 minutes, a 12 mg dose may be given as a rapid IV/IO bolus. The 12 mg dose may be repeated a second time if required. Doses greater than 12 mg should not be administered. Adenosine should only be given by rapid IV/IO bolus, directly into the vein, or into the medication administration port closest to the patient.

℞ Verapamil (Isoptin, Calan)

Class Calcium channel blocker (Class IV antiarrhythmic)

Description

Verapamil is a calcium ion antagonist (calcium channel blocker). Calcium channel blockers cause a relaxation of vascular smooth muscle and slow conduction through the AV node. Verapamil has a greater effect on conduction and a lesser effect on vascular smooth muscle than do other agents in the same class.

Mechanism of Action

Verapamil causes vascular dilation and slows conduction through the AV node. The advantages are twofold. First, verapamil inhibits arrhythmias caused by a reentry mechanism such as with PSVT. Second, it decreases the rapid ventricular response seen with atrial tachyarrhythmias such as atrial flutter and fibrillation. Verapamil also reduces myocardial oxygen demand because of its negative inotropic effects and causes coronary and peripheral vasodilation.

Pharmacokinetics

Onset: 5 minutes (IV)

Peak Effects: 5–15 minutes (IV)

Duration: 10–60 minutes (IV)

Half-Life: 2–8 hours (IV)

Indications

Verapamil should be given only to narrow-complex tachycardias including:

- Stable, narrow-complex tachycardias if rhythm remains uncontrolled or unconverted by adenosine or vagal maneuvers or if SVT is recurrent
- Control ventricular rate in patients with atrial fibrillation or atrial flutter

Contraindications

Verapamil should not be administered to any patient with severe hypotension or cardiogenic shock. In addition, verapamil should not be administered to patients with ventricular tachycardia in the prehospital setting. Before attempting to treat a patient experiencing atrial flutter or atrial fibrillation, it is essential that the paramedic ensure that the patient does not have **Wolff-Parkinson-White syndrome.**

Precautions

Verapamil can cause systemic hypotension and should be avoided in patients with heart failure. Thus, it is essential that the blood pressure be constantly monitored following verapamil administration. Calcium chloride can be used to prevent the hypotensive effects of calcium channel blockers and in the management of calcium channel blocker overdosage.

Side Effects

Verapamil can cause nausea, vomiting, dizziness, headache, bradycardia, heart block, hypotension, and asystole.

Interactions/Incompatibilities

Verapamil should not be administered to patients receiving intravenous β-blockers because of an increased risk of congestive heart failure, bradycardia, and asystole.

Dosage

In the treatment of paroxysmal supraventricular tachycardia, a 2.5–5 mg IV/IO dose should be given initially during a 2-minute interval. A repeat dose of 5–10 mg can be given in 15–30 minutes if the narrow-complex rhythm persists and there have not been any adverse responses to the initial dose. The total dose of verapamil should not exceed 20–30 mg.

℞ Diltiazem (Cardizem)

Class Calcium channel blocker (Class IV antiarrhythmic)

Description

Diltiazem is a calcium-ion antagonist (calcium channel blocker). Calcium channel blockers cause a relaxation of vascular smooth muscle and slow conduction through the AV node. Diltiazem has a nearly equal effect on vascular smooth muscle and AV conduction.

Mechanism of Action

Diltiazem causes vascular dilation and slows conduction through the AV node. It slows the rapid ventricular rate associated with atrial fibrillation and atrial flutter. It is also used in the treatment of angina because of its negative inotropic effect and because it dilates the coronary arteries.

Pharmacokinetics

Onset: 3 minutes
Peak Effects: 7 minutes
Duration: 1–3 hours
Half-Life: 2 hours

Indications

Diltiazem should be given only to narrow-complex tachycardias including:

- Stable, narrow-complex tachycardias if rhythm remains uncontrolled or unconverted by adenosine or vagal maneuvers or if SVT is recurrent
- Control ventricular rate in patients with atrial fibrillation or atrial flutter

Contraindications

Diltiazem should not be administered to any patient with severe hypotension, congestive heart failure, and/or cardiogenic shock. In addition, diltiazem should not be administered to patients with ventricular tachycardia (wide-complex tachycardia) in the prehospital setting. Before attempting to treat a patient experiencing atrial flutter or atrial fibrillation, it is essential that the paramedic ensure that the patient does not have Wolff-Parkinson-White syndrome.

Precautions

Diltiazem can cause systemic hypotension. Thus, it is essential that the blood pressure be constantly monitored following diltiazem administration. Calcium chloride can be used to prevent the hypotensive effects of calcium channel blockers and in the management of calcium channel blocker overdosage. Diltiazem should be kept refrigerated; however, it can be kept at room temperature for 1 month but must be discarded if unused.

Side Effects

Diltiazem can cause nausea, vomiting, dizziness, headache, bradycardia, heart block, hypotension, and asystole.

Interactions/Incompatibilities

Diltiazem should not be administered to patients receiving intravenous β-blockers because of an increased risk of congestive heart failure, bradycardia, and asystole.

Dosage

In the treatment of rapid narrow-complex tachycardia, a 15–20 mg intravenous bolus (0.25 mg/kg) of diltiazem should be administered over 2 minutes. Additional bolus doses of 20–25 mg (0.35 mg/kg) can be administered in 15 minutes as needed. A maintenance infusion of 5–15 mg/hr can be administered for rate control (titrated to the desired rate).

℞ Amiodarone (Cordarone)

Class Antiarrhythmic agent (Class III antiarrhythmic)

Description

Amiodarone is a potent antiarrhythmic agent and the first-line antiarrhythmic agent given during cardiac arrest because it has been clinically demonstrated to improve the rate of ROSC and hospital admission in adults with refractory ventricular fibrillation and pulseless ventricular tachycardia. It can also be used in supraventricular tachycardias.

Mechanism of Action

Amiodarone prolongs the action potential duration in all cardiac tissues. It affects sodium, potassium, and calcium channels and has α- and β-adrenergic blocking properties.

Pharmacokinetics

Onset: 2–3 days (oral)

Peak Effects: 3–7 hours (oral)

Duration: Varies

Half-Life: 40–55 days

Indications

Amiodarone is used in life-threatening cardiac arrhythmias such as ventricular tachycardia and ventricular fibrillation. It can also be used for the following conditions:

- Stable, irregular, narrow-complex tachycardia (atrial fibrillation)
- Stable, regular, narrow-complex tachycardia
- To control rapid ventricular rate due to accessory pathway

Contraindications

Amiodarone is contraindicated in breast-feeding patients in cardiogenic shock and those with severe sinus node dysfunction resulting in marked sinus bradycardia, second- or third-degree AV block, symptomatic bradycardia, or known hypersensitivity.

Precautions

Amiodarone should be used with caution in patients with latent or manifest heart failure because failure may be worsened by its administration.

Side Effects

Paramedics should monitor the patient's ECG and be alert for hypotension, bradycardia, increased ventricular beats, prolonged PR interval, QRS complex, and QT interval. The patient should also be monitored for signs of pulmonary toxicity such as dyspnea and cough.

Interactions/Incompatibilities

Amiodarone may react with warfarin, digoxin, procainamide, quinidine, and phenytoin.

Dosage

Ventricular fibrillation or pulseless ventricular (adults). Initial dose is 300 mg IV/IO. May be repeated at 150 mg as necessary for recurrent or refractory arrhythmias.

Narrow-complex tachycardias. Amiodarone should be dosed at 150 mg IV/IO over 10 minute and repeated as necessary. This can be followed by a 1 mg/min infusion over 6 hours, followed by a 0.5 mg/min infusion as needed. The total 24-hour dose should not exceed 2.2 gm.

℞ Phenytoin (Dilantin)

Class Antiarrhythmic and anticonvulsant (Class IB antiarrhythmic)

Description

Phenytoin is an anticonvulsant and antiarrhythmic that depresses spontaneous ventricular depolarization.

Mechanism of Action

Phenytoin (Dilantin) is used frequently in the treatment of epilepsy but also has antiarrhythmic properties. It has proved effective in the management of arrhythmias caused by digitalis toxicity or tricyclic antidepressant medication overdoses. It depresses spontaneous depolarization of ventricular tissues and appears to improve atrioventricular conduction. Its use in the management of status epilepticus is discussed in Chapter 10.

Pharmacokinetics

Onset: 3–5 minutes
Peak Effects: 1–2 hours
Duration: Variable
Half-Life: 22 hours

Indication

Phenytoin is used in life-threatening arrhythmias resulting from digitalis toxicity or tricyclic antidepressant overdose. Ventricular arrhythmias in the setting of acute myocardial infarction should first be treated with other agents.

Contraindications

Phenytoin is contraindicated in cases of bradycardia and high-grade heart block. It should not be administered to patients who take the medication chronically for seizures until the blood level has been determined.

Precautions

Intravenous administration of phenytoin should not exceed 50 mg/min. Signs of central nervous system depression or hypotension may occur. Elderly patients are at increased risk of developing side effects from phenytoin administration. Extravasation should be avoided. Any patient receiving intravenous phenytoin should have continuous cardiac monitoring as well as frequent monitoring of vital signs.

Side Effects

Phenytoin can cause drowsiness, dizziness, headache, hypotension, arrhythmias, itching, rash, nausea, and vomiting.

Interactions/Incompatibilities

Phenytoin must never be diluted in dextrose-containing solutions such as D_5W. It should be diluted in normal saline or other non-glucose-containing crystalloids.

Dosage

The recommended dose of phenytoin is 100 mg over 5 minutes to a maximum loading dose of 1000 mg, until the arrhythmia is suppressed, or until symptoms of central nervous system depression appear. In the emergency setting, phenytoin should be given by slow IV/IO bolus or IV infusion with constant ECG monitoring.

℞ Edrophonium Chloride (Tensilon)

Class Antiarrhythmic and cholinesterase inhibitor

Description

Edrophonium belongs to a class of medications referred to as anticholinesterase agents. It is used in the treatment of paroxysmal supraventricular tachycardia refractory to first-line agents.

Mechanism of Action

Edrophonium inhibits the actions of the enzyme *acetylcholinesterase*. This enzyme plays an important role in neurophysiology because it deactivates the neurotransmitter of the parasympathetic nervous system, acetylcholine. Physostigmine, an emergency medication used in the management of atropine-type poisonings and tricyclic antidepressant overdoses, is chemically similar to edrophonium. The neurophysiology of the parasympathetic nervous system is discussed in more detail in the following section on parasympatholytics. Edrophonium has proven effectiveness in the management of PSVTs that do not respond to vagal maneuvers. The inhibition of acetylcholinesterase by edrophonium serves to enhance the acetylcholine secreted by the vagus nerve on the heart. This increased parasympathetic effect has been successful in slowing and eventually terminating PSVTs. With the introduction of adenosine and the calcium channel blockers (verapamil), edrophonium has fallen into relative disuse.

Pharmacokinetics

Onset: 30–60 seconds (IV), 2–10 minutes (IM)
Peak Effects: Variable

Duration: 5–10 minutes (IV), 5–30 minutes (IM)

Half-Life: 1–2 hours

Indication

Edrophonium is used for PSVT refractory to vagal maneuvers and adenosine.

Contraindications

Edrophonium should not be administered to patients with a history of hypersensitivity to the medication. It should not be used in patients who are hypotensive or bradycardic because it can worsen these conditions.

Precautions

The respiratory pattern should be carefully monitored during and following administration of edrophonium. Also, the patient should be constantly monitored for signs of bradycardia. Atropine sulfate should be readily available in those cases of bradycardia causing hemodynamic problems. Edrophonium should be used with caution in the elderly.

Side Effects

Edrophonium can cause dizziness, weakness, sweating, increased salivation, constricted pupils, hypotension, bradycardia, abdominal cramps, nausea, and vomiting.

Interactions/Incompatibilities

Edrophonium should not be administered in dextrose solutions because it tends to crystallize in the tubing. The chances of developing a significant bradycardia are enhanced when edrophonium is administered to patients taking digitalis.

Dosage

The standard dosage is 5 mg initially intravenously. If unsuccessful after 10 minutes or so, a second dose of 10 mg may be administered. Physicians frequently order the administration of a test dose of 0.1–0.5 mg, particularly to elderly patients, before the administration of the full dose. Edrophonium should be administered intravenously only.

℞ Magnesium Sulfate

Class Antiarrhythmic

Description

Magnesium sulfate is a salt that dissociates into the magnesium cation (Mg^{2+}) and the sulfate anion when administered. Magnesium is an essential element in numerous biochemical reactions that occur within the body.

Mechanism of Action

Magnesium is an essential element in many of the biochemical processes that occur in the body. It acts as a physiological calcium channel blocker and blocks neuromuscular transmission. A decreased magnesium level (hypomagnesemia) is associated with cardiac arrhythmias, symptoms of cardiac insufficiency, and sudden death. Hypomagnesemia can cause refractory ventricular fibrillation. Administration of magnesium sulfate in the emergency setting appears to reduce the incidence of ventricular arrhythmias that may follow an acute myocardial infarction. It also appears to decrease the complications associated with acute myocardial infarction. Magnesium sulfate has been used for years in the management of preterm labor and the hypertensive disorders of pregnancy (preeclampsia and eclampsia). Its usage in obstetrics is discussed in Chapter 11.

Pharmacokinetics

Onset: Immediate (IV/IO), 1 hour (IM)

Peak Effects: Varies

Duration: 1 hour

Half-Life: Not applicable

Indications

Magnesium sulfate is used in *torsade de pointes* (irregular, polymorphic ventricular tachycardia associated with QT interval prolongation).

Contraindications

Magnesium sulfate should not be administered to patients who are in shock, who have persistent severe hypertension, who have third-degree AV block, who routinely undergo dialysis, or who are known to have a decreased calcium level (hypocalcemia).

Precautions

Magnesium sulfate should be administered slowly to minimize side effects. Any patient receiving intravenous magnesium sulfate should have continuous cardiac monitoring and frequent monitoring of vital signs. If possible, the knee and biceps deep tendon reflexes should be checked prior to beginning magnesium therapy. It should be used with caution in patients with known renal insufficiency. Hypermagnesemia (elevated magnesium level) can occur following magnesium sulfate administration. Calcium salts (calcium chloride or calcium gluconate) should be available as an antidote for magnesium sulfate in case serious side effects occur.

Side Effects

Magnesium sulfate can cause flushing, sweating, bradycardia, decreased deep tendon reflexes, drowsiness, respiratory depression, arrhythmias, hypotension, hypothermia, itching, and rash.

Interactions/Incompatibilities

Magnesium sulfate can cause cardiac conduction abnormalities if administered in conjunction with digitalis.

Dosage

Torsade de pointes. Magnesium can be diluted in 10 mL of D_5W for treatment of torsade. Alternatively, 1–2 g of magnesium sulfate can be diluted in 100 mL of D_5W or normal saline and administered over 15 minutes as an IV/IO piggyback.

PARASYMPATHOLYTICS

Medications that inhibit the actions of the parasympathetic nervous system are referred to as *parasympatholytics*. Sometimes they are referred to as *anticholinergics*. To fully understand the role and actions of the parasympatholytics, we must first review the parasympathetic nervous system.

The parasympathetic, or *cholinergic*, system plays a major role in the maintenance of homeostasis. Parasympathetic stimulation induces peristalsis and causes pupillary constriction and a decrease in the heart rate. The primary nerve of the parasympathetic nervous system is the *vagus nerve*. The vagus nerve descends from the brain along the carotid arteries. It then innervates the heart and the digestive system. Paramedics should be familiar with the manual method of vagal stimulation, carotid sinus massage. Carotid sinus massage is used to slow the heart rate in paroxysmal supraventricular tachycardia.

When the vagus nerve is stimulated, it causes acetylcholine to be released from the presynaptic nerve endings. It then activates acetylcholine receptors on the target organs. These receptors cause the heart rate to slow. Then, after only a fraction of a second, cholinesterase is released, which deactivates acetylcholine. Several medications act on these junctions. The primary medication of this type is atropine sulfate. Atropine binds to the acetylcholine receptors, thus inhibiting activation. Besides increasing the heart rate, atropine is used frequently as a preoperative medication because it decreases digestive secretions, especially salivation. Certain chemicals, especially the organophosphate insecticides, tend to block, in an irreversible manner, the action of cholinesterase. Excessive levels of acetylcholine can cause serious problems.

℞ Atropine Sulfate

Class Anticholinergic

Description

Atropine is a parasympatholytic (anticholinergic) that is derived from parts of the *Atropa belladonna* plant.

Mechanism of Action

Atropine sulfate is a potent parasympatholytic and is used to increase the heart rate in hemodynamically significant bradycardias. Hemodynamically significant bradycardias are those slow heart rates accompanied by hypotension, shortness of breath, chest pain, altered mental status, congestive heart failure, and shock. Atropine acts by blocking acetylcholine receptors, thus inhibiting parasympathetic stimulation. Although it has positive chronotropic properties, it has little or no inotropic effect. It plays an important role as an antidote in organophosphate poisonings.

Pharmacokinetics

Onset: Immediate
Peak Effects: 2–4 minutes
Duration: 4 hours
Half-Life: 2–3 hours

Indications

Atropine is used in hemodynamically significant bradycardia with a pulse.

Contraindications

There are no contraindications in emergency situations. Atropine is no longer recommended in the treatment of cardiac arrest including pulseless electrical activity (PEA) and asystole.

Precautions

Atropine should be used cautiously in the presence of coronary artery disease as the increased heart rate may worsen ischemia. Atropine may actually worsen the bradycardia associated with second-degree Mobitz II and third-degree AV blocks. Transcutaneous pacing should be available. A maximum dose of 3 mg of atropine should not be exceeded except in the setting of organophosphate poisoning.

Side Effects

Atropine sulfate can cause blurred vision, dilated pupils, dry mouth, tachycardia, drowsiness, and confusion.

Interactions/Incompatibilities

There are few interactions in the prehospital setting.

Dosage

Hemodynamically significant bradycardia. An initial dose of 0.5 mg should be administered intravenously (doses less than 0.5 mg can cause paradoxical slowing of the heart rate). Atropine can be repeated every 3 to 5 minutes until a maximum dose of 3 mg has been administered.

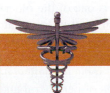

CASE PRESENTATION

Paramedics are called to a local shopping mall for a medical emergency. Reportedly, a patient collapsed and is unconscious, but breathing. On arrival the patient is found lying on the floor in the center court with a pillow under her head. The patient appears to be in her early 60s.

Physical Examination

CNS:	The patient is conscious, slow to respond to verbal commands, and disoriented to person, place, and time
Resp:	Respirations are 12 and shallow; lung sounds clear bilaterally; trachea is midline; no signs of trauma
CVS:	Weak, regular, slow carotid pulse and radial pulses are present; skin is pale, cool, and diaphoretic; no complaint of chest pain
ABD:	Soft and nontender
Muscl/Skel:	Patient able to move extremities slightly, with delay, on command; weak bilateral hand grip; no obvious injuries

(continued)

Case Presentation (continued)

Vital Signs

Pulse:	36/min, regular, weak
Resp:	12/min, shallow
BP:	72/56 mmHg
SpO$_2$:	86 percent
ECG:	Sinus bradycardia
Hx:	Unknown; patient was in the mall alone and is unable to give a history or answer questions
Past Hx:	Unknown; no Medic Alert

Treatment

Oxygen was administered by non-rebreather mask at 100% and well tolerated by the patient. An IV of normal saline was established. The patient was given 0.5 mg of atropine. Following the atropine the patient's pulse rate increased slightly to 42/min and her blood pressure was 80/62. At this point the pacing pads were placed on the patient as a precautionary measure. A second dose of atropine 0.5 mg was given, and the heart rate improved to 68/min with a blood pressure of 108/82. The patient's level of consciousness improved. The patient was moved to the ambulance and transported to the hospital.

En route to the hospital the patient stated that she was shopping alone when she felt faint. She sat down to let the faintness pass. She does not remember what happened prior to fainting. She remembers waking and seeing the paramedics with her.

Atropine should be given as an IV bolus in emergency situations or endotracheally when an IV cannot be placed.

CARDIAC GLYCOSIDES

Digitalis, the principal medication in the cardiac glycoside class, is one of the oldest medications known to humans. For hundreds of years it has been used in the treatment of congestive heart failure. Digitalis and the related cardiac glycosides increase the force (inotropic effect) of the myocardial contraction. When given to patients in congestive heart failure, it significantly increases cardiac output, reducing left ventricular diameter; decreases venous pressure; and hastens reduction of peripheral and pulmonary edema. In recent years digitalis has also proved effective in the management of patients with atrial flutter and atrial fibrillation. In these patients rapid atrial rates produce accelerated ventricular rates, which can be reduced by digitalis therapy.

Several digitalis preparations are available:

Digitoxin. Digitoxin is the longest acting cardiac glycoside. It must not be confused with the shorter acting digoxin.

Digoxin (Lanoxin). Digoxin is the most commonly prescribed form of digitalis.

Ouabain. Ouabain has a rapid rate of onset and a relatively short duration of effect. Its use is reserved for cases in which rapid digitalization is required.

Deslanoside (Cedilanid-D). Deslanoside is the most rapidly acting digitalis preparation.

Cardiac glycosides have profound effects on cardiac function and rhythm. The therapeutic index (therapeutic dose/toxic dose) is low, which means that the possibility of digitalis toxicity should always be considered in patients with this medication. Signs of digitalis toxicity include cardiac arrhythmias (PVCs, PSVT with 2:1 block, and so on), nausea, vomiting, headache, visual disturbances (yellow vision), and drowsiness. Almost any arrhythmia can be associated with digitalis toxicity.

Digitalis is a potent and potentially toxic medication. Extreme care must be used whenever it is administered. Constant monitoring of vital signs and ECG is essential. In almost all cases digitalization should be deferred until the patient is in the emergency department and under the care of the emergency physician.

℞ Digoxin (Lanoxin)

Class Cardiac glycoside (Class V antiarrhythmic)

Description

Digoxin is a moderately rapid-acting cardiac glycoside used in the management of congestive heart failure and to control the heart rate in atrial fibrillation and atrial flutter.

Mechanism of Action

Digoxin is a cardiac glycoside effective in the treatment of congestive heart failure and rapid atrial arrhythmias. It increases the force of the cardiac contraction through its effects on the sodium–potassium ATPase system. Digoxin significantly increases the stroke volume, thus increasing the cardiac output. It also decreases AV nodal conduction, thus slowing the heart rate. Therapeutic effects begin in about half an hour and peak at 24 hours.

Pharmacokinetics

Onset: 5–30 minutes
Peak Effects: 1–5 hours
Duration: 3–4 days
Half-Life: 34–44 hours

Indications

In the emergency setting, digoxin is used in the following conditions:

- Stable, narrow-complex regular tachycardias if rhythm remains uncontrolled or unconverted by adenosine or vagal maneuvers or if SVT is recurrent.
- To control ventricular rate in patients with atrial fibrillation or atrial flutter.

Contraindications

Digoxin should not be given to any patient showing any of the signs or symptoms of digitalis toxicity. It also should not be administered to patients in ventricular fibrillation.

Precautions

Patients receiving digoxin should be constantly monitored for signs and symptoms of digitalis toxicity. Extreme care should be used when administering digoxin to patients with myocardial infarction, because they are prone to digitalis toxicity.

Digitalis toxicity is potentiated in patients with hypokalemia, hypomagnesemia, and hypercalcemia. Digitalis crosses the placenta and thus can affect the fetal heart in much the same manner as the mother's.

Side Effects

Digoxin can cause numerous side effects. Noncardiac side effects include anorexia, nausea, vomiting, abdominal pain, diarrhea, fatigue, depression, drowsiness, yellow vision, headache, dizziness, hallucinations, sweating, itching, and rash. Cardiac side effects include arrhythmias, bradycardias, tachycardias, various degrees of heart block, hypotension, and cardiac arrest.

Interactions/Incompatibilities

Many medications have potential interaction problems with digoxin. Quinidine and the calcium channel blockers (verapamil, nifedipine, and diltiazem) can increase serum digoxin levels. The administration of digoxin concomitantly with beta-blockers can cause severe bradycardia. Diuretics can cause potassium depletion, which can lead to digitalis toxicity.

Dosage

The dosage is 0.25 mg slow IV every 2 hours up to a total loading dose of 1.5 mg. Alternatively, a total dose of 0.5–1.0 mg (50% given as the initial dose and then 25% in subsequent doses at 6–8 hours).

ANTICOAGULANTS

Medications that inhibit blood clot formation (anticoagulants) play an important role in emergency medicine. Many significant medical problems result from either embolic or thrombotic events. These include acute coronary syndrome, acute embolic and thrombotic strokes, pulmonary embolism, and deep venous thrombosis. Deep venous thrombosis is a risk factor for the development of pulmonary embolisms and other thrombotic events.

Several medications are available that inhibit coagulation. The most common of these is warfarin sodium (Coumadin). Warfarin takes several days to achieve therapeutic blood levels. Thus, its role in emergency medicine is rather limited.

Low-molecular-weight heparin (enoxaparin) has become increasingly popular in emergency medicine. Normal heparin has a molecular weight of 5000 to 30 000 Da, whereas low-molecular-weight heparin has a molecular weight of 1000 to 10 000 Da. Because of this, low-molecular-weight heparin has greater bioavailability, is easier to dose, and has fewer effects on platelet function.

Another common anticoagulant, heparin, can be administered only parenterally. Thus, it is easily administered and rapidly effective. The half-life of heparin is short and any bolus must be followed by a continuous infusion until the condition is resolved or the patient is switched to oral warfarin. For the most part, anticoagulant therapy should be guided by blood coagulation studies (prothrombin time [PT] and partial thromboplastin times [PTT]). These are unavailable in the prehospital setting. However, in certain cases, the benefits gained from early coagulation may exceed any risks of administering the medications without baseline coagulation studies.

Platelet aggregation inhibitors, including aspirin, now play a major role in reducing morbidity and mortality associated with acute coronary syndrome (ACS) and the treatment of acute coronary syndrome including percutaneous coronary intervention (PCI).

Platelet Inhibitors

Platelet aggregation inhibitors are medications that antagonize or impair any mechanism leading to blood platelet aggregation. They generally fall into four categories:

- *Cyclooxygenase inhibitors.* Cyclooxygenase (COX) is an enzyme that plays a role in inflammation. Medications that inhibit COX are referred to as anti-inflammatory medications. Of these, the prototype is aspirin.

- *Heparin.* Heparin is a naturally occurring anticoagulant that is released from mast cells. It is one of the oldest parenteral anticoagulants. Standard heparin, often referred to as unfractionated heparin (UFH), is derived from pigs. It can be given only intravenously and requires frequent monitoring of blood clotting parameters. More recently, fractionated heparin, called low-molecular weight heparin (LMWH), has become more frequently used. LMWH consists of smaller molecules, can be given subcutaneously, and does not require frequent laboratory monitoring like UFH. The most common LMWH is enoxaparin (Lovenox).

- *Adenosine diphosphate (ADP) inhibitors.* The ADP inhibitor medications inhibit platelet aggregation by selectively binding to adenlyate cyclase–coupled ADP receptors on the surface of platelets. This binding results in inhibition of platelet aggregation and binding of fibrinogen to the GP IIb-IIIa receptor on activated platelets. This binding is usually irreversible. The major drugs in this class are ticlopidine (Ticlid) and clopidogrel (Plavix).

- *Glycoprotein IIb/IIIa inhibitors.* This class of medications inhibits platelet aggregation by preventing fibrinogen from binding to glycoprotein IIb-IIIa receptors on activated platelets. This is thought to prevent thrombus formation that results from plaque rupture or damage to inner lining of the blood vessels. The major drugs in this class are abciximab (ReoPro), tirofiban (Aggrastat), and eptifibatide (Integrilin).

Rx Aspirin

Class Platelet aggregation inhibitor and anti-inflammatory agent

Description

Aspirin is an anti-inflammatory agent and an inhibitor of platelet function. This makes it a useful agent in the treatment of various thromboembolic diseases such as acute myocardial infarction.

Mechanism of Action

Aspirin blocks the formation of the substance thromboxane A_2, which causes platelets to aggregate and arteries to constrict. This results in an overall reduction in mortality associated with myocardial infarction. It also appears to reduce the rate of nonfatal reinfarction and nonfatal stroke.

Pharmacokinetics

Onset: 5–30 minutes
Peak Effects: 15–120 minutes
Duration: 1–4 hours
Half-Life: 15–20 minutes

Indications

Aspirin is used for new chest pain suggestive of acute coronary syndrome and signs and symptoms suggestive of recent stroke. Several studies have shown that early aspirin administration (within 3 hours of acute coronary syndrome symptom onset) is associated with a significantly decreased risk of death. However, other studies have shown that aspirin is underused in prehospital care in the treatment of chest pain and acute coronary syndrome.

Contraindications

Aspirin is contraindicated in patients with known hypersensitivity to the medication. It is relatively contraindicated in patients with active ulcer disease and asthma.

Precautions

Aspirin can cause gastrointestinal upset and bleeding. Enteric-coated aspirin, if available, should be used in patients who have a tendency for gastric irritation and bleeding with aspirin. Aspirin should be used with caution in patients who report allergies to the nonsteroidal anti-inflammatory (NSAID) class of medications. Doses higher than recommended can actually interfere with possible benefits.

Side Effects

Aspirin can cause heartburn, gastrointestinal bleeding, nausea, vomiting, wheezing, and prolonged bleeding.

Interactions/Incompatibilities

When administered together, aspirin and other anti-inflammatory agents may cause an increased incidence of side effects and increased blood levels of both medications. Administration of aspirin with antacids may reduce the blood levels of the medication by decreasing absorption.

Dosage

The recommended dosage for aspirin is 160–325 mg taken as soon as possible after the onset of chest pain. Baby aspirin (81 mg) is often preferred because it can be chewed and swallowed and is often a little more palatable. Chewable preparations are more rapidly absorbed. Aspirin is often given as part of a thrombolytic therapy protocol. Aspirin suppositories (300 mg) are available for patients who are nauseated or vomiting.

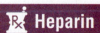 **Heparin**

Class Anticoagulant (unfractionated)

Description

Heparin is a rapid-acting anticoagulant prepared from bovine lung tissue or porcine intestinal mucosa.

Mechanism of Action

Heparin is an indirect inhibitor of thrombin and the inhibitory actions of antithrombin III–thrombin complex, blocking the conversion of prothrombin to thrombin and preventing the conversion of fibrinogen to fibrin.

Pharmacokinetics

Onset: Immediate

Peak Effects: 2–3 minutes

Duration: 2–6 hours

Half-Life: 90 minutes

Indications

Unfractionated heparin (UFH) is used to inhibit clot formation in acute coronary syndrome (ACS). It is also used as an adjunct in fibrinolysis. UFH is also used to prevent pulmonary embolism and deep venous thrombosis in patients predisposed to such problems.

Contraindications

Heparin is contraindicated in patients with known hypersensitivity to the medication, to pork products, and to beef products.

Precautions

Do not use heparin in patients with active major bleeding or thrombocytopenia. Use with caution in the elderly or any patient with increased risk of bleeding. Heparin should be used with caution in chronic alcoholism, in patients with a history of atrophy or anaphylaxis, and during pregnancy (especially the last trimester).

Side Effects

Reported central nervous system side effects include confusion and dizziness. Cardiovascular side effects include edema, chest pain, and irregular heartbeat. Irritation, pain, erythema, or bruising may occur at the injection site. Other side effects are bleeding complications, angioedema, rash, and urticaria.

Interactions/Incompatibilities

Interactions with heparin have been reported with nonsteroidal anti-inflammatory medications, warfarin, and antiplatelet agents. Intravenous nitroglycerin may decrease anticoagulation activities. Protamine antagonizes the effects of heparin.

Dosage

Adult dose (acute STEMI and unstable angina). 60 U/kg IV (maximum 4000 units) followed by 12 U/kg/hr (maximum 1000 U/hr). This is often given with alteplase (rtPA).

Adult dose (NSTEMI and unstable angina). 60 to 70 U/kg IV (maximum, 5000 U) as initial bolus followed by a 12- to 15-U/kg/h infusion.

Pediatric dose. 50 units/kg followed by IV infusion based on laboratory values and body mass.

Rx Enoxaparin (Lovenox)

Class Anticoagulant (fractionated)

Description

Enoxaparin (Lovenox) is a low-molecular-weight heparin (LMWH) derivative.

Mechanism of Action

Enoxaparin accelerates the formation of antithrombin III–thrombin complex and deactivates thrombin. It also prevents the conversion of fibrinogen to fibrin.

Pharmacokinetics

Onset: 3–5 hours
Peak Effects: 3–5 hours
Duration: Varies
Half-Life: 4.5 hours

Indications

Enoxaparin (LMWH) is used to inhibit clot formation in acute coronary syndrome (ACS) including STEMI, NSTEMI, and unstable angina. It is also used to prevent pulmonary embolism and deep venous thrombosis in patients predisposed to such problems.

Contraindications

Enoxaparin is contraindicated in patients with known hypersensitivity to the medication, to pork products, or to heparin.

Precautions

Do not use enoxaparin in patients with active major bleeding or thrombocytopenia. Use with caution in the elderly or any patient with increased risk of bleeding.

Side Effects

Reported central nervous system side effects include confusion and dizziness. Cardiovascular side effects include edema, chest pain, and irregular heartbeat. Irritation, pain, erythema, or bruising may occur at the injection site. Other side effects are bleeding complications, angioedema, rash, and urticaria.

Interactions/Incompatibilities

Interactions with enoxaparin have been reported with nonsteroidal anti-inflammatory medications, warfarin, and antiplatelet agents.

Dosage

Adult dose (STEMI). The recommended dose of enoxaparin in STEMI is a single IV bolus of 30 mg plus a 1 mg/kg SC dose followed by 1 mg/kg administered SC every 12 hours (maximum 100 mg for the first two doses only).

Adult dose Unstable angina (UA)/non-ST segment elevation myocardial infarction (NSTEMI). The recommended dose of enoxapairin in UA/NSTEMI is 1 mg/kg administered SC every 12 hours in conjunction with oral aspirin therapy (100–325 mg once daily).

Pediatric dose. 1 mg/kg SQ.

℞ Clopidogrel (Plavix)

Class Platelet aggregation inhibitor (ADP inhibitor)

Description

Clopidogrel (Plavix) is an adenosine diphosphate (ADP) platelet aggregation inhibitor in the thienopyradine class of medications.

Mechanism of Action

Clopidogrel inhibits platelet aggregation by selectively binding to adenlyate cyclase-coupled ADP receptors on the surface of platelets resulting in inhibition of platelet aggregation and binding of fibrinogen to the GP IIb-IIIa receptor on activated platelets.

Pharmacokinetics

Onset: 2 hours
Peak Effects: 3–7 days
Duration: 7–10 days
Half-Life: 7–8 hours

Indications

Clopidogrel is indicated for the treatment of acute coronary syndrome (ACS) and is also useful in recent myocardial infarction, stroke, or established peripheral vascular disease.

Contraindications

Clopidogrel is contraindicated in patients with a hypersensitivity to the drug. It should also not be used in the presence of a hemostatic disorder or active pathological bleeding such as bleeding peptic ulcer or intracranial bleeding.

Precautions

Clopidogrel should be used with caution in patients taking nonsteroidal anti-inflammatory (NSAID) medications.

Side Effects

Increased risk of bleeding, fever, allergic reactions, myalgias, arthralgias, bronchospasm, and skin rash.

Interactions/Incompatibilities

Nonsteroidal anti-inflammatory drugs increase risk of gastrointestinal bleeding.

Dosage

Clopidogrel is dosed as follows:

- *Acute coronary syndrome.* Non-ST-segment elevation ACS (UA/NSTEMI): 300 mg loading dose followed by 75 mg once daily, in combination with aspirin (75–325 mg once daily)
- *STEMI:* 75 mg once daily, in combination with aspirin (75–325 mg once daily), with or without a loading dose and with or without thrombolytics
- *Recent MI, recent stroke, or established peripheral arterial disease:* 75 mg once daily

℞ Abciximab (Reopro)

Class Platelet aggregation inhibitor (Glycoprotein IIb/IIIa inhibitor)

Description

Abciximab (ReoPro) is a glycoprotein IIb/IIIa receptor antagonist.

Mechanism of Action

Anciximab inhibits platelet aggregation by blocking the glycoprotein IIb/IIIa receptors (integrin receptors) on activated platelets.

Pharmacokinetics

Onset: 1–2 minutes
Peak Effects: 2 hours
Duration: 1–2 days
Half-Life: 10–30 minutes

Indications

Abciximab is indicated as an adjunct to percutaneous coronary intervention (PCI) for the prevention of cardiac ischemic complications in patients undergoing PCI and in patients with unstable angina (UA) not responding to conventional medical therapy when PCI is planned within 24 hours.

Contraindications

Abciximab is contraindicated in patients with active internal bleeding, recent (within 6 weeks); gastrointestinal (GI) or genitourinary (GU) bleeding of clinical significance; history of stroke within 2 years or stroke with a significant residual neurological deficit; bleeding disorders; recent (within 6 weeks) major surgery or trauma, intracranial neoplasm, arteriovenous malformation, or aneurysm; severe uncontrolled hypertension; presumed or documented history of vasculitis; use of intravenous dextran before percutaneous coronary intervention, or intent to use it during intervention; known hypersensitivity to any component of this product or to mouse proteins.

Precautions

Abciximab should be used with caution in patients who have an increased risk of bleeding. Allergic reactions have been reported with abciximab.

Side Effects

Increased risk of bleeding, nausea, vomiting, abdominal pain, anemia, pain, sweating.

Interactions/Incompatibilities

Dextran

Dosage

- *UA/NSTEMI with planned PCI in < 24 hours:* 0.25 mg/kg IV bolus administered 10–60 minutes prior to PCI, followed by a continuous infusion of 0.125 mcg/kg/minute for 12 hours (maximum dose is 10 mcg/min).

℞ Eptifibatide (Integrilin)

Class Platelet aggregation inhibitor (Glycoprotein IIb/IIIa inhibitor)

Description

Eptifibatide (Integrilin) is a glycoprotein IIb/IIIa receptor antagonist.

Mechanism of Action

Eptifibatide inhibits platelet aggregation by blocking the glycoprotein IIb/IIIa receptors (integrin receptors) on activated platelets.

Pharmacokinetics

Onset: Immediate
Peak Effects: Following bolus
Duration: Brief
Half-Life: 2.5 hours

Indications

Eptifibatide is indicated in patients with acute coronary syndrome (ACS) including UA/NSTEMI. It is used for patients who will undergo PCI as well as those who will be managed medically. It is usually administered in combination with aspirin and heparin.

Contraindications

Eptifibatide is contraindicated in patients with a known hypersensitivity to the drug, active internal bleeding or history of bleeding within previous 30 days, severe uncontrolled hypertension (systolic BP > 200 mmHg and/or diastolic BP > 110 mmHg), major surgical procedure within 6 weeks, history of hemorrhagic stroke or other stroke within 30 days, concurrent use of other glycoprotein IIb/IIIa receptor antagonists, platelet count < 100 000/mm^3, severe renal insufficiency or dependency on renal dialysis.

Precautions

Eptifibatide should be used with caution in patients who have an increased risk of bleeding or renal insufficiency.

Side Effects

Increased risk of bleeding and hypotension.

Interactions/Incompatibilities

Increased risk of bleeding with other anticoagulants.

Dosage

Acute Coronary Syndrome. 180 mcg/kg as a bolus dose, followed by 2 mcg/kg/min until hospital discharge or surgical intervention (up to 72 hours).

Percutaneous Coronary Intervention. 180 mcg/kg as a bolus dose, immediately before PCI, followed by 2 mcg/kg/min infusion followed by a second bolus of 180 mcg/kg is given 10 min after first bolus; infusion should continue for 18–24 hours or hospital discharge (minimum of 12 hours).

℞ Tirofiban (Aggrastat)

Class Platelet aggregation inhibitor (Glycoprotein IIb/IIIa inhibitor)

Description

Tirofiban (Aggrastat) is a glycoprotein IIb/IIIa receptor antagonist.

Mechanism of Action

Tirofiban inhibits platelet aggregation by blocking the glycoprotein IIb/IIIa receptors (integrin receptors) on activated platelets.

Pharmacokinetics

Onset: Immediate
Peak Effects: Following bolus
Duration: Brief
Half-Life: 2 hours

Indications

Tirofiban is indicated in patients with acute coronary syndrome (ACS) including UA/NSTEMI. It is used for patients who will undergo PCI as well as those who will be managed medically. It is usually administered in combination with aspirin and heparin.

Contraindications

Tirofiban is contraindicated in patients with known hypersensitivity to any component of the product; active (internal) bleeding or a history of abnormal bleeding tendencies; a history of intracranial hemorrhage or neoplasm, arteriovenous malformation, or aneurysm; patients who developed thrombocytopenia following prior exposure to tirofiban; known coagulation disorder, platelet disorder or history of thrombocytopenia; stroke within 30 days prior to hospitalization or any history of hemorrhagic stroke; major surgical procedure or severe physical trauma within the previous month; history, symptoms or findings suggestive of aortic dissection; severe uncontrolled hypertension; acute pericarditis; cirrhosis or other clinically significant liver disease; and angina caused by obvious provoking factors (arrhythmia, severe anemia, hyperthyroidism, or hypotension).

Precautions

Tirofiban should be used with caution in patients who have an increased risk of bleeding or renal insufficiency.

Side Effects

Increased risk of bleeding and hypotension.

Interactions/Incompatibilities

Increased risk of bleeding with other anticoagulants.

Dosage

Tirofiban should be administered intravenously, at an initial rate of 0.4 mcg/kg/min for 30 minutes and then continued at 0.1 mcg/kg/min.

Fibrinolytics

A myocardial infarction begins with the formation of a blood clot (thrombus) in a coronary artery. This clot results in complete occlusion of the artery and subsequent interruption of blood flow to the area of the myocardium supplied by that artery. Usually, the coronary artery is already partially obstructed by atherosclerosis. These obstructions are often the narrowest (or tightest) portions of the artery and the site of thrombus formation.

Following arterial occlusion, the portion of the myocardium supplied by the obstructed artery becomes ischemic. At this point the ischemia can be reversed with minimal permanent injury to the muscle if the blood supply can be restored. However, if the occlusion continues, the myocardium will become injured and will eventually die. There is a window of 6 hours after the onset of pain to restore perfusion to the injured myocardium. There are several ways perfusion can be restored, including percutaneous coronary intervention (PCI), percutaneous transluminal coronary angioplasty (PTCA), coronary artery bypass grafting (CABG), and fibrinolytic therapy. PTCA requires access to a cardiac catheterization lab and subsequent coronary arteriogram to identify the occlusion. Then, a special balloon catheter is introduced into the diseased artery. The balloon is placed at the site of the occlusion and filled, resulting in dilation of the occlusion. This process is time consuming and not available in every hospital. Likewise, CABG requires an initial arteriogram followed by major surgery to bypass the obstruction. Fibrinolytic therapy, unlike the other procedures, does not require coronary angiography and can be performed in any community hospital and, in some places, in the prehospital setting. Generally speaking, PCI, when available, is the preferred therapy.

Fibrinolytic therapy is the administration of a medication to dissolve the blood clot in the coronary artery causing an acute myocardial infarction. Aspirin, and other types of platelet inhibitors, are widely used in treatment of ischemic heart disease and acute coronary syndrome. These have proven effective in reducing mortality following myocardial infarction.

In the absence of contraindications, fibrinolytic therapy is recommended for STEMI if symptom onset has been within 12 hours of presentation and percutaneous coronary intervention (PCI) is not available within 90 minutes of first medical contact. In patients presenting within 2 hours of symptom onset or when delays to PCI are anticipated, fibrinolytic therapy is recommended.

℞ Streptokinase (Streptase)

Class Fibrinolytic

Description

Streptokinase is a potent fibrinolytic. It is derived from the bacteria Group C, β-hemolytic streptococci.

Mechanism of Action

Streptokinase acts with plasminogen (present in the blood) to produce a so-called activator complex. This activator complex converts plasminogen to the enzyme plasmin. Plasmin then digests fibrin and fibrinogen, resulting in the dissolution of clots that cause coronary occlusion.

Pharmacokinetics

Onset: <1 hour
Peak Effects: 80 minutes
Duration: 2–36 hours
Half-Life: 83 minutes

Indication

Streptokinase is used for acute coronary syndrome.

Contraindications

Streptokinase is absolutely contraindicated in the following cases:
1. Any prior intracranial hemorrhage.
2. Known structural cerebral vascular lesion (e.g., AVM).
3. Known malignant intracranial neoplasm (primary or metastatic).
4. Ischemic stroke within 3 months EXCEPT acute ischemic stroke within 3 hours.
5. Suspected aortic dissection.
6. Active bleeding or bleeding diathesis (excluding menses).
7. Significant closed head trauma or facial trauma within 3 months.

It is relatively contraindicated (i.e., the risks must be weighed against the potential benefits) in the following cases:
1. History of chronic, severe, poorly controlled hypertension.
2. Severe uncontrolled hypertension on presentation (SBP > 180 mmHg or DBP > 110 mmHg). This could be an absolute contraindication in low-risk patients with myocardial infarction.

3. History of prior ischemic stroke > 3 months, dementia, or known intracranial pathology not covered in contraindications.
4. Traumatic or prolonged (> 10 minutes) CPR or major surgery (< 3 weeks).
5. Recent (within 2 to 4 weeks) internal bleeding.
6. Noncompressible vascular punctures.
7. For streptokinase/anistreplase: prior exposure (> 5 days ago) or prior allergic reaction to these agents.
8. Pregnancy.
9. Active peptic ulcer.
10. Current use of anticoagulants: the higher the Internationalized Normalized Ratio (INR), the higher the risk of bleeding.

Precautions

Streptokinase may be ineffective if administered within 12 months of prior streptokinase or anistreplase therapy. Anaphylaxis can occur with streptokinase therapy. Emergency resuscitative medications and equipment should be immediately available. Reperfusion arrhythmias are common once the occluded artery opens. Antiarrhythmic medications should be immediately available.

Side Effects

Streptokinase can cause bleeding, allergic reactions, anaphylaxis, fever, nausea, and vomiting.

Interactions/Incompatibilities

Streptokinase should be used with caution in patients on anticoagulation therapy.

Dosage

Streptokinase should be administered at 1.5 million units over 1 hour. This is typically part of a streptokinase protocol in which aspirin, an antihistamine, and a corticosteroid are administered before administering streptokinase. The antihistamine and corticosteroid are given to prevent a possible allergic reaction to the medication.

Streptokinase must be reconstituted immediately prior to administration. The manufacturer's recommendations for reconstitution, which accompany the medication, should be followed explicitly. Streptokinase should be administered intravenously, preferably through an IV pump.

℞ Anistreplase (Eminase, Apsac)

Class Fibrinolytic

Description

Anistreplase is a potent fibrinolytic. It is a derivative of the plasminogen-streptokinase activator complex and is derived from the bacteria Group C, β-hemolytic streptococci.

Mechanism of Action

Anistreplase is an inactive derivative that is activated when administered. Plasmin is produced from plasminogen (present in the blood). Plasmin then digests fibrin and fibrinogen, resulting in the dissolution of clots that cause coronary occlusion.

Pharmacokinetics

Onset: Immediate
Peak Effects: 45 minutes
Duration: 6–48 hours
Half-Life: 105–120 minutes

Indication

Anistreplase is used for acute coronary syndrome.

Contraindications

Anistreplase is absolutely contraindicated in the following cases:

1. Any prior intracranial hemorrhage.
2. Known structural cerebral vascular lesion (e.g., AVM).
3. Known malignant intracranial neoplasm (primary or metastatic).
4. Ischemic stroke within 3 months EXCEPT acute ischemic stroke within 3 hours.
5. Suspected aortic dissection.
6. Active bleeding or bleeding diathesis (excluding menses).
7. Significant closed head trauma or facial trauma within 3 months.

It is relatively contraindicated (i.e., the risks must be weighed against the potential benefits) in the following cases:

1. History of chronic, severe, poorly controlled hypertension.
2. Severe uncontrolled hypertension on presentation (SBP > 180 mmHg or DBP > 110 mmHg). This could be an absolute contraindication in low-risk patients with myocardial infarction.
3. History of prior ischemic stroke > 3 months, dementia, or known intracranial pathology not covered in contraindications.
4. Traumatic or prolonged (> 10 minutes) CPR or major surgery (< 3 weeks).
5. Recent (within 2 to 4 weeks) internal bleeding.
6. Noncompressible vascular punctures.
7. For streptokinase/anistreplase: prior exposure (> 5 days ago) or prior allergic reaction to these agents.
8. Pregnancy.
9. Active peptic ulcer.
10. Current use of anticoagulants: the higher the Internationalized Normalized Ratio (INR), the higher the risk of bleeding.

Precautions

Anistreplase may be ineffective if administered within 12 months of prior streptokinase or anistreplase therapy. Anaphylaxis can occur with anistreplase therapy. Emergency resuscitative medications and equipment should be immediately available. Reperfusion arrhythmias are common once the occluded artery opens. Antiarrhythmic medications should be immediately available.

Side Effects

Anistreplase can cause bleeding, allergic reactions, anaphylaxis, fever, nausea, and vomiting.

Interactions/Incompatibilities

Anistreplase should be used with caution in patients on anticoagulation therapy.

Dosage

Anistreplase (30 units) should be injected slowly over 4 to 5 minutes in a one-time dose. This is typically part of an Eminase protocol in which aspirin, an antihistamine, and a corticosteroid are administered before administering anistreplase. The antihistamine and corticosteroid are given to prevent a possible allergic reaction to the medication.

Anistreplase must be reconstituted immediately prior to administration and used within 30 minutes of reconstitution. The manufacturer's recommendations for reconstitution, which accompany the medication, should be followed exactly. When mixing the medication, the paramedic must be careful not to shake it. Instead, it should be gently rolled in the vial to mix it.

Anistreplase should be administered by slow intravenous bolus.

℞ Alteplase, Tissue Plasminogen Activator (Activase)

Class Fibrinolytic

Description

Alteplase (r-tPA) is a potent fibrinolytic. It is a tissue plasminogen activator produced through recombinant DNA technology.

Mechanism of Action

Alteplase is an enzyme that converts plasminogen (present in the blood) to the enzyme plasmin. It also produces a limited amount of fibrinogen in the absence of fibrin. When administered, alteplase binds to the fibrin in a thrombus and converts the plasminogen into plasmin. Plasmin then digests fibrin and fibrinogen, causing the dissolution of clots that cause coronary occlusion.

Pharmacokinetics

Onset: 5–10 minutes
Peak Effects: 5–10 minutes
Duration: Varies
Half-Life: 26.5 minutes

Indication

Alteplase is used for acute coronary syndrome. Alteplase is also approved for the treatment of acute ischemic stroke.

Contraindications

Alteplase is absolutely contraindicated in the following cases:

1. Any prior intracranial hemorrhage.
2. Known structural cerebral vascular lesion (e.g., AVM).

3. Known malignant intracranial neoplasm (primary or metastatic).
4. Ischemic stroke within 3 months EXCEPT acute ischemic stroke within 3 hours.
5. Suspected aortic dissection.
6. Active bleeding or bleeding diathesis (excluding menses).
7. Significant closed head trauma or facial trauma within 3 months.

It is relatively contraindicated (i.e., the risks must be weighed against the potential benefits) in the following cases:

1. History of chronic, severe, poorly controlled hypertension.
2. Severe uncontrolled hypertension on presentation (SBP > 180 mmHg or DBP > 110 mmHg). This could be an absolute contraindication in low-risk patients with myocardial infarction.
3. History of prior ischemic stroke > 3 months, dementia, or known intracranial pathology not covered in contraindications.
4. Traumatic or prolonged (> 10 minutes) CPR or major surgery (< 3 weeks).
5. Recent (within 2 to 4 weeks) internal bleeding.
6. Noncompressible vascular punctures.
7. For streptokinase/anistreplase: prior exposure (> 5 days ago) or prior allergic reaction to these agents.
8. Pregnancy.
9. Active peptic ulcer.
10. Current use of anticoagulants: the higher the Internationalized Normalized Ratio (INR), the higher the risk of bleeding.

Precautions

Alteplase does not appear to have the problem with readministration associated with streptokinase or anistreplase. Anaphylaxis can occur with alteplase therapy but is very rare. Emergency resuscitative medications and equipment should be immediately available. Reperfusion arrhythmias are common once the occluded artery opens. Antiarrhythmic medications should be immediately available.

Side Effects

Alteplase can cause bleeding, allergic reactions, anaphylaxis, fever, nausea, and vomiting.

Interactions/Incompatibilities

Alteplase should be used with caution in patients on anticoagulation therapy.

Dosage

Alteplase should be administered at a total dose of 100 mg. A loading dose of 15 mg is administered as an IV bolus over 1 to 2 minutes. This is followed by an infusion of 0.75 mg/kg (up to 50 mg) IV over the first 30 minutes, then 0.5 mg/kg (up to 35 mg) IV over 60 minutes. The infusion must be carefully administered via a controlled IV pump.

℞ Tenecteplase (TNKase)

Class Fibrinolytic

Description

Tenecteplase (TNKase) is a DNA recombinant human tissue-type plasminogen activator (tPA) that acts as a catalyst in the cleavage of plasminogen to plasmin.

Mechanism of Action

Tenecteplase causes an increase in the formation of plasmin by increasing the conversion of plasminogen to plasmin. It is effective in degrading the fibrin matrix of a clot and is thus an effective fibrinolytic.

Pharmacokinetics

Onset: < 5 minutes
Peak Effects: Varies
Duration: Varies
Half-Life: 20–24 minutes

Indication

Tenecteplase is used for acute coronary syndrome.

Contraindications

Tenecteplase is absolutely contraindicated in the following cases:

1. Any prior intracranial hemorrhage.
2. Known structural cerebral vascular lesion (e.g., AVM).
3. Known malignant intracranial neoplasm (primary or metastatic).
4. Ischemic stroke within 3 months EXCEPT acute ischemic stroke within 3 hours.
5. Suspected aortic dissection.
6. Active bleeding or bleeding diathesis (excluding menses).
7. Significant closed head trauma or facial trauma within 3 months.

It is relatively contraindicated (i.e., the risks must be weighed against the potential benefits) in the following cases:

1. History of chronic, severe, poorly controlled hypertension.
2. Severe uncontrolled hypertension on presentation (SBP > 180 mmHg or DBP > 110 mmHg). This could be an absolute contraindication in low-risk patients with myocardial infarction.
3. History of prior ischemic stroke > 3 months, dementia, or known intracranial pathology not covered in contraindications.
4. Traumatic or prolonged (> 10 minutes) CPR or major surgery (< 3 weeks).
5. Recent (within 2 to 4 weeks) internal bleeding.
6. Noncompressible vascular punctures.
7. For streptokinase/anistreplase: prior exposure (> 5 days ago) or prior allergic reaction to these agents.

8. Pregnancy.
9. Active peptic ulcer.
10. Current use of anticoagulants: the higher the Internationalized Normalized Ratio (INR), the higher the risk of bleeding.

Precautions

Tenecteplase does not appear to have the problems with readministration associated with streptokinase or anistreplase. Emergency resuscitative medications and equipment should be immediately available. Antiarrhythmic medications should be readily available.

Side Effects

Tenecteplase can cause bleeding, allergic reactions, anaphylaxis, fever, nausea, and vomiting.

Interactions/Incompatibilities

None in ACLS setting.

Dosage

Adult dose. Tenecteplase is administered as a single weight-based dose over 5 seconds (it should be reconstituted with 10 mL of sterile water or saline):

Patient Weight (kg)	TNKase (mg)	Volume TNKase to be administered (mL)
< 60 kg	30	6
≥ 60 to < 70	35	7
≥ 70 to < 80	40	8
≥ 80 to < 90	45	9
≥ 90	50	10

Pediatric dose. Not indicated.

℞ Reteplase Recombinant (Retavase)

Class Fibrinolytic

Description

Reteplase is a DNA recombinant human tissue-type plasminogen activator (tPA) that acts as a catalyst in the cleavage of plasminogen to plasmin.

Mechanism of Action

Reteplase causes an increase in the formation of plasmin by increasing the conversion of plasminogen to plasmin. It is effective in degrading the fibrin matrix of a clot and is thus an effective fibrinolytic.

Pharmacokinetics

Onset: < 5 minutes
Peak Effects: Varies
Duration: Varies
Half-Life: 13–16 minutes

Indications

Reteplase is used for acute coronary syndrome.

Contraindications

Reteplase is absolutely contraindicated in the following cases:

1. Any prior intracranial hemorrhage.
2. Known structural cerebral vascular lesion (e.g., AVM).
3. Known malignant intracranial neoplasm (primary or metastatic).
4. Ischemic stroke within 3 months EXCEPT acute ischemic stroke within 3 hours.
5. Suspected aortic dissection.
6. Active bleeding or bleeding diathesis (excluding menses).
7. Significant closed head trauma or facial trauma within 3 months.

It is relatively contraindicated (i.e., the risks must be weighed against the potential benefits) in the following cases:

1. History of chronic, severe, poorly controlled hypertension.
2. Severe uncontrolled hypertension on presentation (SBP > 180 mmHg or DBP > 110 mmHg). This could be an absolute contraindication in low-risk patients with myocardial infarction.
3. History of prior ischemic stroke > 3 months, dementia, or known intracranial pathology not covered in contraindications.
4. Traumatic or prolonged (> 10 minutes) CPR or major surgery (< 3 weeks).
5. Recent (within 2 to 4 weeks) internal bleeding.
6. Noncompressible vascular punctures.
7. For streptokinase/anistreplase: prior exposure (> 5 days ago) or prior allergic reaction to these agents.
8. Pregnancy.
9. Active peptic ulcer.
10. Current use of anticoagulants: the higher the Internationalized Normalized Ratio (INR), the higher the risk of bleeding.

Precautions

Reteplase does not appear to have the problems with readministration associated with streptokinase or anistreplase. Anaphylaxis can occur with reteplase therapy, but it is very rare. Emergency resuscitative drugs and equipment should be immediately available. Antiarrhythmic medications should be readily available.

Side Effects

Reteplase can cause bleeding, allergic reactions, anaphylaxis, fever, nausea, and vomiting.

Interactions/Incompatibilities

None in ACLS setting.

Dosage

Adult dose. 10 units IV over 2 minutes. Repeat 10 units IV (over 2 minutes) in 30 minutes (20 units total dose).

Pediatric dose. Not indicated.

ALKALINIZING AGENTS

Alkalinizing medications, such as sodium bicarbonate, are used to buffer the acids present in the body during and after cardiac arrest and other serious conditions. Normal body pH is 7.4 (7.35 to 7.45). During hypoxia, the serum pH may fall quickly. Sodium bicarbonate will help correct metabolic (usually lactic acid) acidosis until hypoxia is corrected. The following reaction illustrates the role of sodium bicarbonate in acid–base balance:

Bicarbonate combines with the strong acids, usually lactic acid, and forms a weak, volatile acid (carbonic acid). This acid then is broken down into carbon dioxide and water. The two end products are then removed via the lungs and the kidneys, respectively.

Excessive administration of sodium bicarbonate may cause metabolic alkalosis, which may be worse than the metabolic acidosis being treated. Primary treatment of metabolic acidosis in the setting of hypoxia or cardiac arrest includes adequate oxygenation and blood pressure support.

 Sodium Bicarbonate

Class Alkalinizing agent

Description

Sodium bicarbonate is a salt that provides bicarbonate to buffer metabolic acidosis, which can accompany several disease processes.

Mechanism of Action

For many years sodium bicarbonate was the cornerstone of ACLS care. Controlled studies have shown that sodium bicarbonate was ineffective in the treatment of cardiac arrest. In many instances it has actually been associated with many adverse reactions. Sodium bicarbonate is occasionally used in the treatment of certain types of medication overdose. The most common example is medications in the tricyclic class of antidepressants. Overdosage of these medications has serious effects including life-threatening cardiac arrhythmias. TCA excretion from the body is enhanced by making the urine more alkaline (raising the pH). Sodium bicarbonate is sometimes administered to increase the pH of the urine to speed excretion of the medication from the body.

Pharmacokinetics

Onset: Immediate

Peak Effects: < 15 minutes

Duration: 1–2 hours

Half-Life: Not applicable

Indications

Sodium bicarbonate is rarely used in the prehospital setting and not recommended for cardiac arrest. Sodium bicarbonate is sometimes used in selected poisonings and overdoses.

Contraindications

When used in the management of the situations described earlier, there are no absolute contraindications.

Precautions

Sodium bicarbonate can cause metabolic alkalosis when administered in large quantities. It is important to calculate the dosage based on patient weight and size.

Side Effects

There are few side effects when sodium bicarbonate is used in the emergency setting.

Interactions/Incompatibilities

Most catecholamines and vasopressors (e.g., dopamine and epinephrine) can be deactivated by alkaline solutions such as sodium bicarbonate. Sodium bicarbonate should not be administered in conjunction with calcium chloride. A precipitate can form, which may clog the IV line.

Dosage

The usual dose of sodium bicarbonate is 1 mEq/kg body weight initially followed by 0.5 mEq/kg of body weight every 10 minutes. When possible, the dosage of sodium bicarbonate should be based on the results of arterial blood gas studies. Sodium bicarbonate should be administered only as an IV bolus.

CARDIAC PAIN MANAGEMENT (ANALGESICS)

Medications that have proved to be effective in alleviating pain are referred to as analgesics. Although they may be administered in many different types of emergencies, they are used most often for the treatment of emergencies involving the cardiovascular system, especially myocardial infarction. Additional analgesics are covered in detail in Chapter 15. This section covers morphine and nitrous oxide.

Morphine is derived from the opium plant. It has impressive analgesic and hemodynamic effects. Nitronox, a 50 percent mixture of oxygen and nitrous oxide that can be easily inhaled by the patient, is entirely different from the other analgesic agents discussed. Its analgesic effects are also very potent yet disappear within a few minutes after the cessation of administration. Thus, Nitronox can be given for many types of pain in the field without fear of impairing subsequent physical examination in the emergency department. In addition to its analgesic effects, Nitronox delivers oxygen to the patient, which makes it useful in cardiac emergencies.

Class Narcotic analgesic

Description

Morphine is a central nervous system depressant and a potent analgesic. It is commonly used in emergency medicine and EMS.

Mechanism of Action

Morphine sulfate is a central nervous system depressant that acts on opiate receptors in the brain, providing both analgesia and sedation. It increases peripheral venous capacitance and decreases venous return. Morphine also decreases myocardial oxygen demand. This action is due to both the decreased systemic vascular resistance and the sedative effects of the medication. Patient apprehension and fear can significantly increase myocardial oxygen demand and in some cases can conceivably increase the size of myocardial infarction.

Pharmacokinetics

Onset: Immediate (IV), 15–30 minutes (IM)
Peak Effects: 20 minutes (IV), 30–60 minutes (IM)
Duration: 2–7 hours
Half-Life: 1–7 hours

Indications

Morphine is used for severe pain associated with myocardial infarction, kidney stones, and so forth. Its use in pulmonary edema and congestive heart failure has been limited in favor of more vasoactive agents (e.g., nitroglycerin, ACE inhibitors).

Contraindications

Morphine should not be used in patients who are volume depleted or severely hypotensive because of the hemodynamic effects described earlier. Morphine should not be administered to any patient with a history of hypersensitivity to the medication or to patients with undiagnosed head injury or abdominal pain.

Precautions

Morphine is a narcotic derivative of opium. It has a high tendency for addiction and abuse and is thus covered under the Controlled Substances Act of 1970. It is classified as a Schedule II medication. Consequently, there are special considerations involved in the handling of the medication. Morphine causes severe respiratory depression in high doses. This is especially true in patients who already have some form of respiratory impairment. The narcotic antagonist naloxone (Narcan) should be readily available whenever morphine is administered.

Side Effects

Morphine can cause nausea, vomiting, abdominal cramps, blurred vision, constricted pupils, altered mental status, headache, and respiratory depression.

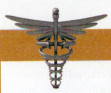

At 1300 hours an ALS unit is dispatched to a mobile home park to aid a 61-year-old male complaining of chest pain. The patient is conscious and breathing.

On arrival paramedics are met at the door by the patient's wife. She states that she and her husband had attended church. During the service, he began to feel short of breath. She noticed that he was sweating heavily and appeared pale. She drove him home. The patient took two nitroglycerin sprays (0.4 mg) with no relief. Initially, he would not let her call the ambulance. Finally, he agreed that she could call the ambulance.

As paramedics approach the patient, they see a man sitting in a reclining chair. The patient appears in obvious distress.

Physical Examination

CNS:	The patient is conscious, alert, and oriented $\times$ 4; appears in obvious distress
Resp:	Respirations are 24 and shallow; lung sounds clear bilaterally; trachea is midline; no signs of trauma
CVS:	Carotid and radial pulses are present and weak; skin is pale, cool, and diaphoretic
ABD:	Soft and nontender
Muscl/Skel:	Patient able to move extremities on command; no weaknesses to hand grip

Vital Signs

Pulse:		96/min, regular, weak
Resp:		24/min, shallow
BP:		144/94 mmHg
SpO$_2$:		88 percent
ECG:		Regular sinus rhythm with ST elevation
Hx:	**P**	No provoking factors
	Q	Squeezing pain
	R	Radiating to left shoulder and jaw
	S	8/10, worst pain ever
	T	Started suddenly about 2 hours ago
Past Hx:		The patient's wife states that her husband has had several episodes of chest pain in the past month but has not seen his doctor during that time. He was diagnosed with angina 2 years ago. He has nitroglycerin spray, which he has used more often this month than ever in the past. Nitroglycerin is the patient's only prescription home medication. The patient has no recent history of operations, ulcers, or hypertension.

Treatment

Oxygen was administered via a nasal cannula at 2 lpm and tolerated by the patient. The patient was hooked up to the ECG monitor, and a regular sinus rhythm with ST elevation was noted. The ST elevation was confirmed in MCL leads 1 and 6. An intravenous line with an 18-gauge catheter was established and run TKO. Paramedics administered nitroglycerin spray (0.4 mg) from their medication kit. The patient stated that the pain

(continued)

Case Presentation (continued)

was not relieved by the oxygen or the nitroglycerin. The base hospital ordered 2.5 mg of morphine IV. The morphine was given, and transport to the hospital was started. En route the patient stated that the chest pain was 6/10 and a second dose of 2.5 mg of morphine was given, with moderate relief. A second 18-gauge IV was started and run TKO. ASA 325 mg was given by mouth. The patient stated the pain was now 2/10. He was pale, cool, and diaphoretic but appeared less anxious. The base hospital was contacted and advised of the patient findings. The base hospital physician agreed with the findings of the paramedics and prepared to follow through with the fibrinolytic protocol on the patient's arrival at the hospital pending evaluation of a 12-lead ECG.

Interactions/Incompatibilities

The CNS depression associated with morphine can be enhanced when administered with antihistamines, antiemetics, sedatives, hypnotics, barbiturates, and alcohol.

Dosage

There are many different approaches to the administration of morphine. An initial dose in the range of 2 to 10 mg intravenously is standard. This dose can be augmented with additional doses of 2 mg every few minutes and can be continued until the pain is relieved or until signs of respiratory depression occur.

To attain desired effects, IM injection usually requires 5 to 15 mg based on the patient's weight. However, morphine is routinely given intravenously in emergency medicine and is often administered with an antiemetic agent such as promethazine (Phenergan) to help prevent the nausea and vomiting that often accompany morphine administration. The antiemetics also tend to potentiate morphine's effects. Morphine can also be given intramuscularly and subcutaneously.

℞ Nitrous Oxide (Nitronox, Entonox)

Class Analgesic and anesthetic gas

Description

Nitronox is a blended mixture of 50 percent nitrous oxide and 50 percent oxygen that has potent analgesic effects. The Entonox unit consists of one tank that contains both nitrous oxide and oxygen. The Entonox tank must be shaken to mix the gases prior to use.

Mechanism of Action

Nitrous oxide is a CNS depressant with analgesic properties. In the prehospital setting it is delivered in a fixed mixture of 50 percent nitrous oxide and 50 percent oxygen. When inhaled, it has potent analgesic effects. These effects quickly dissipate, however, within 2 to 5 minutes after cessation of administration. The Nitronox unit consists of one oxygen and one nitrous oxide cylinder. The gases are fed into a blender that combines them at the appropriate concentration. The mixture is then delivered to a modified demand valve for administration to the patient. Nitronox must be self-administered. It is effective in treating many varieties of pain encountered in the prehospital setting including pain from many types of trauma. The high concentration of oxygen delivered along with the nitrous oxide will increase the oxygen tension in the blood, thus reducing hypoxia.

Pharmacokinetics

Onset: 2–5 minutes
Peak Effect: 205 minutes
Duration: 2–5 minutes
Half-Life: Unknown

Indications

Nitrous oxide is used for pain of musculoskeletal origin (particularly fractures), burns, suspected ischemic chest pain, and states of severe anxiety including hyperventilation.

Contraindications

Nitronox should not be used with any patient who cannot comprehend verbal instructions or who is intoxicated with alcohol or other medications. It should not be administered to any patient with a head injury who exhibits an altered mental status. Nitronox should not be administered to any patient with COPD because the high concentration of oxygen (50 percent) might result in respiratory depression. Nitrous oxide tends to diffuse into closed spaces more readily than either carbon dioxide or oxygen. Many COPD patients have air-containing blebs in their lungs, and nitrous oxide can concentrate in these blebs causing them to swell. Swollen blebs may rupture, causing a pneumothorax.

Nitronox should not be administered to patients with a thoracic injury suspicious of pneumothorax, because the gas may accumulate in the pneumothorax, increasing its size. Also, patients with severe abdominal pain and distension, suggestive of bowel obstruction, should not receive Nitronox. Nitrous oxide can concentrate in pockets of an obstructed bowel, possibly leading to rupture.

Precautions

Nitronox should only be used in areas that are well ventilated. When the gas is used in the patient compartment of an ambulance, it is recommended that a scavenging system be in place. Nitrous oxide exists in a liquid state inside the gas cylinder. Heat present in the air, the cylinder wall, or the various regulators and lines causes the liquid to vaporize. This vaporization process makes the cylinder tank and lines cool to touch. Following prolonged use, frost may develop on the cylinder, regulator, or lines. In very cold environments, generally less than 21°F (6°C), the liquid may be slow to vaporize, and administration may be impossible.

Side Effects

The nitrous oxide–oxygen mixture can cause dizziness, light-headedness, altered mental status, hallucinations, nausea, and vomiting.

Interactions/Incompatibilities

Nitrous oxide can potentiate the effects of other central nervous system depressants such as narcotics, sedatives, hypnotics, and alcohol.

Dosage

Nitronox should only be self-administered. Continuous administration may take place until the pain is significantly relieved or the patient drops the mask. The patient care record should document the duration of medication administration.

DIURETICS

One of the most common cardiovascular emergencies that emergency personnel are called on to treat is congestive heart failure. Congestive heart failure occurs when the heart loses its ability to pump blood effectively. When this occurs, the venous vessels leading to the heart become engorged. Failure of the left side of the heart causes a buildup of blood in the pulmonary circulation. Failure of the right side of the heart results in congestion of the peripheral circulation, which usually manifests as peripheral edema. Common signs of right heart failure include jugular venous distension, ascites, and pedal (ankle or pretibial) edema.

In the treatment of congestive heart failure, the primary objectives are to increase the cardiac output and to reduce pulmonary and peripheral edema. Although the inotropic effects of digitalis preparations will increase cardiac output, the rate of onset is relatively slow, making this medication less than ideal in acute pulmonary edema. In acute heart failure the most effective therapy is to reduce venous filling pressure. Venous filling pressure can be reduced mechanically by applying rotating tourniquets, which are placed on three of the extremities to decrease venous return. Phlebotomy (drawing blood out of the circulatory system) can also be employed. Although the role of diuretics in the treatment of acute congestive heart failure diminished, they still are important emergency medications.

℞ Furosemide (Lasix)

Class Diuretic

Description

Furosemide is a potent diuretic that inhibits sodium and chloride reabsorption in the kidneys and causes venous dilation.

Mechanism of Action

Furosemide is a loop diuretic that inhibits the reabsorption of both sodium and chloride in the kidneys. It is extremely useful in the treatment of congestive heart failure and pulmonary edema. The effects of furosemide are twofold. First, following administration furosemide causes venous dilation. This effect usually occurs within 5 minutes and causes a reduction in preload, thus decreasing cardiac work. The second effect of furosemide is the diuretic effect, which begins 5 to 15 minutes after administration.

Pharmacokinetics

Onset: 5–10 minutes (vasodilation), 5–30 minutes (diuresis)
Peak Effects: 30 minutes (vasodilation), 20–60 minutes (diuresis)

Duration: 2 hours (vasodilation), 6 hours (diuresis)
Half-Life: 30 minutes

Indications

Furosemide is used as an adjunct to nitroglycerin and ACE inhibitors in congestive heart failure and pulmonary edema.

Contraindications

Usage in pregnancy should be limited to life-threatening situations in which the benefits of furosemide outweigh the risks. Furosemide has been known to cause fetal abnormalities. It should not be administered to patients with a known allergy to the sulfa class of medications.

Precautions

Dehydration, electrolyte depletion, and hypotension can result from excessive doses of potent diuretics. Thus, blood pressure should be frequently monitored when furosemide is administered. Furosemide should be protected from light.

Side Effects

Furosemide can cause headache, dizziness, hypotension, volume depletion, potassium depletion, arrhythmias, diarrhea, nausea, and vomiting.

Interactions/Incompatibilities

Furosemide should not be administered in the same line as inamrinone (Inocor) because a chemical reaction can occur between the two, causing the formation of a precipitate in the intravenous line. Administration of furosemide with other diuretics can lead to severe volume depletion and electrolyte imbalance.

Dosage

The standard dosage of furosemide is 40 mg given by slow IV push in patients already on chronic oral furosemide therapy and 20 mg intravenously in patients who are not taking the medication orally on a regular basis. Dosages as high as 80 to 120 mg intravenously may be indicated in severe cases. Furosemide should be given intravenously in emergency situations.

℞ Bumetanide (Bumex)

Class Diuretic

Description

Bumetanide is a potent diuretic with a rapid rate of onset and a short duration of action.

Mechanism of Action

Like furosemide, bumetanide is a loop diuretic that inhibits the reabsorption of sodium chloride in the kidneys and thus causes a net diuresis; 1 mg of bumetanide has the diuretic potency of 40 mg of furosemide.

Pharmacokinetics

Onset: 1–2 minutes
Peak Effects: 15–30 minutes
Duration: 3.5–4.0 hours
Half-Life: 60–90 minutes

Indications

Bumetanide is used as an adjunct to nitroglycerin and ACE inhibitors in congestive heart failure and pulmonary edema.

Contraindications

Usage in pregnancy should be limited to life-threatening situations in which the benefits of using bumetanide outweigh the risks.

Precautions

Dehydration and electrolyte depletion can result from excessive doses of potent diuretics. Patients who have experienced allergic reactions to furosemide have not experienced those same reactions when administered bumetanide, which suggests that this medication may be used in patients with furosemide allergy who are in need of rapid diuresis.

Side Effects

Bumetanide can cause muscle cramps, dizziness, hypotension, headache, nausea, and vomiting.

Interactions/Incompatibilities

Bumetanide can potentiate the effects of the various antihypertensive agents and should be used with caution in patients taking these agents.

Dosage

The usual initial dose of bumetanide is 0.5 to 1.0 mg given during a period of 1 to 2 minutes. A second or third dose can be administered at 2- to 3-hour intervals if required. The total daily dosage should not exceed 10 mg. Bumetanide injection can be given by either the IV or intramuscular route. In the emergency setting, the IV route is preferred.

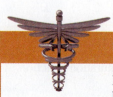

CASE PRESENTATION

Paramedics are called at 0800 hours to a residence to help a woman having difficulty breathing. Dispatch states that the woman is conscious and breathing. On arrival paramedics find a 71-year-old female sitting in a recliner in the living room. She is in severe respiratory distress. Paramedics immediately place the chair into the upright position.

Physical Examination

CNS: The patient is conscious, alert, and oriented × 4; appears in obvious respiratory distress and is very restless

Resp: Respirations are 40 and shallow; lung sounds are diminished bilaterally with loud crackles audible; two- to three-word dyspnea; trachea is midline; no signs of trauma

CVS: Carotid and radial pulses are weak and regular; skin is pale, lips are blue, and the patient is cool and diaphoretic to touch

ABD: Soft and nontender

Muscl/Skel: Patient able to move extremities on command; no weaknesses to hand grip

Vital Signs

Pulse: 120/min, regular, weak

Resp: 40/min, shallow, bilateral loud crackles

BP: 180/108 mmHg

SpO$_2$: 80 percent

ECG: Sinus tachycardia

Hx: The patient's husband states that his wife has been complaining of mild SOB for the past 2 days. She has not been able to lie down to sleep because it increases the difficulty of breathing. Therefore she has been sitting in the recliner to sleep. This morning her breathing is worse. She is having difficulty speaking now. He was not sure what to do and finally called the ambulance.

Past Hx: The patient has a history of congestive heart failure and is currently taking Lasix 20 mg twice per day, Slo-K (potassium), and digoxin.

Treatment

Oxygen was administered by non-rebreather mask at 15 lpm and not well tolerated by the patient. An IV of normal saline was initiated and run TKO. The patient was hooked up to the ECG monitor, and a sinus tachycardia was noted. Nitroglycerin spray was administered, with no relief. The nitroglycerin spray was administered two more times with a slight improvement in symptoms. Following the nitrospray, paramedics applied a continuous positive airway pressure (CPAP) mask and began CPAP therapy at 5 cm/H$_2$O. The patient's signs and symptoms continued to improve and the SpO$_2$ increased to 91%. Paramedics administered 40 mg of Lasix (double the patient's home daily dose of Lasix as per their standing orders). At the hospital the patient was started on intravenous nitroglycerin and lisinopril (an ACE inhibitor) with significant improvement.

NATRIURETIC PEPTIDES

Natriuretic peptides are a group of naturally occurring substances that counteract the effects of the renin–angiotensin system. Thus, they cause vasodilation, stimulating the kidneys to increase sodium excretion (natriuresis) and water loss. They appear to be effective in the management of congestive heart failure because they decrease preload and promote sodium and water loss.

Three types of natriuretic peptides have been identified:

- *Atrial natriuretic peptide (ANP).* ANP is produced in the atria. The identification of ANP was the first indication that the heart also has some endocrine functions.
- *Brain natriuretic peptide (BNP).* BNP is synthesized in the ventricles but named BNP as is was first identified in the porcine brain.
- *C-type natriuretic peptide (CNP).* CNP is produced in the brain.

Both ANP and BNP are released in response to atrial and ventricular stretch, respectively. They cause vasorelaxation, inhibition of aldosterone secretion in the adrenal cortex, and inhibition of renin secretion in the kidney. Both ANP and BNP will cause natriuresis and a reduction in intravascular volume. These effects are amplified by antagonism of antidiuretic hormone (ADH). The physiological effects of CNP are different from those of ANP and BNP. CNP has a hypotensive effect, but no significant diuretic or natriuretic actions.

℞ Nesiritide (Natrecor)

Class Natriuretic peptide

Description

Nesiritide is a genetically engineered form of a naturally occurring substance called B-type (brain) natriuretic peptide (hBPN). It represents a new class of medications.

Mechanism of Action

Nesiritide causes vasodilation through relaxation of vascular smooth muscle. It also causes diuresis and loss of sodium in the kidney (natriuretic effect).

Pharmacokinetics

Onset: 15 minutes
Peak Effects: Varies
Duration: > 60 hours (dose related)
Half-Life: 18 minutes

Indications

Nesiritide is used for the treatment of acutely decompensated congestive heart failure (CHF) in patients who have dyspnea at rest or with minimal physical activity.

Contraindications

Nesiritide should not be administered to people with known hypersensitivity to the medication. It should not be used in patients who have a blood pressure of <90 mmHg and cardiogenic shock. It should not be used in patients with CHF secondary to valvular heart disease.

Precautions

Use with caution in patients receiving angiotensin-converting enzyme inhibitors. Safety in pediatrics and pregnancy has not been established. All physiological monitors should be in place prior to administering nesiritide.

Side Effects

Nesiritide has been associated with headaches, back pain, catheter pain, fever, injection site pain, and leg cramps. Hypotension has been reported as well as arrhythmias.

Interactions/Incompatibilities

None reported.

Dosage

Adult dose. Initial bolus of 2 mcg/kg over 60 seconds followed by continuous infusion of 0.01 mcg/kg/min. Maximum dose is 0.03 mcg/kg/min. Blood pressure must be constantly monitored.

Pediatric dose. Not indicated.

ANTIANGINAL AGENTS

A common manifestation of advanced cardiovascular disease is angina pectoris, which results from a narrowing of the coronary arteries due to the buildup of atherosclerotic plaques, or coronary artery vasospasm. In exercise and other stressful situations, the amount of blood that can be carried by the coronary arteries may not be sufficient to meet the oxygen demands of the myocardium. This results in myocardial hypoxia, causing the classic pain syndrome called angina pectoris. Sublingual nitroglycerin usually gives immediate relief by dilating the coronary arteries and decreasing cardiac work. In recent years there have been trials in which nitroglycerin has been administered to patients suffering myocardial infarction in the hope of decreasing the extent of myocardial damage. Nitroglycerin is often administered to patients complaining of chest pain to rule out angina as the cause. When cardiac pain is not relieved by nitroglycerin, morphine and other potent analgesics are administered.

Nitroglycerin is usually administered sublingually (SL) or topically. Recently, however, it has been given intravenously in certain cases of unstable angina and STEMI.

Calcium-ion *antagonists,* such as nifedipine (Procardia), diltiazem Cardizem), have proved effective in the management of angina, especially when there is coronary artery vasospasm.

℞ Nitroglycerin (Nitrostat)

Class Nitrate

Description

Nitroglycerin is a potent smooth muscle relaxant used in the treatment of angina pectoris.

Mechanism of Action

Nitroglycerin is a rapid smooth muscle relaxant that reduces cardiac work and, to a lesser degree, dilates the coronary arteries. This results in increased coronary blood flow and improved perfusion of the ischemic myocardium. Relief of ischemia causes reduction and alleviation of chest pain. Pain relief following nitroglycerin administration usually occurs within 1 to 2 minutes, and therapeutic effects can be observed up to 30 minutes later. Nitroglycerin also causes vasodilation, which decreases preload; decreased preload leads to decreased ventricular filling, which leads to reduced oxygen demand.

Pharmacokinetics

Onset: 1–3 minutes (SL)

Peak Effects: 5–10 minutes (SL)

Duration: 20–30 minutes (SL)

Half-Life: 1–4 minutes

Indications

Nitroglycerin is used for chest pain associated with acute coronary syndrome and acute pulmonary edema (unless accompanied by hypotension). It is also a first-line therapy for acute congestive heart failure.

Contraindications

Nitroglycerin is contraindicated in patients who are hypotensive or who may have increased intracranial pressure. It should not be administered to patients in shock.

Precautions

Patients taking nitroglycerin may develop a tolerance for the medication, which necessitates increasing the dose. Headache is a common side effect of nitroglycerin administration and results from vasodilation of cerebral vessels. Nitroglycerin deteriorates quite rapidly once the bottle is opened. When a bottle of nitroglycerin is opened, it should be dated. Nitroglycerin should also be protected from light. Blood pressure and the other vital signs should always be monitored during nitroglycerin administration.

Side Effects

Nitroglycerin can cause headache, dizziness, weakness, tachycardia, hypotension, orthostasis, skin rash, dry mouth, nausea, and vomiting.

Interactions/Incompatibilities

Nitroglycerin can cause severe hypotension when administered to patients who have recently ingested alcohol. It can cause orthostatic hypotension when used in conjunction with beta-blockers.

Dosage

One tablet (0.4 mg) is administered sublingually for routine chest pain. This dose can be repeated in 3 to 5 minutes as required. Usually, more than three tablets should not be administered in the prehospital setting. Nitroglycerin should be administered sublingually. Care should be taken to ensure that it is not swallowed. IV nitroglycerin is used in the emergency department and intensive care units, but the sublingual route is adequate for most prehospital situations. Nitroglycerin is also available in patches and in ointment form for transdermal administration.

℞ Nitroglycerin Paste

Class Nitrate

Description

Nitroglycerin paste contains a 2 percent solution of nitroglycerin in a special absorbent paste. When placed on the skin, nitroglycerin is absorbed into the systemic circulation. In many cases it may be preferred over nitroglycerin tablets because of its longer duration of action.

Pharmacokinetics

Onset: 30 minutes (topical)
Peak Effects: Varies
Duration: 3–6 hours (topical)
Half-Life: 1–4 minutes

Mechanism of Action

Nitroglycerin is a rapid smooth muscle relaxant that reduces cardiac work and, to a lesser degree, dilates the coronary arteries. This results in increased coronary blood flow and improved perfusion of the ischemic myocardium. Relief of ischemia causes reduction and alleviation of chest pain. Pain relief following transcutaneous nitroglycerin administration usually occurs within 5 to 10 minutes, and therapeutic effects can be observed up to 30 minutes later. Nitroglycerin also causes vasodilation, which decreases preload; decreased preload leads to decreased cardiac work. This feature, in conjunction with coronary vasodilation, reverses the effects of angina pectoris. It is also a first-line therapy for acute congestive heart failure.

Indications

Nitroglycerin paste is used for chest pain associated with angina pectoris and chest pain associated with acute myocardial infarction.

Contraindications

Nitroglycerin paste is contraindicated in patients with increased intracranial pressure. It should not be administered to patients who are hypotensive or in shock.

Precautions

Patients taking the medication routinely may develop a tolerance and require an increased dose. Headache is a common side effect of nitroglycerin administration and occurs as a result of vasodilation of the cerebral vessels.

Postural syncope sometimes occurs following the administration of nitroglycerin; it should be anticipated and the patient kept supine when possible. It is important to monitor blood pressure constantly.

Side Effects

Nitroglycerin can cause headache, dizziness, weakness, tachycardia, hypotension, orthostasis, skin rash, dry mouth, nausea, and vomiting.

Interactions/Incompatibilities

Nitroglycerin can cause severe hypotension when administered to patients who have recently ingested alcohol. It can cause orthostatic hypotension when used in conjunction with beta-blockers.

Dosage

Generally 1/2 to 1 inch (1.25 to 2.50 cm) of the Nitro-Bid Ointment is applied. Measuring applicators are supplied.

℞ Nitroglycerin Spray

Class Nitrate

Description

Nitroglycerin spray is a special preparation of nitroglycerin in an aerosol form that delivers precisely 0.4 mg of nitroglycerin per spray.

Mechanism of Action

Nitroglycerin is a rapid smooth muscle relaxant that reduces cardiac work and, to a lesser degree, dilates the coronary arteries. This results in increased coronary blood flow and improved perfusion of the ischemic myocardium. Relief of ischemia causes reduction and alleviation of chest pain. Pain relief following nitroglycerin administration usually occurs within 1 to 2 minutes, and peak effects occur within 4 minutes. Therapeutic effects can be observed up to 30 minutes later. Nitroglycerin also causes vasodilation, which decreases preload; decreased preload leads to decreased cardiac work. This feature, in conjunction with coronary vasodilation, reverses the effects of angina pectoris.

Pharmacokinetics

Onset: 1–3 minutes (SL)
Peak Effects: 5–10 minutes (SL)
Duration: 20–30 minutes (SL)
Half-Life: 1–4 minutes

Indications

Nitroglycerin spray is used for chest pain associated with angina pectoris and chest pain associated with acute myocardial infarction. It is also a first-line therapy for acute congestive heart failure.

Contraindications

Nitroglycerin is contraindicated in patients who are hypotensive, who are in shock, or who may have increased intracranial pressure.

Precautions

Patients taking nitroglycerin routinely may develop a tolerance for the medication. Headache is a common side effect of nitroglycerin administration and results from dilation of cerebral blood vessels. This effect should be anticipated. The blood pressure should be monitored during nitroglycerin therapy.

Side Effects

Nitroglycerin can cause headache, dizziness, weakness, tachycardia, hypotension, orthostasis, skin rash, dry mouth, nausea, and vomiting.

Interactions/Incompatibilities

Nitroglycerin can cause severe hypotension when administered to patients who have recently ingested alcohol. It can cause orthostatic hypotension when used in conjunction with beta-blockers.

Dosage

One spray (0.4 mg) should be sprayed under the tongue at the onset of an attack of angina. No more than three sprays are recommended in a 25-minute period. (The spray should not be inhaled.) Nitroglycerin spray should be applied to the sublingual mucous membranes in the manner described earlier for nitroglycerin tablets (Nitrostat).

℞ Nitroglycerin Infusion (Tridil)

Class Nitrate

Description

Nitroglycerin infusion is a preparation of nitroglycerin that can be administered parenterally.

Mechanism of Action

Nitroglycerin is an antianginal/cardiac workload–reducing agent. It appears to reduce myocardial oxygen demand due to a reduction in left ventricular preload and afterload because of venous and arterial dilation (venous vasodiliation is more pronounced). Nitroglycerin causes a more efficient redistribution of blood flow within the myocardium.

Pharmacokinetics

Onset: Immediate
Peak Effects: 1–2 minutes
Duration: 3–5 minutes
Half-Life: 1–4 minutes

Indications

Nitroglycerin infusion is used in the treatment of angina, hypertensive emergencies, and as a treatment adjunct in acute coronary syndrome. Nitrates play a major role in the management of acute congestive heart failure.

Contraindications

Nitroglycerin is contraindicated in patients who are hypotensive, who are in shock, or who may have increased intracranial pressure.

Precautions

Patients taking nitroglycerin routinely may develop a tolerance for the medication. Headache is a common side effect of nitroglycerin administration and results from dilation of cerebral blood vessels. This effect should be anticipated. Nitroglycerin infusion can cause a significant drop in blood pressure. Because of this, the blood pressure should be continuously monitored during nitroglycerin therapy. Nitroglycerin infusion should only be administered via an infusion pump.

Side Effects

Nitroglycerin can cause headache, dizziness, weakness, tachycardia, hypotension, orthostasis, skin rash, dry mouth, nausea, and vomiting.

Interactions/Incompatibilities

Nitroglycerin can cause severe hypotension when administered to patients who have recently ingested alcohol. It can cause orthostatic hypotension when used in conjunction with beta-blockers.

Dosage

Infuse 5 mcg/minute by intravenous route and titrate to effect by 5 mcg/min every 3–5 minutes up to 20 mcg/min. Then, titrate by 10–20 mcg/min.

ANTIHYPERTENSIVES

A dangerously elevated blood pressure is a hypertensive emergency. Hypertension is a chronic disease. Generally speaking, it is not recommended that parenteral medications be administered to lower the blood pressure. Suddenly lowering the blood pressure can lead to stroke, cardiac ischemia, and similar problems. That said, there are selected instances, although rare, when parenteral medications should be administered to lower the blood pressure. The primary indication is a *hypertensive emergency*. Hypertensive emergencies are characterized by severe elevations in BP ($>$ 180/120 mmHg) complicated by evidence of impending or progressive target organ dysfunction. They require immediate BP reduction (not necessarily to normal) to prevent or limit target organ damage. Examples of hypertensive emergencies include hypertensive encephalopathy, intracerebral hemorrhage, acute myocardial infarction, acute left ventricular failure with pulmonary edema, unstable angina pectoris, dissecting aortic aneurysm, or eclampsia. The initial goal of therapy in hypertensive emergencies is to reduce mean arterial BP by no more than 25% (within minutes to 1 hour), then, if stable, to 160/100 to 110 mmHg within the next 2 to 6 hours. Excessive falls in pressure that may precipitate renal, cerebral, or coronary ischemia should be avoided.

Hypertensive urgencies are those situations associated with severe elevations in BP without progressive target organ dysfunction. Examples include upper levels of stage II hypertension associated with severe headache, shortness of breath, epistaxis, or severe anxiety. The majority of these patients present as noncompliant or inadequately treated hypertensives, often with little or no evidence of target organ damage. Some patients with hypertensive urgencies may benefit from treatment with an oral, short-acting agent such as captopril, labetalol, or clonidine followed by several hours of observation. However, there is no evidence to suggest that failure to aggressively lower BP in the prehospital setting or the emergency department is associated with any increased short-term risk to the patient who presents with severe hypertension.

Several different classes of drugs can be used for hypertensive emergencies. These include the calcium channel blockers (e.g., nicardipine, clevidipine), beta-blockers (e.g., labetalol, esmolol), the angiotensin-converting enzyme (ACE) inhibitors (e.g., enalaprilat, captopril), and direct vasodilators (e.g., sodium nitroprusside, hydralazine).

In summary, hypertension is a chronic disease. An elevated blood pressure is not uncommon in the emergency setting. Elevated blood pressure should only be treated if there are significant end-organ changes (i.e., altered mental status). In cases where the blood pressure must be lowered, labetalol, sodium nitroprusside, or other similar agents should be used. In addition to the medications discussed here, several of the beta-blockers discussed earlier in this chapter can be used for the treatment of hypertensive emergencies. The medication should be initiated at a low dose and increased until the blood pressure is controlled. Nifedipine (Procardia) was used for many years in the acute treatment of hypertensive emergencies. However, complications (i.e., stroke) were reported and the popular press published several articles on the adverse effects of nifedipine. Because of this, it is no longer used in this setting.

Calcium Channel Blockers

The following medications block the slow calcium channels in muscle cells thus decreasing intracellular calcium. This leads to a reduction in muscle contraction in the heart and blood vessels. The cardiac effects include a decrease in calcium available for each beat and results in a subsequent decrease myocardial contractility (which makes them effective in angina). Calcium channel blockers also affect the smooth muscles that encircle the blood vessels (arteries primarily). Here, a decrease in calcium results in less contraction of the vascular smooth muscle and an increase in arterial diameter (vasodilation). This vasodilation decreases peripheral vascular resistance, while a decrease in cardiac contractility decreases cardiac output. As blood pressure is a function of cardiac output and peripheral vascular resistance, blood pressure drops following administration of these agents.

℞ Nicardipine (Cardene)

Class Calcium channel blocker

Description

Nicardipine is a calcium channel blocker that is highly selective for vascular smooth muscle and used in the treatment of severe hypertension.

Mechanism of Action

Nicardipine causes relaxation of the smooth muscles that encircle the peripheral blood vessels, principally the arterioles. This relaxation results in peripheral vasodilation, a decrease in peripheral vascular resistance, and a decrease in both the systolic and diastolic blood pressure. Nicardipine has less effect on cardiac muscle than other calcium channel blockers.

Pharmacokinetics

Onset: 5–10 minutes (IV)

Peak Effects: 10–20 minutes (IV)

Duration: 15–30 minutes (can exceed 4 hours)

Half-Life: 34 minutes

Indications

Nicardipine is used in the treatment of hypertensive emergency.

Contraindications

Nicardipine is contraindicated in patients with known hypersensitivity to the medication. It should not be administered to patients who are hypotensive.

Precautions

Nicardipine can cause a significant drop in blood pressure. Thus, blood pressure should be frequently monitored. Nicardipine should be used with caution in patients with heart failure. It should not be administered to patients receiving IV β-blockers.

Side Effects

Nicardipine can cause nausea, vomiting, dizziness, headache, bradycardia, heart block, hypotension, and asystole.

Interactions/Incompatibilities

Nicardipine should not be administered to patients receiving intravenous β-blockers because of an increased risk of congestive heart failure, bradycardia, and asystole. It should be administered with caution to patients receiving intravenous cimetidine.

Dosage

Nicardipine, administered via an infusion pump, is initiated at a dose of 5 mg/hour. If the desired blood pressure reduction is not achieved at this dosage, the infusion rate may be increased by 2.5 mg/hour every 5–15 minutes up to a maximum of 15 mg/hour, until the desired blood pressure reduction is achieved.

℞ Clevidipine (Cleviprex)

Class Calcium channel blocker

Description

Clevidipine is a calcium channel blocker that is highly selective for vascular smooth muscle and used in the treatment of severe hypertension.

Mechanism of Action

Clevidipine causes relaxation of the smooth muscles that encircle the peripheral blood vessels, principally the arterioles. This relaxation results in peripheral vasodilation, a decrease in peripheral vascular resistance, and a decrease in both the systolic and diastolic blood pressure. Clevidipine has less effect on cardiac muscle than other calcium channel blockers.

Pharmacokinetics

Onset: 2–4 minutes (IV)
Peak Effects: 5–8 minutes (IV)
Duration: 5–15 minutes
Half-Life: 0.5 minute

Indications

Clevidipine is used in the treatment of hypertensive emergency.

Contraindications

Clevidipine is contraindicated in patients with known hypersensitivity to the medication. It should not be administered to patients who are hypotensive.

Precautions

Clevidipine can cause a significant drop in blood pressure. Thus, blood pressure should be frequently monitored. Clevidipine should be used with caution in patients with heart failure. It should not be administered to patients receiving IV β-blockers.

Side Effects

Clevidipine can cause nausea, vomiting, dizziness, headache, bradycardia, heart block, hypotension, and asystole.

Interactions/Incompatibilities

Clevidipine should not be administered to patients receiving intravenous β-blockers because of an increased risk of congestive heart failure, bradycardia, and asystole.

Dosage

Clevidipine, administered via an infusion pump, is initiated at a dose of 1 to 2 mg/hr and may be titrated to achieve desired BP reductions by doubling the dose as often as every 90 seconds. The rate of clevidipine titration may become less rapid as BP nears the goal, with dose increases every 5 to 10 minutes at a rate of 1 to 2 mg/hr. Dosage should not exceed 32 mg/hr based on available studies.

℞ Nifedipine (Procardia, Adalat)

Class Calcium channel blocker

Description

Nifedipine is a calcium channel blocker that is used in the treatment of hypertension. It is also used as a tocolytic (to suppress labor).

Mechanism of Action

Nifedipine causes relaxation of the smooth muscles that encircle the peripheral blood vessels, principally the arterioles. This relaxation results in peripheral vasodilation, a decrease in peripheral vascular resistance, and a decrease in both the systolic and diastolic blood pressure. Nifedipine is also effective in reducing coronary artery spasm in angina. Nifedipine can be used in hypertension associated with pregnancy if hydralazine is not available.

Pharmacokinetics

Onset: 1–5 minutes (SL), 5–20 minutes [by mouth (PO)]
Peak Effects: 20–30 minutes (SL), 1–2 hours (PO)
Duration: 2–4 hours
Half-Life: 2–5 hours

Indications

Nifedipine is used in the treatment of chronic hypertension and angina pectoris (although rarely). It is sometimes used to suppress labor (tocolytic).

Contraindications

Nifedipine is contraindicated in patients with known hypersensitivity to the medication. It should not be administered to patients who are hypotensive.

Precautions

Nifedipine can cause a significant drop in blood pressure. Thus, blood pressure should be frequently monitored. Nifedipine should be used with caution in patients with heart failure. It should not be administered to patients receiving IV β-blockers.

Side Effects

Nifedepine can cause nausea, vomiting, dizziness, headache, bradycardia, heart block, hypotension, and asystole.

Interactions/Incompatibilities

Nifedepine should not be administered to patients receiving intravenous β-blockers because of an increased risk of congestive heart failure, bradycardia, and asystole.

Dosage

Typically, 10–20 mg capsules orally. It is no longer recommended in emergency care of hypertensive problems.

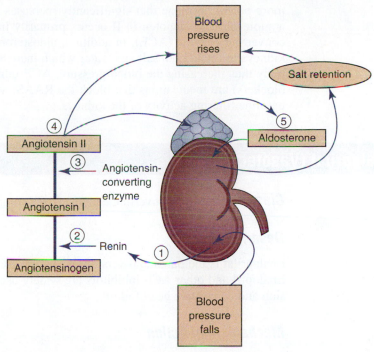

● **FIGURE 7–8** Renin-angiotensin.

Angiotensin-Converting Enzyme (ACE Inhibitors)

The renin-angiotensin–aldosterone system (RAAS) plays an important role in blood pressure regulation (see Figure 7–8). The important components of the RAAS system are:

- *Renin.* A hormone secreted by the juxtaglomerular apparatus in the kidney. It is secreted when the arterial blood pressure falls, the body's sodium and chloride levels decrease, and through activation of β_1-adrenergic receptors. When released, renin breaks down the enzyme *angiotensinogen* (secreted by the liver) to angiotensin I.

- *Angiotensin I.* Angiotensin I is a peptide that causes vasoconstriction thus increasing blood pressure. It also causes the release of the hormone aldosterone from the adrenal cortex. Angiotensin is cleaved to form angiotensin II by angiotensin-converting enzyme (ACE).

- *Angiotensin II.* Angiotensin II is an active peptide and potent vasoconstrictor. It acts on angiotensin II receptors and causes vasoconstriction and the release of aldosterone (thus elevating blood pressure).

- *Angiotensin-converting enzyme (ACE).* ACE is an important enzyme, found throughout the body—but predominantly in the lungs, that cleaves angiotensin I to angiotensin II to regulate extracellular fluid volume. It also degrades some vasodilatory peptides such as bradykinin.

- *Aldosterone.* Aldosterone is a hormone by the adrenal glands that causes the retention of sodium in the distal nephron of the kidney. This serves to further increase blood pressure.

When the blood pressure drops for any reason, renin is released causing the conversion of **angiotensinogen** into angiotensin I. Angiotensin I is not a strong regulator of blood pressure. Thus, most angiotensin I is converted to angiotensin II—a more potent hormone that significantly increases blood pressure. The conversion of angiotensin I to angiotensin II occurs primarily in the lungs by way of angiotensin-converting enzyme (ACE). In addition, aldosterone release by the RAAS causes the kidneys to retain both salt and water which increases the total amount of water in the body thus increasing the blood pressure. ACE inhibitors (and angiotensin II receptor blockers) are medications that block the RAAS system and lower blood pressure the baseline filtering activity of the kidneys.

℞ Enalaprilat (Vasotec)

Class Angiotensin-converting enzyme (ACE) inhibitor

Description

Enalaprilat is the parenteral version of the oral ACE inhibitor enalopril (Vasotec). Enalopril and other ACE inhibitors are widely used in medicine to treat hypertension and congestive heart failure.

Mechanism of Action

Enalaprilat causes relaxation of the smooth muscles that encircle the peripheral blood vessels, principally the arterioles blocking a angiotensin-converting enzyme (ACE) causing relaxation of the peripheral blood vessels thus lowering blood pressure (both systolic and diastolic). This effect also serves to reduce afterload on the heart making it an effective treatment for non-valvular congestive heart failure.

Pharmacokinetics

Onset: 15–30 minutes (IV)
Peak Effects: 1–2 hours (IV), may occur up to 4 hours after dosing
Duration: 6–12 hours
Half-Life: 1–2 days

Indications

Enalaprilat is used in the treatment of hypertension and congestive heart failure. Anaphylactic reactions and angioedema have been reported.

Contraindications

Enalaprilat is contraindicated in pregnancy, patients with angioedema (swelling of the tongue and mouth) and in patients with known hypersensitivity to the medication. It should not be administered to patients who are hypotensive. Anaphylactic reactions and angioedema have been reported. Enalaprilat should be avoided in acute myocardial infarction.

Precautions

Enalaprilat can cause a significant drop in blood pressure. Thus, blood pressure should be frequently monitored.

Side Effects

The most common side effects seen with enalaprilat include cough and headache. Less frequent side effects include joint pain (arthralgias), diarrhea, dizziness, syncope, fatigue, fever, hypotension, nausea, and a skin rash.

Interactions/Incompatibilities

Enalaprilat should be used cautiously in patents taking lithium and diuretics.

Dosage

The dose in hypertension is 1.25–5 mg (typically 1.25 mg) every six hours administered intravenously over a five minute period. A clinical response is usually seen within 15 minutes. Peak effects after the first dose may not occur for up to four hours after dosing. The peak effects of the second and subsequent doses may exceed those of the first. The dose for afterload reduction for acute congstive heart failure is similar.

Captopril (Capoten)

Class Angiotensin-converting enzyme (ACE) inhibitor

Description

Captopril is the prototypical ACE inhibitor and widely-used in medicine to treat hypertension and congestive heart failure. It has a shorter onset of action than enalaprilat.

Mechanism of Action

Captopril causes relaxation of the smooth muscles that encircle the peripheral blood vessels, principally the arterioles blocking angiotensin-converting enzyme (ACE) causing relaxation of the peripheral blood vessels thus lowering blood pressure (both systolic and diastolic). This effect also serves to reduce afterload on the heart making it an effective treatment for non-valvular congestive heart failure.

Pharmacokinetics

Onset: 5–6 minutes
Peak Effects: 1–2 hours
Duration: 2–12 hours
Half-Life: 2 hours

Indications

Captopril is used in the treatment of hypertension and congestive heart failure. Anaphylactic reactions and angioedema have been reported.

Contraindications

Captopril is contraindicated in pregnancy, patients with angioedema (swelling of the tongue and mouth) and in patients with known hypersensitivity to the medication. It should not be administered to patients who are hypotensive. Anaphylactic reactions and angioedema have been reported. Captopril should be avoided in acute myocardial infarction.

Precautions

Captopril can cause a significant drop in blood pressure. Thus, blood pressure should be frequently monitored.

Side Effects

The most common side effects seen with captopril include cough and headache. Less frequent side effects include joint pain (arthralgias), diarrhea, dizziness, syncope, fatigue, fever, hypotension, nausea, and a skin rash.

Interactions/Incompatibilities

Captopril should be used cautiously in patents taking lithium and diuretics.

Dosage

Captopril is primarily given sublingually at a dose of 12.5–25 mg if the BP is between 90–110 mm.

℞ Sodium Nitroprusside (Nitropress, Nipride)

Class Antihypertensive and vasodilator

Description

Sodium nitroprusside is a potent vasodilation agent used in the management of hypertensive emergencies when a prompt reduction in blood pressure is required.

Mechanism of Action

Sodium nitroprusside acts by dilating both peripheral arteries and peripheral veins. This reduction in peripheral vascular resistance results in an immediate reduction in blood pressure, which is generally proportional to the rate of medication administration. Sodium nitroprusside administration is usually accompanied by an increase in heart rate.

Although not approved for this use, sodium nitroprusside is occasionally used in the management of severe congestive heart failure. The dilation of the peripheral veins results in decreased blood return to the heart (preload). In addition, the dilation of the peripheral arteries reduces the pressure against which the heart has to pump (afterload). This results in a net increase in cardiac output in patients with severe congestive heart failure (see Figure 7–9).

Because sodium nitroprusside is such a potent agent, the blood pressure, pulse rate, respiratory status, and EKG should be constantly monitored during medication administration. The initiation of sodium nitroprusside for antihypertensive therapy almost always requires ICU admission.

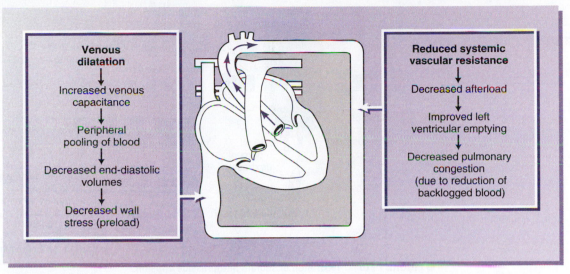

● **FIGURE 7–9** Actions of sodium nitroprusside.

Pharmacokinetics

Onset: < 1 minute

Peak Effects: 1–5 minutes

Duration: 1–10 minutes

Half-Life: 2.7–7.0 days

Indication

Hypertensive emergency in which a prompt reduction (in 1 hour) in blood pressure is essential.

Contraindications

None when used in the management of life-threatening hypertensive crisis.

Precautions

Once the sodium nitroprusside infusion is prepared, it should be immediately wrapped in an opaque material, usually aluminum foil, to protect it from light. Once exposed to light, the medication is quickly inactivated. Sodium nitroprusside should not be used in children or pregnant women in the prehospital setting. The dosage should be reduced somewhat in elderly patients. The constant monitoring of blood pressure and pulse is essential throughout sodium nitroprusside administration.

Side Effects

Sodium nitroprusside can cause dizziness, headache, hypotension, chest pain, dyspnea, palpitations, nausea, and vomiting. It can also cause cyanide toxicity—especially in higher doses.

Interactions/Incompatibilities

The effects of sodium nitroprusside can be potentiated when administered with other antihypertensive agents.

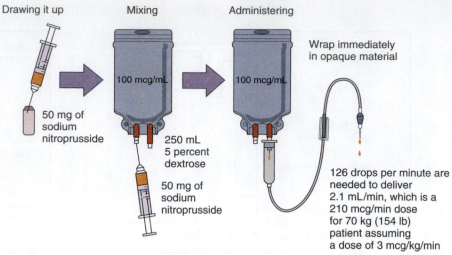

Drawing it up   Mixing   Administering

Wrap immediately in opaque material

100 mcg/mL   100 mcg/mL

50 mg of sodium nitroprusside

250 mL 5 percent dextrose

50 mg of sodium nitroprusside

126 drops per minute are needed to deliver 2.1 mL/min, which is a 210 mcg/min dose for 70 kg (154 lb) patient assuming a dose of 3 mcg/kg/min

● **FIGURE 7–10**   Preparation of sodium nitroprusside infusion.

Dosage

The standard dose is 50 mg of sodium nitroprusside diluted in 500 mL of D_5W. This will give a concentration of 100 mcg/mL. The initial dose should be 0.25 mcg/kg/min (see Figure 7–10). The typical dosage range is from 0.25 to 3 mcg/kg/min (higher doses can be used but are more commonly associated with thiocyanate toxicity). Sodium nitroprusside should only be diluted in D_5W or normal saline and administered by slow IV infusion using a minidrip administration set (preferably through an IV pump). *This medication should never be given by IV bolus.*

℞ Hydralazine (Apresoline)

Class Antihypertensive and vasodilator

Description

Hydralazine is a potent vasodilating agent used to lower blood pressure in cases of hypertensive crisis.

Mechanism of Action

Hydralazine, like sodium nitroprusside, relaxes vascular smooth muscle, primarily in the arterial system, thus causing decreased arterial pressure (diastolic greater than systolic), decreased peripheral resistance, and increased cardiac output. Hydralazine causes postural hypotension to a lesser degree than does sodium nitroprusside. The effects of hydralazine are usually seen within 5 to 10 minutes after the initiation of therapy.

Pharmacokinetics

Onset: 5–15 minutes (IV), 10–40 minutes (IM)

Peak Effects: < 80 minutes

Duration: 2–6 hours

Half-Life: 2–8 hours

Indications

Hydralazine is used in hypertensive emergency in which a prompt reduction in blood pressure is required and hypertension complicating pregnancy (preeclampsia and eclampsia).

Contraindications

Hydralazine should not be administered to patients with a known history of hypersensitivity to the medication, coronary artery disease, or rheumatic heart disease involving the mitral valve.

Precautions

The administration of hydralazine may cause angina pectoris or ECG changes because of the increased cardiac output. This medication should not be used in the prehospital phase of emergency medical care of children because of limited experience with the medication in these cases. The blood pressure, pulse rate, respiratory status, and ECG should be monitored at all times during hydralazine therapy. Headache, nausea, and vomiting have been known to occur following hydralazine therapy and should be expected.

Side Effects

Hydralazine can cause headache, dizziness, altered mental status, tachycardia, arrhythmias, orthostasis, chest pain, nausea, and vomiting.

Interactions/Incompatibilities

The effects of hydralazine can be potentiated when administered with other antihypertensive agents.

Dosage

The usual dosage of hydralazine in the management of hypertensive crisis is 10–20 mg given by slow IV bolus (or 10–40 mg IM). This dose can be repeated in 4–6 hours if required. The blood pressure and ECG should be continuously monitored. Parenteral hydralazine should be administered by slow IV bolus. When necessary, however, the medication can be administered by intramuscular injection.

OTHER CARDIOVASCULAR MEDICATIONS

The following agent does not readily fit into the classes of medications discussed thus far.

℞ Calcium Chloride

Class Calcium supplement

Description

Calcium chloride provides elemental calcium in the form of the cation (Ca^{2+}). Calcium is required for many physiological activities.

Mechanism of Action

Calcium chloride replaces calcium in cases of hypocalcemia. Calcium chloride causes a significant increase in the myocardial contractile force and appears to increase ventricular automaticity. Although frequently used for many years in the management of cardiac arrest, especially that resulting from asystole and electromechanical dissociation, recent studies have presented data that seriously question the role of calcium chloride, even in these situations. Calcium chloride is an antidote for magnesium sulfate and can minimize some of the side effects of calcium channel blocker usage.

Pharmacokinetics

Onset: Immediate
Peak Effects: Unknown
Duration: Varies
Half-Life: Not applicable

Indications

Calcium chloride is used in acute hyperkalemia (elevated potassium), acute hypocalcemia (decreased calcium), and calcium channel blocker toxicity (nifedipine, verapamil, and diltiazem).

Contraindications

Caution is warranted when calcium chloride is administered to patients receiving digitalis, because it may precipitate digitalis toxicity.

Precautions

It is extremely important to flush the IV line between administrations of calcium chloride and sodium bicarbonate to avoid precipitation. Calcium chloride can cause tissue necrosis at the injection site. It should always be administered through an IV that is patent and running well.

Side Effects

Calcium chloride can cause bradycardia, arrhythmias, syncope, nausea, vomiting, and cardiac arrest.

Interactions/Incompatibilities

Calcium chloride will interact with sodium bicarbonate and form a precipitate. In addition, calcium chloride can cause elevated digoxin levels, and possibly digitalis toxicity, when administered to patients receiving digitalis preparations.

Dosage

The standard dose for calcium chloride is 2 to 4 mg/kg intravenously. This dose may be repeated every 10 minutes as required. Calcium chloride should only be given intravenously in the emergency setting.

CHAPTER REVIEW

Summary

All of the medications discussed in this chapter are of value only when used in conjunction with other treatment modalities. Without appropriate cardiopulmonary resuscitation, the medications used in the management of cardiac arrest are not effective. As mentioned, the dosages presented in this chapter are based on nationally accepted regimens. Paramedics should become familiar with the routine dosages and protocols used in their areas.

Key Words

adrenergic receptors Receptors specific to norepinephrine- and epinephrine-like substances.

adrenergic system The part of the nervous system that prepares the body to deal with various stresses, whether real or imagined. Also referred to as the sympathetic nervous system.

anaerobic metabolism The process of generating energy without the aid of oxygen.

antagonist A medication or other substance that blocks a physiological response or that blocks the action of another medication or substance.

catecholamine A class of hormones that act on the autonomic nervous system. They include epinephrine, norepinephrine, and similar compounds.

cholinergic system A division of the autonomic nervous system that is responsible for controlling vegetative functions. Also called the parasympathetic nervous system.

concomitant Occurring at the same time.

dopaminergic receptor Receptor in the renal and splanchnic vessels that maintains vasodilation.

endogenous Coming from inside the body.

homeostasis The natural tendency of the body to maintain a relatively constant internal environment.

hypoxic drive Respiratory control system commonly present in patients with chronic obstructive pulmonary disease whereby respirations are dependent on changes in the concentration of oxygen as opposed to changes in the concentration of carbon dioxide.

lactic acid An organic acid normally present in tissue. One form of lactic acid in muscle and blood is a product of the change of the carbohydrates glucose and glycogen to energy during physical exercise.

neurotransmitter A substance that is released from the axon terminal of a presynaptic neuron on excitation and that travels across the synaptic cleft to either excite or inhibit the target cell. Examples include acetylcholine, norepinephrine, and dopamine.

pheochromocytoma A tumor of the adrenal gland that causes too much release of two hormones (epinephrine and norepinephrine). Signs include high blood pressure, headache, sweating, high blood sugar level, nausea, vomiting, and fainting spells.

pulse oximetry An assessment modality that measures the oxygen saturation level of the blood through a noninvasive sensor placed on a finger or earlobe.

stroke volume The amount of blood ejected by the heart in one cardiac contraction.

sympathomimetic A medication or substance that causes effects such as those of the sympathetic nervous system (also called adrenergic).

torsade de pointes   A form of ventricular tachycardia in which the morphology of the QRS appears to change (the axis rotates). It is often medication induced but may be the result of low potassium levels in the blood (hypokalemia) or profound slow heart beat (bradycardia).

Wolff-Parkinson-White syndrome   A disorder of the heart characterized by early contraction of the heart muscle.

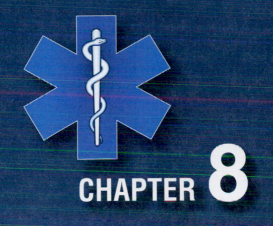

CHAPTER 8

MEDICATIONS USED IN THE TREATMENT OF RESPIRATORY EMERGENCIES

OBJECTIVES

After completing this chapter, the reader should be able to:

- Discuss the devices commonly used to administer oxygen in the field.
- Discuss pulse oximetry and end-tidal carbon dioxide detection and describe the prehospital use of both.
- Discuss the pathophysiology and prehospital management of asthma and status asthmaticus.
- Describe and list the indications, contraindications, and dosages for the following bronchodilators used in respiratory emergencies: epinephrine 1:1000, albuterol, levalbuterol, racemic epinephrine, terbutaline, isoetharine, metaproterenol, and aminophylline.
- Describe and list the indications, contraindications, and dosages for the following anticholinergics: atropine and ipratropium.
- Describe and list the indications, contraindications, and dosages for magnesium sulfate.
- Describe and list the indications, contraindications, and dosages for the following corticosteroids: methylprednisolone and hydrocortisone.

INTRODUCTION

Oxygen is among the most commonly used medications in the management of respiratory emergencies. In addition to oxygen, however, several pharmacological agents have proved quite effective in relieving respiratory distress. In this chapter medications commonly used in the prehospital treatment of respiratory emergencies are discussed. These medications include the following:

Gases

Oxygen

Beta Agonists

Epinephrine 1:1000
Albuterol/salbutamol (Proventil, Ventolin)
Levalbuterol (Xopenex)
Racemic epinephrine (microNefrin, Vaponefrin)

Terbutaline (Brethine, Bricanyl)
Isoetharine (Bronkosol)
Metaproterenol (Alupent)

Xanthines

Aminophylline (Somophyllin)

Anticholinergics

Atropine sulfate
Ipratropium (Atrovent)

Mineral

Magnesium sulfate

Corticosteroids

Methylprednisolone (Solu-Medrol)
Hydrocortisone (Solu-Cortef)

Sympathomimetics are among the most frequently used agents in the treatment of respiratory emergencies. The principal sympathomimetics include epinephrine, isoetharine, terbutaline, metaproterenol, levalbuterol, and albuterol. In treating cardiovascular emergencies it is highly desirable to activate β_1-adrenergic receptors. When treating patients in respiratory distress, however, it is desirable to activate β_2-receptors. Unfortunately, most of the agents that activate β_2-receptors also have some effect on β_1-receptors. When activated, β_1-receptors cause an increase in heart rate and myocardial contractile force, whereas β_2-receptors cause peripheral vasodilation and, most important, bronchodilation. Common side effects of these medications include palpitations, anxiety, and dizziness. Considerable effort has been devoted to isolation of pharmacological agents that act principally on β_2-receptors. Currently, levalbuterol and albuterol are the sympathomimetic agents most frequently used in the prehospital phase of emergency medical care. They are chemically related to epinephrine but tend to be more selective than epinephrine for β_2-receptors.

Another agent occasionally used in the management of respiratory emergencies is aminophylline. Aminophylline, chemically unrelated to the catecholamines, belongs to a class of medications called xanthines. A commonly encountered medication within the xanthines class is caffeine. Aminophylline causes relaxation of the bronchiole smooth musculature and bronchodilation.

Although not discussed in detail here, corticosteroids play a major role in the treatment of respiratory diseases. Asthma and many cases of **chronic obstructive pulmonary disease (COPD)** have inflammation as the underlying cause. Although the β-agonists help reverse bronchospasm, they do little for the underlying inflammation. Corticosteroids have a very long rate of onset (1 to 4 hours), and thus their effects are not usually seen in the prehospital setting.

Some systems have added neuromuscular-blocking agents to their paramedic medication lists. These medications are very effective in providing muscle relaxation for endotracheal intubation. However, because they remove a patient's protective reflexes and cause apnea, they should be used only by personnel with experience in their use.

OXYGEN

Oxygen administration is an important aspect of patient care. It is essential in cases that involve suspected **hypoxia** of any cause, chest pain due to myocardial ischemia, asthma, and cardiorespiratory arrest.

Oxygen Administration

Administering oxygen to a hypoxic patient raises his or her oxygen level by increasing the

- Inspired percentage of oxygen
- Oxygen concentration at the alveolar level
- Arterial oxygen levels
- Amount of oxygen delivered to the patient's cells

Oxygen administration corrects hypoxia and reduces the volume of respiration necessary to oxygenate the blood. It also reduces the myocardial work demanded to maintain a given arterial oxygen tension.

There are no absolute contraindications to oxygen administration. However, recent studies have shown that high-levels of oxygen can be toxic resulting in oxidative stress. Oxygen should only be used to treat hypoxia and then only enough administered to maintain the patient in a normoxic range. Hyperoxia should be avoided.

Oxygen Devices

Devices commonly used to administer oxygen in the field include the nasal cannula, the simple face mask, the non-rebreather mask, and, to a lesser extent, the Venturi mask.

Nasal Cannula

The *nasal cannula* is a frequently used device that is comfortable and is easily tolerated by the patient. It can deliver oxygen concentrations ranging from 24 to 44 percent. The oxygen flow rates for the nasal cannula vary from 1 to 6 lpm.

Simple Face Mask

The *simple face mask* delivers an oxygen concentration of 40–60 percent. Flow rates administered through the simple face mask range from 8 to 12 lpm. No fewer than 6 lpm should be administered through this device, because expired carbon dioxide can accumulate in the mask. Flow rates in excess of 8 lpm are needed to "wash out" any expired carbon dioxide.

The simple face mask provides oxygen to patients who are suffering from moderate hypoxia. Disadvantages include that it may feel confining to the patient, it muffles the patient's speech, and it requires a tight face seal. Because the mask covers the patient's face, it should be used with caution in cases that involve nausea or vomiting. With the pediatric patient, a flow rate of 6–8 lpm is generally considered acceptable.

Non-rebreather Mask

When the patient inhales, the 100 percent oxygen contained in the reservoir is drawn into the mask and the patient's respiratory passages. Ambient air is prevented from entering the mask by the rubber flap that closes over the inlet-outlet ports during inspiration. When the patient exhales, the flapper valve is open to allow the expired air an exit. A one-way valve situated between the mask and the reservoir prevents the expired air from entering the reservoir bag.

The *non-rebreather mask* delivers the highest concentration of oxygen. When supplied at a flow rate of 15 lpm, it can deliver an 80–100 percent oxygen concentration. No fewer than 8 lpm of oxygen should be administered through this device. Because the non-rebreather mask is a relatively closed system, it restricts the inspiration of ambient air. Therefore, its reservoir bag should not be allowed to deflate totally or be allowed to kink. Otherwise, the patient might suffocate.

The non-rebreather mask is similar to the simple face mask in that it requires a tight seal. A tight seal may be difficult to obtain with some patients because they find the mask confining. This device should be employed with caution in nauseated patients. Its main application lies in the treatment of severely hypoxic patients—those suffering respiratory compromise, shock, acute myocardial infarction, trauma, or carbon monoxide poisoning.

Venturi Mask

With the *venturi mask*, relatively precise concentrations of oxygen can be provided. This device is not commonly used in prehospital care and is used in the treatment of COPD patients. To control the amount of ambient air taken in by a patient, some Venturi masks are supplied with dial selection, and others come with interchangeable caps. These devices deliver oxygen concentrations of 24, 28, 35, or 40 percent. The liter flow depends on the oxygen concentration desired.

Ventilation

In the field, paramedics are called on in many cases to provide ventilatory support. Situations will range from those that involve apneic patients to less obvious cases in which patients are experiencing depressed respiratory function.

When a patient is unconscious, his or her respiratory center may not function at a satisfactory level. A significant decrease in the patient's rate or depth of breathing will lead to decreased respiratory minute volume, hypercarbia, hypoxia, and a lowered **pH**. If not corrected, respiratory or cardiac arrest may occur. To achieve effective ventilatory support, an adequate rate and volume of air must be delivered—at least 800 mL of air at a rate of 12–20 breaths per minute.

Non-invasive ventilation, continuous positive-pressure ventilation (CPAP), and bi-level positive airway pressure (BiPAP), are now commonly used in the emergency setting and have proven to be highly effective. In addition to oxygen, these devices provide continuous positive airway pressure (CPAP) which serves to keep alveoli expanded and improve the lung's ventilatory efficiency.

Pulse Oximetry

Pulse oximetry is now widely used in emergency care. The pulse oximeter is a quick and accurate tool that can objectively determine the oxygenation status of the patient. The pulse oximeter provides immediate and continuous evaluation of oxygen delivery to body tissues. It quantifies the effects of interventions including oxygen therapy, medication, suctioning, and ventilatory assistance. In addition, oximetry often detects problems with oxygenation before blood pressure, pulse, and respirations would reveal such a problem. Pulse oximetry, when available, should be used in virtually any patient care situation. In fact, it has been referred to as the fifth vital sign. It should be used during the patient assessment process to determine the patient's baseline value. It should also be used to guide patient care and to monitor the patient's response to paramedic interventions. Normal SpO_2 varies between 96 and 100 percent. Readings between 91 and 95 percent indicate mild hypoxia and warrant further evaluation and judicious supplemental oxygen administration. Readings between 86 and 91 percent indicate moderate hypoxia. These patients should receive 100 percent supplemental oxygen. Readings of 85 percent or lower indicate severe hypoxia and warrant immediate intervention, including the administration of 100 percent oxygen, ventilatory assistance, or both. The goal of therapy is to maintain the SpO_2 in the normal (> 96 percent) range.

The incidence of false readings with pulse oximetry is small. When it does occur, the oximeter generates an error signal or a blank screen. Causes of false readings include carbon monoxide poisoning, high-intensity lighting, and certain hemoglobin abnormalities. The absence of a pulse in an extremity will give a false reading. In hypovolemia and in severely anemic patients, the pulse oximetry reading may be misleading. Although the SpO_2 reading may be normal, the total amount of hemoglobin available to carry oxygen may be so markedly decreased that the patient will remain hypoxic at the cellular level.

Pulse oximetry is now an important part of emergency care, including prehospital care. Like the electrocardiogram (ECG) monitor, it provides important information related to the patient. It is important to remember that it is only an additional tool. It does not replace other assessment or monitoring skills. Prehospital care providers cannot depend solely on pulse oximetry reading to guide care; they must always consider and treat the whole patient. The reliability and validity of the pulse oximeter are well documented.

Capnography

Capnography is the measurement of exhaled carbon dioxide concentrations. The devices that make such measurements are called capnometers or end-tidal carbon dioxide ($ETCO_2$) detectors. Their use in prehospital care has increased significantly, most commonly to assess proper placement of an endotracheal tube. The absence of carbon dioxide from the exhaled air strongly indicates that the tube is in the esophagus; its presence indicates proper tracheal placement. Capnography can be used to ensure proper tube placement following insertion and to monitor tube placement during ventilation and cardiopulmonary resuscitation (CPR).

Capnometers are available either as disposable colorimetric devices or as electronic monitors. They are attached either in-line or alongside the endotracheal tube and the ventilation device. A color change in the colorimetric device or a light on the electronic monitor confirms proper tube placement. On the colorimetric device, the low CO_2 content of inspired air makes the device purple, whereas the higher CO_2 content of expired air makes it yellow. Some electronic devices now combine pulse oximetry, $ETCO_2$ detection, blood pressure, pulse rate, respiratory rate, and temperature monitors in one unit.

Although capnography is accurate, the $ETCO_2$ level falls precipitously during cardiac arrest. Therefore, these patients may not cause a color change on the capnometer detector despite proper placement of the endotracheal tube.

Capnography is being used with increasing frequency to monitor nonintubated patients as well. $ETCO_2$ is proportional to pulmonary perfusion and thus, in turn, to systemic perfusion. It can provide important information with regard to patient condition, especially in cases of bronchospastic disease (asthma, COPD) where it can help with early determinations of whether a patient's respiratory status is changing. Likewise, capnography can also monitor perfusion status and provide an early indication of impending shock. As with pulse oximetry, you should use a capnometer only in conjunction with other methods of assessing endotracheal placement. It does not replace actually visualizing the endotracheal tube's passage through the vocal cords.

ASTHMA

Asthma is a common respiratory illness that affects many people. Whereas deaths from other respiratory diseases have been steadily declining, deaths from asthma have significantly increased during the past decade or so. Most of the increased asthma deaths have occurred in patients who are 45 years of age or older. Approximately 50 percent of patients who die from asthma do so before reaching the hospital. Thus, emergency medical service (EMS) personnel are frequently called on to treat patients suffering an asthma attack. Prompt recognition, followed by appropriate treatment, can significantly improve the patient's condition and enhance chances of survival.

Pathophysiology of Asthma and COPD

Asthma is a chronic inflammatory disorder of the airways. In susceptible individuals, this inflammation causes symptoms usually associated with widespread but variable airflow obstruction. The major characteristic of asthma is reversible lower airway obstruction. This obstruction is caused by edema, mucus, and smooth muscle spasm; typically, all three factors are involved. An obstruction narrows the diameter of the smaller, smooth muscle–walled bronchioles. The natural dilation of the airways during inhalation allows air to enter these narrowed airways. However, contraction of the airways on exhalation and the obstruction caused by asthma combine to prevent air from escaping.

Air becomes trapped behind the obstruction, preventing continued ventilation of the alveoli, and oxygen–carbon dioxide exchange may be severely impaired. Hypoxemia and hypercarbia result, with the degree of respiratory distress increasing with the severity of obstruction and number of airways involved.

Asthma may be triggered by one of many different factors. These items, commonly referred to as triggers or inducers, vary from one individual to the next. In allergic individuals, environmental **allergens** are a major cause of inflammation. These allergens may occur both indoors and outdoors. In addition to allergens, asthma may be triggered by cold air, exercise, foods, irritants, and certain medications. Often a specific trigger cannot be identified.

Within minutes of exposure to the offending trigger, a two-phase reaction occurs. The first phase of the reaction is characterized by the release of chemical mediators such as histamine. These mediators cause contraction of the bronchial smooth muscle and leakage of fluid from peribronchial capillaries. This results in both bronchoconstriction and bronchial **edema**. These two factors can significantly decrease expiratory airflow, causing the typical "asthma attack." Often, the asthma attack resolves spontaneously in 1 to 2 hours or may be aborted by the use of inhaled bronchodilator medications such as albuterol. However, within 6 to 8 hours after exposure to the trigger, a second reaction occurs. This late phase is characterized by inflammation of the bronchioles as cells of the immune system (eosinophils, neutrophils, and lymphocytes) invade the mucosa of the respiratory tract. This leads to additional edema and swelling of the bronchioles and a further decrease of expiratory airflow.

The second phase of the reaction does not typically respond to inhaled beta agonist medications such as epinephrine or albuterol. Instead, anti-inflammatory agents such as corticosteroids are often required. It is important to point out that the severe inflammatory changes seen in an acute asthma attack do not develop over a few hours or even a few days. The inflammation often begins several days or several weeks before the onset of the actual asthma attack.

Status Asthmaticus

Status asthmaticus is defined as a severe, prolonged asthma attack that cannot be broken by repeated doses of epinephrine or albuterol. It is a serious medical emergency that requires prompt recognition, treatment, and transport. The patient suffering from status asthmaticus frequently has a greatly distended chest from continual air trapping. Breath sounds, and often wheezing, may be absent. The patient is usually exhausted, severely acidotic, and dehydrated. Paramedics should recognize that respiratory arrest is imminent and be prepared for endotracheal intubation. Transport should be immediate, with aggressive treatment continued en route.

Management of Asthma

Treatment of asthma is designed to correct hypoxia, reverse any **bronchospasm**, and treat inflammatory changes associated with the disease. Oxygen should be initially administered at a high concentration (100 percent). Intravenous access should be established, and the patient should be placed on an ECG monitor. Initial treatment should be directed at reversing any bronchospasm present. The most commonly used medications are inhaled beta agonist preparations such as albuterol (Ventolin, Proventil) (see Table 8–1). These medications can be easily administered with a small-volume, oxygen-powered nebulizer (Figure 8–1). The patient's response to these medications should be monitored and documented.

TABLE 8–1

Medications Used in the Treatment of Asthma

Mechanism of Action	Medication
Bronchodilators	
Nonspecific agonists	Epinephrine
	Ephedrine
Beta$_2$ specific agonists	
Inhaled (short-acting)	Albuterol (Ventolin, Proventil)
	Levalbuterol (Xopenex)
	Metaproterenol (Alupent)
	Terbutaline (Brethine)
Inhaled (long-acting)	Salmeterol (Serevent)
Methylxanthines	Theophylline (Theo-Dur, Slo-Bid)
	Aminophylline
Anticholinergics	Atropine
	Ipratropium (Atrovent)
Anti-Inflammatory Agents	
Glucocorticoids	
Inhaled	Beclomethasone (Beclovent)
	Fluticasone (Flovent)
	Triamcinolone (Azmacort)
Oral	Prednisone (Deltasone)
Injected	Methyprednisolone (Solu-Medrol)
	Dexamethasone (Decadron)
Leukotriene antagonists	Zafirlukast (Accolate)
	Zileuton (Zyflo)
Mast-Cell Membrane Stabilizer	Cromolyn (Intal)

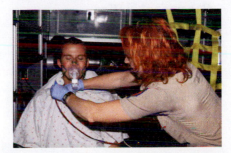

● **FIGURE 8–1** Inhaled β-agonist therapy has become the mainstay for emergency asthma treatmemt. © Bryan E. Bledsoe

In addition to beta agonists, early administration of corticosteroids should be considered. Although the inhaled beta agonists will help with bronchoconstriction, they will do little for the underlying inflammation, which is the principal problem. If paramedics anticipate a long transport time, medical control may request the administration of methylprednisolone or similar corticosteroid. However, the beneficial effects of corticosteroid administration will probably not be detected until 6–8 hours following administration.

If symptoms are severe and do not improve with administration of the inhaled beta agonists, the intravenous administration of aminophylline may be indicated. If the patient is not currently taking a theophylline preparation, paramedics administer a loading dose of 5–6 mg/kg of aminophylline over 20 to 30 minutes. This dose should be followed by a maintenance infusion of 0.8–1.0 mg/kg/hr. Both the inhaled beta agonists and aminophylline may increase heart rates and/or cause tremors, nausea, and vomiting.

Epinephrine

Class Sympathetic agonist

Description

Epinephrine is a naturally occurring catecholamine. It is a potent α- and β-adrenergic stimulant; however, its effect on β-receptors is more profound.

Mechanism of Action

Epinephrine acts directly on α- and β-adrenergic receptors. Its effect on β-receptors is much more profound than its effect on α-receptors. The effects of epinephrine include increased heart rate, cardiac contractile force, systemic vascular resistance, and increased blood pressure. It also causes bronchodilation due to its effects on β_2-adrenergic receptors. It is occasionally used to treat the bronchoconstriction accompanying asthma and COPD and is also effective in treating bronchoconstriction associated with anaphylaxis.

Epinephrine's effects usually appear within 90 seconds of administration, and they are usually of short duration. Occasionally the medication must be readministered in 15 to 30 minutes if needed. Epinephrine 1:1000 is given intramuscularly to ensure a steady and prolonged action. Inhaled β-agonists are preferred over epinephrine in the treatment of bronchospasm because they have fewer undesirable side effects.

Pharmacokinetics

Onset: 3–10 minutes (IM)
Peak Effects: 20 minutes (IM)
Duration: 20–30 minutes (IM)
Half-Life: Not applicable

Indications

Epinephrine is used in bronchial asthma, exacerbation of some forms of COPD, allergic reactions, and anaphylaxis.

Contraindications

Because of the cardiac effects seen with the administration of epinephrine, it should not be administered to patients with underlying cardiovascular disease or hypertension. Patients with profound anaphylactic reactions, characterized by hypotension and shock, are usually peripherally vasoconstricted, which will delay absorption of the medication from the subcutaneous site of injection. In these cases, epinephrine 1:10 000 should be administered intravenously.

Precautions

Epinephrine should be protected from light. Also, as with the other catecholamines, it tends to be deactivated by alkaline solutions. Any patient receiving epinephrine 1:1000 should be carefully monitored for changes in blood pressure, pulse, end-tidal CO_2, and ECG. Palpitations, anxiety, nausea, and headache are fairly common side effects.

Side Effects

Epinephrine can cause palpitations, anxiety, tremulousness, headache, dizziness, nausea, and vomiting. Because of its strong inotropic and chronotropic properties, epinephrine increases myocardial oxygen demand. Even in low doses it can cause myocardial ischemia. These effects should be kept in mind when administering epinephrine in the emergency setting.

Interactions

The effects of epinephrine can be intensified in patients who are taking antidepressants.

Dosage

The standard dose of epinephrine 1:1000 ranges from 0.3 to 0.5 mg administered intramuscularly, depending on the patient's weight and overall medical condition; 0.3 mg is the usual starting dose for adults. The dose for pediatric patients is 0.01 mg/kg administered intramuscularly. In the prehospital phase of emergency medical care, epinephrine 1:1000 should be administered only intramuscularly or subcutaneously (except in the case of pediatric cardiac arrest).

Albuterol (United States) (Proventil) Salbutamol (Canada) (Ventolin)

Class Sympathetic agonist

Description

Albuterol is a sympathomimetic that is selective for β_2-adrenergic receptors.

Mechanism of Action

Albuterol is a selective β_2-agonist with a minimal number of side effects. It causes prompt bronchodilation and has a duration of action of approximately 5 hours.

Pharmacokinetics

Onset: 5–15 minutes (inhaled)
Peak Effects: 1.0–1.5 hours
Duration: 3–6 hours
Half-Life: < 3 hours

Indications

Albuterol is used in bronchial asthma and reversible bronchospasm associated with chronic bronchitis and emphysema.

Contraindications

Albuterol should not be administered to any patient with a known history of hypersensitivity to the medication.

Precautions

As with any sympathomimetic, the patient's vital signs must be monitored. Caution should be used when administering albuterol to elderly patients and those with cardiovascular disease or hypertension. Lung sounds should be auscultated before and after each treatment. Ideally, the patient's peak flow rate should be measured both before and after medication administration.

Side Effects

Albuterol can cause palpitations, anxiety, dizziness, headache, nervousness, tremor, hypertension, arrhythmias, chest pain, nausea, and vomiting.

Interactions

The possibility of developing unpleasant side effects increases when albuterol is administered with other sympathetic agonists. β-blockers may blunt the pharmacological effects of albuterol.

Dosage

Albuterol can be administered by metered-dose inhaler or small-volume nebulizer. A common initial dose is two sprays when using a metered-dose inhaler. Each spray delivers 90 mcg of albuterol. When using a small-volume nebulizer, the standard adult dose is 2.5 mg (0.5 mL of a 0.5 percent solution diluted in 2.5 mL of normal saline). This amount is typically delivered over 5 to 15 minutes. Albuterol (Ventolin) is also available in the Rotahaler form. A special 200 mcg Rotacap is placed in the device and inhaled by the patient. Albuterol should only be administered by inhalation.

℞ Levalbuterol (Xopenex)

Class Sympathetic agonist

Description

Levalbuterol is a sympathomimetic that is selective for β₂-adrenergic receptor.

Mechanism of Action

Levalbuterol is a selective β_2-adrenergic agonist that causes relaxation of bronchial smooth muscle, thus decreasing airway resistance and increasing vital capacity. Levalbuterol is a chemical variant of albuterol with greater affinity for the β_2-adrenergic receptors.

Pharmacokinetics

Onset: 5–15 minutes
Peak Effects: 1–1.5 hours
Duration: 3–6 hours
Half-Life: 3.3 hours

Indications

Levalbuterol is used in the treatment of bronchospasm associated with reversible obstructive airway disease (asthma, chronic bronchitis, emphysema).

Contraindications

Levalbuterol is contraindicated in patients with known hypersensitivity to the medication.

Precautions

Levalbuterol should be used with caution in patients with cardiac ischemia. Try one treatment, measuring peak flow before and after treatment. Lung sounds should be auscultated before and after each treatment.

Side Effects

Tremors, anxiety, dizziness, headache, insomnia, nausea, palpitations, tachycardia, and hypertension have been associated with levalbuterol administration.

Interactions

The possibility of developing unpleasant side-effects increase when levalbuterol is administered with other sympathetic agonists. β-blockers may blunt the pharmacologic effects of levalbuterol.

Dosage

Adult dose. A standard nebulizer dose is 0.63 mg in 3.0 mL normal saline every 6 to 8 hours.

Pediatric dose. Children less than 12 years old is 0.31 mg in 3.0 mL normal saline three times a day.

℞ Racemic Epinephrine (S2, microNefrin, Vaponefrin)

Class Sympathetic agonist

Description

Racemic epinephrine is slightly different chemically from the epinephrine compounds that have been discussed previously. Compounds that differ only in their chemical arrangement are called **isomers**. This particular form is frequently used in children to treat croup.

Mechanism of Action

Racemic epinephrine stimulates both α- and β-adrenergic receptors. However, racemic epinephrine has a slight preference for β_2-adrenergic receptors and causes bronchodilation. It also has some effect in relieving the subglottic edema associated with croup. Racemic epinephrine should only be administered by inhalation.

Pharmacokinetics

Onset: < 5 minutes

Peak Effects: 5–15 minutes

Duration: 1–3 hours

Half-Life: Not applicable

Indication

Racemic epinephrine is used to treat croup (laryngotracheobronchitis).

Contraindications

Racemic epinephrine should not be used in the management of epiglottitis.

Precautions

Racemic epinephrine can result in tachycardia and possibly arrhythmias. Vital signs should be monitored. Many patients develop "rebound worsening" 30 to 60 minutes after the initial treatment and after the effects of racemic epinephrine have worn off. Thus, all children who receive racemic epinephrine should be transported to the hospital. Most hospitals have an institutional policy that requires all children who have received racemic epinephrine to be admitted for at least 24 hours in case rebound worsening occurs.

Dosage

A standard dose is 0.25 to 0.75 mL racemic epinephrine diluted with 2 mL normal saline (2.25 percent) and administered via a standard aerosol nebulizer. It should only be used initially and not repeated. Racemic epinephrine should be given only by inhalation, generally by small-volume nebulizer, diluted with 2 to 3 mL of normal saline.

℞ Terbutaline (Brethine, Bricanyl)

Class Sympathetic agonist

Description

Terbutaline is a synthetic sympathomimetic that is selective for β_2-adrenergic receptors.

Mechanism of Action

Terbutaline, because of its effects on β_2-adrenergic receptors, causes immediate bronchodilation with minimal cardiac effects. Its onset of action is similar to that of epinephrine. Terbutaline is also used to suppress preterm labor.

Pharmacokinetics

Onset: < 5 minutes (SC), 5–30 minutes (inhaled)

Peak Effects: 30–60 minutes (SC), 1–2 hours (inhaled)

Duration: 1.5–4.0 hours (SC), 3–4 hours (inhaled)

Half-Life: 3–4 hours

Indications

Terbutaline is used in bronchial asthma and reversible bronchospasm associated with chronic bronchitis and emphysema.

Contraindications

Terbutaline should not be administered to any patient with a history of hypersensitivity to the medication.

Precautions

As with any sympathomimetic, the patient's vital signs must be monitored. Caution should be used when administering terbutaline to elderly patients and those with cardiovascular disease or hypertension. Lung sounds should be auscultated before and after each treatment. Ideally, the patient's peak flow rate should be measured both before and after medication administration.

Side Effects

Terbutaline can cause palpitations, anxiety, dizziness, headache, nervousness, tremor, hypertension, arrhythmias, chest pain, nausea, and vomiting.

Interactions

The possibility of developing unpleasant side effects increases when terbutaline is used with other sympathetic agonists. β-blockers may blunt the pharmacological effects of terbutaline.

Dosage

The standard dose is two inhalations, 1 minute apart, from a metered-dose inhaler. Terbutaline can also be administered by subcutaneous injection. The usual dose is 0.25 mg. This dose can be repeated in 15 to 30 minutes if needed. Terbutaline should only be administered by inhalation or by subcutaneous injection as described herein.

Rx Isoetharine (Bronkosol)

Class Sympathetic agonist

Description

Isoetharine is a sympathomimetic similar in chemical structure to epinephrine. It exhibits a slight specificity for β_2-adrenergic receptors, thus reducing the potential for cardiac toxicity.

Mechanism of Action

Isoetharine is a β-agonist with slight selectivity for β_2-adrenergic receptors, causing pulmonary bronchodilation. Its onset of action is similar to that of epinephrine. However, it has a longer duration of effect.

Pharmacokinetics

Onset: Immediate
Peak Effects: 5–15 minutes
Duration: 1–4 hours
Half-Life: Not applicable

Indications

Isoetharine is used in bronchial asthma and reversible bronchospasm associated with chronic bronchitis and emphysema.

Contraindications

Isoetharine should not be administered to any patient with a history of hypersensitivity to any of the ingredients.

Precautions

As with any sympathomimetic, the patient's vital signs must be monitored. Caution should be used when administering isoetharine to elderly patients and those with cardiovascular disease or hypertension. Lung sounds should be auscultated before and after each treatment. Ideally, the patient's peak flow rate should be measured both before and after medication administration.

Side Effects

Isoetharine can cause palpitations, anxiety, dizziness, headache, nervousness, tremor, hypertension, arrhythmias, chest pain, nausea, and vomiting.

Interactions

The possibility of developing unpleasant side effects increases when isoetharine is administered with other sympathetic agonists. β-blockers may blunt the pharmacological effects of isoetharine.

Dosage

There are three major ways to administer isoetharine, each with different dosages. They are as follows:

Method of Administration	Usual Dose	Dilution
Metered-dose inhaler	2 inhalations	Undiluted
Oxygen aerosolization	0.5 milliliters	1:3 with saline
Intermittent positive-pressure breathing	0.5 milliliters	1:3 with saline

Isoetharine should be administered only by one of the methods listed.

℞ Metaproterenol (Alupent)

Class Sympathetic agonist

Description

Metaproterenol is a sympathomimetic that is selective for β_2-adrenergic receptors.

Mechanism of Action

Metaproterenol is a selective β_2-agonist and is an effective bronchodilator. Its duration of effect is up to 4 hours.

Pharmacokinetics

Onset: 1 minute
Peak Effects: 1 hour
Duration: 1–5 hours
Half-Life: Not applicable

Indications

Metaproterenol is used in bronchial asthma and reversible bronchospasm associated with chronic bronchitis and emphysema.

Contraindications

Metaproterenol should not be used in patients with cardiac arrhythmias or significant tachycardia.

Precautions

As with any sympathomimetic, the patient's vital signs must be monitored. Caution should be used when administering metaproterenol to elderly patients and those with cardiovascular disease or hypertension. Lung sounds should be auscultated before and after each treatment. Ideally, the patient's peak flow rate should be measured both before and after medication administration.

Side Effects

Metaproterenol can cause palpitations, anxiety, dizziness, headache, nervousness, tremor, hypertension, arrhythmias, chest pain, nausea, and vomiting.

Interactions

The possibility of developing unpleasant side effects increases when metaproterenol is administered with other sympathetic agonists. β-blockers may blunt the pharmacological effects of metaproterenol.

Dosage

Metaproterenol may be administered by metered-dose inhaler. Each spray contains 0.65 mg of metaproterenol. The usual single dose is two to three inhalations, a minute apart, as needed. Metaproterenol may also be administered by small-volume nebulizer. The typical adult dose is 0.2–0.3 mL of metaproterenol diluted in 2.5 mL of normal saline. This dose is usually administered over 5 to 15 minutes. Metaproterenol should be administered by inhalation only in the emergency setting.

℞ Aminophylline (Somophyllin)

Class Xanthine

Description

Aminophylline is a xanthine bronchodilator that sometimes proves effective in cases in which sympathomimetics have not been effective.

Mechanism of Action

Aminophylline achieves its bronchodilation effects via a different mechanism than the sympathomimetics. It relaxes bronchial smooth muscle but does not act on adrenergic receptors. Aminophylline also stimulates the respiratory center in the brain. This effect is particularly useful in the treatment of infants with apnea. In addition to bronchodilation, aminophylline has mild diuretic properties, increases the heart rate and cardiac output, and may precipitate arrhythmias. Because of its mild diuretic and inotropic effects, aminophylline can be used (although rarely) in the management of congestive heart failure and pulmonary edema. In prehospital emergency care, aminophylline is usually given by slow IV infusion. Some systems also carry aminophylline suppositories for use in special situations.

Pharmacokinetics

Onset: 15 minutes
Peak Effects: 15 minutes
Duration: Varies
Half-Life: 4 hours

Indications

Aminophylline is used in bronchial asthma, reversible bronchospasm associated with chronic bronchitis and emphysema, congestive heart failure, and pulmonary edema.

Contraindications

Aminophylline should not be administered to any patient with a history of hypersensitivity to the medication. It should not be used in patients who have uncontrolled cardiac arrhythmias.

Precautions

Extreme caution should be used when administering aminophylline to any patient with a history of cardiovascular disease or hypertension. Any patient receiving aminophylline should have a cardiac monitor. One should be alert for any signs of cardiac irritability, especially premature ventricular contractions (PVCs) and tachycardia. Hypotension can occur following rapid administration.

Side Effects

Aminophylline can cause tachycardia, arrhythmias, palpitations, chest pain, nervousness, headache, seizures, nausea, and vomiting.

Interactions

Aminophylline should not be administered to patients who are on chronic theophylline therapy (Slo-Bid, Theo-Dur, and so on) until the amount of medication in the blood has been obtained (theophylline level). Concomitant use with β-blockers and medications of the erythromycin class of antibiotics may lead to theophylline toxicity.

Dosage

Two major regimens are used in administering aminophylline. The first is for use in patients in whom fluid overload or edema does not appear to be present (i.e., acute bronchial asthma): Place 250 or 500 mg in 90 or 80 mL of 5 percent dextrose, respectively. This can be done with a 100 mL IV bag or with a Buretrol- or Volutrol-type administration set. This solution is then infused over 20 to 30 minutes. This mechanism of slow infusion tends to reduce the chances of arrhythmias. In patients with congestive heart failure, or for whom any additional fluid might be dangerous, a more concentrated infusion is prepared: Place 250 or 500 mg (2 to 5 mg/kg) in 20 mL of 5 percent dextrose in water. This solution is then infused over 20 to 30 minutes using a Buretrol- or Volutrol-type administration set. Parenteral aminophylline should only be given by slow intravenous (IV) infusion by one of the regimens discussed earlier.

℞ Atropine Sulfate

Class Anticholinergic

Description

Atropine is a parasympatholytic (anticholinergic) that is derived from parts of the *Atropa belladonna* plant.

Mechanism of Action

Atropine sulfate is a potent parasympatholytic. It is used in the treatment of respiratory emergencies, because it causes bronchodilation and drying of respiratory tract secretions. Atropine acts by blocking acetylcholine receptors, thus inhibiting parasympathetic stimulation. With the release of ipratropium, atropine has fallen into relative disuse in the treatment of reactive airway disease.

Pharmacokinetics

Onset: 5–30 minutes (inhaled)

Peak Effects: 1–4 hours (inhaled)

Duration: 2–4 hours (inhaled)

Half-Life: 2–3 hours

Indications

Atropine is used in bronchial asthma and reversible bronchospasm associated with chronic bronchitis and emphysema.

Contraindications

Atropine sulfate should not be used in patients hypersensitive to the medication. It is not indicated for the acute treatment of bronchospasm, for which rapid response is required.

Precautions

The patient's vital signs must be monitored during therapy with atropine. Caution should be used when administering atropine to elderly patients and those with cardiovascular disease or hypertension. Lung sounds should be auscultated before and after each treatment. Ideally, the patient's peak flow rate should be measured both before and after medication administration.

Side Effects

Atropine can cause palpitations, anxiety, dizziness, headache, nervousness, rash, nausea, and vomiting.

Interactions

There are few interactions in the prehospital setting.

Dosage

Atropine is usually administered with a β-agonist. Typically, 0.5 to 1.0 mg of atropine is placed in 2 to 3 mL of normal saline. This dose is administered by small-volume nebulizer with or without a β-agonist.

How Supplied

Atropine is supplied in ampules and vials containing 1.0 mg in 1 mL of solution.

Ipratropium (Atrovent)

Class Anticholinergic

Description

Ipratropium is an anticholinergic (parasympatholytic) bronchodilator that is chemically related to atropine.

Mechanism of Action

Ipratropium is a parasympatholytic used in the treatment of respiratory emergencies. It causes bronchodilation and dries respiratory tract secretions. Ipratropium acts by blocking acetylcholine receptors, thus inhibiting parasympathetic stimulation.

Pharmacokinetics

Onset: Varies
Peak Effects: 1.5–2.0 hours
Duration: 4–6 hours
Half-Life: 1.5–2.0 hours

Indications

Ipratropium is used in bronchial asthma and reversible bronchospasm associated with chronic bronchitis and emphysema.

Contraindications

Ipratropium should not be used in patients hypersensitive to the medication. It is not indicated for the acute treatment of bronchospasm, for which rapid response is required.

Precautions

The patient's vital signs must be monitored during therapy with ipratropium. Caution should be used when administering it to elderly patients and those with cardiovascular disease or hypertension. Lung sounds should be auscultated before and after each treatment. Ideally, the patient's peak flow rate should be measured both before and after medication administration.

Side Effects

Ipratropium can cause palpitations, anxiety, dizziness, headache, nervousness, rash, nausea, and vomiting.

Interactions

There are few interactions in the prehospital setting.

Dosage

Ipratropium is usually administered with a β-agonist. Typically, 500 mcg of Atrovent is placed in a small-volume nebulizer. A β-agonist can be added if desired. This solution is then administered by small-volume nebulizer with or without a β-agonist. Atrovent is also available in a metered-dose inhaler.

℞ Magnesium Sulfate

Class Mineral, electrolyte

Description

Magnesium sulfate is a salt that dissociates into the magnesium cation (Mg^{2+}) and the sulfate anion when administered. Magnesium is an essential element in numerous biochemical reactions that occur within the body.

Mechanism of Action

Magnesium acts as a physiological calcium channel blocker and blocks neuromuscular transmission. Magnesium sulfate has been used for years in the management of preterm labor and the hypertensive disorders of pregnancy (preeclampsia and eclampsia). Its usage in obstetrics is discussed in Chapter 11.

Pharmacokinetics

Onset: Immediate (IV), 1 hour (IM)
Peak Effects: Varies
Duration: 1 hour
Half-Life: Not applicable

Indications

Magnesium sulfate is used in severe bronchospasm, in severe refractory ventricular fibrillation or pulseless ventricular tachycardia, after myocardial infarction for prophylaxis of arrhythmias, and in torsade de pointes (multiaxial ventricular tachycardia).

Contraindications

Magnesium sulfate should not be administered to patients who are in shock, who have persistent, severe hypertension, who have a third-degree atrioventricular (AV) block, who routinely undergo dialysis, or who are known to have a decreased calcium level (hypocalcemia).

Precautions

Magnesium sulfate should be administered slowly to minimize side effects. Any patient receiving intravenous magnesium sulfate should have continuous cardiac monitoring as well as frequent monitoring of vital signs. If possible, the knee and biceps deep tendon reflexes should be checked prior to magnesium therapy.

It should be used with caution in patients with known renal insufficiency. Hypermagnesemia (elevated magnesium) can occur following magnesium sulfate administration. Calcium salts (calcium chloride or calcium gluconate) should be available as an antidote for magnesium sulfate in case serious side effects occur.

Side Effects

Magnesium sulfate can cause flushing, sweating, bradycardia, decreased deep tendon reflexes, drowsiness, respiratory depression, arrhythmias, hypotension, hypothermia, itching, and rash.

Interactions

Magnesium sulfate can cause cardiac conduction abnormalities if administered in conjunction with digitalis.

Dosage

The standard dosage is 2 g over 2 to 5 minutes.

℞ Methylprednisolone (Solu-Medrol)

Class Corticosteroid and anti-inflammatory

Description

Methylprednisolone is a synthetic steroid with potent anti-inflammatory properties.

Mechanism of Action

Corticocosteroids have multiple actions in the body. They have potent anti-inflammatory properties and inhibit many of the substances that cause inflammation (cytokines, interleukin, interferon) and also inhibit the synthesis of pro-inflammatory enzymes. The pharmacological actions of the steroids are vast and complex. In general medical practice, steroids have a wide range of uses. Effective as anti-inflammatory agents, they are used in the management of allergic reactions, asthma, and anaphylaxis. Methylprednisolone is considered an intermediate-acting steroid with a plasma half-life of about 3–4 hours.

Pharmacokinetics

Onset: Varies
Peak Effects: 4–8 days (IM)
Duration: 1–5 weeks (IM)
Half-Life: 3.5 hours

Indications

Methylprednisolone is used in severe anaphylaxis, asthma or COPD, and urticaria (hives).

Contraindications

There are no major contraindications to the use of methylprednisolone in the acute management of severe anaphylaxis.

Precautions

A single dose of methylprednisolone is all that should be given in the prehospital phase of care. Long-term steroid therapy can cause gastrointestinal bleeding, prolonged wound healing, and suppression of adrenocortical steroids.

Side Effects

Methylprednisolone can cause fluid retention, congestive heart failure, hypertension, abdominal distension, vertigo, headache, nausea, malaise, and hiccups.

Interactions

There are few interactions in the prehospital setting.

Dosage

The standard dosage of methylprednisolone in the management of severe anaphylaxis is 125–250 mg administered intravenously. Methylprednisolone may be administered intravenously or intramuscularly, but the intravenous route is preferred in emergency medicine.

℞ Hydrocortisone (Solu-Cortef)

Class Corticosteroid and anti-inflammatory

Description

Hydrocortisone is a potent corticosteroid with anti-inflammatory properties.

Mechanism of Action

Corticocosteroids have multiple actions in the body. They have potent anti-inflammatory properties and inhibit many of the substances that cause inflammation (cytokines, interleukin, interferon) and also inhibit the synthesis of pro-inflammatory enzymes. The pharmacological actions of the steroids are vast and complex. Hydrocortisone is considered a short-acting steroid with a plasma half-life of 90 minutes. Like the other adrenocorticosteroids, it is effective as an adjunct in the management of severe anaphylaxis.

Pharmacokinetics

Onset: Immediate
Peak Effects: 4–8 hours
Duration: 1.0–1.5 days
Half-Life: 90 minutes

Indications

Hydrocortisone is used in severe anaphylaxis, asthma or COPD, and urticaria (hives).

Contraindications

There are no major contraindications to the use of hydrocortisone in the acute management of anaphylaxis.

Precautions

A single dose of hydrocortisone is all that should be given in the prehospital phase of care. Long-term steroid therapy can cause gastrointestinal bleeding, prolonged wound healing, and suppression of adrenocortical steroids.

Side Effects

Hydrocortisone can cause fluid retention, congestive heart failure, hypertension, abdominal distension, vertigo, headache, nausea, malaise, and hiccups.

Interactions

There are few interactions in the prehospital setting.

Dosage

The standard dosage of hydrocortisone in the management of severe anaphylaxis is 40–250 mg administered intravenously.

Route

The IV route is preferred in emergency medicine. However, hydrocortisone can be administered intramuscularly when an IV cannot be started.

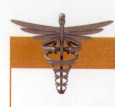

EMS is called to a residence to help a female patient complaining of shortness of breath. The patient is conscious and breathing. En route dispatch informs the paramedics that the patient has a history of COPD and uses an inhaler. On arrival paramedics are met by the patient's son, who takes them to the bedroom where the patient is sitting up in bed. The patient, an 88-year-old woman, is in obvious respiratory distress. She is leaning forward and struggling to breathe.

Physical Examination

CNS:	The patient is conscious, alert, and oriented × 4; she is able to answer questions with short answers only (less than 4 words); patient is clearly frightened
Resp:	Respirations are 42 and shallow; patient is wheezing; wheezes are heard throughout all lung fields on expiration; trachea is midline; no signs of trauma
CVS:	Carotid and radial pulses are present and weak; skin is warm and dry
ABD:	Soft and nontender
Muscl/Skel:	Patient able to move extremities on command; no weaknesses to hand grip

Vital Signs

Pulse:	120/min, irregular, weak
Resp:	42/min, shallow
BP:	152/110 mmHg
SpO$_2$:	88 percent
EtCO$_2$:	51 mmHg
ECG:	Sinus rhythm with unifocal PVCs at 4 to 6 per minute
Hx:	Patient has emphysema and was recently hospitalized for it and then discharged 2 days ago. She has had a cold for the past 2 weeks and states that changes in weather cause her "lungs to act up." She has been getting progressively worse, and her son states that the inhaler that she uses ran out this afternoon. She has no chest pain and denies any recent trauma.
PHx:	She has had emphysema, which seems to get worse during the winter months, for 20 years. She has been hospitalized numerous times for "breathing problems." The patient had a "heart attack" 2 years ago. Medications include Ventolin and Advair inhalers, synthroid, and verapamil; she has no allergies.

Treatment

Oxygen was administered by nasal cannula at 6 lpm, and 5 mg of albuterol (Ventolin) was administered by an oxygen-powered nebulizer. With coaching, the patient relaxed and her breathing improved slightly. The patient was hooked up to the ECG monitor and a sinus tachycardia was noted. En route to the hospital, a second dose of 5 mg of albuterol and 500 mcg of ipratropium bromide (Atrovent) were administered via a nebulizer. On arrival at the hospital, the patient was able to speak normally and the wheezing had diminished significantly. The SpO$_2$ had increased to 96 percent. Her prescription for the inhalers was refilled, and after an overnight stay in the hospital she was released.

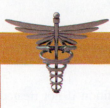

At 1830 hours paramedics are called to a rural residence 45 minutes from the hospital to aid a 45-year-old woman complaining of shortness of breath. She is conscious and breathing. On arrival paramedics are met by the patient's husband, who leads them to the living room. There, paramedics find a patient leaning forward in a chair. The patient is using home oxygen by nasal cannula and an oxygen-powered nebulizer. The patient appears very anxious and in severe respiratory distress.

Physical Examination

CNS:	The patient is conscious, alert, and oriented $\times$ 4; in extreme respiratory distress
Resp:	Respirations are 36 and shallow; wheezes are heard unaided by stethoscope; there are tight, barely audible wheezes in the apices bilaterally and no sounds heard in the bases; trachea is midline; no signs of trauma
CVS:	Carotid and radial pulses are present and weak; skin is pale and cool
ABD:	Soft and nontender
Muscl/Skel:	Patient able to move extremities on command; no weaknesses to hand grip

Vital Signs

Pulse:	140/min, regular, weak
Resp:	36/min, shallow
BP:	144/94 mmHg
SpO$_2$:	82 percent
ECG:	Sinus tachycardia
Hx:	Patient has a 20-year history of asthma and was taking albuterol by inhaler twice a day, Becloforte twice a day, and home oxygen by nasal cannula at 4 lpm as needed and during sleep. The patient was talking to her granddaughter on the phone. She became very upset during the telephone call and then became short of breath. The patient put on her oxygen (which provided no relief) and also took one dose (2.5 mg) of albuterol with an oxygen-powered nebulizer (which also provided no relief).

Treatment

Paramedics administered 5 mg of Ventolin and 500 mcg of Atrovent by nebulizer mask as per standing orders, and the patient was coached to take a breath and hold it. The patient was very agitated, and the coaching had little effect. An IV was initiated and run TKO. The patient was hooked up to the ECG monitor and a sinus tachycardia was noted. The base hospital was contacted, and the paramedics were directed to administer 125 mg of Solu-Medrol IV push and to continue administering Ventolin. The patient's condition deteriorated en route to the hospital. Although the patient was conscious, she was fatigued and unable to follow verbal commands. The base hospital was contacted, and the paramedics were directed to sedate and intubate the patient. The procedure was explained to the patient; 100 mcg of fentanyl (Sublimaze) and 2.5 mg of midazolam (Versed) were administered IV. Sellick's maneuver was applied to occlude the esophagus, at which point 1.5 mg/kg of succinylcholine (Anectine) was given IV. Once the jaw relaxed, the patient was intubated and bilateral breath sounds were confirmed. The patient was admitted to the intensive care unit on arrival at the hospital.

CHAPTER REVIEW

Summary

Respiratory emergencies are a serious and potentially fatal condition if not treated immediately. Prompt recognition of the signs and symptoms of respiratory distress is essential. Oxygen is the primary medication for treating any respiratory problem. Many types of medical problems, especially asthma and anaphylaxis, respond only to the medications discussed in this chapter.

Key Words

allergens   A foreign substance that can cause an allergic response in the body but is harmful only to some people.

bronchospasm   An abnormal contraction of the bronchi, resulting in narrowing and blockage of the airway. A cough with wheezing is the usual symptom. Bronchospasm is the main feature of asthma and bronchitis.

capnography   A system for measuring the concentration of exhaled carbon dioxide.

chronic obstructive pulmonary disease (COPD)   A pulmonary disease characterized by a decreased ability of the lungs to perform the function of ventilation.

edema   An abnormal pooling of fluid in the tissues.

hypoxia   A state in which insufficient oxygen is available to meet the oxygen requirements of the cells.

isomers   Compounds that have the same number of atoms yet have different structural properties.

pH   A scientific method of expressing the acidity or alkalinity of a solution. It is the logarithm of the hydrogen ion concentration divided by 1. The higher the pH, the more alkaline the solution. The lower the pH, the more acidic the solution.

pulse oximetry   An assessment modality that measures the oxygen saturation level of the blood through a noninvasive sensor placed on a finger or earlobe.

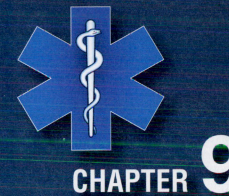

CHAPTER 9

MEDICATIONS USED IN THE TREATMENT OF ALLERGIC REACTIONS AND ANAPHYLAXIS

OBJECTIVES

After completing this chapter, the reader should be able to:

- Define the terms *allergic reaction* and *anaphylaxis* and distinguish the similarities and differences between the two.
- Discuss the role of histamine in allergic reactions.
- List the major types of histamine receptors and their related effects.
- List common causes of allergic reactions and anaphylaxis.
- Describe the difference between epinephrine 1:1000 and 1:10 000.
- Discus the role and effects of epinephrine in the treatment of allergic reactions.
- Discuss the role of antihistamine therapy in allergic reactions.
- Describe the role and importance of corticosteroids in allergic reactions.
- Detail the treatment of a mild-moderate allergic reaction.
- Detail the treatment of anaphylaxis.

INTRODUCTION

An **allergic reaction** is an exaggerated response by the immune system to a foreign substance. Allergic reactions can range from mild skin rashes to severe, life-threatening reactions that involve virtually every body system. The most severe type of allergic reaction is called **anaphylaxis**. Anaphylaxis is a life-threatening emergency that requires prompt recognition and specific treatment by EMS professionals. The emergency treatment of anaphylaxis is one area of prehospital care where advanced life support measures often mean the difference between life and death. Anaphylaxis can develop within seconds and cause death just minutes after exposure to the offending agent. Fortunately, there are several emergency medications available that can reverse the adverse effects of anaphylaxis.

The first complete description of anaphylaxis was reported in 1902 by Portier and Richet—French immunologists who were attempting to immunize dogs against the toxin of the deadly sea anemone (sea flower). They were injecting small, non-lethal quantities of the toxin into the animals in hopes of stimulating immunity to the toxin. However, when the animals received secondary injections of sub-lethal quantities of the toxin, at a time when it might be expected that they would be immune, the dogs developed shock and died. Richet called this dramatic and unexpected phenomenon *anaphylaxis,* which means the opposite of *"phylaxis,"* or protection.

Anaphylaxis results from exposure to a particular substance that sets off a biochemical chain of events that can ultimately lead to shock and death. The exact incidence of anaphylaxis is unknown. However, an estimated 400 to 800 deaths annually in the United States are attributed to anaphylaxis. Injected penicillin and bee and wasp (***Hymenoptera***) stings are the two most common causes of fatal anaphylaxis. Approximately 100 to 500 deaths per year are attributed to the parenteral administration of parenteral medications. Approximately 25 to 40 persons die each year from *Hymenoptera* stings.

The immune system is the principal body system involved in allergic reactions. However, other body systems are also affected by an allergic reaction. These include the *cardiovascular system,* the *respiratory system,* the *nervous system,* and the *gastrointestinal system,* among others. Certainly, the *integumentary system* (skin) is involved in allergic reactions. To fully appreciate the complexity of allergic and anaphylactic reactions, it is first necessary to review the anatomy and physiology of the immune system as it relates to the immune response.

The initial exposure of an individual to an antigen is referred to as **sensitization**. Sensitization results in an immune response. Subsequent exposure induces a much stronger secondary response. Some individuals can become hypersensitive (overly sensitive) to a particular antigen. **Hypersensitivity** is an unexpected and exaggerated reaction to a particular antigen. In many instances, hypersensitivity is used synonymously with the term **allergy**. Generally speaking, there two types of hypersensitivity reactions, delayed and immediate. However, these are often broken down into four categories (see Table 9–1).

Delayed and Immediate Hypersensitivity

Delayed hypersensitivity is a result of **cellular immunity** and therefore does not involve antibodies. Delayed hypersensitivity usually occurs in the hours and days following exposure and is the sort of allergy that occurs in normal people. Delayed hypersensitivity most commonly results in a skin rash and is often due to exposure to certain drugs and chemicals. The rash associated with poison ivy is an example of delayed hypersensitivity.

When people use the term *allergy,* they are usually referring to **immediate hypersensitivity** reactions. Examples of immediate hypersensitivity reactions include hay fever, drug allergies, food allergies, eczema, and asthma. Some persons have an allergic tendency. This allergic tendency is usually genetic, meaning it is passed from parent to child and is characterized by the presence of large quantities of **IgE antibodies**. An

TABLE 9–1

Gell and Coombs Classification of Hypersensitivity Reactions

Type	Classification	Mediator	Examples
I	Immediate hypersensitivity reactions	Immunoglobulin E (IgE)	Common allergies
			Asthma
II	Cytotoxic hypersensitivity reactions	i\Immunoglobulin G (IgG)	Thrombocytopenia
		Immunoglobulin M (IgM)	
III	Immune-complex reactions	Circulating antigen-antibody	Serum sickness
		Complexes	Systemic lupus erythematosis
IV	Delayed hypersensitivity reactions	Cell mediated (T cells)	Poison ivy, oak
			Chronic transplant rejection

antigen that causes release of the IgE antibodies is referred to as an **allergen**. Common allergens include:

- Drugs
- Foods and food additives
- Animals
- Insects (*Hymenoptera* stings) and insect parts
- Fungi and molds
- Radiology contrast materials
- Latex (rubber gloves, condoms)

Allergens can enter the body through various routes. These include oral ingestion, inhalation, topically, and through injection or envenomation. The vast majority of anaphylactic reactions result from injection or envenomation. However, recent increases in processed foods and similar problems have led to an increase in food allergies. Allergic reactions to certain foods (e.g., peanuts) can be life threatening.

Parenteral penicillin injections are the most common cause of fatal anaphylactic reactions. Insect stings are the second most frequent cause of fatal anaphylactic reactions. Insects in the order *Hymenoptera* are the most frequent offending insects. There are three families in this order: fire ants *(Formicoidea);* wasps, yellow jackets, and hornets *(Vespidae);* and the honey bees *(Apoidea)*. All produce a unique venom, although there are similar components in each. Honeybees often will leave their stinger embedded in the victim following a sting.

Following exposure to a particular allergen, large quantities of IgE antibodies are released. These antibodies attach to the membranes of **basophils** and **mast cells**—specialized cells of the immune system that contain chemicals that assist in the immune response. When the allergen binds to IgE attached to the basophils and mast cells, these cells release histamine, heparin, and other substances into the surrounding tissues. Histamine and other substances are stored in **granules** found within the basophils and mast cells. In fact, because of this feature, basophils and mast cells are often called **granulocytes**. The process of releasing these substances from the cells is called **degranulation**. This release results in what people call an *allergic reaction* that can be very mild or very severe.

The principal chemical mediator of an allergic reaction is histamine. **Histamine** is a potent substance that causes bronchoconstriction, increased intestinal motility, vasodilation, and increased vascular permeability. Increased vascular permeability causes the leakage of fluid from the circulatory system into the surrounding tissues. A common manifestation of severe allergic reactions and anaphylaxis is angioneurotic edema. **Angioneurotic edema**, also called *angioedema,* is marked edema of the skin and usually involves the head, neck, face, and upper airway. Histamine acts by activating specialized histamine receptors present throughout the body.

There are four classes of histamine receptors. H_1 receptors, when stimulated, cause bronchoconstriction and contraction of the intestines. H_2 receptors cause peripheral vasodilation and secretion of gastric acids. Other histamine types are detailed in Table 9-2. The goal of histamine release is to minimize the body's exposure to the antigen. Bronchoconstriction decreases the possibility of the antigen entering through the respiratory tract. Increased gastric acid production helps destroy an ingested antigen. Increased intestinal motility serves to move the antigen quickly though through the gastrointestinal system with minimal absorption of the antigen into the body. Vasodilation and capillary permeability help remove the allergen from the circulation where it has the potential to do the most harm.

Anaphylaxis usually occurs when a specific allergen is injected directly into the circulation. This is the reason anaphylaxis is more common following injections of drugs and diagnostic agents and following bee stings. When the allergen enters the circulation, it is distributed widely throughout the body. The allergen interacts with both basophils and mast cells, resulting in the massive dumping of histamine and other substances associated with anaphylaxis. The principal body systems affected by anaphylaxis are the cardiovascular system, the respiratory system, and gastrointestinal systems, and the skin. Histamine causes widespread peripheral vasodilation as well as increased permeability of the capillaries. Increased capillary permeability results in marked loss of plasma from the circulation. People sustaining anaphylaxis can actually die from circulatory shock.

Also released from the basophils and mast cells is a substance called **slow-reacting substance of anaphylaxis (SRS-A)**. This causes spasm of the bronchial smooth muscle, resulting in an asthma-like attack and occasionally asphyxia. SRS-A potentiates the effects of histamine, especially on the respiratory system.

Treatment

The treatment of allergic reactions and anaphylaxis generally follows a step-wise approach. Because these reactions significantly impact the respiratory and cardiovascular systems, medications that act upon these systems are among the first used (cardiovascular medications were discussed in Chapter 7 and respiratory medications were discussed in Chapter 8).

Allergic Reactions

Mild to moderate allergic reactions (those without respiratory or cardiovascular compromise) can be treated with sympathomimetics and antihistamines. The most commonly used sympathomimetic is epinephrine 1:1000. Epinephrine 1:1000 contains 1 milligram of epinephrine in 1 milliliter of solvent. The typical dose is 0.3–0.5 milligrams IM. The IM route is preferred over the subcutaneous (SQ) route because blood flow to the subcutaneous tissues is often unpredictable during allergic reactions that make epinephrine absorption also unpredictable. Patients who receive IM epinephrine will have transient tachycardia, tremors and anxiety following administration. These will usually clear in 20–30 minutes.

The second-line therapy in allergic reactions is antihistamines. Antihistamines block various histamine receptors. There are four types of known histamine receptors and these are detailed in Table 9–2.

Most common antihistamines block H_1 receptors, H_2 receptors, or both. They vary in their selectivity for the various receptor types. The most commonly used antihistamine is diphenhydramine (Benadryl) that blocks both H_1 and H_2 receptors. Some of the medications used to treat gastritis and peptic ulcer disease are also antihistamines (e.g., cimetidine [Tagamet], ranitidine [Zantac], and famotidine [Pepcid]). These have

TABLE 9–2

Types of Histamine Receptors

Receptor Type	Major Tissue Locations	Major Biological Effects
H_1	Smooth muscle, endothelial cells	Acute allergic reactions
H_2	Gastric parietal cells	Secretion of gastric acid
H_3	Central nervous system	Modulation of neurotransmission
H_4	Mast cells, eosinophils, T cells	Regulate immune response

a propensity to block H_2 receptors over H_1 receptors thus decreasing gastric acid secretion without causing the sedation seen with diphenhydramine. However, they do have some H_1 effects and can be used in the treatment of acute allergic reactions. Patients who are wheezing or coughing may benefit from inhaled β-agonist therapy. Finally, in selected cases, corticosteroids are used to further treat allergic reactions and the inflammatory processes that occur. Typically, an oral agent such as prednisone is administered. Occasionally, injectable corticosteroids such as methylprednisolone (Solu-Medrol), dexamethasone (Decadron), and hydrocortisone (Solu-Cortef) are also administered (either IV or IM depending on the drug).

Anaphylaxis

Anaphylaxis requires a much more intense response and treatment. Because bronchospasm is common, oxygen should be administered to all hypoxic patients. Histamines and the other agents of anaphylaxis increase capillary permeability allowing fluid to leave the intravascular space and enter the interstitial space (causing edema, urticaria). Thus, these patients can rapidly develop intravascular volume depletion requiring emergent IV fluid therapy to maintain blood pressure and perfusion. Then, and concomitantly, other medications are required as well.

Epinephrine

Epinephrine is a sympathetic agonist. It causes an increase in heart rate, an increase in the strength of the cardiac contractile force, and peripheral vasoconstriction. It can also reverse some of the bronchospasm associated with anaphylaxis. Epinephrine also reverses much of the capillary permeability caused by histamine. It acts within minutes of administration. In severe anaphylaxis, characterized by hypotension and/or severe airway obstruction, administer epinephrine 1:10 000 intravenously. Epinephrine 1:10 000 contains 1 mg of epinephrine in 10 milliliters (mL) of solvent. The effects of intravenous epinephrine wear off in 3–5 minutes, so repeat boluses may be required. In severe cases of sustained anaphylaxis, medical direction may order the preparation and administration of an epinephrine drip.

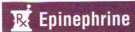 **Epinephrine**

Class Sympathetic agonist

Description

Epinephrine is a naturally occurring catecholamine. It is a potent α- and β-adrenergic stimulant; however, its effect on β-receptors is more profound.

Mechanism of Action

Epinephrine acts directly on α- and β-adrenergic receptors. Its effect on β-receptors is much more profound than its effect on α-receptors. The effects of epinephrine include the following:

- Increased heart rate
- Increased cardiac contractile force
- Increased systemic vascular resistance
- Increased blood pressure
- Decreased capillary permeability

Epinephrine has been the mainstay in the treatment of allergic reactions and anaphylaxis.

When given IV in anaphylaxis epinephrine's effects usually appear within 90 seconds of administration, and they are usually of short duration. Therefore, it must be administered every 3 to 5 minutes to maintain therapeutic levels or an epinephrine drip started. When given IM, the onset of effect is slower and the duration of effect is prolonged.

Pharmacokinetics

Onset: < 2 minutes (IV)

Peak Effects: < 5 minutes (IV)

Duration: 5–10 minutes (IV)

Half-Life: 5 minutes (IV)

Indications

Allergic reactions (1:1000) and anaphylaxis (typically 1:10 000).

Contraindications

Epinephrine 1:10 000 is contraindicated in patients who do exhibit signs of cardiovascular collapse (anaphylaxis). With simple allergic reactions and asthma, the 1:1000 dilution should be used and is administered intramuscularly.

Precautions

Epinephrine, like all catecholamines, should be protected from light. It can be deactivated by alkaline solutions such as sodium bicarbonate. Thus, it is essential that the IV line be adequately flushed between administrations of epinephrine and sodium bicarbonate.

Side Effects

Epinephrine can cause palpitations, anxiety, tremulousness, headache, dizziness, nausea, and vomiting. Because of its strong inotropic and chronotropic properties, epinephrine increases myocardial oxygen demand. Even in low doses it can cause myocardial ischemia. When administering epinephrine in the emergency setting, these effects should be kept in mind.

Interactions/Incompatibilities

Epinephrine is pH dependent and can be deactivated when administered with highly alkaline solutions such as sodium bicarbonate. The effects of epinephrine can be intensified in patients who are taking antidepressants.

Dosage

Epinephrine can be administered intramuscularly, intravenously, intraosseously, or endotracheally. Common doses include the following:

Anaphylaxis (adults). The dose of epinephrine in anaphylaxis is 0.05–0.1 mg (5% to 10% of the epinephrine dose used routinely in cardiac arrest) of a 1:10 000 solution intravenously or via an intraosseous device. Higher dosages may be ordered by medical control. The endotracheal dose should be increased to at least 2–2.5 times the intravenous dose but is generally ineffective. If repeated boluses are required, consider an epinephrine infusion at 5–15 mcg/min based on severity of reaction and in addition to crystalloid infusion.

Allergic reaction (adult). The initial dose of epinephrine in mild to moderate allergic reactions is 0.1–0.3 mg of the 1:1000 solution IM. This can be repeated in 15–20 minutes as required.

Severe anaphylaxis or severe asthma (children). Intravenous epinephrine should be used only for life threatening, severe anaphylaxis and severe asthma. Less severe cases should be treated with epinephrine 1:1000 intramuscularly or with an inhaled β-agonist. In severe anaphylaxis or asthma the initial dose should be 0.01 mg/kg intravenously. The dose may be repeated every 5–15 minutes as required. An epinephrine drip may be required in severe cases.

Antihistamines

Antihistamines are second-line agents in the treatment of anaphylaxis. They should only be given following the administration of epinephrine. Antihistamines block the effects of histamine by blocking histamine receptors. They do not displace histamine from the receptors. They only block additional histamine from binding. They also help reduce histamine release from mast cells and basophils. Most antihistamines are non-selective and block both H_1 and H_2 receptors. Others are more selective for either H_1 or H_2 receptors.

Diphenhydramine (Benadryl) is probably the most frequently used antihistamine in the treatment of allergic reactions and anaphylaxis. It is non-selective and acts on both H_1 and H_2 receptors. The standard dose of diphenhydramine is 25–50 mg intravenously or intramuscularly. It should be administered slowly when given intravenously. The pediatric dose of diphenhydramine is 1–2 milligrams per kilogram (mg/kg) of body weight. Other non-selective antihistamines frequently used are hydroxyzine (Atarax, Vistaril) and promethazine (Phenergan). Hydroxyzine is a potent antihistamine, but it can be administered only intramuscularly. Promethazine can be administered intravenously or intramuscularly, but does not appear to be as potent as diphenhydramine. Promethazine has significant side effects that limit its use in EMS and emergency medicine.

Selective histamine blockers are primarily H_2 blockers used to treat ulcer disease. Blockage of the H_2 receptors decreases gastric acid secretion. However, H_2 receptors are also present in the peripheral blood vessels. Administration of H_2 blockers conceivably will reverse some of the vasodilation associated with anaphylaxis. The two most frequently used H_2 blockers are cimetidine (Tagamet) and ranitidine (Zantac). Typically, 300 mg of cimetidine or 50 mg of ranitidine are administered by slow IV push (over 3–5 minutes). (Some recent studies have questioned the effectiveness of H_2 blockers in the treatment of allergic reactions.) Also, these agents are more expensive than the non-selective antihistamines.

℞ Diphenhydramine (Benadryl)

Class Antihistamine

Description

H_1 receptor antagonist

Mechanism of Action

Diphenhydramine is an H_1 receptor antagonist blocking histamine release. It also has considerable anticholinergic activity

Pharmacokinetics

Onset: 10–15 minutes (IV)
Peak Effects: 1 hour
Duration: 6–8 hours
Half-Life: 1–4 hours

Indications

Allergic reactions and anaphylaxis. It is also effective in extrapyramidal symptoms.

Contraindications

Do not use in patients with a known hypersensitivity to the drug.

Precautions

Use with caution in patients with asthma, narrow-angle glaucoma, benign prostatic hypertrophy.

Side Effects

Drowsiness, dizziness, headache, fatigue, palpitations, euphoria, and urinary frequency have been reported.

Interactions/Incompatibilities

Furosemide

Dosage

25–50 mg IV or IM

Route

IV, IM, PO

Corticosteroids

Corticosteroids are important in the treatment and prevention of anaphylaxis. Although they are of little benefit in the initial stages of treatment they help suppress the inflammatory response associated with these emergencies. Commonly used corticosteroids include methylprednisolone (Solu-Medrol), hydrocortisone (Solu-Cortef), and dexamethasone (Decadron).

℞ Methylprednisolone (Solu-Medrol)

Class Corticosteroid and anti-inflammatory

Description

Methylprednisolone is a synthetic steroid with potent anti-inflamatory properties.

Mechanism of Action

Corticocosteroids have multiple actions in the body. They have potent anti-inflammatory properties and inhibit many of the substances that cause inflammation (cytokines, interleukin, interferon) and also inhibit the synthesis of pro-inflammatory enzymes. The pharmacological actions of the steroids are vast and complex. In general medical practice, steroids have a wide range of uses. Effective as anti-inflammatory agents, they are used in the management of allergic reactions, asthma, and anaphylaxis. Methylprednisolone is considered an intermediate-acting steroid with a plasma half-life of about 3 to 4 hours.

Pharmacokinetics

Onset: Varies
Peak Effects: 4–8 days (IM)
Duration: 1–5 weeks (IM)
Half-Life: 3.5 hours

Indications

Methylprednisolone is used in severe anaphylaxis, asthma or COPD, and urticaria (hives).

Contraindications

There are no major contraindications to the use of methylprednisolone in the acute management of severe anaphylaxis.

Precautions

A single dose of methylprednisolone is all that should be given in the prehospital phase of care. Long-term steroid therapy can cause gastrointestinal bleeding, prolonged wound healing, and suppression of adrenocortical steroids.

Side Effects

Methylprednisolone can cause fluid retention, congestive heart failure, hypertension, abdominal distension, vertigo, headache, nausea, malaise, and hiccups.

Interactions/Incompatibilities

There are few interactions in the prehospital setting.

Dosage

The standard dosage of methylprednisolone in the management of severe anaphylaxis is 125–250 mg administered intravenously. Methylprednisolone may be administered intravenously or intramuscularly, but the intravenous route is preferred in emergency medicine.

Hydrocortisone (Solu-Cortef)

Class Corticosteroid and anti-inflammatory

Description

Hydrocortisone is a potent corticosteroid with anti-inflammatory properties.

Mechanism of Action

Corticocosteroids have multiple actions in the body. They have potent anti-inflammatory properties and inhibit many of the substances that cause inflammation (cytokines, interleukin, interferon) and also inhibit the synthesis of pro-inflammatory enzymes. The pharmacological actions of the steroids are vast and complex. Hydrocortisone is considered a short-acting steroid with a plasma half-life of 90 minutes. Like the other adrenocorticosteroids, it is effective as an adjunct in the management of severe anaphylaxis.

Pharmacokinetics

Onset: Immediate
Peak Effects: 4–8 hours
Duration: 1.0–1.5 days
Half-Life: 90 minutes

Indications

Hydrocortisone is used in severe anaphylaxis, asthma or COPD, and urticaria (hives).

Contraindications

There are no major contraindications to the use of hydrocortisone in the acute management of anaphylaxis.

Precautions

A single dose of hydrocortisone is all that should be given in the prehospital phase of care. Long-term steroid therapy can cause gastrointestinal bleeding, prolonged wound healing, and suppression of adrenocortical steroids.

Side Effects

Hydrocortisone can cause fluid retention, congestive heart failure, hypertension, abdominal distension, vertigo, headache, nausea, malaise, and hiccups.

Interactions/Incompatibilities

There are few interactions in the prehospital setting.

Dosage

The standard dosage of hydrocortisone in the management of severe anaphylaxis is 40–250 mg administered intravenously.

Route

The IV route is preferred in emergency medicine. However, hydrocortisone can be administered intramuscularly when an IV cannot be started.

℞ Dexamethasone (Decadron)

Class Corticosteroid and anti-inflammatory

Description

Dexamathasone is a potent corticosteroid with anti-inflammatory properties.

Mechanism of Action

Corticocosteroids have multiple actions in the body. They have potent anti-inflammatory properties and inhibit many of the substances that cause inflammation (cytokines, interleukin, interferon) and also inhibit the synthesis of pro-inflammatory enzymes. The pharmacological actions of the steroids are vast and complex. Dexametasone is considered an intermediate long-acting steroid with a plasma half-life of 3+ hours. Like the other adrenocorticosteroids, it is effective as an adjunct in the management of severe anaphylaxis.

Pharmacokinetics

Onset: Immediate
Peak Effects: 1–2 hours
Duration: 2.75 days
Half-Life: 3–4.5 hours

Indications

Dexamethasone is used in severe anaphylaxis, asthma or COPD, and urticaria (hives).

Contraindications

There are no major contraindications to the use of dexamethasone in the acute management of anaphylaxis.

Precautions

A single dose of dexamathasone is all that should be given in the prehospital phase of care. Long-term steroid therapy can cause gastrointestinal bleeding, prolonged wound healing, and suppression of adrenocortical steroids.

Side Effects

Dexamethasone can cause fluid retention, congestive heart failure, hypertension, abdominal distension, vertigo, headache, nausea, malaise, and hiccups.

Interactions/Incompatibilities

There are few interactions in the prehospital setting.

Dosage

The standard dosage of dexamethasone in the management of severe anaphylaxis is 4 to 10 mg administered intravenously.

Route

The IV route is preferred in emergency medicine. However, dexamethasone can be administered intramuscularly when an IV cannot be started.

Vasopressors

Severe and prolonged anaphylactic reactions may require the use of potent vasopressors to support blood pressure. Use these medications in conjunction with first line therapy and adequate fluid resuscitation. Commonly used agents include dopamine, norepinephrine, and epinephrine. These medications are prepared as infusions and are continuously administered to support blood pressure and cardiac output.

Beta$_2$-Agonists

Many patients with severe allergic reactions and anaphylaxis will develop bronchospasm, laryngeal edema, or both. In these cases, an inhaled beta agonist can be useful. The most frequently used beta agonists in prehospital care is albuterol (Ventolin, Proventil) or levalbuterol (Xopenex). Although usually used in the treatment of asthma, these agents will help reverse some of the bronchospasm and laryngeal edema associated with anaphylaxis. Give the adult patient 2.5 mg of albuterol in 3 milliliters mL of normal saline via a hand-held nebulizer. Children (between ages 2 and 12) should receive 0.63 or 1.25 mg of albuterol based on their weight. Other beta agonists, such as metaproterenol (Alupent) or levalbuterol (Xopenex) may be used instead of albuterol.

Other Agents

Other drugs occasionally used in the treatment of anaphylaxis include aminophylline and cromolyn sodium. Aminophylline is a bronchodilator unrelated to the beta-agonists. It can be administered by slow intravenous infusion to treat the bronchospasm associated with anaphylaxis. Although cromolyn sodium (Intal) is not used in the treatment of allergic reactions and anaphylaxis, it is used in their prevention. Cromolyn sodium helps to stabilize the membranes of the mast cells, thus reducing the amount of histamine and other mediators released when these cells are stimulated.

CHAPTER REVIEW

Summary

Allergic reactions can be problematic and even life threatening. The longer treatment is delayed, the more inflammation will occur and the more difficult the emeregncy will be to treat. Anaphylaxis is a severe allergic reaction and life threatening. The primary drug in the treatment of allergic reactions is epinephrine. Following that, antihistamines, inhaled beta agonists, and corticosteroids play an important role. Prompt recognition of the signs and symptoms of allergic reactions is essential.

Key Words

allergen   A substance that is foreign to the body and can cause an allergic reaction in certain people.

allergic reaction   A hypersensitivity reaction to a particular allergen.

allergy   A hypersensitivity to a substance that causes the body to react to any contact with that substance.

anaphylaxis   An extreme and life-threatening extreme sensitivity to an antigen, causing secretion of histamine and other mediators.

angioneurotic edema   The rapid swelling of subcutaneous tissues and submucosal tissues following exposure to an allergen and certain medications.

basophils   A type of white blood cell that contains granules that stain readily with basic dyes.

cellular immunity   A type of immunity resulting from a cell-mediated immune response. Also called *cell-mediated immunity*.

degranulation   A cellular process whereby granulocytes release chemicals to help manage an invading infection or allergen.

delayed hypersensitivity   An inflammatory reactions initiated by mononuclear leukocytes (cell-mediated).

granules   A small particle of a given substance.

granulocytes   A group of white cells that have granules in their cytoplasm (eosinophils, basophils, neutrophils).

histamine   A chemical found in humans and other mammals that is released as part of the body's immune response, causing physiological changes including dilation of the blood vessels, contraction of smooth muscle (as in the airways), and increased gastric acid secretion. The itching and sneezing typical of respiratory allergies are caused by the release of histamine.

Hymenoptera   An order of insects including bees, wasps and ants.

hypersensitivity   Overly sensitive; another term for allergy.

IgE antibody   One of the five major classes of immunoglobulins (antibodies). It is present primarily in the skin and mucous membranes.

immediate hypersensitivity   Allergic reaction that involves release of histamine and other mediators from basophils and mast cells.

mast cells   A cell found in connective tissue that contains numerous basophilic granules and releases substances such as heparin and histamine in response to injury or inflammation of bodily tissues.

sensitization   To make hypersensitive or reactive to an antigen especially by a second or repeated exposure.

slow-reacting substance of anaphylaxis (SRS-A)   An inflammatory agent released by mast cells in the anaphylactic reaction, inducing a slow, prolonged contraction of certain smooth muscles and acting as an important mediator of allergic bronchial asthma.

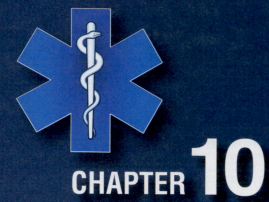

CHAPTER 10

MEDICATIONS USED IN THE TREATMENT OF METABOLIC-ENDOCRINE EMERGENCIES

OBJECTIVES

After completing this chapter, the reader should be able to:

- Define the term *hormone*.
- Discuss the function and location of the pancreas.
- List two functions of the pancreas.
- Discuss the function of glucagon.
- Define *diabetes mellitus*.
- Discuss the function of insulin and its relation to glucose metabolism.
- Compare and contrast type I and type II diabetes mellitus.
- Compare and contrast diabetic ketoacidosis and hyperosmolar hyperglycemic state.
- Detail the pathophysiology and treatment of hypoglycemia.
- Describe and list the indications, contraindications, and dosages for insulin, glucagon, dextrose, and thiamine.

INTRODUCTION

Glands that secrete **hormones** directly into the blood, without the aid of ducts, are called **endocrine glands**. A hormone is a chemical substance produced by an organ or specialized cells that regulates or controls the activities of another organ. Hormones are typically released directly into the bloodstream where they are transported to the target issues. With the exception of the pancreas, they rarely cause emergency disorders. Occasionally the thyroid, the endocrine gland that controls metabolic rate, begins secreting excess thyroid hormones. This disorder, called hyperthyroidism, is characterized by increased heart rate, loss of body weight, insomnia, dry skin, hair loss, and nervousness. A rare but severe form of thyroid dysfunction is called *thyroid storm*. Thyroid storm causes fever, tachycardia, dehydration, and a change in mental status. Although this chapter is devoted to metabolic-endocrine emergencies, we primarily discuss the pancreatic disorder **diabetes mellitus**.

DIABETES MELLITUS

The disease diabetes mellitus is marked by inadequate insulin activity in the body. Insulin is critical to maintaining normal blood glucose levels. Glucose is important for all cells, but it is especially important for brain cells. In fact, glucose is the only substance that brains cells can readily and efficiently use as an energy source. In addition, insulin enables the body to store energy as glycogen, protein and fat.

The pancreas is located in the retroperitoneal space, within the folds of the small intestine. Within the pancreas is an area called the *islets of Langerhans*. The islets of Langerhans have three types of cells that secrete three different hormones. The alpha (α) cells secrete the hormone *glucagon*. The beta (β) cells secrete *insulin*. A third hormone, called *somatostatin,* is secreted from the delta (γ) cells. Insulin is required for the passage of glucose into the cells. Without insulin the blood glucose level rises. Glucagon causes stored carbohydrates, especially glycogen, to be broken down to glucose. When the blood sugar level falls, glucagon is released, which then causes a release of stored carbohydrates. Somatostatin inhibits the secretion of both insulin and glucagon as well as growth hormone.

Diabetes mellitus is a group of endocrine/metabolic diseases that is characterized by elevated blood glucose levels (**hyperglycemia**) that results from defects in insulin secretion, insulin action, or both. The chronic hyperglycemia of diabetes is associated with long-term cell and tissue damage, dysfunction, and failure of various organs, especially the eyes, kidneys, nerves, heart, and blood vessels.

Several pathophysiological processes have been associated with the development of diabetes. These range from the autoimmune destruction of the β-cells of the pancreas with subsequent insulin deficiency to abnormalities that result in resistance to insulin action. The fundamental basis of the abnormalities in carbohydrate, fat, and protein metabolism in diabetes is deficient action of insulin on target tissues. Deficient insulin action results from inadequate insulin secretion and/or diminished tissue responses to insulin at one or more points in the complex pathways of hormone action. Impairment of insulin secretion and defects in insulin action often coexist, and it is often unclear which abnormality is the primary cause of the hyperglycemia.

Symptoms of marked hyperglycemia include polyuria, polydipsia, weight loss, sometimes with polyphagia, and blurred vision. Impairment of growth and susceptibility to certain infections may also accompany chronic hyperglycemia. Acute, life-threatening consequences of uncontrolled diabetes are hyperglycemia with **ketoacidosis** or the hyperosmolar hyperglycemic state.

The long-term complications of diabetes include retinopathy with potential loss of vision; kidney damage (nephropathy) leading to renal failure; peripheral nerve damage (neuropathy) with risk of foot ulcers, amputations, and joint destruction (Charcot joints); and autonomic neuropathy causing gastrointestinal, genitourinary, and cardiovascular symptoms and sexual dysfunction. Patients with diabetes have an increased incidence of atherosclerotic cardiovascular, peripheral arterial, and cerebrovascular disease. Hypertension and abnormalities of lipid metabolism are often found in people with diabetes (see Table 10–1).

REGULATION OF BLOOD GLUCOSE LEVELS

Homeostasis of blood glucose is remarkably effective. Fasting blood glucose (after an overnight fast) is usually between 80 and 100 mg/dL (4.4–5.5 mmol/L) blood. In the first hour or so after a meal blood glucose may increase to about 120–140 mg/dL (6.6–7.7 mmol/L) before falling toward the baseline level.

TABLE 10–1

Typical Findings in Diabetic-Induced Altered Mental Status

Hypoglycemia

Scene Size-up	Primary Assessment	Signs and Symptoms	Vitals/Physical Exam	History	Causes	Management
Presence of syringes, insulin, glucometers, lower extremity prosthetic devices	Chief complaint may reveal patient or family awareness of diabetic condition; may complain of confusion, restlessness, weakness Acute onset Airway compromise (vomitus, tongue)	Weakness/uncoordination Lethargy/confusion Headache Irritable, nervous behavior Hunger, thirst, polyuria Malaise Abdominal pain May appear intoxicated Coma (severe cases)	**Vitals** Weak or full, rapid pulses Cold clammy skin Diaphoresis Pupils normal to dilated	History of diabetes, cardiac, renal, or vascular disease Obesity, endocrine problems; exertion, infection Slow healing wounds, poor peripheral perfusion, scarring of fingers; provisional amputations	Patient has taken too much insulin Patient has overexerted, thus reducing glucose levels	Check blood sugar level Administer dextrose as per protocol/standing order

Hyperglycemia (DKA/HHNKS)

Scene Size-up	Primary Assessment	Signs and Symptoms	Vitals/Physical Exam	History	Causes	Management
Presence of syringes, insulin, glucometers, lower extremity prosthetic devices	Chief complaint may reveal patient or family awareness of diabetic condition; may complain of confusion, restlessness, weakness Gradual onset "Fruity" smell of ketones on patient's breath Airway compromise	Polyuria, polydypsia, polyphagia Nausea, vomiting Tachycardia Deep, rapid respirations Warm, dry skin Fruity odor on breath Abdominal pain Falling blood pressure Fever (occasionally) Decreased level of consciousness	**Vitals** Weak, rapid pulses Kussmaul respirations Low blood pressure in later stages Poor skin turgor, pallor, delayed capillary refill related to dehydration **Physical** Injection sites; medical alert jewelry Slow healing wounds, poor peripheral perfusion Scarring of fingers; Provisional amputations	History of diabetes, cardiac disease, renal disease, vascular disease, obesity, endocrine problems Family history of diabetes	Patient has not taken insulin Patient has overeaten, flooding the body with carbohydrates Patient has infection that disrupts glucose/insulin balance	Check blood sugar level Fluids Insulin

A blood glucose level lower than baseline (often defined as less than 80 mg/dL (4.0 mmol/L)) reflects **hypoglycemia**, or low blood sugar.

TYPES OF DIABETES

Generally, diabetes mellitus can be divided into several categories. The two most common are type I and type II diabetes mellitus. Type I diabetes usually begins in the early years. Patients who have type I diabetes must take insulin. Type II diabetes usually begins later in life and tends to be associated with age, genetics, and obesity. Type II diabetes can often be controlled without using insulin. It is important for paramedics to understand the difference between these two forms of diabetes.

Type I Diabetes Mellitus

Type I diabetes mellitus is characterized by a very low production of insulin by the pancreas. In many cases, no insulin is produced at all. Type I diabetes is commonly called juvenile onset diabetes because it usually occurs during childhood or adolescence. The term *insulin dependent diabetes mellitus* (IDDM) is also used because patients require regular insulin injections to maintain glucose homeostasis. However, some patients with type II diabetes will also require insulin. This type of diabetes is less common than type II diabetes. Diabetes is regularly among the ten leading causes of death in North America, and type I diabetes accounts for most diabetes-related deaths.

Heredity is an important factor in determining which persons will be predisposed to development of type I diabetes. The cause of type I diabetes is often unclear. However, viral infection, production of autoantibodies directed against beta cells, and genetically determined early deterioration of beta cells are all possible causes. The immediate cause of the disease is destruction of beta cells.

In untreated type I diabetes, blood glucose levels rise because, without adequate insulin, cells cannot take up the circulating sugar. Hyperglycemia in the range of 120–140 mg/dL (6.6–7.7 mmol/L) is not uncommon. As glucose spills into the urine, large amounts of water are lost through osmotic diuresis. Catabolism of fat becomes significant as the body switches to fatty acids as the primary energy source. Overall, this pathophysiology accounts for the constant thirst (polydipsia), excessive urination (polyuria), ravenous appetite (polyphagia), weakness and weight loss associated with untreated type I diabetes. Ketosis can occur as the result of fat catabolism, and it may proceed to frank diabetic ketoacidosis, a medical emergency addressed later.

Type II Diabetes Mellitus

Type II diabetes is associated with a moderate decline in insulin production accompanied by a markedly deficient response to the insulin that is present in the body. Type II diabetes is sometimes called adult-onset diabetes or non-insulin-dependent diabetes mellitus (NIDDM) although some type II diabetics require insulin. However, more and more children are developing type II diabetes mellitus because of childhood obesity. Thus, the term type II diabetes mellitus is preferred.

Heredity plays a major role in predisposition. In addition, obese persons are more likely to develop type II diabetes, and obesity probably plays a role in the development of the disease. Increased weight (and increased size of fat cells) causes a relative deficiency in the number of insulin receptors per cell, which makes fat cells, as well as muscle and liver cells, less responsive to insulin. This type of diabetes is far more common than type I diabetes, accounting for about 80 percent of cases of diabetes mellitus.

Untreated type II diabetes typically presents with a higher level of hyperglycemia (due to longstanding hyperglycemia) and fewer major signs of metabolic disruption. For instance, insulin stores, although inadequate for most body processes, are usually sufficient to keep the body from switching to fats as the primary energy source (thus avoiding the production of ketones). Thus, DKA is uncommon in these patients. However, a complication called hyperosmolar hyperglycemic nonketotic state (HHNKS) can occur and will present as a medical emergency. This is discussed below.

Medical treatment of type II diabetes is less intrusive than that required for type I diabetes. Initial therapy often consists of dietary change and increased exercise in an attempt to improve body weight. If nonpharmacological therapy is insufficient to bring blood glucose levels down to the normal range, oral hypoglycemic agents may be prescribed. Many of these medications stimulate insulin secretion by beta cells, however, control may eventually require use of insulin.

DIABETIC KETOACIDOSIS (DIABETIC COMA)

Diabetic coma is a general term describing the alteration in mental status often seen with hyperglycemia. Diabetic coma can be caused by *diabetic ketoacidosis (DKA)* or **hyperosmolar hyperglycemic nonketotic state (HHNKS)**. It is often difficult to distinguish these two conditions in the prehospital setting.

DKA is a serious, potentially life-threatening complication associated with type I diabetes. It occurs when there is a profound insulin deficiency coupled with increased glucagon activity. DKA may be the initial presentation of severe diabetes. It can result from patient noncompliance with insulin injections or as the result of physiological stress caused by surgery or serious infection. Some of the major characteristics of diabetic emergencies are listed in Table 10-1.

Pathophysiology: In the initial phase of DKA, profound hyperglycemia exists because of lack of insulin. Body cells cannot take in glucose. The compensatory mechanism for low glucose levels with cells, **gluconeogenesis**, only contributes more blood glucose. The consequent loss of glucose in the urine, accompanied by loss of water through osmotic diuresis, produces significant dehydration.

As the body switches to a fat-based metabolism, the blood level of ketones rises. The ketone load accounts for much of the observed acidosis. By the time the characteristic decrease in pH from about 7.4 to about 6.9 has occurred, the patient is hours from death if left untreated.

Signs and Symptoms: The onset of clinically obvious DKA is often slow, lasting from 12 to 24 hours. In the initial phase, signs of diuresis appear, including increased urine production and dry, warm skin and mucous membranes. The individual often has excessive hunger and thirst, coupled with a progressive sense of general malaise. Volume depletion induces tachycardia and feelings of physical weakness.

As ketoacidosis develops, a major compensatory mechanism for acidosis appears: the rapid, deep breathing pattern termed **Kussmaul respirations**, which helps expel carbon dioxide (CO_2) from the body. The breath itself may have a fruity or acetone-like smell as some blood acetone (ketones) is expelled through the lungs. The blood profile includes not only hyperglycemia and an acidic pH, but also electrolyte abnormalities. Low bicarbonate levels reflect loss of acid–base buffer. Low potassium levels may be found secondary to diuresis, with marked hypokalemia increasing the risk for cardiac arrhythmias or death. Over time, mental function declines, and frank coma may occur. Fever is not characteristic of DKA. If present, it is a sign of infection.

Assessment and Management: The approach used with the patients suffering from DKA is essentially the same as with any other patient who has mental impairment or is unconscious. First, complete your primary assessment or airway, breathing, and circulation. Then, complete a focused history and secondary assessment. Look for a MedicAlert bracelet on the patient and/or insulin in the refrigerator. Obtain a history from anyone present. The sweet, fruity odor of ketones occasionally can be detected on the breath. Complete a rapid blood glucose level. It is not uncommon for patients with ketoacidosis to have blood glucose levels well in excess of 250–300 mg/dL or more.

Focus field management on maintenance of the ABCs and fluid resuscitation to counteract dehydration. Administer 1–2 liters of normal saline or follow local protocol. If the transport time is likely to be lengthy, medical direction may request paramedics administer intravenous or subcutaneous regular insulin. Rapid transport to the appropriate facility is essential to ensure definitive care.

HYPEROSMOLAR HYPERGLYCEMIC NONKETOTIC STATE (HHNKS)

Hyperosmolar hyperglycemic nonketotic state is a serious complication associated with type II diabetes. Typically, both insulin and glucagon activity are present. Hyperosmolar hyperglycemic nonketotic state develops when two conditions occur: Sustained hyperglycemia causes osmotic diuresis sufficient to produce marked dehydration, and water intake is inadequate to replace lost fluids. Renal dialysis, high-osmolarity feeding supplements, infection, and certain medications can also be associated with development of this condition.

Pathophysiology: As sustained hyperglycemia ensues, glucose spills into the urine, causing osmotic diuresis and resultant dehydration. The level of hyperglycemia can be much higher than the levels seen in ketoacidosis (often up to 600 mg/dl or more). However, insulin activity in patients with hyperosmolar hyperglycemic nonketotic state prevents significant production of ketone bodies. Inadequate fluid replacement results in characteristic signs and symptoms.

The mortality rate for hyperosmolar hyperglycemic nonketotic state is higher than for ketoacidosis. The higher mortality rate may be due to the lack of early signs and symptoms that bring patients with ketoacidosis to the attention of family or health care professionals. The mortality rate of hyperosmolar hyperglycemic nonketotic state is also high because it primarily affects the elderly.

Signs and Symptoms: The onset of hyperosmolar hyperglycemic nonketotic state is even slower than that of ketoacidosis, with development often occurring over several days. Early signs include increased urination and increased thirst. Subsequent volume depletion can result in orthostatic hypotension when the patient gets out of bed, along with other signs, such as dry skin and mucous membranes as well as tachycardia. The patient may become lethargic and confused and enter frank coma. Kussmaul respirations are rarely seen because of the lack of acidosis.

Assessment and Management: The approach used with the patient suffering from hyperosmolar hyperglycemic nonketotic state is essentially the same as with any other patient who has mental impairment or is unconscious. It is often difficult in the field to distinguish diabetic ketoacidosis from hyperosmolar hyperglycemic nonketotic state. Therefore, the prehospital treatment of both emergencies is identical.

HYPOGLYCEMIA (INSULIN SHOCK)

Hypoglycemia, or low blood sugar, is a medical emergency. It can occur when a patient takes too much insulin, eats too little to match an insulin dose, or overexerts and uses almost all available blood glucose. As the period of hypoglycemia lengthens, there is a rise in the risk that brain cells will be permanently damaged or die due to lack of glucose. Brain cells can adapt to use fats as an energy source. However, this adaptation requires hours to develop, and the switch to fat-based metabolism cannot correct any damage already occurred. This is why every second counts in treating hypoglycemia.

Pathophysiology: Hypoglycemia, or insulin shock, reflects high insulin and low blood glucose. Regardless of the reason for low blood sugar, insulin causes almost all remaining blood glucose to be taken up by cells. Because of the high level of insulin, glucagon may be ineffective in raising blood glucose levels. In prolonged fasts, almost half the glucose normally produced through gluconeogenesis is of renal origin. This activity is stimulated by epinephrine. A diabetic patient with kidney failure may be predisposed to hypoglycemia because of lack of renal gluconeogenesis.

Signs and Symptoms: The signs and symptoms of hypoglycemia are many and varied. Altered mental status is the most important. In the earliest stages of hypoglycemia, the patient may appear restless or impatient or complain of excessive hunger. As blood glucose falls lower, he may display inappropriate anger (even rage) or display a bizarre behavior. Sometimes, the patient may be placed in police custody for such behavior or be involved in an automobile accident.

Physical signs may include diaphoresis and tachycardia. If blood glucose falls to a critically low level, the patient may have a hypoglycemia seizure or become comatose.

In contrast to diabetic ketoacidosis, hypoglycemia can develop quickly. A clear change in mental status can occur without warning. Always consider hypoglycemia when encountering a patient with bizarre behavior.

TABLE 10–2

Insulin Types

Rapid Acting			
Lispro (Humalog)	< 15 minutes	0.5–3.0 hours	3–5 hours
Aspart (Novolog)	< 15 minutes	0.5–3.0 hours	3–5 hours
Glulisine (Apidra)	< 15 minutes	0.5–3.0 hours	3–5 hours
Short Acting			
Regular (Novolin R or Humulin R)	0.5–1.0 hour	2–4 hours	4–8 hours
Intermediate Acting			
NPH (Novolin N or Humulin N)	2–4 hours	4–10 hours	10–18 hours
Long Acting			
Glargine (Lantus)	4–6 hours	Same throughout day	24 hours
Detemor (Levemir)	2–3 hours	6–8 hours	Dose-dependent
Combinations			
Humulin or Novolin 70/30	0.5–1.0 hour	2–10 hours	10–18 hours
Novolog Mix 70/30	< 15 minutes	1–2 hours	10–18 hours

Assessment and Management: In suspected cases of hypoglycemia, perform the primary assessment quickly. Look for MedicAlert bracelet. Determine the blood glucose level. If the blood sugar level is less than 80 mg/dl (4.4 mmol/l), start an IV of normal saline. Next, administer 50 mL (25 g) of 50 percent dextrose intravenously. If the patient is conscious and able to swallow, complete glucose administration with available glucose paste/gels, or orange juice or sugared sodas if the patient is able to follow commands.

When an IV cannot be established, hypoglycemic patients may improve following the administration of glucagon. This is a much slower process and will work only if there are adequate stores of glucagon available. Glucagon must be reconstituted immediately prior to administration. The adult dose of 1 mg intramuscularly or subcutaneously is usually adequate.

INSULIN

Patients with type I diabetes mellitus require insulin to control their blood glucose level. Insulin may also be given to type II diabetics. Four sources of insulin are available:

- Beef insulin: from bovine pancreas (no longer available in the United States)
- Pork insulin: from porcine pancreas (no longer available in the United States)
- Human insulin: from recombinant deoxyribonucleic acid (DNA)
- Human insulin: from an enzymatic conversion of pork insulin through which the pork insulin molecule becomes identical to the insulin produced by the human pancreas

CASE PRESENTATION

At 2130 hours on a Saturday evening, paramedics are called to respond to a residence to aid a patient who is unconscious and unresponsive. Dispatch reports that the caller is unable to "wake up" his wife. The husband meets the paramedics as they arrive. He says that his wife is a diabetic and that the ambulance has been called several times before. Paramedics find the patient lying in bed in the master bedroom. The man says that his wife has been sick for a couple of days now and has been in bed for most of that time. Paramedics try to awaken the patient by gently shaking her, but there is no response. There is no evidence of trauma or of a fall. The patient is a 40-year-old woman who is unconscious and unresponsive. She is breathing adequately and has both a radial and a carotid pulse. Both, however, are weak.

Physical Examination

CNS:	The patient is unconscious and unresponsive
Resp:	Respirations are 24 per minute and shallow; lungs are clear bilaterally, with equal air entry; trachea is midline; no signs of trauma
CVS:	The radial and carotid pulses are present but weak; skin is pale and quite diaphoretic
ABD:	Soft and nontender in all four quadrants; no sign of vomiting
Muscl/Skel:	No apparent injuries; no pitting edema

(continued)

Vital Signs

Pulse:	112/minute
Resp:	24/minute, shallow
BP:	118/78 mmHg
SpO₂:	92 percent
ECG:	Sinus tachycardia
Past Hx:	The patient's husband states that the patient has been diabetic for most of her life. He also shows paramedics the insulin vials in the refrigerator (Humulin N and Humulin R). The patient has had a low-grade fever for 2 days and has not been eating because of nausea. She is also alcoholic.

Treatment

To confirm your diagnosis of hypoglycemia, paramedics decide to take a blood glucose reading. While one paramedic prepares to check the level, another administers oxygen by nasal cannula. An IV is initiated with an 18-gauge catheter and, prior to connecting the IV tubing, paramedics draw a red-top blood tube for analysis. They also use the hub of the needle to obtain a blood sample for glucose testing. An IV of normal saline is initiated and run at 125 mL/hour. The blood glucose reading is 40 mg/dL (2.2 mmol/L). At this time paramedics administer 100 mg of thiamine IV because of the history of alcoholism and 50 mL (25 g) of $D_{50}W$. Following administration of the $D_{50}W$, a fluid bolus of 20 mL of normal saline is administered to flush the IV line. Almost immediately following the $D_{50}W$ administration, the patient begins to make sounds and move about. The patient awakens and is surprised to see the paramedics. After a few minutes she is alert and oriented, although still a little lethargic. Paramedics decide to transport her to the hospital for assessment and monitor both vital signs and blood glucose levels en route. During the transport she tells paramedics that although she has not been eating normally, she was taking her regular amount of insulin.

Insulin is not effective when taken orally because the gastrointestinal (GI) tract breaks down the protein molecule before it reaches the bloodstream. All insulin, however, may be given by subcutaneous (SC) injection. Absorption of SC insulin varies according to the injection site and the vascular supply and degree of tissue hypertrophy at the injection site. Regular (unmodified) insulin may be given intravenously (IV) or intramuscularly (IM) as well.

After absorption into the bloodstream, insulin is distributed throughout the body. Insulin-response tissues are located in the liver, adipose tissue, and muscle. Insulin is metabolized primarily in the liver and to a lesser extent in the kidneys and muscle tissue; it is excreted in the feces and urine.

The exact times for onset, peak, and duration are not absolute. They may vary not only from patient to patient but from injection to injection in the same patient. If insulin absorption is altered, the onset of action, peak concentration level, and duration of action are also altered. If insulin absorption occurs more rapidly, the onset of action and peak concentration times occur more rapidly. Conversely, if insulin absorption is prolonged, onset of action and peak concentration are delayed, and duration of action is prolonged.

Insulin is an anabolic, or building, hormone. It promotes the storage of glucose as glycogen, increases protein and fat synthesis, and inhibits the breakdown of glycogen, protein, and fat.

Insulin is used for type I diabetes mellitus. It may also be required for patients with type II diabetes mellitus when other methods of maintaining normal blood glucose level are ineffective. Patients with type II diabetes mellitus may find the usual methods of maintaining a normal blood glucose level ineffective during times of emotional or physical stress (such as surgery and infection) or contraindicated because of pregnancy or hypersensitivity. These patients may need insulin to control blood glucose levels more stringently. Insulin is also indicated for two of the comas that are complications of diabetes: diabetic ketoacidosis (more common with type I diabetes mellitus) and hyperosmolar hyperglycemic nonketotic state (more common with type II diabetes mellitus).

Sometimes insulin is prescribed for patients who do not have diabetes mellitus. Because insulin stimulates cellular uptake of potassium, it may be administered with hypertonic glucose to patients with severe hyperkalemia. The administration of insulin and glucose produces a shift of serum potassium into cells and lowers the serum potassium level for a short time.

All insulin has the same effect in the body. The advantages or disadvantages of a particular kind of insulin reflect the differences in onset of action, peak concentration, and duration of action, as well as concentration, source, and purity. Many different insulin preparations are available; several are available in more than one concentration.

℞ Insulin (Humulin, Novolin)

Class
Hormone and antihyperglycemic

Description

Insulin is a protein secreted by the β cells of the islets of Langerhans. It is responsible for promoting the uptake of glucose by the cells. In diabetics, in whom insulin secretion has diminished, supplemental insulin must be obtained by injection. Older forms of insulin are derived from animals (bovine and porcine). However, animal insulin is not identical to human insulin. Consequently, many patients develop antibodies to animal insulin, rendering it less effective. Human insulin can be manufactured through genetic engineering (recombinant DNA technology). Genetically engineered insulin (Humulin, Novolin) is chemically identical to the insulin hormone secreted by the pancreas. Patients do not develop antibodies to human insulin as they do to animal insulin. There are various types of insulin with varying onsets of action and duration effect so that therapy may be tailored for the patient's condition.

Mechanism of Action

Insulin, when administered, is distributed throughout the body. It combines with insulin receptors present on the cell membranes, which promotes glucose entry into the cell and lowers the blood glucose level.

Pharmacokinetics

Onset: 0.5–1.0 hour
Peak Effects: 2–3 hours
Duration: 5–7 hours
Half-Life: 13 hours

Indications

Insulin is used in diabetic ketoacidosis, hyperglycemia, and hyperkalemia.

Contraindications

Insulin should be administered only when hyperglycemia or ketoacidosis has been confirmed. A blood glucose approximation should be obtained in all diabetic emergencies. Every emergency medical service unit carrying insulin and 50 percent dextrose should also carry an electronic glucose determination device for approximating blood glucose levels. Based on the results of the blood glucose test, and in conjunction with the physical examination, the differential field diagnosis between hypoglycemia and ketoacidosis can usually be made. If there is any doubt about the etiology of diabetic coma, glucose should be administered. Insulin is almost always administered in the emergency department and not during the prehospital phase of emergency medical care.

Precautions

Repeated measurements of the blood glucose level, including possible administration of glucose, are necessary.

Side Effects

Insulin may cause hypoglycemia. Few side effects are seen with the modern human analog insulin products.

Interactions

Certain medications, such as the corticosteroids, can increase the blood glucose level. Patients receiving these medications may require a higher dose of insulin. The signs and symptoms of hypoglycemia may be masked in patients receiving β-blockers. Paramedics must always determine the blood glucose level.

Dosage

A standard dose for diabetic coma is 5–10 units of regular insulin IV followed by an infusion at 0.1 unit per kilogram per hour; 5–20 units of regular insulin can be administered subcutaneously or intramuscularly if there is not an immediate need for intravenous insulin. In an emergency setting insulin should be given intravenously, intramuscularly, or subcutaneously.

GLUCAGON

Unlike insulin and the oral antidiabetic agents, which decrease the blood glucose level, glucagon increases it. This hyperglycemic agent is a hormone normally produced by the α cells of the islets of Langerhans in the pancreas. After SC, IM, or IV injection, glucagon is absorbed rapidly. It cannot be taken orally because it is a protein, and it would be destroyed in the GI tract. Glucagon is distributed throughout the body, although its effect occurs primarily in the liver. The exact metabolic fate of glucagon is unknown, although it is degraded extensively in the liver. Glucagon is removed from the body by the liver and the kidneys.

Glucagon regulates the rate of glucose production through **glycogenolysis**, gluconeogenesis, and **lipolysis**. A glucagon deficiency results in hypoglycemia. Although glucagon stimulates insulin secretion, insulin indirectly antagonizes glucagon's action through a negative feedback system.

Glucagon is used for emergency treatment of severe hypoglycemia. It is also used as an antidote for β-blocker overdose. Glucagon is ineffective in poorly nourished or starving patients.

℞ Glucagon

Class Hormone and antihypoglycemic

Description

Glucagon is a protein secreted by the α cells of the pancreas. Glucagon for parenteral administration is extracted from beef and pork pancreas. It is used to increase the blood glucose level in cases of hypoglycemia in which an IV cannot be immediately placed.

Mechanism of Action

Glucagon is a hormone secreted by the pancreas. When released it causes a breakdown of stored glycogen to glucose. It also inhibits the synthesis of glycogen from glucose. Both actions tend to cause an increase in circulating blood glucose. In hypoglycemia the administration of glucagon increases blood glucose levels. The medication of choice in the management of insulin-induced hypoglycemia is still $D_{50}W$. A return to consciousness is seen almost immediately following the administration of glucose. A return to consciousness following the administration of glucagon usually takes from 5 to 20 minutes. Glucagon is effective only if there are sufficient stores of glycogen in the liver. Glucagon exerts a positive inotropic action on the heart and decreases renal vascular resistance.

Pharmacokinetics

Onset: 5–20 minutes
Peak Effects: 30 minutes
Duration: 1–2 hours
Half-life: Variable

Indications

Glucagon is used in hypoglycemia and β-blocker and calcium-channel blocker overdose.

Contraindications

Glucagon should not be administered to patients with a known hypersensitivity to the medication.

Precautions

Glucagon is only effective if there are sufficient stores of glycogen within the liver. In an emergency situation intravenous glucose is the agent of choice. Glucagon should be administered with caution to patients with a history of cardiovascular or renal disease.

Side Effects

Although side effects are rare, glucagon can cause hypotension, dizziness, headache, nausea, and vomiting.

Interactions

Few interactions with glucagon are reported in the emergency setting.

Dosage

A standard initial dose is 0.25 to 0.5 mg administered intravenously. If an IV cannot be obtained, 1 mg of glucagon can be administered intramuscularly.

Route

Glucagon can be administered intravenously, intramuscularly, or subcutaneously.

Dextrose in Water ($D_{50}W$, $D_{25}W$, $D_{10}W$)

Class Carbohydrate

Description

Dextrose is used to describe the six-carbon sugar *d-glucose,* which is the principal form of carbohydrate used by the body.

Mechanism of Action

Dextrose supplies supplemental glucose in cases of hypoglycemia. Serious brain injury can occur if hypoglycemia is prolonged. Thus, in hypoglycemia the rapid administration of glucose is essential. When the hypoglycemic patient is comatose, glucose cannot be given by mouth and should be given as an IV $D_{50}W$ solution. Studies have shown that less-concentrated dextrose solutions ($D_{25}W$ or $D_{10}W$) are as effective as $D_{50}W$ and do not cause labile blood glucose levels after administration.

Pharmacokinetics

Onset: < 1 minute
Peak Effects: Varies
Duration: Varies
Half-Life: Not applicable

Indication

Dextrose is used in hypoglycemia and coma of unknown origin.

Contraindications

There are no major contraindications to the IV administration of $D_{50}W$ to a patient with suspected hypoglycemia. Even if a patient were suffering from ketoacidosis, the amount of glucose present in 50 mL of 50 percent dextrose would not adversely affect the clinical outcome; 50 percent dextrose should be used with caution in patients with increased intracranial pressure because the dextrose load may worsen cerebral edema.

Precautions

It is important to use a blood glucose monitor and draw a sample of blood before initiating an IV infusion and giving 50 percent dextrose. Localized venous irritation may occur when smaller veins are used. Infiltration of 50 percent dextrose may result in tissue necrosis.

Side Effects

Side effects can include tissue necrosis and phlebitis at the injection site.

Interactions

There are no interactions in the emergency setting.

Dosage

The standard dosage of 50 percent dextrose in hypoglycemia is 25 g (50 mL of a 50 percent solution) administered intravenously. If an initial dose is ineffective, a second dose of 25 g may also be given; 50 percent dextrose should be diluted 1:1 with sterile water for pediatric administration (thus forming $D_{25}W$). The pediatric dose is 0.5–1.0 g/kg of body weight by slow, intravenous bolus.

Route

Dextrose is given only intravenously. Concentrated glucose solutions can cause venous irritation if administered for an extended period.

THIAMINE

Thiamine is a vitamin that is essential in the conversion of glucose to energy. In medicine, thiamine is used primarily to prevent and treat thiamine deficiency syndromes such as beriberi, Wernicke's encephalopathy, and peripheral neuritis associated with pellagra. Thiamine malabsorption may occur in patients with alcoholism, cirrhosis, or GI disease, requiring supplements. In most cases thiamine administration does not result in adverse reactions or toxicity. Various nonspecific reactions that have been reported include nausea, anxiety, sweating, and sensations of warmth. Allergic reactions, ranging from itching and urticaria to cardiovascular failure and death, have occurred with parenteral administration.

℞ Thiamine

Class Vitamin

Description

Thiamine is an important vitamin commonly referred to as vitamin B_1. It is required for the conversion of pyruvic acid to acetyl coenzyme A.

Mechanism of Action

A vitamin is a substance that the body cannot manufacture but that is required for metabolism. Most of the vitamins required by the body are obtained through the diet. Thiamine is required for the conversion of pyruvic acid to acetyl coenzyme A.

Without this step, a significant amount of the energy available in glucose cannot be obtained. The brain is extremely sensitive to thiamine deficiency. Chronic alcohol intake interferes with the absorption, intake, and use of thiamine. A significant percentage of alcoholics have thiamine deficiency. During extended periods of fasting, neurological symptoms owing to thiamine deficiency may occur. These symptoms include Wernicke's encephalopathy and Korsakoff's psychosis. Wernicke's encephalopathy is an acute and reversible encephalopathy characterized by an unsteady gait, eye muscle weakness, and mental derangement. Korsakoff's psychosis is a significant memory disorder and may be irreversible. A comatose patient, especially one who is suspected to be alcoholic, should receive IV thiamine in addition to the administration of 50 percent dextrose or naloxone.

Pharmacokinetics

Onset: Rapid

Peak Effects: Varies

Duration: Varies

Half-Life: Not applicable

Indication

Thiamine is used for coma of unknown origin, especially if alcohol may be involved, and delirium tremens.

Contraindications

There are no contraindications to the administration of thiamine in the emergency setting.

Precautions

A few cases of hypersensitivity to thiamine have been reported. Thiamine should never be administered as part of a "coma cocktail." "Coma cocktails" involve the empiric administration of 50 percent dextrose, thiamine, and naloxone (and in some cases, flumazenil) to unresponsive patients in an attempt to correct the cause of their unresponsiveness and awaken them. "Coma cocktails" are a poor prehospital practice. Therapy should always be guided by objective data such as patient assessment findings and blood glucose determination.

Side Effects

Few side effects are reported with thiamine usage. However, hypotension, dyspnea, and respiratory failure have been reported with its use.

Interactions

There are no interactions in the emergency setting.

Dosage

The emergency dose of thiamine is 100 mg administered intravenously or intramuscularly.

Route

Thiamine can be given either intravenously or intramuscularly. The intravenous route is preferred in emergency medicine.

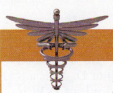

At 1630 hours on a Thursday afternoon, paramedics are called to respond to a suburban residence to aid a patient who is unresponsive. The emergency medical dispatcher reports that the caller is a 9-year-old girl who just came home from school and cannot wake up her mother.

Paramedics are met by the young girl as they arrive at the small frame residence. Tearfully she tells them that her mother is a diabetic and that the ambulance has been called several times before. As paramedics enter the residence, they notice that someone had been preparing a meal. They find the mother lying on the floor in the living room. The girl tells them that her mother's name is Tanya. Paramedics call to Tanya and gently shake her shoulder, but there is no response. There is no evidence of trauma or of a fall. The patient is a 30-year-old woman who is unconscious and unresponsive. She is breathing adequately and has both a radial and a carotid pulse. Both, however, are weak.

Physical Examination

CNS:	The patient is unconscious and unresponsive
Resp:	Respirations are 30 per minute and shallow; lungs are clear bilaterally, with equal air entry; trachea is midline; no signs of trauma
CVS:	Radial and carotid pulses present but weak; skin is pale and quite diaphoretic
ABD:	Soft and nontender in all four quadrants; no sign of vomiting
Muscl/Skel:	No apparent injuries; no pitting edema

Vital Signs

Pulse:	112/min
Resp:	30/min, shallow
BP:	118/78 mmHg
SpO$_2$:	92 percent
ECG:	Sinus tachycardia
Past Hx:	Her daughter states that the patient has been a diabetic for as long as she can remember. She also shows you insulin vials in the refrigerator (Humulin N and Humulin R). The daughter does not know when her mother last ate. However, they usually eat at 5 P.M.

Treatment

Based on physical findings, the patient history obtained from the daughter, and the presence of insulin in the refrigerator, paramedics suspect that the patient is hypoglycemic. To confirm, they decide to determine the blood glucose level. While one paramedic prepares to do this, another administers oxygen by non-rebreather mask at 15 lpm. By medical control protocol, they are able to begin definitive advanced life support procedures. Paramedics perform venipuncture with an 18-gauge catheter and, prior to connecting the IV tubing, draw a red-top blood tube for analysis. They also use the hub of the needle to obtain a blood sample for glucose testing. An IV of D$_5$W

(continued)

Case Presentation (continued)

(normal saline is also acceptable) is initiated and run at 125 mL/hour rate. The blood glucose reading is 40 mg/dL (2.2 mmol/L). At this time 50 mL (25 g) of $D_{50}W$ is administered. Following administration of the $D_{50}W$, a fluid bolus of 25 mL of D_5W is administered to flush the IV line.

Almost immediately following the $D_{50}W$ administration, the patient begins to make sounds and move about. The patient awakens and is surprised to see the paramedics. She is very apologetic and somewhat embarrassed. She insists that she is fine now and refuses transport to the hospital. After paramedics are sure that the patient is conscious, alert, and in no further danger, they inform her of the risks of refusing transport. She acknowledges the risks and signs the release form. Paramedics aseptically discontinue the IV, apply an adhesive strip, and leave the scene.

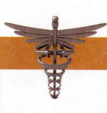

CASE PRESENTATION

Late in the afternoon on a warm September day, paramedics are dispatched to a residence to help a patient "not feeling well." The emergency medical dispatcher reports that the patient is a 60-year-old man who is reportedly conscious and alert. On arrival paramedics are directed into the patient's bedroom by his wife. The patient is lying in bed, propped up by two pillows. The patient says he has been feeling ill for over 48 hours. He also reports that he has had rather severe abdominal pain accompanied by nausea and vomiting. However, he has been able to tolerate some clear liquids. He has not been able to keep down any food. He denies any diarrhea or any other problems and is sure that this is the flu.

Physical Examination

CNS:	The patient is conscious, alert, and oriented × 4
Resp:	Respirations are 32/minute, deep and labored; lungs are clear bilaterally, with equal air entry; trachea is midline; no signs of trauma
CVS:	Both radial and carotid pulses are present but weak; skin is slightly pale and dry
ABD:	Soft and nontender in all four quadrants
Muscl/Skel:	No apparent injuries; no pitting edema

Vital Signs

Pulse:	140/min
Resp:	32/min, shallow, labored
BP:	92/54 mmHg
SpO$_2$:	94 percent
ECG:	Sinus tachycardia
Past Hx:	Past medical history includes insulin-dependent diabetes mellitus (type I). His wife states that the patient has not taken insulin since he has been sick.

Treatment

Oxygen is administered by nasal cannula at 2 lpm. The rapid, deep respirations are consistent with Kussmaul respirations. One paramedic prepares an IV of normal saline while another performs venipuncture with a 16-gauge catheter. Blood is drawn for a red-top tube and the hub of the needle is used to obtain a blood sample for glucose testing. The IV of normal saline is connected to the catheter and run at 150 mL/hr. The blood glucose reading exceeds 400 mg/dL (22.2 mmol/L). Paramedics suspect the patient is in early diabetic ketoacidosis. Care provided during transport to the hospital is primarily supportive and includes monitoring of vital signs and fluid replacement.

At the emergency department the patient's blood glucose reading is 880 mg/dL (48.88 mmol/L). His serum ketones are positive at 1:16 dilution. An arterial blood gas reveals a pH of 7.16, pCO_2 of 30 Torr, and pO_2 of 190 Torr (on 40 percent mask), which is generally consistent with a partially compensated metabolic acidosis. He is started on an insulin drip and admitted to the hospital. A chest X-ray reveals a right lower lobe pneumonia, which the emergency department physician feels contributed to the development of diabetic ketoacidosis. Following a 3-day course of antibiotics and aggressive fluid therapy, the patient is discharged.

CHAPTER REVIEW

Summary

Diabetes mellitus is probably the most common metabolic-endocrine emergency seen in the prehospital phase of emergency medical care. Hypoglycemia, if not immediately treated, can result in serious and permanent brain damage. It is important to remember that acute metabolic-endocrine disorders can cause a wide range of signs and symptoms, from bizarre behavior to coma.

Prehospital medication administration should be guided by available data. Paramedics should always determine the blood glucose level. If it is low, 50 percent dextrose should be administered. If alcoholism is suspected, administration of thiamine should be considered. If narcotic abuse is possible, administration of naloxone is considered. The "coma cocktail" is a thing of the past. Prehospital care should be based on physical exam findings and the patient's medical history.

Key Words

diabetes mellitus   An endocrine disorder characterized by inadequate insulin production by the β cells of the islets of Langerhans in the pancreas.

endocrine glands   Glands that secrete hormones directly into the blood.

gluconeogenesis   Biochemical process that produces glucose from noncarbohydrate sources; it serves to raise blood glucose levels in hypoglycemia.

glycogenolysis   Biocehmical process whereby glycogen, present in the liver and muscle, is broken down into glucose as a result of stimulation by epinephrine or glucagon.

hormones   Chemical substances released by a gland that control or affect other glands or body systems.

hyperglycemia   A complication of diabetes characterized by excessive levels of blood glucose.

hyperglycemic hyperosmolar nonketotic state   A complication of diabetes characterized by a severe hyperglycemia, hyperosmolarity, and dehydration in the absence of significant ketoacidosis.

hypoglycemia   A complication of diabetes characterized by low levels of blood glucose. It often occurs from too high a dose of insulin or from inadequate food intake following a normal insulin dose. Sometimes called *insulin shock,* hypoglycemia is a true medical emergency.

ketoacidosis   A complication of diabetes due to decreased insulin secretion or intake. It is characterized by high levels of glucose in the blood, metabolic acidosis, and, in advanced stages, coma. Ketoacidosis is often called *diabetic coma.*

Kussmaul respirations   A very deep, gasping respiratory pattern found in diabetic coma.

lipolysis   Biochemical breakdown of lipids (fats) for energy; often producing ketones as a by-product.

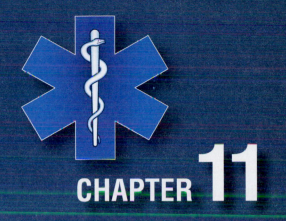

CHAPTER 11

MEDICATIONS USED IN THE TREATMENT OF NEUROLOGICAL EMERGENCIES

OBJECTIVES

After completing this chapter, the reader should be able to:

- Describe the treatment for a patient with a blunt or penetrating head injury.
- List three acute, nontraumatic neurological disorders.
- Describe and list the indications, contraindications, and dosages for the following medications used in the treatment of seizures: diazepam, lorazepam, midazolam, phenytoin, fosphenytoin, and phenobarbital.

INTRODUCTION

Emergencies involving the nervous system can be devastating. In addition, they are also difficult to manage. Signs and symptoms of neurological disorders can range from slight headache to coma. They may be temporary or permanent and prompt recognition and treatment are essential.

NEUROLOGICAL TRAUMA

Head injuries are an all-too-common result of automobile and motorcycle collisions. Although encased within the protective skull, the brain is quite susceptible to injury. Following craniocerebral trauma, cerebral edema occurs within 24 hours.

The primary treatment of patients with blunt or penetrating head injury is supportive. Airway management is of paramount importance, and continuous monitoring of blood pressure to detect occult blood loss in major trauma is mandatory. Pharmacological agents that have been used in the management of neurological emergencies include *mannitol,* an osmotic diuretic that is also useful in reducing brain edema. However, it is seldom used in prehospital care.

High-dose methylprednisolone (Solu-Medrol) was previously recommended as an emergency treatment for acute spinal cord injury. This recommendation is not supported by the literature and is no longer practiced in emergency medicine.

℞ Mannitol (Osmotrol)

Class Osmotic diuretic

Description

Mannitol is a six-carbon sugar compound that has osmotic diuretic properties.

Mechanism of Action

Mannitol is an osmotic diuretic that inhibits sodium and water absorption in the kidneys. It promotes movement of fluid from the intracellular into the extracellular space. Because it dehydrates brain tissue, mannitol has proved effective in the management of cerebral edema and reduces intracranial pressure.

Pharmacokinetics

Onset: 15 minutes

Peak Effects: 3–8 hours

Duration: Varies

Half-Life: 100 minutes

Indications

Mannitol is used for acute cerebral edema and blood transfusion reactions.

Contraindications

Mannitol should not be used in any patient with acute pulmonary edema or severe pulmonary congestion. It should not be used in any patient who is profoundly hypovolemic.

Precautions

Rapid administration of mannitol can cause a transitory increase in intravascular volume and can result in congestive heart failure. The diuresis that accompanies mannitol therapy can cause sodium depletion.

One problem in the use of mannitol in the prehospital phase of emergency medical care is crystallization of the drug. The more concentrated the solution, the more tendency it has to crystallize at low temperatures. Crystallization begins as temperatures approach 45°F. Any time a concentrated solution of mannitol is used, usually 15 percent or greater, an in-line filter should be present. It is important to remember that microscopic crystals appear long before those that can be seen by the naked eye. If mannitol solution crystallizes, it should be warmed slowly in boiling water until the crystals disappear. It should be removed from emergency medical service vehicles that are not parked in heated areas during colder weather.

Side Effects

Mannitol can cause chills, headache, dizziness, lethargy, mental status change, chest pain, nausea, and vomiting.

Interactions

Mannitol should not be administered with whole blood or packed red blood cells because it can damage the red blood cells.

Dosage

The typical adult dose of mannitol is 1.5–2.0 g/kg of body weight administered intravenously. This dose can be given as a slow IV bolus or IV infusion. The slower rate of infusion helps eliminate the chances of inducing circulatory overload and congestive heart failure.

Route

Mannitol should be given intravenously.

NONTRAUMATIC NEUROLOGICAL EMERGENCIES

There are many acute nontraumatic neurological disorders. Drugs, poisonings, and metabolic derangements can precipitate neurological emergencies. Little can be done for stroke and brain tumors in the prehospital phase of emergency medical care. Seizures attributable to epilepsy and other disorders can be managed in the field, however.

Seizures

One of the most common neurological emergencies paramedics attend is for the complaint of seizures. While most of these seizures are resolved prior to EMS arrival, some patients are still actively seizing and require immediate treatment. These patients may be experiencing **status epilepticus**, a continuous seizure that lasts for more than 30 minutes or a series of seizures without full recovery of consciousness between seizures. However, more recent research has demonstrated that seizures lasting more than 5 minutes can cause nervous system injury. *Status epilepticus* constitutes a serious threat to life and should be terminated as quickly as possible.

Seizures are a state of hyperactivity of either a section of the brain (partial seizure) or all of the brain (generalized seizure). They may or may not be accompanied by convulsions. Therefore, although the medications used to treat seizures are often called anticonvulsants, they are more appropriately referred to as antiseizure or antiepileptic medications. The goal of seizure management is to balance the elimination of the seizures against the side effects of the medications used to treat them. Controlling seizures is a lifelong process for most patients and requires diligent compliance with medication dosing regimens.

Partial (or focal) seizures erupt from a specific focus and are described in terms of alterations in consciousness or behavior. These may be further divided into simple or complex partial seizures based on the specific area of the brain in which the focus is located. Complex partial seizures are also known as psychomotor seizures and are characterized by repetitive movements.

Generalized seizures involve both hemispheres of the brain and are described in terms of visible motor activity. Grand mal seizures involve periods of muscle rigidity (tonic stage) followed by twitching (clonic stage) and then flaccidity and a gradual return to consciousness (postictal stage). Petit mal seizures are also generalized but do not have obvious convulsions. They involve brief losses of consciousness that may occur hundreds of times a day. They are also called absence seizures and are treated differently from other types of seizures. Finally, *status epilepticus*, as detailed above, is a life-threatening condition characterized by uninterrupted grand mal seizures lasting more than 30 minutes or by two or more tonic-clonic seizures without an intervening lucid period. The preferred therapy for each type of seizure differs.

Seizures are treated through several general mechanisms. The most common is a direct action on the sodium and calcium ion channels in the neural membranes. Phenytoin (Dilantin) and carbamazepine (Tegretol) both inhibit the influx of sodium into the cells, thus decreasing the cell's ability to depolarize and propagate seizures. Valproic acid and ethosuximide act similarly, but they interact with calcium channels in the thalamus, where absence seizures typically begin. These two medications are useful because they are specific to hyperactive neurons and therefore have few side effects. Other medications, such as benzodiazepines and barbiturates, interact with the GABA receptor-chloride ion channel complex.

Anitseizure medications include several pharmacological classes including:

Benzodiazepines: diazepam (Valium), lorazepam (Ativan), and midazolam (Versed)

Barbiturates: phenobarbital (Luminal)

Hydantoins: phenytoin (Dilantin), fosphenytoin (Cerebyx)

Succinimides: ethosuximide (Zarontin)

GABA analogs: gabapentin (Neurontin)

Miscellaneous medications: valproic acid (Depakote)

Benzodiazepines are the most common prehospital medications used to treat seizures. However, phenytoin (Dilantin) and phenobarbital are also effective.

Benzodiazepines

Benzodiazepines produce many effects, including daytime and preanesthetic sedation, sleep inducement, relief of anxiety and tension, skeletal muscle relaxation, and anticonvulsant activity. In the prehospital setting, benzodiazepines are primarily used as skeletal muscle relaxants, for preprocedure sedation (such as cardioversion), and for anticonvulsant activity.

Benzodiazepines are absorbed well from the gastrointestinal (GI) tract and distributed widely in the body. In the prehospital setting, benzodiazepines are almost always given parenterally. All benzodiazepines are metabolized in the liver and excreted primarily in the urine. Onset of action when administered IV is 1 to 5 minutes, with peak immediate and duration of 15 minutes to 1 hour.

The principal sites of action for benzodiazepines are the cerebral cortex and the limbic, thalamic, and hypothalamic levels of the **central nervous system** (CNS).

In most cases benzodiazepines are preferred over barbiturates because of their effectiveness and safety. Benzodiazepines offer many advantages, including fewer adverse reactions, decreased potential for abuse, fewer drug interactions, a wide margin of safety between therapeutic and toxic dosages that makes overdoses less likely, and a reduced risk of physical and psychological dependence with therapeutic dosages.

℞ Diazepam (Valium)

Class Anticonvulsant and sedative

Description

Diazepam is a benzodiazepine that is frequently used as an anticonvulsant, sedative, and hypnotic.

Mechanism of Action

Benzodiazepines bind to specific sites on gamma-aminobutyric acid (GABA) Type A receptors within the brain. GABA is the major inhibitory neurotransmitter of the central nervous system. Benzodiazepines have no direct effect on the GABA receptors, but do potentiate the effects of GABA within the brain. Increased GABA levels cause sedation. Through this mechanism, the benzodiazepines display their hypnotic, anxiolytic, and anticonvulsant effects. Their usefulness, however, is limited by a broad range of side effects including compromised sedation, ataxia, amnesia, alcohol and barbiturate potentiation, tolerance development, and abuse potential.

In emergency medicine, diazepam is principally used for its anticonvulsant properties. It suppresses the spread of seizure activity through the motor cortex of the brain. It does not appear to abolish the abnormal discharge focus, however. Diazepam, one of the most frequently prescribed medications in the United States, is used in the management of anxiety and stress. It is effective in treating the tremors and anxiety associated with alcohol withdrawal. It is also an effective skeletal muscle relaxant, which makes it an effective adjunct in orthopedic injuries. It is a good premedication for minor operative procedures and cardioversion because it induces amnesia, which diminishes the patient's recall of such procedures.

Pharmacokinetics

Onset: 1–5 minutes (IV), 15–30 minutes (IM)
Peak Effects: 15 minutes (IV), 30–45 minutes (IM)
Duration: 15–60 minutes
Half-Life: 20–50 hours

Indications

Diazepam is used in major motor seizures, *status epilepticus,* premedication before cardioversion, skeletal muscle relaxant, and acute anxiety states.

Contraindications

Diazepam should not be administered to any patient with a history of hypersensitivity to the drug.

Precautions

Because diazepam is a relatively short-acting drug, seizure activity may recur. In such cases, an additional dose may be required. Flumazenil (Romazicon), a benzodiazepine antagonist, should be available to use as antidote if required. Injectable diazepam can cause local venous irritation. To minimize irritation, it should only be injected into relatively large veins and should not be given faster than 1 mL/min.

Side Effects

Diazepam can cause respiratory depression, hypotension, drowsiness, headache, amnesia, blurred vision, nausea, and vomiting.

Interactions

Diazepam is incompatible with many medications. Whenever diazepam is given intravenously in conjunction with other medications, the IV line should be adequately flushed. The effects of diazepam can be addictive when used in conjunction with other CNS depressants and alcohol.

Dosage

In the management of seizures, the usual dose of diazepam is 5–10 mg IV. In many instances it may be necessary to give diazepam directly into the vein, because the seizure activity will prevent the insertion of an indwelling catheter. When given directly into a vein, it is essential that a large vein, preferably in the antecubital fossa, be used. In acute anxiety reactions, the standard dosage is 2–5 mg administered intramuscularly.

To induce amnesia prior to cardioversion, a dosage of 5–15 mg of diazepam is given intravenously. Peak effects are seen in 5–10 minutes. Diazepam should be given intravenously by slow IV push. It can be injected intramuscularly, but absorption via this route is variable. When an IV line cannot be started, parenteral diazepam can be administered rectally with a similar onset of action.

Diazepam can be given rectally when an IV or IO line cannot be established. It is commercially available in a gel for rectal administration (Diastat). It is occasionally prescribed for home administration in the treatment of chronic seizures.

℞ Lorazepam (Ativan)

Class Anticonvulsant and sedative

Description

Lorazepam is a benzodiazepine that is used as an anticonvulsant, sedative, and hypnotic.

Mechanism of Action

Lorazepam is a benzodiazepine with the same mechanism of action as diazepam. It has a shorter half-life than that of diazepam, however it has a longer duration of action than diazepam when used in the treatment of seizures. It is used in the management of anxiety and stress. It is a good premedication for minor operative procedures and cardioversion because it induces **amnesia**, which diminishes the patient's recall of such procedures. Lorazepam is often used in pediatrics as an anticonvulsant because of its shorter half-life. Like diazepam, lorazepam suppresses the spread of seizure activity through the motor cortex of the brain. It does not appear to abolish the abnormal discharge focus.

Pharmacokinetics

Onset: 1–5 minutes (IV), 15–30 minutes (IM)
Peak Effects: 15–20 minutes (IV), 2 hours (IM)
Duration: 6–8 hours
Half-Life: 10–20 hours

Indications

Lorazepam is used in major motor seizures, in *status epilepticus,* as premedication before cardioversion, and for acute anxiety states.

Contraindications

Lorazepam should not be administered to any patient with a history of hypersensitivity to the drug.

Precautions

Lorazepam should be diluted with normal saline or D_5W prior to intravenous administration. Because lorazepam is a relatively short-acting drug, seizure activity may recur. In such cases, an additional dose may be required. Flumazenil (Romazicon), a benzodiazepine antagonist, should be available to use as an antidote if required. Lorazepam must be stored at 35–45 degrees F. They can be stored without refrigeration as long as they are replaced every 60–90 days.

Side Effects

Lorazepam can cause hypotension, drowsiness, headache, amnesia, respiratory depression, blurred vision, nausea, and vomiting.

Interactions

The effects of lorazepam can be additive when used in conjunction with other CNS depressants and alcohol.

Dosage

The usual dose of lorazepam is 0.5–2 mgs when given intravenously. The dose can be increased to 1–4 mg when given intramuscularly. It can be given rectally when an IV cannot be placed. The medication should be drawn up into a syringe. A small, red, rubber pediatric feeding tube can be attached to the syringe. The feeding tube should be inserted 2–4 cm into the rectum and the drug administered. Often it is necessary to hold the buttocks together to help the patient retain the drug.

℞ Midazolam (Versed)

Class Sedative, anticonvulsant, and hypnotic

Description

Midazolam is a benzodiazepine with strong hypnotic and amnestic properties.

Mechanism of Action

Benzodiazepines bind to specific sites on GABA Type A receptors within the brain. GABA is the major inhibitory neurotransmitter of the central nervous system. Benzodiazepines have no direct effect on the GABA receptors, but do potentiate the effects of GABA within the brain. Increased GABA levels cause sedation. Through this mechanism, the benzodiazepines display their hypnotic, anxiolytic, and anticonvulsant effects. Their usefulness, however, is limited by a broad range of side effects including compromised sedation, ataxia, amnesia, alcohol and barbiturate potentiation, tolerance development, and abuse potential.

Midazolam is a potent but short-acting benzodiazepine used widely in medicine as a sedative, anticonvulsant, and hypnotic. It is three to four times more potent than diazepam. Its onset of action is approximately 3–5 minutes when administered intravenously and 15 minutes when administered intramuscularly. Midazolam has marked amnestic properties. Like the other benzodiazepines, it has no effect on pain.

Pharmacokinetics

Onset: 3–5 minutes (IV), 15 minutes (IM)
Peak Effects: 20–60 minutes
Duration: < 2 hours (IV), 1–6 hours (IM)
Half-Life: 1–4 hours

Indications

Midazolam is used as a premedication before cardioversion and other painful procedures. It is also an effective anticonvulsant.

Contraindications

Midazolam should not be administered to any patient with a history of hypersensitivity to the drug. It should not be used in patients who have narrow-angle glaucoma. Midazolam should not be administered to patients in shock, with depressed vital signs, or who are in alcoholic coma.

Precautions

Emergency resuscitative equipment must be available prior to the administration of midazolam. Vital signs must be continuously monitored during and after drug administration. Midazolam has more potential than the other benzodiazepines to cause respiratory depression and respiratory arrest. Flumazenil (Romazicon), a benzodiazepine antagonist, should be available to use as an antidote if required.

Side Effects

Midazolam can cause laryngospasm, bronchospasm, dyspnea, respiratory depression and arrest, drowsiness, amnesia, altered mental status, bradycardia, tachycardia, premature ventricular contractions, and retching.

Interactions

The effects of midazolam can be accentuated by CNS depressants such as narcotics and alcohol.

Dosage

When used for sedation, midazolam must be administered cautiously, because the amount of medication required to achieve sedation varies from individual to individual. Typically, 1–2.5 mg are administered by slow IV injection. Higher doses may be required when used as an anticonvulsant. Usually, it is best to dilute midazolam with normal saline or D$_5$W prior to IV administration. Midazolam can be administered intramuscularly at a dose of 0.07–0.08 mg/kg (average adult dose of 5 mg). Recently, many centers have been administering midazolam intranasally or by mouth to sedate children prior to painful procedures.

Hydantoins

Phenytoin and phenytoin sodium are the most commonly prescribed anticonvulsant agents. In the prehospital setting, phenytoin may be used as a second-line drug for the treatment of seizures and as a second-line antiarrhythmic.

Hydantoin anticonvulsants are usually absorbed slowly, rapidly distributed, and extensively protein bound. They are metabolized in the liver and excreted in the urine.

In most cases, the hydantoin anticonvulsants can stabilize nerve cells against hyperexcitability. Phenytoin's primary site of action appears to be the motor cortex, where the drug inhibits the spread of seizure activity. Phenytoin also exhibits antidysrhythmic properties similar to those of quinidine or procainamide. Because of its clinical efficacy and relatively low toxicity, phenytoin is the most commonly prescribed anticonvulsant.

℞ Phenytoin (Dilantin)

Class Anticonvulsant and antiarrhythmic

Description

Phenytoin is a long-acting anticonvulsant. It is also used as an antidysrhythmic because it depresses spontaneous ventricular depolarization.

Mechanism of Action

Phenytoin produces a voltage- and frequency-dependent blockade of sodium channels in rapidly discharging nerve cells. Thus, it stops sustained repetitive firing such as that occurring during a seizure. Because of this it prevents the spread of seizure discharge.

Phenytoin is an effective anticonvulsant. Its onset of action, however, is longer than that of diazepam. In most emergency situations the seizure should first be controlled with benzodiapzepines. If seizure activity recurs, phenytoin can be administered. Phenytoin also is used to treat dysrhythmias caused by digitalis toxicity. This use of the drug is discussed in Chapter 7.

Pharmacokinetics

Onset: 3–5 minutes
Peak Effects: 1–2 hours
Duration: Varies
Half-Life: 22 hours

Indications

Phenytoin is used in major motor seizures, *status epilepticus*, and arrhythmias caused by digitalis toxicity.

Contraindications

Phenytoin should not be given to any patient with a history of hypersensitivity to the drug. It is contraindicated in cases of bradycardia and high-grade heart block. It should not be administered to patients who take the drug chronically for seizures until the blood level has been determined.

Precautions

Intravenous administration of phenytoin should not exceed 50 mg/min. Signs of central nervous system depression or hypotension may occur. Elderly patients are at increased risk of developing side effects from phenytoin administration. Extravasation should be avoided. Any patient receiving intravenous phenytoin should have continuous cardiac monitoring as well as frequent monitoring of vital signs.

Side Effects

Phenytoin can cause drowsiness, dizziness, headache, hypotension, dysrhythmias, itching, rash, nausea, and vomiting.

Interactions

Phenytoin must never be diluted in dextrose-containing solutions such as D_5W. It should be diluted in normal saline or other non-glucose-containing crystalloids.

Dosage

The loading dose of phenytoin is typically 10–20 mg/kg. This dose should be administered no faster than 50 mg/min. Phenytoin should be diluted with normal saline, because dilution with 5 percent dextrose may result in precipitation of the drug. In emergency medicine phenytoin should be administered intravenously only.

 Fosphenytoin (Cerebyx)

Class Anticonvulsant

Description

Fosphenytoin is a prodrug of phenytoin. It is converted to phenytoin after parenteral administration. Unlike phenytoin, fosphenytoin can be given by intramuscular injection when IV access is unavailable.

Mechanism of Action

Fosphenytoin is an effective anticonvulsant with properties similar to those of phenytoin. Like phenytoin, it suppresses seizure activity in the brain. Since fosphenytoin is a prodrug of phenytoin, it is administered in a dosing form called "phenytoin equivalents." This is the amount of fosphenytoin necessary to achieve the desired phenytoin levels.

Pharmacokinetics

Onset: < 15 minutes (IM)

Peak Effects: 30 minutes (IM)

Duration: Varies

Half-Life: 15 minutes to convert to phenytoin (phenytoin half-life: 22 hours)

Indications

Fosphenytoin is used in major motor seizures. Like phenytoin, it has unlabeled use as an antiarrhythmic, particularly for digitalis-induced arrhythmias.

Contraindications

Hypersensitivity to the phenytoin (hydantoin) class of medications. Fosphenytoin should not be used in seizures caused by hypoglycemia, bradycardia, or complete or partial heart block.

Precautions

Use with caution in patients with impaired kidney function, alcoholism, hypotension, heart block, bradycardia, respiratory depression, or severe heart disease. An ECG monitor and a pulse oximeter should be used whenever administering fosphenytoin. Vital signs should be checked regularly during administration.

Side Effects

Side effects associated with fosphenytoin include dizziness, somnolence, drowsiness, bradycardia, heart block, blurred vision, and hypotension. These are reduced with slower administration.

Interactions

Alcohol decreases the effects of fosphenytoin.

Dosage

The IV loading dose is 15–20 mg phenytoin-equivalent (PE) per kilogram administered at 100–150 mg/minute. IV maintenance dose is 4–6 mg PE/kg per day. IM administration is possible if IV access cannot be attained.

Barbiturates

The long-acting barbiturate phenobarbital is also one of the most widely employed anticonvulsants. Phenobarbitol is used in the long-term treatment of **epilepsy** and is prescribed selectively for acute treatment of *status epilepticus*.

The barbiturate anticonvulsants are metabolized in the liver, and metabolites and unchanged medications are excreted in the urine. Phenobarbitol provides an onset of action within 30 minutes after oral administration. Peak anticonvulsant effect occurs in 8–12 hours. The onset after IV administration occurs within 5–15 minutes, with peak anticonvulsant effect within 30 minutes. Phenobarbitol has an extremely long half-life of 2–6 days.

℞ Phenobarbital (Luminal)

Class Anticonvulsant and barbiturate

Description

Phenobarbital belongs to a class of medications called *barbiturates*. It is used as a sedative and an anticonvulsant.

Mechanism of Action

Phenobarbital increases the action of the inhibitory neurotransmitter of GABA in the brain. It also appears to inhibit the release of glutamate (an excitatory neurotransmitter) from nerve endings. It is through these actions that phenobarbital exerts its sedative and anticonvulsant properties.

Barbiturates have many uses in medicine. They are central nervous system depressants and are used as anticonvulsants and in the management of insomnia and anxiety. Phenobarbital is an effective anticonvulsant of relatively low toxicity. It depresses the sensory cortex, decreases motor activity, alters cerebellar function, and causes drowsiness, sedation, and hypnosis.

Pharmacokinetics

Onset: 5–15 minutes (IV)
Peak Effects: 30 minutes (IV)
Duration: 4–6 hours (IV)
Half-Life: 2–6 days

Indications

Phenobarbital is used in major motor seizures, *status epilepticus,* and acute anxiety states.

Contraindications

Phenobarbital should not be administered to any patient with a history of hypersensitivity to barbiturates.

Precautions

Respiratory depression and hypotension can occur following IV administration of phenobarbital. Constant monitoring of respiratory pattern and blood pressure is essential. Administration of phenobarbital to children may result in hyperactive behavior.

Side Effects

Phenobarbital can cause drowsiness, altered mental status, agitation, hypoventilation, apnea, bradycardia, hypotension, syncope, headache, nausea, and vomiting.

Interactions

Phenobarbital may enhance the sedative effects of other sedatives including alcohol, narcotics, antihistamines, and antidepressants.

Dosage

The standard dosage of phenobarbital in the management of *status epilepticus* is 100–250 mg given slowly by IV.

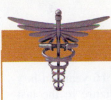

At 14:30 hours paramedics are called with fire department first responders to a motor-cycle collision. On arrival they find an 18-year-old male, unhelmeted rider. Bystanders state that he lost control of the motorcycle on a corner and slid head first into the cement retaining wall.

The patient is unconscious and unresponsive to deep pain. He is lying on his left side. His head is being supported by a bystander, who states that the patient has been uncon-scious and unresponsive since he arrived.

Physical Examination

CNS: The patient is unconscious and unresponsive; pupils are bilaterally constricted; abnormal flexion (decorticate posture) bilaterally

Resp: Respirations are 30 per minute and deep; lungs are clear bilaterally with equal air entry; trachea is midline; no signs of trauma to the neck or chest

CVS: Both radial and carotid pulses are present and weak; skin is pale and diaphoretic

ABD: Soft and nontender in all four quadrants

Muscl/Skel: No other injuries noted

Vital Signs

Pulse: 50/min

Resp: 30/min, deep

BP: 160 by palpation

SpO$_2$: 87 percent

ECG: Sinus bradycardia

Past Hx: The patient's history is unknown.

Treatment

Fire department first responders assist with spinal immobilization while a paramedic inserts an oropharyngeal airway and begins to ventilate the patient with a bag-valve-mask device and 100 percent oxygen. The patient is moved to an ALS ambulance follow-ing rapid immobilization and stabilization on a long spine board. During transport the patient's condition remains largely unchanged except as follows: (1) Respiration rate increases to 36 per minute, (2) blood pressure increases to 210/120 mmHg, (3) oxygen saturation (as measured by pulse oximetry) increases to 91 percent, and (4) pupils become uneven (right > left). Because of the critical nature of this patient's injuries, the following procedures were completed: endotracheal intubation with in-line c-spine stabilization, IV line × 2, 14-gauge catheter (per trauma protocol), normal saline TKO, and mannitol 1.5 g/kg. Total scene time was 10 minutes, and transport time to the hospital was 8 minutes. There were no changes in patient condition en route. On arrival at the hospital the patient was immediately taken to CT, where an epidural hematoma was visualized. The patient was taken emergently to surgery, where the epidural hematoma was decompressed. The patient was transferred to the neurology ICU, where he remains.

At 0900 hours paramedics are called to the local high school to help a 16-year-old boy with reported seizures. Dispatch reports that the boy has had one seizure in the last 10 minutes and is now into his second seizure. The boy has a history of epilepsy and takes medication for it. He is unconscious and unresponsive. Three minutes later paramedics arrive at the school and are met by a very frantic teacher, who leads them to a classroom. There they find the patient lying on the floor. The desks have been moved away from the patient, and the patient has been placed in the recovery position. The patient appears to be postictal now.

Physical Examination

CNS: The patient is unconscious and unresponsive

Resp: Respirations are 32 per minute and shallow; trachea is midline; no external signs of trauma

CVS: Both the radial and carotid pulses are present but are rapid and weak; skin is pale and diaphoretic

ABD: Soft and nontender in all four quadrants; no signs of vomiting; patient has been incontinent of urine

Muscl/Skel: No injuries detected

Vital Signs

Pulse: 120/min

Resp: 36/min, shallow

BP: 124/82 mmHg

SpO$_2$:   90 percent

ECG: Sinus tachycardia

Past Hx: The teacher states that the patient has epilepsy. She shows paramedics a prescription bottle of Dilantin from the patient's coat pocket. The patient had the first seizure at 0850, and the second started at 0900. She does not know if he has been sick or experienced any recent trauma.

Treatment

One paramedic performs oropharyngeal suction to remove some frothy sputum from the patient's mouth and then ventilates the patient with a bag-valve-mask unit with 100 percent oxygen. Following contact with the base hospital, another paramedic is preparing to give lorazepam (Ativan) IV push. An 18-gauge IV is initiated in the right antecubital fossa and secured in place with tape and roller gauze in case the patient has another seizure. The patient's blood glucose level is checked from the blood in the IV hub, and it is 100 mg/dL (5.6 mmol/L). He then begins to seize, and paramedics administer lorazepam 2–4 mg IV push. If that does not terminate the seizure, a repeat dose of 2–4 mg may be given. Paramedics administer the first dose of lorazepam, and the seizure subsides in 1 minute. Within 5 minutes the patient is in the postictal stage. He is transported to the hospital without incident and without further seizure. At the hospital the patient's phenytoin level is checked to see if it was too low. The phenytoin level obtained from the blood is 3.4 mg/L (therapeutic level is 10–20 mg/L). IV phenytoin is administered, and the patient is admitted to the intensive care unit. He does well, with no additional seizures, and is released with an increased daily dosage of phenytoin.

CHAPTER REVIEW

Summary

In the management of acute head injury, mannitol has proved effective in reducing cerebral edema. Airway management and ventilation are important aspects of acute head injury management. It is important to remember that stabilization of the cervical spine, maintenance of the airway, and supplemental delivery of oxygen are of primary importance.

In a general motor seizure, as occasionally occurs, the primary treatment is that of protecting the patient from injury. It is important to remember that most epileptic patients are already taking orally one or two anticonvulsant medications. The judicious use of the parenteral agents discussed in this chapter is therefore indicated. It is helpful to the emergency physician to obtain blood samples from seizure patients prior to the administration of an anticonvulsant. Some authorities believe that a significant percentage of patients who have general motor seizures do so because they fail to follow instructions on ordered medications. Blood studies taken before the administration of anticonvulsants will aid the physician in making a diagnosis.

Key Words

amnesia A loss of memory.

benzodiazepine A class of medications frequently used to relieve anxiety and insomnia and to induce sedation.

central nervous system The central portion of the nervous system, namely the brain and spinal cord.

epilepsy A group of nervous system disorders characterized by the presence of seizures.

seizures A sudden change in nervous function. The symptoms can range from a slight alteration in mental status to violent, generalized, uncontrollable contraction of muscles.

status epilepticus A state of repeated seizures without an intervening period of consciousness.

CHAPTER 12

MEDICATIONS USED IN THE TREATMENT OF OBSTETRICAL AND GYNECOLOGICAL EMERGENCIES

OBJECTIVES

After completing this chapter, the reader should be able to:

- List three obstetrical and gynecological emergencies that require intervention with pharmacological agents.
- Describe and list the indications, contraindications, and dosages for oxytocin.
- List the signs and symptoms of hypertensive disorders of pregnancy.
- Distinguish among gestational hypertension, preeclampsia, and eclampsia.
- Describe and list the indications, contraindications, and dosages for magnesium sulfate.
- Describe the management of a patient in preterm labor.
- Describe and list the indications, contraindications, and dosages for terbutaline.
- Define the following terms: *abruptio placenta, eclampsia, ectopic pregnancy, placenta previa, postpartum hemorrhage, preeclampsia,* and *spontaneous abortion.*

INTRODUCTION

Special Considerations in Pregnancy

Any time you administer medications to a woman of childbearing years, you must consider the possibility that she is pregnant. Treating pregnant patients clearly means treating two patients. Although emphasis appropriately seems to center on the mother during care, you must understand that many medications that affect the mother also affect the fetus. A medication's possible benefits to the mother must clearly outweigh the potential risks to the fetus. For example, some situations such as cardiac arrest, justify giving the mother medications that may harm the fetus because the medication's potential harm to the fetus is clearly outweighed by the fetus's certain death if the mother dies.

Pregnancy presents two particular pharmacological problems: changes in the mother's anatomy and physiology, and the potential for medications to harm the fetus. Because the mother is supporting the fetus entirely, her heart rate, cardiac output, and blood volume all increase. This altered maternal physiology can affect the onset and duration of action of many medications. During the first trimester of pregnancy the

TABLE 12–1

American FDA Pregnancy Categories

Category	Description
A	Adequate studies in pregnant women have not demontrated a risk to the fetus in the first trimester or later trimesters.
B	Animal studies have not demonstrated a risk to the fetus, but there are not adequate studies in pregnant women. OR Adequate studies in pregnant women have not demonstrated a risk to the fetus in the first trimester and there is no risk in the last trimester, but animal studies have demonstrated adverse effects.
C	Animal studies have demonstrated adverse effects. There are no adequate studies in pregnant women; however, benefits may be acceptable despite the potential risks. OR No adequate animal studies or adequate studies of pregnant women have been done.
D	Fetal risk has been demonstrated in certain circumstances; benefits could outweigh the risks.
X	Fetal risk has been demonstrated. This risk outweighs a possible benefit to the mother. Avoid using in pregnant or potentially pregnant patients.

ingestion of some medications (teratogenic medications) may potentially deform, injure, or kill the fetus. During the last trimester, medications adminstered to the mother may have unwanted effects on the fetus. Others may not be metabolized or excreted, possibly resulting in toxic accumulations. Additionally, a breast-feeding mother's milk may pass some medications on to her infant.

Under some conditions, of course, the health and safety of the mother and fetus demand the use of medications during pregnancy. Examples include pregnancy-induced diabetes, hypertension, and seizure disorders. To help health care providers determine when medications are needed during pregnancy, the American Food and Drug Administration (FDA) has developed the classification system shown in Table 12–1, which is also observed in Canada. Always consult medical direction for any questions about medication safety in pregnancy.

Prehospital care for most obstetrical and gynecological emergencies is supportive. There are three complications, however, that necessitate intervention with pharmacological agents. These are the hypertensive disorders of pregnancy, severe vaginal bleeding, and preterm labor. Magnesium sulfate has proved effective in controlling the convulsions associated with eclampsia. Oxytocin, a medication chemically identical to the hormone oxytocin, is effective in causing uterine contraction and will control many cases of postpartum vaginal bleeding. Terbutaline, a β_2-agonist, is effective in the suppression of preterm labor.

HYPERTENSIVE DISORDERS OF PREGNANCY

Paramedics should be aware of several pregnancy-associated problems known collectively as *hypertensive disorders of pregnancy* (formerly called *toxemia of pregnancy*). These disorders are characterized by hypertension, weight gain, edema, protein in the urine, and, in late stages, seizures. Hypertensive disorders of pregnancy occur in approximately 5 percent of pregnancies. They are thought to be caused by abnormal vasospasm in the mother, which results in increased blood pressure and other associated symptoms. The hypertensive disorders of pregnancy generally include the following:

Gestational hypertension (GH). GH is characterized by a blood pressure of 140/90 level or greater in pregnancy in a patient who was previously normotensive. GH is the early stage of the disease process. It is important to remember that blood pressure usually drops in pregnancy, and a blood pressure reading of 130/80 may be elevated.

Preeclampsia. Patients who have **preeclampsia** have hypertension, abnormal weight gain, edema, headache, protein in the urine, epigastric pain, and, occasionally, visual disturbances. If untreated, preeclampsia may progress to the next stage, eclampsia.

Eclampsia. **Eclampsia** is the most serious manifestation of the hypertensive disorders of pregnancy. It is characterized by grand mal seizure activity. Eclampsia is often preceded by visual disturbances, such as flashing lights or spots before the eyes. Also, the development of epigastric pain or pain in the right upper abdominal quadrant often indicates impending seizure. Eclampsia can be distinguished from epilepsy by the history and physical appearance of the patient. Patients who become eclamptic are usually edematous and have markedly elevated blood pressure, whereas epileptics usually have a prior history of seizures and are taking anticonvulsant medications.

The hypertensive disorders of pregnancy tend to occur most often with a woman's first pregnancy. They also appear to occur more frequently in patients with preexisting hypertension. Diabetes mellitus is also associated with an increased incidence of this disease process.

Patients who develop GH and preeclampsia are at increased risk for cerebral hemorrhage, the development of renal failure, and pulmonary edema. Patients who are preeclamptic have intravascular volume depletion, because a great deal of their body fluid is in the third space. If eclampsia develops, death of the mother and fetus frequently results. Eclampsia must be treated aggressively. Magnesium sulfate is the medication of choice for controlling the convulsions associated with eclampsia. In addition, it may be necessary to administer an antihypertensive agent, such as those discussed in Chapter 7, to prevent the complications of hypertensive crisis. The decision to administer an antihypertensive in the prehospital phase of emergency medical care rests with the base station physician. Each case should be treated individually.

℞ Magnesium Sulfate

Class Electrolyte

Description

Magnesium sulfate is a central nervous system depressant effective in the management of seizures associated with eclampsia. It is used for the initial therapy of convulsions associated with pregnancy. After cessation of seizure activity, other anticonvulsant agents may be administered. Magnesium is also a smooth muscle relaxant that can reverse some of the vasospasm seen in preeclampsia and eclampsia. This aids in maintaining placental perfusion.

Mechanism of Action

Magnesium sulfate is a salt that dissociates into the magnesium cation (Mg^{2+}) and the sulfate anion when administered. Magnesium is an essential element in numerous biochemical reactions that occur within the body.

Pharmacokinetics

Onset: Immediate (IV), 1 hour (IM)
Peak Effects: Varies
Duration: 30–60 minutes
Half-Life: Not applicable

Indications

Magnesium sulfate is used in eclampsia (seizures accompanying pregnancy) and preterm labor. It can also be used as a tocolytic.

Contraindications

Magnesium sulfate should not be administered to any patient with heart block. It should not be administered to patients who are in shock; who have persistent, severe hypertension; who routinely undergo dialysis; or who are known to have a decreased calcium level (hypocalcemia).

Precautions

Magnesium sulfate, like other central nervous system depressants, can cause hypotension, circulatory collapse, and depression of cardiac and respiratory function. The most immediate danger is respiratory depression. Calcium chloride should be readily available for IV administration as an antidote in case respiratory depression occurs. Magnesium sulfate should be administered slowly to minimize side effects. Any patient receiving intravenous magnesium sulfate should have continuous cardiac monitoring as well as frequent monitoring of vital signs. If possible, the knee and biceps deep tendon reflexes should be checked prior to and during magnesium therapy.

Side Effects

Magnesium sulfate can cause flushing, sweating, bradycardia, decreased deep tendon reflexes, drowsiness, respiratory depression, arrhythmias, hypotension, hypothermia, itching, and rash.

Interactions

Magnesium sulfate can cause cardiac conduction abnormalities if administered in conjunction with digitalis.

Dosage

The standard dosage for the management of convulsions associated with eclampsia is 4–6 g slow IV over 30 min. This is often followed by an infusion at 1–2 g/hr. If an IV cannot be started, magnesium sulfate can be administered intramuscularly at a dose of 4–5 g every 4 hours. Because of the volume of the medication (5–10 mL), the dose should be divided in half and each half administered intramuscularly at a separate site (usually each gluteus).

SEVERE VAGINAL BLEEDING

Vaginal bleeding that occurs during the first trimester of pregnancy is usually due to **spontaneous abortion** or **ectopic pregnancy**. During the third trimester of pregnancy, vaginal bleeding is most frequently caused by either **abruptio placenta** or **placenta previa**.

Bleeding following childbirth is common. Hypovolemic shock can develop when blood loss is in excess of 500 mL. Severe vaginal bleeding can be a life-threatening emergency, necessitating immediate therapy. The management of severe vaginal bleeding is similar to that employed with any other type of severe hemorrhage. Initial treatment should include airway maintenance, administration of supplemental oxygen (if needed), and infusion of intravenous volume expanders. In addition, the intravenous (IV) administration of oxytocin in postpartum hemorrhage can be effective in controlling severe vaginal bleeding.

℞ Oxytocin (Pitocin)

Class Hormone and uterine stimulant

Description

Oxytocin is a naturally occurring hormone that is secreted by the posterior pituitary.

Mechanism of Action

Oxytocin causes contraction of uterine smooth muscle and lactation. Oxytocin is used to induce labor in selected cases and is also effective in inducing uterine contractions following delivery, thereby controlling **postpartum hemorrhage**. When a baby is placed on the breast, the sucking action causes the posterior pituitary to release oxytocin. It is important to remember this inherent mechanism whenever confronted by a patient suffering moderate to severe postpartum bleeding.

Pharmacokinetics

Onset: Immediate (IV), 3–7 minutes (IM)
Peak Effects: Varies
Duration: 1 hour (IV), 2–3 hours (IM)
Half-Life: 3–5 minutes

Indication

Oxytocin is used for postpartum hemorrhage.

Contraindications

In the prehospital setting, oxytocin should be administered only to patients suffering severe postpartum bleeding. Before administration it is essential to verify that the baby *and the placenta* have been delivered and that there is not an additional fetus in the uterus.

Precautions

Excess oxytocin can cause overstimulation of the uterus and possible uterine rupture. Hypertension, cardiac arrhythmias, and anaphylaxis have been reported in conjunction with the administration of oxytocin. Vital signs and uterine tone should be monitored.

Side Effects

Oxytocin can cause hypotension, arrhythmias, tachycardia, seizures, coma, nausea, and vomiting in the mother. When administered prior to delivery, oxytocin can cause fetal hypoxia, fetal asphyxia, fetal arrhythmias, and possibly fetal intracranial bleeding.

Both oxytocin and antidiuretic hormone (ADH) are secreted from the posterior pituitary and are similar in chemical structure. Because of this, oxytocin may have some ADH effects—especially in higher doses. These include water restriction and, to a lesser degree, vasoconstriction.

Interactions

Oxytocin can cause hypertension when administered in conjunction with vasoconstrictors such as norepinephrine.

Dosage

Following are two regimens for the administration of oxytocin in the management of patients with postpartum hemorrhage:

1. 3 to 10 units can be administered intramuscularly following delivery of the placenta or
2. 10–20 units can be placed in either 500 or 1000 mL of D_5W, 0.9 percent normal saline, or lactated Ringer's solution. This should be titrated according to the severity of the bleeding and the uterine response. Oxytocin should only be administered intramuscularly or by slow IV infusion.

PRETERM LABOR

Preterm labor is labor that begins before the age of fetal maturity, usually before 36 weeks. If labor begins early, obstetricians often try to suppress it to allow more time for intrauterine fetal development. Labor can be suppressed by the use of tocolytics. Although many tocolytics are available, β_2-agonists are frequently used. Stimulation of uterine β_2-receptors causes uterine relaxation and suppression of preterm labor. Common β_2-agonists include terbutaline and ritodrine (Yutopar). Terbutaline is used more frequently in the emergency setting. Magnesium sulfate, previously discussed, is also effective in suppressing preterm labor. More recently, calcium channel blockers have been used in the treatment of preterm labor.

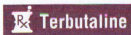 **Terbutaline**

Class Sympathetic agonist and tocolytic

Description

Terbutaline is a synthetic sympathomimetic that is selective for β_2-adrenergic receptors.

Mechanism of Action

Terbutaline, because of its effects on β_2-adrenergic receptors, causes immediate bronchodilation with minimal cardiac effects. It is also used to suppress preterm labor. Stimulation of β_2-adrenergic receptors in the uterus causes uterine relaxation and can suppress labor.

Pharmacokinetics

Onset: < 15 minutes (SC)

Peak Effects: 30–60 minutes (SC)

Duration: 1.5–4.0 hours (SC)

Half-Life: 3–4 hours

Indication

Terbutaline is used for preterm labor.

Contraindications

Terbutaline should not be administered to any patient with a history of hypersensitivity to the medication.

Precautions

As with any sympathomimetic, the patient's vital signs must be monitored. Caution should be used when administering terbutaline to elderly patients and those with cardiovascular disease or hypertension.

Side Effects

Terbutaline can cause palpitations, anxiety, dizziness, headache, nervousness, tremor, hypertension, arrhythmias, chest pain, nausea, and vomiting.

Interactions

The possibility of developing unpleasant side effects increases when terbutaline is used with other sympathetic agonists. β-blockers may blunt the pharmacological effects of terbutaline.

Dosage

Terbutaline should be administered initially by subcutaneous injection. The initial dose should be 0.25 mg administered subcutaneously. This dose can be repeated in 30 minutes to 1 hour as required. A terbutaline drip can be used to provide ongoing suppression of labor. It can be prepared by placing 5 mg of terbutaline in 500 mL of lactated Ringer's solution or normal saline. The drip should be started at 30 mL/hr (5 mcg/min). This can be slowly increased to a maximum dose of 80 mcg/min as required.

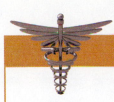

An ALS ambulance is called to a rural hospital to transport a maternity patient to a larger city hospital 1 hour away. Paramedics are asked to bring the monitor in with the stretcher. On arrival at the hospital the nurse attending the patient gives the following information: The patient is an 18-year-old female, gravida 1, para 0, in her third trimester of pregnancy. She came to the hospital by private car after suffering a grand mal seizure at home. She had no prior history of seizures, and her pregnancy had been uneventful to date. She evidently was not in labor prior to the seizure. At present the patient is lying on a hospital bed and is not having contractions, as based on the external fetal monitor. The fetal heart rate is stable. The hospital diagnosis is eclampsia.

Physical Examination

CNS:	The patient is conscious but lethargic
Resp:	Respirations are 24 per minute and shallow; symmetrical chest wall movement with clear bilateral breath sounds
CVS:	Both carotid and radial pulses are present and strong; a systolic flow murmur can be heard; minimal blood loss is noted from the vagina; neck veins are not distended; skin color is normal, warm, and diaphoretic to touch; patient is very edematous
ABD:	Obviously pregnant with no contractions noted
Muscl/Skel:	No apparent injuries
Extremities:	Pedal and finger edema noted

Vital Signs

Pulse:	100/min, regular
Resp:	24/min
BP:	166/112 mmHg
SpO$_2$:	95 percent
ECG:	Normal sinus rhythm

Hospital Treatment

The patient is receiving high-concentration oxygen. A large-bore IV was started in the left forearm. Magnesium sulfate is being infused at a rate of 1 g/hr. The receiving hospital was notified and is expecting the patient.

Treatment

The patient is moved to the ambulance stretcher and then to the ambulance. Oxygen is administered at 15 lpm by non-rebreather mask. The pulse oximeter is applied and shows an SpO$_2$ of 96 percent. The cardiac monitor shows a regular sinus rhythm and is checked frequently by the paramedics who are watching for any ECG changes. The IV of magnesium sulfate initiated in the hospital is continued at 1 g/hr. The interior ambulance lights are dimmed to help prevent additional seizure activity. A prefilled syringe of diazepam is removed from the lock box in case the patient suffers another seizure.

During transport the patient is continually assessed, with special attention to the IV of magnesium sulfate. Deep tendon reflexes are periodically checked to ensure the magnesium effect is not excessive. The trip to the hospital is uneventful. On arrival at the receiving facility, an emergency sonogram is obtained. It shows a fetal age of 37 weeks ($\pm$2 weeks). Labor is induced, and the patient delivers a healthy female infant 18 hours later.

CHAPTER REVIEW

Summary

Most obstetrical and gynecological emergencies are not managed in the field. Prehospital treatment should include stabilization of the airway, administration of supplemental oxygen, and replacement of intravascular volume. In severe postpartum bleeding, the administration of oxytocin is often effective. In the hypertensive disorders of pregnancy, magnesium sulfate may be used during the prehospital phase of emergency medical care to control convulsions. The definitive treatment of preeclampsia and eclampsia is delivery of the fetus.

Key Words

abruptio placenta   A premature separation of the placenta from the uterus before birth. Because it often results in severe bleeding, it is considered to be a serious condition.

eclampsia   The most serious manifestation of the hypertensive disorders of pregnancy. It is characterized by grand mal seizure activity. Eclampsia is often preceded by visual disturbances, such as flashing lights or spots before the eyes. Also, the development of epigastric pain or pain in the right upper abdominal quadrant often indicates impending seizure. Patients who become eclamptic are usually edematous and have markedly elevated blood pressure.

ectopic pregnancy   The implantation of a developing fetus outside the uterus, often in the fallopian tube.

placenta previa   A condition in which the placenta partly or completely covers the opening of the cervix. It is the most common cause of painless bleeding in the third trimester.

postpartum hemorrhage   The loss of 500 mL or more blood in the first 24 hours following delivery.

preeclampsia   A manifestation of the hypertensive disorders of pregnancy characterized by hypertension, abnormal weight gain, edema, headache, protein in the urine, epigastric pain, and, occasionally, visual disturbances. If untreated, preeclampsia may progress to the next stage, eclampsia.

spontaneous abortion   A fetal loss, also called a miscarriage, that occurs of its own accord. Most spontaneous abortions occur before the 12th week of pregnancy. Many occur 2 weeks after conception and are mistaken for menstrual periods.

OBJECTIVES

After completing this chapter, the reader should be able to:

- Discuss the importance of toxicological emergencies in prehospital care.
- Discuss the role of regional poison centers in the management of the poisoned patient.
- Describe the key historical information required in the management of a toxicological emergency.
- Describe the various routes of exposure to toxic substances.
- Describe the general management of the patient exposed to a toxin, including decontamination and elimination.
- Define the term *toxidrome* and describe the common toxidromes encountered in prehospital care.
- Describe the signs, symptoms, and management (including antidotes where appropriate) of the following toxic exposures and overdoses: acetaminophen, anticholinergics, neuroleptics, beta-blockers, calcium channel blockers, carbon monoxide, cyanide, cyclic antidepressants, digoxin/digitalis, ethylene glycol, iron, isopropyl alcohol, lithium, methanol, narcotics and narcotic antagonists, organophosphates and carbamates, salicylates, and selective serotonin reuptake inhibitors (SSRIs).

INTRODUCTION

Toxicology is a rapidly evolving science that can provide the prehospital care provider with a fascinating window into the field of pharmacology and pharmacokinetics. The management of toxin exposure and overdoses represents a constantly expanding aspect of prehospital care. Maintaining clinical competence in managing these patients reflects a significant challenge because new medications and chemicals, each with its own unique toxicological potential, are continuously being introduced. The approach to the poisoned or overdosed patient can be likened to a form of detective work. The clinical clues required to manage these patients are often subtle, and providers must be aware that virtually any patient presentation may be directly or indirectly related to a toxicological problem. Without suspicion, even the most obvious clinical clues can go unnoticed.

In this chapter, the discussion focuses not only on prescription medications but also on nonprescription toxins that may be encountered in prehospital care. There are similarities between many of the agents presented here and those used by terrorists as weapons of mass destruction. The attacks on the United States on September 11, 2001, significantly changed the way prehospital care is practiced in the world. Terrorism has brought once obscure chemical and biological agents to the forefront of medical care. As a result, antidotes and palliative medications are now routinely stocked on ambulances and rescue vehicles. The modern emergency medical service (EMS) provider must be familiar with common antidotes and treatments for many of the chemical and biological weapons available throughout the world.

REGIONAL POISON CENTERS

Once the possibility of a poisoning or overdose has been identified, several resources are available to assist in patient management. Traditionally, a hospital-based medical director has provided guidance and direction for the management of toxicological emergencies. In recent years the emergence of toxicology as a distinct discipline has led to the development of regional poison centers whose role is to provide information and advice to caregivers encountering poisoned patients. Poison information specialists are typically nurses and pharmacists with specialized training in toxicology. They are generally available 24 hours per day to provide telephone advice to prehospital care providers, laypeople, and hospital medical staff. They can serve as an extremely valuable resource to care providers, particularly in rural settings where the decision to transfer a patient to a larger center can be a difficult one. The prehospital care provider should not overlook the potential benefit of consultation with a regional poison center.

PATIENT HISTORY

The history constitutes an essential part of the initial approach to the toxicology patient. Like all detective work, suspicion is the foundation for discovering the truth; the truth in this case is the identity, quantity, and time of exposure to the toxic substance. Despite its importance, the history is frequently confusing and inconsistent in this patient population. The problem is related to factors such as illicit drug use, associated psychiatric illnesses, and in some cases a lack of awareness on the part of both the patient and the care provider that an exposure has actually occurred.

A thorough history includes *what* agent the patient was exposed to, *how much* of the agent, *when* the exposure occurred (time), *how* the exposure occurred (*route of exposure*), *where* (location) the exposure occurred, and any *treatment* the patient may have received prior to the arrival of the prehospital care provider.

The importance of identifying the agent in question is obvious. Knowing which agent is involved can allow the care provider to plan decontamination, provide initial treatment, and anticipate problems before they actually occur. With some toxic agents, immediate management is required in the field, whereas others can have therapy initiated in the emergency department. In the latter cases, it is extremely useful to provide hospital staff with all available information so that they can prepare for the patient's arrival. Some agents have antidotes that can be lifesaving if used appropriately. In circumstances in which the toxic agent cannot be identified or an antidote is not available, management may be limited to supportive care. Searching the scene for pill bottles, poisons, evidence of drug abuse, venomous plants, and animals is paramount. Whenever possible, toxicological evidence, especially pill bottles and medication dispensers, should be transported to the hospital for review by a physician.

The dose or amount of toxin can be very helpful in predicting the occurrence or severity of clinical symptoms. It may also help to determine the need for decontamination procedures and antidote treatment. Making note of the date on prescription medication containers and the number of pills still present can assist in quantifying the dosage.

The time of exposure is important for several reasons. First, it allows an estimation of the degree of toxicity (however, many toxins have delayed symptom onset). Second, it allows some planning for decontamination and management. Finally, some agents (salicylates and acetaminophen) require blood levels to determine the need for treatment. Interpretation of these blood levels often requires knowledge of the time of ingestion. Reviewing the patient's recent activities and time of symptom onset with family members or friends can be very helpful.

Potential routes of exposure include *oral ingestion, inhalation, dermal exposure, injection* (*intra-* or *extravascular*), and *mucosal absorption.* The route of exposure guides treatment (e.g., gastric decontamination would not be indicated in a patient who has had dermal exposure).

The location of the exposure can be helpful in identifying the agent (e.g., an agricultural worker who develops symptoms shortly after spraying organophosphate pesticides on a wheat field). The route of exposure can be crucial in ensuring the safety of the care provider because some toxins can be airborne (e.g., carbon monoxide) or spread through patient contact (e.g., organophosphate pesticides).

Identifying any treatment provided prior to medical attention is also important. The occurrence of vomiting is relevant because it suggests some emptying of residual gastric toxins has already occurred. Although no longer widely used and potentially dangerous, syrup of ipecac is still available and may be administered by laypeople. If administered, the prehospital care provider must anticipate vomiting and take steps to prevent aspiration of gastric contents.

GENERAL APPROACH TO THE POISONED PATIENT

As emphasized earlier, the foundation of managing the poisoned patient is a clinical suspicion supplemented by clues present at the scene and in the presentation of the patient. Generally speaking, the mortality from acute poisonings is less than 1 percent. The initial approach to the poisoned patient includes early attention to *airway, breathing,* and *circulation.* Airway control should occur early where indicated, followed by establishment of vascular access. Because vomiting is a frequent occurrence in the poisoned patient, aspiration is a significant risk and should be anticipated and prevented wherever possible. *Vital signs* must be recorded early because they can provide clues to both the type of toxin and the severity of the overdose. *Cardiac monitoring* is crucial because many toxic exposures are associated with serious arrhythmias. In the setting of tricyclic antidepressant overdose, the presence of a wide QRS complex may guide treatment, as discussed in greater detail later in the chapter. *Blood glucose levels* should be measured in all patients with altered level of consciousness because hypoglycemia can often be misinterpreted as an intoxicated state. As discussed previously, both the patient and care providers must be protected from further exposure to the toxin. Discussion of physical exam findings is deferred to the later review of specific toxidromes.

Decontamination and enhancing *elimination* of toxins in the poisoned patient may have a role in prehospital care. Traditional approaches have included *syrup of ipecac, gastric lavage,* and *activated charcoal* with or without a cathartic agent (an agent that enhances bowel motility and speeds transit through the gut). These are no longer recommended for most poisonings.

Syrup of ipecac acts by inducing vomiting and theoretically decreasing further absorption of remaining toxins from the gastrointestinal tract. Its usage has largely fallen out of favor recently due to a lack of evidence for improved patient outcome as well as significant concerns regarding its safety. The *American Academy of Clinical*

Toxicology's position statement on syrup of ipecac states that it should not be administered routinely in the management of poisoned patients. There is no evidence from clinical studies that ipecac improves the outcome of poisoned patients and its routine administration in the emergency department should be abandoned. There are insufficient data to support or exclude ipecac administration soon after poison ingestion. Ipecac may delay the administration or reduce the effectiveness of activated charcoal, oral antidotes, and whole bowel irrigation.

Gastric lavage is also no longer routinely recommended. The American Academy of Clinical Toxicology issued a position statement regarding gastric lavage. It stated that gastric lavage should not be employed routinely in the management of poisoned patients. There is no certain evidence that its use improves clinical outcomes and it may cause significant morbidity. Gastric lavage should not be considered unless a patient has ingested a potentially life-threatening amount of a poison and the procedure can be undertaken within 60 minutes of ingestion. Even then, clinical benefit has not been confirmed in controlled studies. Unless a patient is intubated, gastric lavage is contraindicated if airway protective reflexes are lost. It is also contraindicated if a hydrocarbon with high aspiration potential or corrosive substance has been ingested. As a rule, gastric lavage is impractical for most prehospital settings because it requires multiple personnel and may be associated with significant complications such as aspiration and esophageal rupture.

Activated charcoal has been shown to be effective in decreasing the toxicity in certain oral ingestions and in agents with enterohepatic circulation. However, charcoal is by no means effective for all orally ingested toxins. As with ipecac and gastric lavage, the routine use of activated charcoal in acute poisoning is rarely indicated. The American Academy of Clinical Toxicology's position paper states that single-dose activated charcoal should not be administered routinely in the management of poisoned patients. There is no evidence that the administration of activated charcoal improves clinical outcome. Unless a patient has an intact or protected airway, the administration of charcoal is contraindicated.

Although cathartic agents may improve elimination somewhat, the resultant frequent and voluminous bowel movements can create a suboptimal patient care environment in the back of an ambulance. To summarize, the mortality rate from acute poisonings is less than 1 percent. Most of the medications and procedures formerly used have proven of little benefit. For the most part, unless a specific antidote is available, the care of most poisoning patients is simply supportive.

TOXIDROMES

A **toxidrome** is a set of clinical signs that are considered diagnostic of certain toxins or classes of toxins. Although not all toxins have their own unique toxidrome, an ability to recognize the common toxidromes can greatly enhance toxin identification and thereby aid patient care in certain circumstances. The clinical reliability of toxidromes is limited in cases of mixed overdoses, for which physical findings can be contradictory.

Perhaps the most common toxidrome encountered in prehospital care is that of the narcotized patient (*narcotic* or *opiate toxidrome*). Whether self-induced or iatrogenic, the classic triad of decreased level of consciousness, respiratory depression, and constricted pupils (miosis) is seen with frequency and, when present, can guide therapy. Although this triad generally holds for the common narcotics, including morphine, heroin, and codeine, it is important to remember that not all narcotics cause pupillary constriction. Meperidine (Demerol) and pentazocine (Talwin), and others may not demonstrate miosis.

Another relatively common toxidrome is that of *anticholinergic* toxicity, as commonly seen with antihistamine (e.g., dimenhydrinate [Dramamine, Gravol], diphenhydramine [Benadryl]) and tricyclic antidepressant (Elavil, Sinequan) overdoses. These patients commonly display both central signs and peripheral antimuscarinic signs. Peripheral signs are typically more common and include dry skin and mucous membranes, thirst, dysphagia, blurred vision, fixed dilated pupils, tachycardia, fine red (scarlatiniform) rash, hyperthermia, abdominal distension with decreased or absent bowel sounds, and urinary urgency or retention. Central signs include lethargy, confusion, restlessness, delirium, hallucinations, ataxia, seizures, and in severe cases cardiopulmonary collapse. Agents that can cause this toxidrome include dimenhydrinate and cyclic antidepressants. A common mnemonic for remembering the clinical signs of anticholinergic syndrome is "*hot* as Hell, *blind* as a bat, *dry* as a bone, *red* as a beet, *mad* as a Hatter."

The *cholinergic toxidrome*, as is classically seen with organophosphate pesticide poisoning, can present with a complex cascade of signs that include muscarinic, nicotinic, and central nervous system (CNS) signs and symptoms. Once again, the multiple clinical signs can be simplified through the use of a mnemonic. The muscarinic symptoms are described by the mnemonic *DUMBELS*, in which the signs include defecation, urination, miosis, bronchorrhea, excitation (muscular), lacrimation, and salivation or seizures. Alternatively, the mnemonic *SLUDGE* is also used. It represents salivation, lacrimation, urination, defecation, gastrointestinal upset, and emesis. The nicotinic symptoms can be summarized by a mnemonic based on the days of the week, *MTWtHF*, which stands for muscle weakness and paralysis, tachycardia, weakness, hypertension, and fasiculations.

The **sympathomimetic syndrome** can present with various symptoms depending on which class of agents is involved. Alpha-adrenergic agents include phenylephrine, methoxamine, and phenylpropanolamine and typically present with hypertension (HTN) and reflex bradycardia secondary to vasoconstriction of resistance vessels. Beta-adrenergic agents include theophylline, caffeine, and metaproterenol and typically present with tachycardia with or without hypotension (secondary to excessive stimulation of the sinus node or vascular smooth muscle dilatation).

The **serotonin syndrome** is a life-threatening condition caused by excessive amounts of the neurotransmitter serotonin. It is most often caused by medications that affect the body's serotonin levels. Among these are the selective serotonin uptake inhibitors (SSRIs) such as the antidepressants fluoxetine (Prozac), sertraline (Zoloft), citalopram (Celexa), escitalopram (Lexapro), and paroxetine (Paxil). Also, the selective serotonin/norepinephrine uptake inhibitors (SNRIs), such as duloxetine (Cymbalta) and venlafaxine (Effexor), have been associated with serotonin syndrome. The triptan class of migraine medications (e.g., Imitrex, Maxalt) can cause serotonin syndrome as well. The signs and symptoms of serotonin syndrome include agitation or restlessness, diarrhea, tachycardia, diaphoresis, hallucinations, confusion, hyperthermia, ataxia, nausea, vomiting, hyperreflexia, and hypertension or hypotension.

The **neuroleptic malignant syndrome** is a similar, yet rare, condition that results from many of the antipsychotic agents (e.g., haloperidol) and some of the antiemetic medications (e.g., prochlorperazine). However, it can be seen with other medication classes such as some of medications used for Parkinson disease. The syndrome is related to abnormal levels of the neurotransmitter dopamine. The signs and symptoms include hyperthermia, muscle rigidity, mental status change, tachycardia, hypertension or hypotension, diaphoresis, tremor, incontinence, tachypnea, and metabolic acidosis.

SPECIFIC TOXIC AGENTS ENCOUNTERED IN PREHOSPITAL CARE

The following sections summarize some of the commonly encountered toxins in prehospital care. The list of agents discussed is by no means comprehensive but emphasizes those that may require specific treatment.

Acetaminophen

Acetaminophen is found in many over-the-counter medications and, as such, is a commonly encountered overdose. The primary concern in this overdose is the potential for irreversible hepatic injury. Therapy is aimed at preventing hepatotoxicity. A specific antidote, *N*-acetylcysteine, is available but is generally reserved for use in the hospital.

Route of Exposure	Oral.
Mechanism of Toxicity	Metabolism is primarily hepatic and can cause hepatotoxicity through the production of toxic metabolites. Ninety percent of acetaminophen is conjugated with glucuronic or sulfuric acid in the liver to form nontoxic compounds that are excreted in the urine. A toxic by-product formed by this process is normally conjugated with hepatic glutathione and subsequently excreted in the urine. When glutathione stores are depleted, as in a massive overdose, hepatotoxicity occurs.
Toxic Dose	*Acute ingestion:* Doses greater than 7.5 g or 140 mg/kg are predictive of hepatotoxicity in an adult. Hepatotoxicity is rare in children. Certain medications such as cimetidine and ethanol are protective in acute overdose because they compete with acetaminophen.
	Chronic ingestion: Variable toxicity can occur at low doses (> 4 g per day), especially in chronic alcoholics who have higher levels of acetaminophen and thus develop toxic metabolites more readily.
	Toxicity can be accurately predicted using serum drug levels (assuming the time of ingestion is known).
Signs and Symptoms	Signs and symptoms are classified into stages (see Table 13–1).
Prehospital Management	Supportive care should be provided, including airway support and careful monitoring. If possible, the time of ingestion should be determined as accurately as possible.
In-Hospital Management	Activated charcoal is still used in certain situations (e.g., early presentation after ingestion). Treatment with *N*-acetylcysteine (NAC) either orally or intravenously is the mainstay of therapy in cases of confirmed toxicity. Toxicity and the need for NAC therapy are determined by measurement of serum levels. These serum levels are most useful if measured 4 hours postingestion but can be used up to 25 hours postingestion. The level is plotted on the Rumack-Matthew nomogram for acetaminophen poisoning. Hepatotoxicity can be prevented with NAC therapy but once present is generally irreversible. NAC therapy is most effective if initiated within 8 hours of ingestion but in some circumstances is used even later. Liver transplant has been performed as a lifesaving measure in rare cases.

Anticholinergics

Anticholinergic properties can be found in many agents including both prescription medications and drugs of abuse. Medications with anticholinergic properties include tricyclic antidepressants, antihistamines, phenothiazines, and antiparkinsonian

TABLE 13–1

Stages of Acetaminophen Toxicity

Stage	Time Postingestion	Characteristics
I	1/2 to 24 hours[a]	Anorexia, nausea, vomiting, malaise, pallor, and diaphoresis
II	24 to 48 hours	Abdominal pain, liver tenderness, elevated liver enzymes, and oliguria
III	48 to 96 hours	Peak liver enzyme abnormalities, jaundice, hypoglycemia, coagulopathies, and encephalopathy
IV	4 days to 2 weeks	Resolution of hepatotoxicity or progressive hepatic failure

[a]Some patients may be completely asymptomatic during stage I.

medications. Dimenhydrinate, an antiemetic, is a medication with anticholinergic properties that is commonly used recreationally, especially among adolescents. Some plants (e.g., Jimson weed) and mushrooms (including the hallucinogenic varieties that are used recreationally) also have anticholinergic properties.

Route of Exposure	Oral, intravenous (IV), or dermal.
Mechanism of Toxicity	As described previously, cholinergic blockade occurs both centrally and peripherally and involves both muscarinic and nicotinic receptors. Different agents have different degrees of effect on the two receptor types and, as such, can have slightly different presentations.
Toxic Dose	Variable.
Signs and Symptoms	See earlier description of anticholinergic toxidrome. (*Remember:* Hot as Hell, blind as a bat, dry as a bone, red as a beet, mad as a Hatter.)
Prehospital Management	Conservative supportive care is the mainstay of therapy. Monitoring of airway, breathing, and circulation supplemented with IV access and cardiac monitoring is indicated in all but the most minor overdoses.
In-Hospital Management	Supportive care should be provided as in prehospital management. Seizures and agitation are treated with benzodiazepines. Arrhythmias can be treated with conventional therapy with the exception that Class Ia medications (quinidine, disopyramide, and procainamide) should be avoided because of the quinidine-like effects of some anticholinergics. The use of physostigmine, a reversible acetylcholinesterase inhibitor, may be indicated. However, it may aggravate arrhythmias and seizures, and as such its use is limited to severe toxicity unresponsive to conventional therapy. Indications may include uncontrollable agitation, hemodynamically unstable arrhythmias, and coma with respiratory depression, malignant hypertension, or refractory hypotension. Physostigmine can potentiate toxicity in tricyclic antidepressant overdose and should be avoided. Toxic symptoms of anticholinergics are generally evident within 4–6 hours of ingestion, and patients asymptomatic at that point can generally be safely discharged.

Neuroleptics

Neuroleptics are a broad class of medications that include the antipsychotics and some tranquilizers. The two most commonly encountered neuroleptic classes are the butyrophenones (such as haloperidol and droperidol) and the phenothiazines (such as chlorpromazine). These agents are typically prescribed to patients with significant psychiatric illness and, as such, are frequently seen in overdose settings. Significant adverse reactions can occur to these agents even when taken at normally prescribed dosages.

Route of Exposure	Oral, IV, or intramuscular (IM).
Mechanism of Toxicity	Act by blocking neurotransmission involving dopaminergic, adrenergic, muscarinic, and histaminic receptors. Therapeutic and toxicologic effects vary from agent to agent depending on the degree of blockage of each receptor subtype.
Toxic Dose	Variable.
Signs and Symptoms	Adverse reactions are common and may occur even in the setting of normal therapeutic dosages. These reactions include the following:

Dystonic reaction, which features involuntary, muscle spasm including torticollis, facial grimacing, opisthotonos (flexion adduction of the arms), oculogyric crisis, and laryngeal spasm. Treatment is diphenhydramine or benztropine.

Akathisia that features restlessness, jittery feeling, and insomnia. May be treated with benztropine, amantadine, or propranolol.

Pseudoparkinsonism featuring resting tremor, rigidity, and masked facies. May be treated with benztropine, diphenhydramine, or amantadine.

Tardive dyskinesia which features lip smacking, tongue protrusion, grimacing, and chewing motion.

Neuroleptic malignant syndrome (NMS) which is a life-threatening condition (10 percent mortality rate) featuring hyperthermia, rigidity, altered mental status, and autonomic instability.

Symptoms of acute overdose are highly variable and can include any of the previously described conditions as well as CNS depression (ranging from sedation to coma), respiratory depression, hypo or hyperthermia, pinpoint pupils (especially phenothiazines), anticholinergic symptoms, hypotension with reflex tachycardia, cardiac arrhythmias, and prolongation of the PR and QT intervals (with resultant ventricular arrhythmias such as *torsade de pointes*).

Prehospital Management	ABCs, cardiac monitoring, naloxone, and chemstrip if altered LOC. Treat hypotension with crystalloid (normal saline) and norepinephrine or phenylephrine as needed. Ventricular arrhythmias should be treated initially with bicarbonate (1–2 mEq/kg IV bolus) followed by lidocaine or phenytoin. Torsade de pointes should be treated initially with magnesium, followed by isoproterenol or overdrive pacing as needed. Seizures should be treated using standard methods including benzodiazapines, phenytoin, or phenobarbital.

In-Hospital Management Consists of supportive care including all the aforementioned methods. Class 1A antiarrhythmics such as quinidine and procainamide should be avoided because they may exacerbate the cardiac toxicity. Cooling or warming techniques may be needed to control extremes of temperature. Management of NMS includes muscle relaxation using benzodiazepines and, if necessary, neuromuscular blockade. Dantrolene and bromocriptine, a dopamine agonist, have been used with mixed results in the treatment of NMS.

℞ Flumazenil (Anexate, Romazicon)

Class Benzodiazepine antagonist

Description

Flumazenil is a benzodiazepine antagonist. It is used to reverse the sedative effects of benzodiazepines, especially respiratory depression.

Mechanism of Action

Flumazenil antagonizes the actions of the benzodiazepines in the central nervous system. Particularly, it inhibits their actions on the gamma-aminobutyric acid–benzodiazepine complex. It is used to reverse the sedative effects of the benzodiazepines.

Pharmacokinetics

Onset: 1–5 minutes
Peak Effects: 6–10 minutes
Duration: 2–4 hours
Half-Life: 54 minutes

Indications

Flumazenil is used for complete and partial reversal of CNS and respiratory depression caused by benzodiazepines including the following agents: diazepam (Valium), midazolam (Versed), lorazepam (Ativan), triazolam (Halcion), temazepam (Restoril), flurazepam (Dalmane), clorazepate (Tranxene), clonazepam (Klonopin), zolpidem (Ambien), estazolam (ProSom), and alprazolam (Xanax). Flumazenil should *not* be used as a diagnostic agent for benzodiazepine overdose. The potential of inducing a life-threatening benzodiazepine withdrawal reaction in patients addicted to benzodiazepines with flumazenil is not worth the perceived benefits.

Contraindications

Flumazenil is contraindicated in patients with a known hypersensitivity to the medication or to benzodiazepines. It should not be administered to patients who have received benzodiazepines to control life-threatening conditions such as status epilepticus. It should not be used in patients with tricyclic antidepressant overdoses.

Precautions

Flumazenil should be administered with caution to patients dependent on benzodiazepines. Benzodiazepine withdrawal can be life threatening. Signs and symptoms of benzodiazepine withdrawal include tachycardia, hypertension, anxiousness, confusion, and seizures. The effects of flumazenil can wear off, resulting in the return of sedation. Following administration, patients should be monitored for signs of resedation and respiratory depression. Flumazenil should never be administered as part of a "coma cocktail." "Coma cocktails" involve the empiric administration of 50 percent dextrose, thiamine, and naloxone (and in some cases, flumazenil) to unresponsive patients in an attempt to correct the cause of their unresponsiveness and awaken them. "Coma cocktails" are a poor prehospital practice. Therapy should always be guided by objective data such as patient assessment findings and blood glucose determination.

Side Effects

Flumazenil can cause fatigue, headache, agitation, nervousness, dizziness, flushing, confusion, convulsions, arrhythmias, nausea, and vomiting.

Interactions

There are few interactions in the emergency setting.

Dosage

The standard dose of flumazenil in benzodiazepine overdose is 0.2 mg (2 mL) administered intravenously over 30 seconds. If the desired level of consciousness is not obtained after waiting 30 seconds, a further dose of 0.3 mg (3 mL) can be administered over another 30 seconds. Further doses of 0.5 mg (5 mL) can be administered over 30 seconds at 1-minute intervals up to a cumulative dose of 3 mg. Flumazenil should only be given intravenously in the emergency setting.

Beta-Blockers

Although intentional overdose on beta-blockers is relatively rare, toxic symptoms occur frequently. True overdoses are often life threatening and difficult to manage because of the profound hemodynamic effects. Glucagon is the primary antidote and is often the only useful treatment modality.

Route of Exposure	Generally oral; occasionally ocular.
Mechanism of Toxicity	Beta-blockers cause blockade of both β_1- and β_2-receptors in the adrenergic nervous system. This blockade can affect several organ systems, most notably the cardiovascular (bradycardia, atrioventricular [AV] block, or vasodilation) and respiratory (bronchospasm or congestive heart failure).
Toxic Dose	The toxic dose is highly variable. Toxicity is more likely in the setting of underlying heart disease.
Signs and Symptoms	Bradycardia, AV blockade, and hypotension are common. Tachycardia has been reported with some β-blockers such as pindolol, and sotalol. Hypotension is a result of negative chronotropy (bradycardia) and negative inotropy (decreased cardiac contractility). Changes in mental status, ranging from confusion to seizures or

coma, have been described. Bronchospasm and congestive heart failure can occur. Beta-blockers can mask the normal adrenergic signs and symptoms of hypoglycemia. In addition, they can impair recovery from hypoglycemia.

Prehospital Management   Supportive care, including airway management, is provided where indicated. Symptomatic patients with abnormal vital signs may respond to atropine or catecholamines (epinephrine) but more frequently require glucagon therapy. Glucagon acts by augmenting heart rate, AV conduction, and myocardial contractility. The required dose for glucagon therapy in this setting is typically 3–10 mg given as a bolus. This dosage is frequently problematic in that few EMS vehicles carry these quantities of glucagon in the field. Cases unresponsive to these pharmacological interventions may be supported with fluid therapy and/or transcutaneous pacing. Seizures can be treated with benzodiazepines (diazepam or lorazepam) or in refractory cases phenytoin or phenobarbital. Bronchospasm can be treated with β_2-agonists and in severe cases aminophylline.

In-Hospital Management   Supportive care should be provided as in prehospital management. Patients often require intensive care unit (ICU) support including continuous glucagon infusion with or without pressor therapy (dopamine or epinephrine).

Calcium Channel Blockers

Calcium channel blocker overdose is becoming one of the most lethal prescription drug ingestions. The clinical presentation of calcium channel blocker overdose can be extremely variable depending on the agent involved but is often clinically similar to beta-blocker toxicity. The effects of calcium channel blockers include peripheral vasodilation, decreased heart rate, decreased contractility, and decreased cardiac conduction. Hyperglycemia and acidosis are common. Although calcium therapy can be useful, major overdoses are often dependent on inotrope therapy (epinephrine or dopamine) and occasionally glucagon.

Route of Exposure   Oral, sublingual, or intravenous.

Mechanism of Toxicity   Virtually any cell utilizing calcium can be affected, most notably myocardium, the sinoatrial (SA) and AV nodes, and the AV nodal conduction pathway. Metabolism occurs in the liver.

Toxic Dose   The toxic dose is variable. The effects are generally more severe in the presence of underlying cardiovascular disease.

Signs and Symptoms   Hypotension, bradycardia, and AV conduction blocks are common. The extent of these effects is dependent on the specific agent ingested. Nonspecific features include lethargy, slurred speech, nausea, vomiting, coma, and respiratory depression.

Prehospital Management   Supportive care is provided as required. In cases of severe toxicity, calcium chloride or calcium gluconate may be given intravenously in a dosage of 10 cc of a 10 percent solution. Calcium therapy is occasionally but not universally effective. Other therapeutic options for cardiac toxicity include atropine and transcutaneous pacing. Intravenous glucagon therapy has also been tried with some success in cases unresponsive to calcium and pressors. Hypotension may be partially responsive to IV fluids and inotropes (dopamine and norepinephrine).

In-Hospital Management Supportive care should be provided as in prehospital management. Prolonged toxicity is common, and observation for extended periods is often required. Severe cases may require ICU admission with assisted ventilation and inotropic therapy.

Carbon Monoxide

Carbon monoxide (CO) exposure, both intentional and accidental, is a common toxicological problem. Death is not infrequent, and long-term neurological sequelae are also common. Oxygen is the mainstay of therapy, and hyperbaric oxygen therapy may be indicated in severe cases.

Route of Exposure Inhalation is the most common route of exposure and is caused by blocked ventilation of furnace, chimney, or automobile exhaust systems. Carbon monoxide exposure is also common in smoke inhalation and can be seen with ingestion or inhalation of paint thinners (containing methylene chloride, which can be metabolized to CO).

Mechanism of Toxicity CO binds hemoglobin to form **carboxyhemoglobin**, thereby reducing the availability of hemoglobin to carry oxygen and thus inducing hypoxemia. It may also impair cellular oxygenation by competing with oxygen for binding sites of enzymes on the **electron transport chain** (cytochrome oxidase). The affinity of hemoglobin for CO is 250× that of O_2. CO also binds directly to both cardiac and skeletal myoglobin, thereby decreasing contractility. In the CNS, CO can induce cerebral edema and necrosis of white matter.

Toxic Dose Variable.

Signs and Symptoms Signs and symptoms depend on levels (levels do not always correspond with symptoms):

< 10 percent:	Generally asymptomatic; smokers often run levels up to 10 percent
10–20 percent:	Headache and dyspnea
20–30 percent:	Headache, fatigue, and visual disturbance
40–50 percent:	Tachycardia and altered level of consciousness; may precipitate angina
> 60 percent:	Coma, seizures, and cherry red skin

CO levels (carboxyhemoglobin levels) can be measured with pule CO-oximetry or exhaled CO monitoring. At levels greater than 25 percent, virtually any organ system can be affected. Pulmonary effects include non-cardiogenic pulmonary edema, congestive heart failure, and aspiration. CNS effects include ataxia, nystagmus, hearing loss, tinnitus, papilledema, retinal hemorrhages, coma, and seizures. Cardiovascular system (CVS) effects include arrhythmias, ST and T wave changes on electrocardiogram (ECG), and occasionally ischemia or infarction. Renal effects include rhabdomyolysis or myoglobinuria and acute renal failure. Although the occurrence of cherry red skin is commonly described in the presence of CO poisoning, it is actually a rare finding and its absence does not rule out CO poisoning. Pallor or cyanosis is seen relatively frequently in CO poisoning.

Prehospital Management   Supportive care supplemented by O_2 (via 100 percent non-rebreather mask) and airway management should be provided as required. Oxygen acts to decrease the half-life of CO:

$t_{1/2}$ room air $= 320$ minutes

$t_{1/2}$ 100 percent $O_2 = 60$–80 minutes

$t_{1/2}$ hyperbaric $O_2 = 20$–30 minutes

The measured O_2 saturation is unreliable in the setting of CO poisoning because the unit cannot differentiate between carboxyhemoglobin and oxyhemoglobin. As such it gives a falsely high saturation reading. The difference between an accurately measured O_2 saturation and the falsely elevated oximetry measurement is known as the saturation gap and is characteristic of CO poisoning. Unfortunately, accurate measurement of the O_2 saturation requires the use of arterial blood gases and therefore is generally not possible in a prehospital care setting.

In-Hospital Management   Supportive care should be provided as in prehospital management. Use of hyperbaric oxygen therapy remains controversial but may offer benefit in patients with severe symptoms and neurological deficits. Indications for hyperbaric O_2 therapy include patients with significant neurological abnormalities, patients with cardiovascular abnormalities, or symptomatic pregnant patients. Some studies suggest symptomatic patients with levels > 20 to 25 percent warrant hyperbaric O_2 therapy. Long-term neurological sequelae occur, and some centers routinely use psychometric testing to monitor neurological function.

Cyanide

Cyanide is a substance with a somewhat notorious history commonly found in many industrial products, medications, and plants. It is found in many manufacturing plants and laboratories and is produced in the burning of some plastics, wool, silk, and furniture. It is found in plant material, including apricot, peach, and cherry pits, and in some poisons. It is an uncommon but potentially deadly toxin; patients who have been exposed to it can be treated using a specific antidote kit that may be life saving if used early.

Route of Exposure   Inhalation, ingestion, intravenous, or dermal contact.

Mechanism of Toxicity   Cyanide binds a key cellular enzyme, cytochrome oxidase, causing cellular asphyxia and thus affecting virtually all organ systems.

Toxic Dose	Highly variable.
Signs and Symptoms	Most commonly present very quickly postexposure as unconscious, noncyanosed patients with hypotension and bradycardia; death occurs in seconds to minutes. In less severe cases or very early postexposure, the patient may have headache, dyspnea, confusion, or seizures with hypotension. Permanent neurological sequelae can occur in survivors. Care providers may detect a bitter almond odor.
Prehospital Management	Recognition of cyanide exposure is the key to management because the window for implementing therapy is extremely short. As always, initial supportive care, including airway, breathing and circulation, is paramount. A specific antidote, known as the Pasadena Cyanide Antidote Kit, is available and is often kept on site at industrial sites using cyanide products. Some EMS systems, particularly in rural settings, carry the antidote kit. The kit contains three different products: amyl nitrite pearls for inhalation, sodium nitrite solution for intravenous use, and sodium thiosulfate for intravenous use. The amyl nitrite pearls can be broken and inhaled immediately by the victim, and the sodium nitrite should be given immediately on establishment of IV or IO access. Both nitrite products work by inducing methemoglobinemia—a form of hemoglobin that scavenges cyanide. Sodium thiosulfate works by converting cyanide to thiocyanate, a much less toxic compound that is gradually excreted in the urine. If the symptoms are relatively mild, sodium thiosulfate should be used alone, because methemoglobinemia can itself be dangerous and is only valuable in truly life-threatening cases of cyanide poisoning. Base physician contact or poison center consultation should come early in the course of managing cyanide poisoning.

An additional antidote for cyanide poisoning is now available. It is easy to administer and has a good safety profile. The antidote is hydroxocobalamin (CyanoKit). Hydroxocobalamin is a precursor to cyanocobalamin (vitamin B_{12}) and removes the cyanide molecule from cytochrome oxidase thus restoring cellular energy production. |
| *In-Hospital Management* | Supportive care should be provided as in prehospital management. Inhalational exposures related to closed-space combustion can often present with concurrent cyanide and carbon monoxide toxicity, and both must be treated aggressively. In cases requiring nitrite therapy, methemoglobin levels must be closely monitored. Intravenous hydroxycobalamin (CyanoKit) can be a useful adjunct because it combines with cyanide to form a nontoxic cyanocobalamin (Vitamin B_{12}) that is excreted renally. Hyperbaric oxygen has no proven role in cyanide poisoning, although it may be indicated in cases of concurrent CO poisoning. For oral cyanide ingestion, charcoal may be beneficial. |

Class Vasodilator/cyanide antidote

Description

Amyl nitrite is a potent vasodilator and an antidote for cyanide poisoning.

Mechanism of Action

Amyl nitrite, which is chemically related to nitroglycerin, has been used for many years in the treatment and symptomatic relief of angina. It is also effective in the emergency management of cyanide poisoning. It is supplied in a glass inhalant that can be broken and inhaled immediately. Amyl nitrite causes the oxidation of hemoglobin to a compound called **methemoglobin**. Methemoglobin reacts with the toxic cyanide ion to form *cyanomethemoglobin,* which can be enzymatically degraded. This serves to remove cyanide from the blood.

Pharmacokinetics

Onset: 10–30 seconds

Peak Effects: 30 seconds

Duration: 3–5 minutes

Half-Life: Not applicable

Indication

Cyanide poisoning.

Contraindications

There are no contraindications to the use of amyl nitrite in the management of cyanide poisoning.

Precautions

Headache and hypotension have been known to occur following the inhalation of amyl nitrite. Amyl nitrite is a medication of abuse and should be kept in a secure place with the narcotics. It has a horrible odor resembling dirty sweat socks. It has some degree of abuse potential (e.g., "locker room").

Side Effects

Amyl nitrite can cause severe headache, weakness, dizziness, flushing, cold sweats, tachycardia, syncope, orthostatic hypotension, nausea, and vomiting.

Interactions

The hypotensive effects of amyl nitrite can be potentiated by antihypertensive agents, β-blockers, and certain antiemetics (phenothiazines).

Dosage

One to two inhalants of amyl nitrite should be crushed and inhaled. It should be repeated every minute or so. This should be maintained until the patient has reached an emergency department. Therapeutic effects diminish after approximately 20 minutes. Amyl nitrite should be administered by inhalation only.

Rx Sodium Nitrite

Class Nitrate/cyanide antidote

Description

Sodium nitrite is a nitrate salt and a part of the Pasadena Cyanide Antidote Kit (Figure 13–1). It is seldom used alone in the treatment of cyanide poisoning; instead, it is usually used with sodium thiosulfate and amyl nitrite. When used together, these compounds are more effective than when used alone.

Mechanism of Action

Sodium nitrite converts hemoglobin to methemoglobin. Methemoglobin has a high affinity for cyanide and can actually draw cyanide from the cells. The methemoglobin–cyanide complex is still toxic (but less so than cyanide bound to cytochrome a_3) and must be detoxified by sodium thiosulfate. The mechanism of action of sodium nitrite is not fully understood.

Pharmacokinetics

Onset: 2–5 minutes
Peak Effects: 30–70 minutes
Duration: Varies
Half-Life: Not applicable

Indications

Cyanide poisoning as a part of the Pasadena Cyanide Antidote Kit.

Contraindications

Sodium nitrite should not be administered to asymptomatic patients following exposure to cyanide. It should not be administered to patients with smoke inhalation and combined carbon monoxide and cyanide poisoning unless hyperbaric oxygen therapy is available and such therapy has already been initiated.

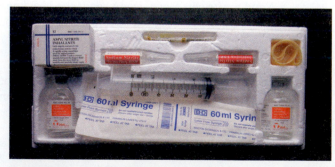

● **FIGURE 13–1**   Cyanide antidote kit. © Jeff Forster

Precautions

Excessive methemoglobinemia may occur, especially when doses larger than those recommended are administered to children. Hypotension is common following rapid administration of sodium nitrite due to its vasodilating properties and can be minimized by slow IV administration. Blood pressure should be monitored carefully during sodium nitrite administration, and the infusion rate slowed if hypotension occurs.

Patients with smoke inhalation and combined carbon monoxide and cyanide poisoning with elevated carboxyhemoglobin levels should not be given sodium nitrite unless treatment in a hyperbaric oxygen chamber is available and such treatment has been initiated.

Side Effects

Excessive methemoglobinemia may occur, especially with doses exceeding those recommended. Hypotension may occur with rapid intravenous infusion.

Interactions

None when used in the setting of cyanide poisoning.

Dosage

Adult dose: Give amyl nitrite until IV access available, and then administer 300 mg (10 mL of 3 percent solution) sodium nitrite IV. Subsequent doses of 150 mg can be administered in 30 minutes as needed or if there is no response to the first dose.

Pediatric dose: 10 mg/kg IV. Fifty percent of the original dose can be administered in 30 minutes as needed.

℞ Sodium Thiosulfate

Class Cyanide antidote

Description

Sodium thiosulfate is a part of the Pasadena Cyanide Antidote Kit. It is seldom used alone in the treatment of cyanide poisoning; instead, it is usually used with sodium nitrite and amyl nitrite. When used together, these compounds are more effective than when used alone.

Mechanism of Action

The major route of detoxification of cyanide in the body is conversion to thiocyanate. The thiocyanate is then removed by the kidneys.

Pharmacokinetics

Onset: 2–5 minutes
Peak Effects: Varies
Duration: Varies
Half-Life: Not applicable

Indications

Cyanide poisoning as a part of the Pasadena Cyanide Antidote Kit.

Contraindications

None when used in the treatment of cyanide poisoning.

Precautions

Sodium thiosulfate is most effective as a cyanide antidote when used in conjunction with nitrites.

Side Effects

Nausea, vomiting, and joint aches are common. Psychosis reported with higher doses. Side effects are mild and of minor importance compared to the risks associated with cyanide poisoning.

Interactions

None when used in the setting of cyanide poisoning.

Dosage

Adult dose: Administer following sodium nitrite and/or amyl nitrite. The initial dose is 12.5 g (50 mL of 25 percent solution) IV over 10 minutes. Repeat half original dose if signs recur.

Pediatric dose: The initial dose in children is 400 (300–500) mg/kg body weight given intravenously as indicated above.

℞ Hydroxocobalamin (Cyanokit)

Class Cyanide antidote

Description

Hydroxocobalamin (CyanoKit) is a cyanide antidote that is a chemical precursor to cyanocobalamin (vitamin B_{12})

Mechanism of Action

Hydroxocobalamin chelates the cyanide ion from cytochrome oxidase (the terminal enzyme in the electron transport chain). Each hydroxocobalamin molecule can bind one molecule of cyanide. The resultant compound, cyanocobalamin (Vitamin B_{12}) is cleared in the urine.

Pharmacokinetics

Onset: 2–15 minutes
Peak Effects: Varies
Duration: Varies
Half-Life: 26–31 hours

Indications

Known or suspected cyanide poisoning.

Contraindications

None when used in the treatment of cyanide poisoning.

Precautions

In addition to hydroxocobalamin, treatment of cyanide poisoning must include immediate attention to airway patency, adequacy of oxygenation and hydration, cardiovascular support, and management of any seizure activity. Consideration should be given to decontamination measures based on the route of exposure. Allergic reactions and a transient increase in blood pressure have been reported.

Side Effects

Chromaturia (red-colored urine), red skin, rash, elevated blood pressure, nausea, and headache have been reported. Side effects are generally mild and of minor importance compared to the risks associated with cyanide poisoning.

Interactions

Other emergency medications should be administered through a different IV line than the line through which hydroxocobalamin is being infused.

Dosage

Adult dose: The starting dose of hydroxocobalamin is 5 g (i.e., both 2.5 g vials) administered as an intravenous (IV) infusion over 15 minutes (approximately 15 mL/min). Depending upon the severity of the poisoning and the clinical response, a second dose of 5 g may be administered by IV infusion for a total dose of 10 g. The rate of infusion for the second dose may range from 15 minutes (for patients *in extremis*) to two hours, as clinically indicated.

Pediatric dose. Safety and effectiveness of hydroxocobalamin has not been established in children. In non-US marketing experience, a dose of 70 mg/kg has been used to treat pediatric patients.

Cyclic Antidepressants (Tricyclics)

Despite the introduction of various new classes of antidepressant agents in recent years, tricyclics continue to be sometimes prescribed—often for specific psychiatric disorders and some non-psychiatric conditions. Unfortunately, the clinical benefit of these agents is often offset by their lethal potential in the setting of overdose. Cardiac toxicity, predominantly in the form of lethal arrhythmias, is the clinical hallmark, and intravenous bicarbonate therapy continues to be an essential part of management. Examples of agents in this class include amitriptyline and nortriptyline.

Route of Exposure	Oral.
Mechanism of Toxicity	Multiple physiological effects lead to clinical toxicity. Blockage of norepinephrine, dopamine, and serotonin reuptake at the presynaptic receptor leads to eventual norepinephrine depletion. Tricyclics also possess some anticholinergic activity, calcium channel blocking activity, and alpha-blocking activity. Cardiac toxicity is

related to antagonism of cardiac fast sodium channels (quinidine-like effects), resulting in prolonged QRS complexes, as well as blockade of potassium efflux, resulting in QT interval prolongation. Metabolism is almost entirely hepatic, with a half-life of approximately 24 hours at therapeutic doses. In the setting of overdose, the half-life can be as much as 72 hours.

Toxic Dose Highly variable.

Signs and Symptoms Symptoms include dizziness, confusion, blurred vision, and dry mouth. Signs can be classified into three categories: cardiovascular, CNS, and anticholinergic. Cardiovascular signs include conduction blocks, hypotension, arrhythmias, and cardiac arrest. CNS signs include delirium, agitation, extrapyramidal signs, myoclonus, seizures, and coma. Anticholinergic signs occur as described previously and include tachycardia, mydriasis, decreased bowel sounds, urinary retention, and hyper- or hypothermia. The earliest and most sensitive sign of cyclic antidepressant overdose is tachycardia. Life-threatening arrhythmias are generally preceded by prolongation of the QRS complex.

Prehospital Management Supportive care, including airway support, should be provided as indicated. Intravenous access and fluid therapy are indicated if hypotension is present. Sodium bicarbonate remains a mainstay of therapy and has the following specific indications: hypotension, ventricular arrhythmias, seizure activity (bicarbonate is not therapeutic for the seizure itself, but seizure activity is considered predictive of impending cardiac arrhythmias, which may be averted with bicarbonate therapy), and wide QRS complexes on cardiac monitor. (The QRS interval requiring bicarbonate therapy remains somewhat controversial—some authors advocate 0.10 seconds, whereas others advocate that it be reserved for complexes > 0.16 seconds; base physician contact is generally indicated where possible.)

Several mechanisms have been postulated for the therapeutic effects of bicarbonate, including increased protein binding of tricyclic antidepressant (TCA) in an alkaline environment (thus there is less free TCA to induce cardiac toxicity), alkalinization increasing the amount of unionized TCA, which appears to be less able to bind the sodium channel, and alkalinization causing free TCA to be pulled out of cardiac tissue. Additionally, some evidence suggests that the sodium in sodium bicarbonate helps to overcome the sodium channel blockade.

Hypotension unresponsive to bicarbonate and IV fluid may require inotrope therapy. Seizure activity unresponsive to bicarbonate therapy may be treated with benzodiazepines such as diazepam or lorazepam. Mechanical hyperventilation (guided by capnography) may be of some value in reducing cardiac and CNS toxicity.

In-Hospital Management Supportive care should be provided as in prehospital management. Cases of suspected toxicity require an observation period of at least 6 hours to rule out serious sequelae.

Digoxin and Digitalis

Although not as widely used as it once was, digoxin remains a relatively common medication that can cause severe illness and death in the setting of overdose. A specific antidote, digitalis-specific Fab fragments, is available but is not commonly used in the prehospital setting. Digoxin has a relatively narrow therapeutic window, and EMS providers should maintain a high index of suspicion for toxicity in cases in which a patient is known to be taking the medication. It is found in several sources, including prescription medications, plants (most notably foxglove), and certain toad venom.

Route of Exposure	Generally oral; can be related to plant exposure (digitalis compounds are derived from plants, most notably the foxglove plant).
Mechanism of Toxicity	Digitalis compounds inhibit the sodium-potassium ATPase, causing potassium efflux and sodium and calcium influx into cells. Toxicity is enhanced in hypokalemia, hypomagnesemia, hypercalcemia, and alkalosis.
Toxic Dose	The toxic dose is highly variable. Patients with underlying heart disease, renal failure, hypothyroidism, and hypoxemia and those using nonsteroidal anti-inflammatory medications (NSAIDs) are more prone to toxicity.
Signs and Symptoms	Symptoms are nonspecific and include fatigue, anorexia, disorientation, confusion, delerium, hallucinations, gastrointestinal upset, visual halos (green or yellow), slowed conduction in SA and AV nodes, increased PR interval, shortened QT intervals, AV block, asystole, ST-T wave scooping, junctional rhythms, and hemodynamic instability. Virtually any cardiac arrhythmia can be seen.
Prehospital Management	Supportive care, including fluids and pressor agents for the treatment of hypotension, should be provided.
In-Hospital Management	Supportive care should be provided as in prehospital management. Electrolyte abnormalities, including hyperkalemia, should be corrected. Calcium should *not* be given. Magnesium therapy may lessen cardiac toxicity. Phenytoin (Dilantin) may be helpful for ventricular arrhythmias. Atropine and pacing may be required for symptomatic bradycardias. Procainamide and quinidine are contraindicated because they may worsen conduction and contractility problems. Digibind (digoxin Fab fragments) can be lifesaving in severe overdose. It acts by directly binding and inactivating digitalis compounds, thereby allowing for rapid excretion by the kidneys. Digibind is indicated in ingestions that are potentially lethal based on the amount of ingested medication (generally 10 mg in an adult), high serum levels (> 12.8–19.2 mmol/L), marked hyperkalemia, malignant arrhythmias, resistant bradycardias, and hypotension. Clinical response to Digibind can occur as early as 20–30 minutes after administration.

Ethylene Glycol

The toxic alcohols include ethylene glycol, methanol, and isopropyl alcohol. In the case of ethylene glycol, which is most commonly found in antifreeze, ingestion is often accidental and may not be recognized until severe toxicity has occurred. Ethylene glycol poisoning is frequently misdiagnosed as ethanol intoxication, often resulting in suboptimal outcomes. Ethanol therapy helps to avert toxicity, but in severe cases dialysis may be required.

Route of Exposure	Generally oral.
Mechanism of Toxicity	Toxic metabolites are formed, causing acidosis and renal damage. Ethylene glycol is metabolized by alcohol dehydrogenase into several toxic metabolites including glycoaldehyde, glycolic acid, glyoxylic acid, and oxalate. These products take some time to accumulate, and thus signs and symptoms may not appear until 6–12 hours after the ingestion. This delay is even more pronounced if ethanol is also ingested because ethanol competes for alcohol dehydrogenase and thereby slows the development of toxic metabolites.
Toxic Dose	The minimal toxic dose is 1–2 mL/kg.
Signs and Symptoms	Toxicity is sometimes divided into three phases.

- Phase I is from 1 to 12 hours postingestion and typically presents with signs of intoxication without the smell of ethanol (which prehospital care providers should be able to recognize). CNS symptoms may include ataxia, seizures, and nystagmus. Nausea and vomiting are common in phase I.
- Phase II occurs from 12 to 36 hours postingestion and consists of cardiopulmonary toxicity including hypertension, tachycardia, and tachypnea. In severe poisoning pulmonary edema, congestive heart failure, and shock may develop.
- Phase III occurs from 24 to 72 hours postingestion and is associated with acute renal toxicity consisting of flank pain, costovertebral angle tenderness, decreased urine output, and acute renal failure.

	Not all patients go through these phases; some can present critically ill early postingestion (i.e., within 12 hours). The fluorescent additive in antifreeze can sometimes be seen excreted in the urine.
Prehospital Management	Supportive care, including airway management, should be provided as required. Intravenous fluid therapy is indicated because dehydration is common and renal perfusion may be compromised. Ethanol therapy is indicated as a means of preventing metabolism to toxic metabolites. Although not widely used in a prehospital care setting, some circumstances (such as long transport times) may warrant the use of oral or IV ethanol therapy. Patients who have been coingesting ethanol have the benefit of having initiated their own therapy. Fomepizole (Antizole) is an antidote for ethylene glycol toxicity. It competes with the enzyme (alcohol dehydrogenase) that breaks ethylene glycol into toxic compounds thus slowing and even preventing the formation of toxic byproducts.
In-Hospital Management	Supportive care should be provided as in prehospital management. Metabolism to toxic metabolites is limited by administering ethanol as a competitive inhibitor of alcohol dehydrogenase. In this way ethanol allows for

excretion of unchanged ethylene glycol without metabolism. The half-life of ethylene glycol is 5 hours, whereas with therapeutic ethanol levels it is increased to approximately 17 hours. Serum ethanol levels are used to determine the need for ethanol therapy, which is usually given intravenously but can be given orally in unusual circumstances. Hemodialysis is indicated in cases of renal failure, in severe metabolic acidosis, or as determined by blood levels. Hypocalcemia can occur and, when present, requires treatment. Magnesium is a cofactor in the conversion to nontoxic metabolites, and magnesium supplementation is sometimes required. Bicarbonate is used in cases of profound acidosis. Pyridoxine is used to help promote conversion of glyoxylic acid to its nontoxic metabolite, glycine. Fomepizole (Antizole) is an antidote for ethylene glycol toxicity. It competes with the enzyme (alcohol dehydrogenase) that breaks down ethylene glycol into toxic compounds thus slowing and even preventing the formation of toxic byproducts.

Iron

Iron overdose is relatively common and tends to be seen most frequently in the pediatric population. Symptoms are highly variable, depending on the time since ingestion. A specific antidote, deferoxamine, is available but is generally reserved for use in the hospital.

Route of Exposure	Oral.
Mechanism of Toxicity	Iron has a direct corrosive effect on gastric and intestinal mucosa that can lead to hemorrhage or perforation. Fluid loss from the gastrointestinal (GI) tract and vasodilation can cause hypotension. Iron is also an intracellular toxin that causes uncoupling of oxidative phosphorylation, leading to impaired generation of ATP and cellular death.
Toxic Dose	The toxic dose is somewhat dependent on the form of iron ingested because it is the elemental amount of iron present that is relevant. Ferrous sulfate tablets contain only 20 percent elemental iron per weight, whereas ferrous fumarate contains 33 percent iron by weight. Taking this into account, 20–60 mg/kg of elemental iron has moderate risk of toxicity, whereas > 60 mg/kg has high risk for toxicity.
Signs and Symptoms	Some authors describe four distinct stages of iron toxicity, and others describe five. The classification based on four stages is presented here.

- Stage 1 (0.5–2 hours postingestion): Severe vomiting and diarrhea (often with blood), lethargy, coma, pallor, tachycardia, hypotension, acidosis, hyperglycemia, hypovolemia, shock, renal failure, and death.
- Stage 2 (2–12 hours postingestion): Relatively asymptomatic period.
- Stage 3 (12–48 hours postingestion): Recurrence of GI symptoms including bloody emesis and diarrhea, GI perforation, coma, seizures, shock, hepatorenal failure, coagulation defects, hypoglycemia, and severe metabolic acidosis.

- Stage 4 (beyond 48 hours postingestion): Pyloric (gastric outlet) strictures. In this stage either death or recovery occurs.

Prehospital Management   Treatment is limited to supportive care including airway support and fluid resuscitation in cases of volume depletion.

In-Hospital Management   Supportive care should be provided as in prehospital management. Iron levels are helpful but do not completely rule out iron toxicity, particularly in the later stages. Levels generally peak 3–5 hours postingestion, and levels drawn outside this window may be misleading. Iron tablets can often be seen on X-ray, and, as such, abdominal X-rays may be helpful. Charcoal does not bind iron and is therefore not indicated. Gastric lavage is of limited value because iron can form concretions or bezoars, which are too large to fit in lavage tubing. Whole-bowel irrigation is the decontamination method of choice. Patients with toxic levels or clinical signs and symptoms are treated with deferoxamine, which works by binding with iron to form a water-soluble compound, ferrioxamine, which is renally excreted. A deferoxamine challenge test is sometimes used in which deferoxamine is administered and a change in urine color (vin-rose) is considered diagnostic of a toxic iron ingestion. Charcoal hemoperfusion and exchange transfusions have been used occasionally with some success. Symptomatology always takes precedence over laboratory values in managing cases of suspected iron overdose.

Isopropyl Alcohol

Isopropyl alcohol, commonly known as rubbing alcohol, is a commonly abused toxic alcohol. Although it is far less toxic than methanol or ethylene glycol, in high doses it can induce hypotension unresponsive to conventional therapy and cardiac ischemia.

Route of Exposure   Oral, skin contact, or inhalation.

Mechanism of Toxicity   Isopropyl alcohol is a CNS depressant and vasodilator. In the liver it is metabolized to acetone, which is subsequently excreted by the kidneys.

Toxic Dose   Toxic dose is 0.5–1 mL/kg of 70 percent isopropyl alcohol (typical concentration).

Signs and Symptoms   Signs of intoxication and CNS depression may appear. It is twice as potent a CNS depressant as ethanol. In severe overdose, hypotension secondary to vasodilation that is largely unresponsive to fluids and pressor therapy can occur. Cardiac ischemia or infarction can occur.

Prehospital Management   Supportive care, including airway management, assisted ventilation, and fluid therapy, should be provided as needed. Ethanol therapy is not indicated.

In-Hospital Management   Supportive care should be provided as in prehospital management. Vasopressor therapy, though of limited value, may be tried. Dialysis is rarely required but may be indicated in cases involving severe, unresponsive hypotension.

Lithium

Lithium is a relatively common medication used in the treatment of certain psychiatric disorders such as bipolar (manic-depressive) disorder. Although overdose is not common, it can be serious. No specific antidote is available, and therapy is generally aimed at enhancing elimination and providing supportive care.

Route of Exposure	Oral.
Mechanism of Toxicity	Lithium replaces sodium, thereby altering cellular processes, membrane structures, response to hormones, and utilization of energy at a cellular level. In the CNS these effects can result in permanent neurological damage. Lithium is excreted almost entirely by the kidneys. Because it decreases renal function, lithium tends to decrease its own clearance and can in fact enhance its own reabsorption by the kidney.
Toxic Dose	The toxic dose is highly variable depending on whether it is an acute or chronic ingestion. Overdose in the setting of chronic ingestion tends to be more severe because serum lithium levels are already high, allowing lithium to enter cells (predominantly CNS) more readily. Toxicity is generally more severe in the setting of poor underlying renal function, diuretic use, and dehydration.
Signs and Symptoms	Signs and symptoms are variable depending on levels. *Low (serum levels less than 1.5 mEq/L):* GI symptoms including nausea, vomiting, and diarrhea. *Moderate (serum levels 1.5–3.0 mEq/L):* Polyuria followed by urinary and fecal incontinence, muscle weakness (which can progress to myoclonic twitches and muscle rigidity with choreoathetoid movements), and neurological symptoms (which can include restlessness, vertigo, slurred speech, blurred vision, and coma). *Severe (serum levels > 3.0 mEq/L):* Seizures, coma, cardiac arrhythmias, hypotension with peripheral vascular collapse, muscle twitching, and spasticity.
Prehospital Management	Supportive care should be provided as indicated. Virtually all patients with lithium overdoses are volume depleted, and aggressive fluid resuscitation using normal saline is indicated. It remains unclear whether the administration of sodium chloride aids elimination.
In-Hospital Management	Whole-bowel irrigation has also been shown to be beneficial. Correction of volume depletion is essential and can take several hours. Hemodialysis is indicated in cases of renal failure, of severe cardiovascular or neurological abnormalities, or with high serum levels.

Methanol

Methanol is found in many solutions including wood alcohol, window washer fluid, paint solvent, and industrial solvents. Ingestion is generally accidental, and small doses can be fatal. Although virtually any organ system can be involved, visual disturbances including blindness remain the clinical hallmark. Toxicity is dependent on the formation of toxic metabolites, and thus toxicity is generally delayed for several hours.

Route of Exposure	Generally oral but can be dermal or by inhalation.
Mechanism of Toxicity	Toxic metabolites, predominantly formaldehyde and formic acid, are formed through the metabolism of methanol by alcohol dehydrogenase. These toxic metabolites have direct toxic effects at a cellular level and result in a profound acidosis that can further accelerate toxicity. Methanol is metabolized by alcohol dehydrogenase to form formaldehyde, which in turn is converted to fomic acid by aldehyde dehydrogenase. Up to 5 percent of ingested methanol may be excreted unchanged by the kidneys and via respiration.
Toxic Dose	Death has been reported with as small a dose as 15–30 mL (1–2 tablespoons).
Signs and Symptoms	An initial latent period ranging from 6 to 30 hours consists of signs of intoxication and gastrointestinal irritation. Some patients may have a prolonged asymptomatic period, particularly if ethanol has been coingested. Caution must be used, because a lack of symptoms early on does not preclude toxicity.
	As toxic metabolites are formed, nausea, vomiting, abdominal pain, and CNS symptoms (ranging from headache and confusion to coma) occur. Ocular toxicity is the hallmark of methanol overdose and can manifest as decreased visual acuity (haziness or "snowfield blindness").
	Death is generally related to profound acidosis and severe CNS effects including cerebral edema. Gastrointestinal bleeding secondary to gastritis can occur.
Prehospital Management	Supportive care, including airway management, should be provided as indicated. As with ethylene glycol, oral or IV ethanol therapy has been utilized in some prehospital care settings.
In-Hospital Management	Diagnosis can be difficult because blood levels are not always available or reliable at the time of presentation. Laboratory investigation generally reveals an anion gap metabolic acidosis, as well as an osmolar gap. Fomepizole (Antizole) is an antidote for methanol poisoning. It competes with the enzyme (alcohol dehydrogenase) that breaks down methanol into toxic compounds thus slowing and even preventing the formation of toxic by-products. Hemodialysis is indicated in the presence of visual symptoms, severe acidosis, high serum levels, or an ingestion of greater than 30 mL. Bicarbonate is reserved for cases of profound acidosis. Folate is a cofactor for the conversion of formate to nontoxic by-products and has a role in therapy.

Narcotics and Opioids

Narcotics and opioids are widely used for both medicinal and therapeutic purposes. Overdoses are common, especially in large urban centers. Recognition of these overdoses is important, because a specific antidote (naloxone) is available in most prehospital settings. In hospital settings, Revex, a long-acting opioid antagonist, may be given.

Route of Exposure	Oral, intravenous, intramuscular, or dermal.
Mechanism of Toxicity	Narcotics and opioids act directly on opiate receptors within the CNS, causing CNS depression. Some opioids have mixed agonist and antagonist properties.
Signs and Symptoms	The classic triad of opioid overdose consists of miosis, respiratory depression, and decreased level of consciousness. Certain types of opioids (e.g., meperidine, morphine, and pentazocine) can present with mydriasis rather than miosis. Occasionally seizures, hypotension, and ventricular arrhythmias can be seen.
Prehospital Management	Supportive care, including airway management, takes priority over naloxone therapy. Track marks (IV) are helpful diagnostically when present and should always be examined. Following assessment and initial stabilization, early use of naloxone (Narcan) may avert the need for invasive airway control. Patients with opioid overdose can rapidly become combative and violent when given naloxone, and precautions need to be taken to ensure that both the patient and care providers are adequately protected from injury. This may include prophylactic use of restraints. Response to naloxone is often effective for diagnosis as well as treatment.
In-Hospital Management	Supportive care and naloxone therapy are provided as described earlier. Long periods of observation are often required to ensure that sedation does not recur. The duration of action of intravenous naloxone is typically 20–120 minutes, which is considerably shorter than the duration of action of most opioids (typically 3–6 hours). In cases of severe, prolonged opioid toxicity, continuous naloxone infusion may be indicated.

℞ Naloxone (Narcan)

Class Narcotic antagonist

Description

Naloxone is an effective narcotic antagonist. It has proved effective in the management and reversal of overdoses caused by narcotics or synthetic narcotic agents.

Mechanism of Action

Naloxone is chemically similar to the narcotics. However, it has only antagonistic properties. Naloxone competes for opiate receptors in the brain. It also displaces narcotic molecules from opiate receptors. It can reverse respiratory depression associated with narcotic overdose.

Pharmacokinetics

Onset: < 2 minutes (IV/IO), 2–10 minutes (IM, ET)
Peak Effects: < 2 minutes (IV/IO), 2–10 minutes (IM, ET)

Duration: 20–120 minutes

Half-Life: 60–90 minutes

Indications

Naloxone is used for the complete or partial reversal of depression caused by narcotics including the following agents: morphine, meperidine (Demerol), heroin, paregoric, hydromorphone (Dilaudid), codeine, oxycodone (Percodan, Percocet), fentanyl, and methadone. It is also used for the complete or partial reversal of depression caused by synthetic narcotic analgesic agents including the following medications: nalbuphine (Nubain), pentazocine (Talwin), and butorphanol (Stadol).

Contraindications

Naloxone should not be administered to a patient with a history of hypersensitivity to the medication.

Precautions

Naloxone should be administered cautiously to patients who are known or suspected to be physically dependent on narcotics. Abrupt and complete reversal by naloxone can cause withdrawal-type effects. This includes newborn infants of mothers with known or suspected narcotic dependence.

Side Effects

Side effects associated with naloxone are rare. However, hypotension, hypertension, ventricular arrhythmias, nausea, and vomiting have been reported.

Interactions

Naloxone may cause narcotic withdrawal in the narcotic-dependent patient. In cases of suspected narcotic dependence, only enough of the medication to reverse respiratory depression should be administered.

Dosage

The standard dosage for suspected or confirmed narcotic or synthetic narcotic overdoses is 1–2 mg administered IV or IO. It can also be administered intra-nasally or by small volume nebulizer. If unsuccessful, then a second dose may be administered 5 minutes later. Failure to obtain reversal after two to three doses indicates another disease process or overdosage on non-opioid medications. An intravenous infusion can be prepared by placing 2 mg of naloxone in 500 mL of D_5W. This gives a concentration of 4 mcg/mL; 100 mL/hr should be infused, thus delivering 400 mcg/hr. In the emergency setting, naloxone should be administered intravenously only. When an IV line cannot be established, intramuscular or subcutaneous (SC) administration can be performed. Naloxone can be administered endotracheally. The dose should be increased to 2.0–2.5 times the intravenous dose. Furthermore, naloxone should be diluted in enough normal saline to provide a total of 10 mL of fluid.

Organophosphates and Carbamates

Organophosphates and carbamates are commonly found in commercial insecticides. Although rare, toxic exposure to these agents is generally serious and often fatal. Diagnosis is frequently difficult because of the subtle nature of many exposures and generalized symptoms. A contaminated piece of clothing may prolong exposure over several days, further confusing the diagnosis. Atropine is widely used and can be highly effective for treatment of poisoning secondary to these agents.

Route of Exposure	Dermal, oral, ocular, or by inhalation.
Mechanism of Toxicity	Organophosphates and carbamides inhibit acetylcholinesterase activity, leading to increased acetylcholine at nerve synapses and an initial overstimulation followed by disruption of transmission in the CNS, parasympathetic nerve endings and some sympathetic nerve endings, somatic nerve endings, and autonomic ganglia.
Toxic Dose	Highly variable; toxicity can occur with minimal exposure. Recurrent exposure secondary to contaminated clothing is common.
Signs and Symptoms	The CNS symptoms include agitation, drowsiness, seizures, cardiorespiratory depression, coma, and death. The mnemonics DUMBELS or SLUDGE can be used to describe the muscarinic signs and symptoms of cholinergic excess, and the mnemonic MTWtHF is used to describe the nicotinic features (see description under "Toxidromes" earlier in this chapter). Miosis is typically present, but in 10 percent of cases mydriasis is present. The history is not always clear in identifying an exposure. A garlic odor may be present.
Prehospital Management	As with all toxicological emergencies, supportive care must be provided immediately. Atropine at a dose of 1 mg every 2–5 minutes (maximum of 100 mg) reverses the cholinergic symptoms. End points for atropine therapy include drying of secretions, reversal of bradycardia, and pupillary mydriasis. It is important to monitor ventilation closely because diaphragmatic weakness is not treated by atropine.
	Extreme care must be taken to avoid contamination of care providers by removal of contaminated clothing and use of gloves and gowns (where available). Contaminated clothing should be removed as soon as practically possible.
	Seizures should be treated with benzodiazepines as needed.
In-Hospital Management	Supportive care should be provided as in prehospital management. Additional therapies include the use of pralidoxime (2-PAM), which acts to regenerate acetylcholinesterase. Charcoal and lavage may be indicated for oral ingestions.

℞ Atropine Sulfate

Class Parasympatholytic

Description

Atropine sulfate is a potent parasympatholytic (anticholinergic). It blocks acetylcholine receptors, thus aiding the management of organophosphate poisonings. Organophosphate poisonings inhibit the enzyme cholinesterase, causing an increase and accumulation of the neurotransmitter acetylcholine. Often, large doses are required to achieve atropinization. Severe poisonings, especially those characterized by paralysis and muscle twitching, require pralidoxime (2-PAM), in addition to atropine.

Mechanism of Action

Atropine sulfate is a potent parasympatholytic and is used to increase the heart rate in hemodynamically significant bradycardias. Hemodynamically significant bradycardias are those slow heart rates accompanied by hypotension, shortness of breath, chest pain, altered mental status, congestive heart failure, and shock. Atropine acts by blocking acetylcholine receptors, thus inhibiting parasympathetic stimulation. Although it has positive chronotropic properties, it has little or no inotropic effect. It plays an important role as an antidote in organophosphate poisonings.

Pharmacokinetics

Onset: Immediate

Peak Effects: 2–4 minutes

Duration: 4 hours

Half-Life: 2–3 hours

Indications

Organophosphate poisoning, bradycardias that are hemodynamically significant.

Contraindications

There are no contraindications to atropine when used in the management of severe organophosphate poisoning.

Precautions

It is important to remove all clothing from a patient who has suffered organophosphate poisoning. The patient must then be completely bathed to remove all residual organophosphate present on the skin. Always be sure to protect the rescuer. Atropine may actually worsen the bradycardia associated with second-degree Mobitz II and third-degree AV blocks. In these cases, go straight to transcutaneous pacing instead of trying atropine.

Side Effects

Atropine sulfate can cause blurred vision, dilated pupils, dry mouth, tachycardia, drowsiness, and confusion.

Interactions

Few in the prehospital setting.

Dosage

One milligram of atropine should be administered initially IV/IO to determine whether or not the patient is tolerant to atropine. If the patient responds to the diagnostic dose, then most likely he or she is not severely poisoned or is not tolerant to atropine. If there is no improvement, a second dose of 2–5 mg may be indicated for an adult (0.05 mg/kg for a child). Doses exceeding 100 mg are sometimes required to treat severe organophosphate poisoning. Atropine should be repeated every 1–5 minutes as the patient's clinical condition dictates. Following the prehospital initial administration of atropine, prompt transportation to an emergency department is indicated. In severe organophosphate poisoning, atropine sulfate is administered intravenously.

℞ Pralidoxime (2-PAM) (Protopam)

Class Cholinesterase reactivator

Description

Pralidoxime is a cholinesterase reactivator.

Mechanism of Action

Pralidoxime is an antidote for severe organophosphate poisonings. It chemically removes the phosphate group from cholinesterase that was transferred from an organophosphate poison. Once cholinesterase is reactivated, it can deactivate acetylcholine. Pralidoxime also detoxifies some organophosphates by direct chemical reaction. It reverses respiratory depression and skeletal muscle paralysis resulting from organophosphate poisoning.

Pralidoxime should be reserved for severe organophosphate poisonings characterized by muscle twitching and paralysis. It should follow atropinization.

Pharmacokinetics

Onset: Varies
Peak Effects: 5–15 minutes (IV/IO), 10–20 minutes (IM)
Duration: Varies
Half-Life: 0.8–2.7 hours

Indication

Severe organophosphate poisoning.

Contraindications

Pralidoxime should not be used in cases of poisoning resulting from inorganic phosphates or the carbamate class of insecticides.

Precautions

Always protect yourself and other rescuers when caring for the victim of organophosphate poisoning.

Intravenous administration should be carried out slowly because tachycardia, laryngospasm, and muscle rigidity have been seen with rapid administration. When used in conjunction with atropine, the effects of atropinization may be seen much earlier than expected. This is especially true if the atropine dose has been large. Excitement and manic behavior have been known to occur immediately following recovery from unconsciousness in a few cases.

Side Effects

Pralidoxime can cause tachycardia, increased salivation, headache, altered mental status, dizziness, blurred vision, nausea, and vomiting.

Interactions

Patients who have sustained organophosphate poisonings should not receive respiratory depressants because these can potentiate the effects of the organophosphates. These medications include narcotics, phenothiazines (antiemetics), antihistamines, and alcohol. Pralidoxime should not be used with theophylline preparations (including aminophylline).

Dosage

One to 2 g of pralidoxime should be placed in 250–500 mL of normal saline and infused over 30 minutes. Pralidoxime can be administered IV or IM. The dose may need to be repeated in 12 hours as the patient's clinical situation dictates.

Salicylates

Salicylate (ASA) overdose is commonly encountered and can be fatal if not treated appropriately. These agents are found in a variety of over-the-counter medications and are frequently confused with other analgesics such as ibuprofen and acetaminophen. The clinical presentation is variable depending on the time since ingestion. Although a specific antidote is not available, therapy is aimed at enhancing elimination and thereby preventing long-term sequelae.

Route of Exposure	Oral; occasionally dermal.
Mechanism of Toxicity	Salicylates cause cellular toxicity through the uncoupling of oxidative phosphorylation and induce anion gap metabolic acidosis.
Metabolism	Salicylates are extensively metabolized by the liver; the kidneys excrete inactive metabolites.
Toxic Dose	*Acute:* Mild-moderate toxicity = 150-300 mg/kg Moderate-severe toxicity = >300 mg/kg *Chronic:* Variable
Signs and Symptoms	*Mild to moderate:* Tachypnea, vomiting, diaphoresis, tinnitus, and acid–base disturbances. The tachypnea is typically early in the course of overdose and can result in an early respiratory alkalosis. *Severe:* CNS abnormalities ranging from confusion and delirium to coma secondary to cerebral edema, hypoglycemia (rare), pulmonary edema, coagulopathies and platelet dysfunction, and occasionally hyperthermia. An anion gap metabolic acidosis is the classic acid–base disturbance in the later stages of toxicity. Renal failure is possible.

Prehospital Management	Supportive care, including airway management, should be provided as required. Hypoglycemia should be ruled out (especially in children).
In-Hospital Management	Toxicity is determined both by clinical criteria and by plotting blood levels taken at least 6 hours postingestion on the Done nomogram. The nomogram is a guideline only and is not useful for chronic toxicity. A single serum salicylate value is not always conclusive, and repeat levels aimed at determining half-lives are sometimes required. When toxicity is suspected by history and physical exam, therapy is initiated regardless of availability of serum levels. Renal excretion of salicylate is enhanced by inducing an alkaline diuresis. This is typically accomplished using an IV solution consisting of sodium bicarbonate mixed in D_5W. Potassium supplementation is often required. Hemodialysis is indicated in severe toxicity associated with renal failure, severe CNS or cardiac dysfunction, or severe acidosis not responsive to the alkaline diuresis.

SSRIs

Selective serotonin reuptake inhibitors (SSRIs) are the newest generation of antidepressant agents and are currently prescribed more frequently than more traditional antidepressants such as tricyclics. The popularity of these agents is largely attributable to their improved safety profile, particularly in the setting of overdose. Prototypical agents include fluoxetine (Prozac), trazodone (Desyrel), sertraline (Zoloft), and paroxetine (Paxil).

Route of Exposure	Oral.
Mechanism of Toxicity	SSRIs block reuptake of serotonin at the presynaptic junction.
Toxic Dose	The toxic dose is variable, but the SSRIs are generally well tolerated even in large overdoses. If used in combination with a monoamine oxidase inhibitor (MAOI), the serotonin syndrome, which is potentially fatal, can occur.
Signs and Symptoms	Overdose with SSRIs is often asymptomatic. Symptoms and signs include agitation, insomnia, CNS excitation, tachycardia, hypertension, and ST depression. Serotonin syndrome can occur when the medication is used in combination with MAOIs due to its serotonergic effects. Serotonin syndrome can include hyperthermia, shivering, tremor, myoclonus, seizures, delirium, agitation, rigidity or hypertonia, autonomic instability, coma, and death.
Prehospital Treatment	Only supportive care is provided; no specific treatment is available.
In-Hospital Treatment	Supportive care is the primary treatment. Serotonin syndrome may require aggressive airway management, assisted ventilation, and pharmacological therapy including IV Dantrolene or oral cyproheptadine. Seizures are treated with benzodiazepines, and hypertension can be treated with nicardipine or sodium nitroprusside.

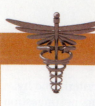

Paramedics are dispatched at 1430 hours on a weekday to a residence in an older neighborhood. En route the call taker provides further information. The patient is a 4-year-old female who is unconscious. On arrival a woman in her late 60s runs out of the house carrying a flaccid, unresponsive 4-year-old child.

Physical Examination

CNS: The child is unresponsive. Her pupils are dilated and unresponsive to light. She is unresponsive to voice and pain.

Resp: Respirations are agonal at 4 per minute and shallow. Her lungs are clear bilaterally with equal air entry. The trachea is midline and there are no signs of trauma.

CVS: The carotid pulse is present, but weak. The radial pulse is absent. Her skin is pale, with cyanotic/gray color to face. Skin is cool and dry.

ABD: Soft and nontender in all four quadrants. There are no signs of vomiting or diarrhea.

Muscl/Skel: No injuries are noted.

Vital Signs

Pulse: 40 per minute

Resp: 4 per minute and shallow

B/P: Unable to obtain

SpO$_2$: error

ECG: 3rd-degree block

Past Hx: The grandmother states that she put her granddaughter down for a nap around 1400 hours. At about 1430 she checked on her granddaughter and found her on the floor of the grandmother's bedroom. The girl was unconscious and unresponsive with an open bottle of heart pills beside her. The grandmother called 911. The prescription is for verapamil (Isoptin) 120 mg. There are 10–12 pills on the floor. The bottle of 60 is empty.

The granddaughter has no previous illnesses and is in good health. She is not taking any medications, nor does she have any allergies.

Treatment

An OPA is inserted and the patient's respirations are assisted by a bag-valve-mask device with 100 percent oxygen via a reservoir bag. The patient is placed on a cardiac monitor, which shows a third-degree block. A weak pulse is still present. An intravenous line is initiated with a 20-gauge catheter in the antecubital fossa.

At the earliest moment, paramedics contact the poison control center for advice.

The patient is given fluid bolus of 20 mL/kg. The patient is approximately 25 kg so a bolus of 500 mL is administered. If perfusion does not improve with the bolus, the paramedics will, in consultation with poison control, administer calcium chloride 10 percent at 10–25 mg/kg diluted to 50 mL and given over 5 minutes. If calcium is not available, paramedics will consider epinephrine 0.01 mg/kg administered slow IV push.

The patient is prepared for transcutaneous pacing. Because this patient weighs more than 15 kg, the adult pads should work. Although this is unusual in children, the paramedics feel it is indicated because of the profound symptoms and may be required if the patient does not respond to medications. The paramedics realize that atropine does not work on third-degree heart blocks.

Outcome

The patient responded to medications and her heart rate increased to 100 with a junctional rhythm. She was transferred to ICU where she battled an aspiration pneumonia and liver failure (secondary to verapamil). She was eventually discharged from hospital with no complications.

CASE PRESENTATION

Early one evening Waterville EMS is called to a residence in an upscale area of the city. Dispatch reports that they are responding to a "man down," unconscious, unresponsive, and not breathing. On arrival a woman in her 20s meets the paramedics and states that her boyfriend is not breathing. Paramedics are led to the living room, where they find a male in his mid-20s lying supine on the floor. There is emesis near the patient.

Physical Examination

CNS:	The patient is unresponsive; Glasgow Coma Scale score is 3; both pupils are pinpoint yet equal
Resp:	Respirations are 6 per minute and very shallow; the airway has residue from vomiting
CVS:	The carotid pulse is slow and weak; the radial pulse is absent; skin is pale; lips are blue
ABD:	Soft and nontender in all four quadrants; the patient has vomited
Muscl/Skel:	No apparent injuries; no pitting edema

Vital Signs

Pulse:	56/min
Resp:	6/min
B/P:	70/52 mmHg
SpO$_2$:	72 percent
ECG:	Sinus bradycardia
Past Hx:	Initially the patient's girlfriend states that she does not know what happened. She states that her boyfriend is very healthy, has no medical problems, and does not take any medication. Paramedics specifically ask about alcohol or recreational medications. The girlfriend emphatically states, "No."

Treatment

Police backup is requested. The initial treatment begins with the ABCs. The airway is suctioned, and an oropharyngeal airway is placed. Ventilation by bag-valve-mask device and 100 percent oxygen by reservoir bag is initiated at 24 breaths per minute. Airway compliance is good. An IV of normal saline is prepared and paramedics perform venipuncture with a 16-gauge catheter. Blood is drawn for a red-top tube, and the hub of the needle is used to obtain a blood sample for glucose testing. The IV of normal saline is connected to the catheter, and the fluid is administered at 100 mL/hr.

As one paramedic starts the IV, she looks for previous needle marks and does not find any. The absence of needle marks does not change the paramedic's assessment. Based on the age of the patient (a male in his mid-20s does not just stop breathing), the slow respirations, and the pinpoint pupils, the paramedic is fairly certain that the patient has taken a narcotic or some designer drug.

(continued)

Case Presentation (continued)

The patient's girlfriend is questioned once again as to whether her boyfriend uses any drugs. The paramedic tells her that her boyfriend's condition is very serious and that she must be absolutely honest. Finally the girlfriend states that her boyfriend uses heroin. She found him on the floor when she came home and then called for the ambulance after she hid the drugs and syringes.

At this point the police arrive and assist the paramedics. The patient is moved to the stretcher and restrained. The paramedics are concerned for their safety because the patient may be aggressive or violent as he comes out of the coma. His airway is still patent, and intubation is not required at this time. Narcan is administered intravenously in 1.0 mg dosages. The paramedics carefully titrate the dose to increase the respiratory rate. The stretcher and patient are moved to the ambulance, and a police officer agrees to accompany the paramedics to the hospital. The patient is not fighting against the bag-valve-mask device or straining against the restraints. The patient's girlfriend gives the paramedics the rest of the drugs and the syringe.

En route to the hospital a paramedic monitors the patient's vital signs closely. Respirations increase to 20 per minute, and the patient is placed on oxygen by non-rebreather mask at 15 lpm. The pulse rate increases to 112 per minute, and blood pressure increases to 124/82 mmHg. The blood glucose reading is 125 mg/dL (7.0 mmol/L). The half-life of Narcan is likely to be less than that of the narcotic. Thus, the patient's level of consciousness may decrease. On arrival at the hospital, the patient is conscious and verbally abusive and has stable vital signs. While awaiting the results of laboratory tests, the patient gets up, sneaks out the back door, and leaves the emergency department unseen.

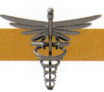

CASE PRESENTATION

Paramedics are called to meet the police at a local motel, where they have found an unconscious person in one of the motel suites. On arrival, several police officers escort paramedics to the room, where they find a 42-year-old male lying supine on the bed. He appears to have been alone in the room, and there is an empty bottle of whiskey lying on the floor next to the bed.

Physical Examination

CNS:	The patient is unresponsive; his pupils are pinpoint and unresponsive to light
Resp:	Respirations are 4 per minute and shallow; lungs are clear bilaterally, with equal air entry; trachea is midline; no signs of trauma
CVS:	The carotid pulse is present but weak; the radial pulse is absent; skin is pale, cool, and dry, with dry mucous membranes
ABD:	Soft and nontender in all four quadrants; no signs of vomiting or diarrhea
Muscl/Skel:	No injuries are noted

Vital Signs

Pulse:	124/min
Resp:	4/min and shallow
BP:	70/40 mmHg
SpO$_2$:	80 percent

ECG:	Sinus tachycardia
Past Hx:	The police state that the patient had called his wife earlier in the evening and had threatened to kill himself. His wife then called the police, who managed to track the patient down to this motel. The patient's wife told the police that the patient had been suffering from depression for the past couple of months and had recently begun to drink heavily. The police found two empty pill bottles in the bathroom. One bottle contained amitriptyline (Elavil), and the other contained meperidine (Demerol). Both prescriptions had been filled recently.

Treatment

An OPA is inserted, and the patient's respirations are assisted by a bag-valve-mask device with 100 percent oxygen via a reservoir bag. The patient is placed on a cardiac monitor, which shows a sinus tachycardia with widened QRS complexes at 0.16 mm width. An intravenous line is initiated with a 16-gauge catheter, and a solution of normal saline is run wide open (20 mL/kg fluid bolus); 100 mEq sodium bicarbonate is administered along with 2 mg naloxone. The patient is prepared for transport to the hospital with the assistance of the police. Following the administration of the sodium bicarbonate, the QRS complexes eventually narrow to 0.12 mm. However, the patient's level of consciousness does not change. Once in the ambulance, the patient is intubated. The patient's condition remains unchanged during transport to the hospital. On arrival at the hospital, the patient is treated and then admitted to the ICU.

CHAPTER REVIEW

Summary

Paramedics must be diligent in the assessment and treatment of suspected overdose. Without a high index of suspicion, even the most obvious clues can go unnoticed. By reviewing the general principles of toxicology, the paramedic will be better prepared to treat these emergencies.

Key Words

carboxyhemoglobin   Hemoglobin complex formed when carbon monoxide binds to the iron structures of hemoglobin.

electron transport chain   Biochemical system in the mitochondria that extracts energy.

methemoglobin   Hemoglobin type where iron structure is altered and cannot transport oxygen.

neuroleptic malignant syndrome   A rare, but life-threatening, idiosyncratic reaction to a neuroleptic medication. The syndrome is characterized by fever, muscular rigidity, altered mental status, and autonomic dysfunction.

serotonin syndrome   Life-threatening condition caused by excessive amounts of the neurotransmitter serotonin.

sympathomimetic syndrome   Toxidrome caused by sympathomimetic medications that reflects excess sympathetic stimulation.

toxidrome   A syndrome caused by a dangerous level of toxins in the body.

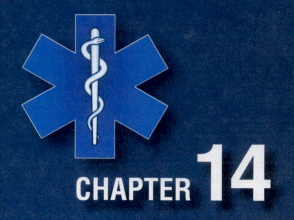

CHAPTER 14

MEDICATIONS USED IN THE TREATMENT OF BEHAVIORAL EMERGENCIES

OBJECTIVES

After completing this chapter, the reader should be able to:

- Define the term *behavioral emergency*.
- List the intrapsychic causes of altered behavior.
- Explain interpersonal and environmental causes of behavioral emergencies.
- Explain organic causes of behavioral emergencies.
- Explain the signs and symptoms of excited delirium.
- Describe the coordinated treatment of a patient with suspected excited delirium.
- Describe and list the indications, contraindications, and dosages for the following medications used in behavioral emergencies: haloperidol, chlorpromazine, ziprasidone, olanzapine, diazepam, lorazepam, midazolam, and hydroxyzine.

INTRODUCTION

Behavioral emergencies rarely require pharmacological intervention during the prehospital phase of emergency medical care. There are situations, however, in which emergency personnel may be called on to administer a sedative or similar agent. Among these are acute anxiety reactions and paranoid psychoses. Occasionally, it may be necessary to administer a sedative to friends or family of a patient who has been severely injured or who has recently died.

UNDERSTANDING BEHAVIORAL EMERGENCIES

A *behavioral emergency* is an intrapsychic, environmental, situational, or organic alteration that results in behavior that cannot be tolerated by the patient or other members of society. It usually requires immediate attention.

Intrapsychic Causes

Intrapsychic causes of altered behavior arise from problems within the person. Such behavior usually results from an acute stage of an underlying psychiatric condition. A wide range of behaviors can be manifested, including depression, withdrawal, catatonia, violence, suicidal acts, homicidal acts, paranoid reactions, phobias, hysterical conversion, disorientation, and disorganization. In the field, behavioral emergencies resulting from intrapsychic causes are less common than those resulting from other causes, such as alcohol or medication abuse.

Interpersonal and Environmental Causes

Interpersonal and **environmental causes** of behavioral emergencies result from reactions to stimuli outside the person. They often result from overwhelming and stressful incidents, such as the death of a loved one, rape, or a disaster. The change in behavior can frequently be linked to a specific incident or series of incidents. The range of behavior manifested is broad, and a patient's specific symptoms often relate to the type of incident that precipitated them.

Organic Causes

An **organic cause** of altered behavior results from a disturbance in the patient's physical or biochemical state. Such disturbances include medication or substance abuse, alcohol abuse, trauma, medical illness, and dementia. The area of the brain affected by the disturbance determines the type of behavior change. It is important to consider the possibility of organic disease in *all* behavioral emergencies. As a result, physical assessment of patients with aberrant behavior is extremely important. It may uncover unsuspected causes of the altered behavior, such as medication or alcohol abuse, hypoxia, hypoglycemia, head injury, or meningitis. Common agents used in the acute treatment of behavioral emergencies include haloperidol (Haldol), chlorpromazine (Thorazine, Largactil), ziprasidone (Geodon), olanzapine (Zyprexa, Zyprexa Zydis), diazepam (Valium), lorazepam (Ativan), midazolam (Versed), and hydroxyzine (Vistaril, Atarax).

Many cases of suspected behavioral problems have a metabolic and treatable cause. These include hypoxia, hypoglycemia, drug intoxication or overdose, stroke, brain injury, and dementia. It is important for EMS personnel to first consider possible medical causes for patients with a behavioral complaint before assuming the problem is of a psychiatric or behavioral origin.

Excited Delirium

It has been long recognized that certain patients die in the course of being restrained or arrested. Most of those who die are either psychotic from a mental illness or are intoxicated with drugs—usually stimulants. This condition has been defined and now called **excited delirium (ExDS)**. ExDS is characterized by the triad of delirium, psychomotor agitation, and physiological excitation. It was originally described in 1985 and initially found to result from cocaine intoxication and had four components: hyperthermia, delirium with agitation, respiratory arrest, and death. Patients with ExDS can display significant physical strength (similar to PCP intoxication) and can develop cardiopulmonary arrest. Risk factors for ExDS include: young age, males, obesity, and history of stimulant abuse—most commonly cocaine and amphetamines. However, all stimulants including MDMA (ecstasy) and LSD (acid) can cause the condition. Other conditions associated with ExDS include psychiatric illness, alcohol withdrawal, head trauma, or a combination of these. Initially considered somewhat controversial, ExDS was recently recognized as a new and novel disease by the *American College of Emergency Physicians (ACEP)*. Diagnosis should be considered in patients who exhibit the triad of delirium, psychomotor agitation, and physiological excitation. ExDS is most commonly seen in conjunction with abuse of stimulant drugs. It has been estimated that approximately 8-14% of people with ExDS die.

Prehospital care includes control of the airway and stabilization of cardiopulmonary status. Hyperthermia, the most life-threatening complication of ExDS, requires rapid intervention. While the exact physiologic cause of severe hyperthermia in stimulant abuse remains unclear, evidence points to an increase in the neurotransmitters norepinephrine, dopamine, and serotonin. These agents play an important role in controlling the hypothalamus—the major control center for body temperature. Prompt lowering of the body's core temperature is necessary to prevent permanent injury to the brain and other essential structures.

It has been proposed that many deaths that occur in ExDS are due to fatal arrhythmias. Also, profound acidosis is typically seen in these patients and may be one of the causes of the fatal arrhythmias described. In one study, five patients with excited delirium were found to have a pH that ranged from 6.25 to 6.81 (normal 7.35–7.45). Four of these patients subsequently died. An elevated serum lactate (the anion of lactic acid), which is associated with the lactic acidosis, is often seen in ExDS.

Generally the excited delirium symptoms are well underway when EMS and police arrive, although there are a few case reports of calm patients suddenly exploding into excited delirium.

In restraining the patient, you may find the patient has extraordinary strength and it will take a coordinated effort of several officers to control the patient. The major concern is that once the patient is controlled, there may be period of sudden tranquility, which is often the first sign of a respiratory arrest. When this occurs immediate attention must be placed on the adequacy of ventilations and the patient's cardiac rhythm. If hypoventilation or arrhythmia are observed the patient must be treated immediately.

The primary treatment of excited delirium involves control of the excitatory cascade through the use of sedatives such as diazepam (Valium), lorazepam (Ativan), or midazolam (Versed). Though many of these patients have been reported to develop profound metabolic acidosis, the routine or prophylactic use of sodium bicarbonate has not been adequately studied and is not recommended at this time. The focus of treatment is the chemical sedation of the patient and rapid transport to the hospital.

One important point of excited delirium is that the longer the patient remains in this state, the greater the chance of death. **Therefore it is very important that EMS and police work quickly to restrain and sedate the patient followed by rapid transport.**

There are some basic steps for EMS and police to follow in excited delirium incidents.

1. EMS and law enforcement will work in a coordinated approach.
2. EMS will be dispatched immediately in situations where law enforcement believes excited delirium is present.
3. The first arriving law enforcement officers will contain the patient in a safe area.
4. Once sufficient numbers of personnel are present (EMS/ law enforcement), the patient must then be controlled and restrained physically and chemically (as required) as soon as possible.
5. Law enforcement will determine the most appropriate method of controlling the patient by:
   a. Physical restraint
   b. Conducted energy weapon (TASER)
6. EMS and law enforcement will work to physically restrain the patient, ensuring that the patient is placed either supine or in the recovery position.
7. Once patient is restrained, EMS must immediately assess the patient for Airway, Breathing, and Circulation.
8. EMS may, as required, provide further patient care as required including the sedation of the patient using a benzodiazepine.
9. EMS will immediately transport the patient in the recovery position.

10. A law enforcement officer will accompany the patient to the hospital.
11. During transport, EMS will:
    a. Continually assess and monitor the patient.
    b. Continuously communicate with the patient.
    c. If the patient was TASERed, assure the patient that he or she was TASERed and not shot.
    d. Minimize the amount of time the patient stays on his/her stomach.
12. EMS will contact the receiving hospital with as much notice as possible.

℞ Haloperidol (Haldol)

Class Antipsychotic and neuroleptic

Description

Haloperidol is a frequently used major tranquilizer.

Mechanism of Action

Haloperidol is a major tranquilizer of the butyrophenone class that has proved effective in the management of acute psychotic episodes. It has pharmacological properties similar to those of the phenothiazine class of medications (e.g., chlorpromazine [Thorazine]). Haloperidol appears to block dopamine receptors in the brain associated with mood and behavior. However, its precise mechanism of action is not clearly understood. Haloperidol has weak anticholinergic properties.

Pharmacokinetics

Onset: 30–45 minutes

Peak Effects: 10–20 minutes

Duration: Varies

Half-Life: 3–35 hours

Indication

Haloperidol is used in acute psychotic episodes.

Contraindications

Haloperidol should not be administered in cases in which other medications, especially sedatives, may be present. It should not be used in the management of dysphoria caused by pentazocine (Talwin) because it may promote sedation and anesthesia.

Precautions

Haloperidol may impair mental and physical abilities. Occasionally, orthostatic hypotension may be seen in conjunction with haloperidol use. Caution should be used when administering haloperidol to patients taking anticoagulants. Extrapyramidal or dystonic reactions have been known to occur following the administration of haloperidol, especially in children. Diphenhydramine (Benadryl) should be readily available.

Although haloperidol has not received a "black box" warning from the FDA, paramedics should know that there have been reported adverse cardiovascular efforts, most notably several cases of prolonged QT/QTc and some cases of torsade de pointes. Most, but not all complications, were associated with much higher doses than those used in prehospital care.

Side Effects

Haloperidol can cause extrapyramidal symptoms (EPS), insomnia, restlessness, drowsiness, seizures, respiratory depression, dry mouth, constipation, hypotension, and tachycardia.

Interactions

Antihypertensive medications may increase the likelihood of a patient developing hypotension with haloperidol administration. Haloperidol should be used with caution in patients taking lithium, because irreversible brain damage (encephalopathic syndrome) has been reported when these two medications are used together.

Dosage

Doses of 2–5 mg administered intramuscularly are fairly standard in the management of an acute psychotic episode with severe symptoms.

℞ Droperidol (Inapsine)

Class Antiemetic and antipsychotic

Description

Droperidol is a butyrophenone derivative that is structurally and pharmacologically related to haloperidol.

Mechanism of Action

Droperidol antagonizes the emetic effects of morphine-like analgesics and other drugs that act on the chemoreceptor trigger zone (CTZ). Its mild alpha-adrenergic blocking properties and direct vasodilation effects may cause hypotension. It acts at the subcortical level to produce sedation and reduce anxiety and minor activities without necessarily inducing sleep.

Pharmacokinetics

Onset: 3–10 minutes

Peak Effects: 30 minutes

Duration: 2–4 hours

Half-Life: 2 hours

Indications

Droperidol is indicated in the treatment of nausea and vomiting in patients refractory to first-line antiemetics. It can be used to produce a tranquilizing effect and as an antipsychotic.

Contraindications

Droperidol is contraindicated in patients with a known hypersensitivity to the drug. Safe usage during pregnancy and in children less than 2 years of age has not been established.

Precautions

Droperidol has received a "black box" warning from the FDA because of reported adverse cardiovascular effects. Most notably, several cases of prolonged QT/QTc intervals and some cases of torsade de pointes have been associated with droperidol administration. Most, but not all complications, were associated with much higher doses than those used in prehospital care.

Droperidol should be used with caution in elderly, debilitated, and other poor-risk patients, including those with Parkinson's disease, hypotension, liver disease, kidney disease, and cardiac disease (including arrhythmias).

The dosage of droperidol should be decreased in patients who have received other central nervous system (CNS) depressants. Monitor the vital signs and ECG closely. Be aware of possible postural hypotension.

Side Effects

CNS side effects include drowsiness, extrapyramidal symptoms, dystonia, dizziness, restlessness, anxiety, hallucinations, and depression. Cardiovascular side effects reported include hypotension and tachycardia. Other reported side effects include chills, shivering, laryngospasm, and bronchospasm.

Interactions

None reported.

Dosage

Usual dose is 2.5 to 10.0 mg intravenously (IV) or intramuscular (IM).

℞ Chlorpromazine (Thorazine)

Class Antipsychotic and neuroleptic

Description

Chlorpromazine is an antipsychotic of the phenothiazine type and neuroleptic used in the management of severe psychotic episodes.

Mechanism of Action

Chlorpromazine is a member of the phenothiazine class of medications. Phenothiazine medications are thought to block dopamine receptors in the brain that are associated with behavior and mood. Chlorpromazine is also effective in the management of mild alcohol withdrawal and intractable hiccoughs. It is also effective in treating nausea and vomiting, although more appropriate agents are available.

Pharmacokinetics

Onset: 3–5 minutes
Peak Effects: 30–60 minutes
Duration: 4–6 hours
Half-Life: 6 hours

Indications

Chlorpromazine is used in acute psychotic episodes, intractable hiccoughs, and nausea and vomiting.

Contraindications

Chlorpromazine should not be administered to patients in comatose states or who have recently taken a large amount of sedatives. Chlorpromazine should not be administered to patients who may have recently taken hallucinogens because it tends to promote seizures.

Precautions

Chlorpromazine may impair mental and physical abilities. Occasionally, orthostatic hypotension may be seen in conjunction with chlorpromazine use. Extrapyramidal or dystonic reactions have been known to occur following the administration of chlorpromazine, especially in children. Diphenhydramine should be readily available.

Side Effects

Chlorpromazine can cause dry mouth, constipation, blurred vision, dry eyes, sedation, headache, drowsiness, hypotension, and tachycardia.

Interactions

Antihypertensive medications may increase the likelihood of a patient developing hypotension with chlorpromazine administration.

Dosage

The standard dose of chlorpromazine in the management of an acute psychotic episode is 25 to 50 mg administered intramuscularly. Intractable hiccoughs will usually respond to a 25 mg dose of chlorpromazine. Paramedics should only administer chlorpromazine intramuscularly.

℞ Ziprasidone (Geodon)

Class Antipsychotic

Description

Ziprasidone is an antipsychotic unrelated to the phenothiazines or butyrophenone classes of antipsychotics. It is a direct agonist/antagonist of the dopamine and serotonin receptors. It may also block the uptake of serotonin and norepinephrine.

Mechanism of Action

Ziprasidone's mechanism of action is unknown, but is probably related to inhibition of synaptic uptake of serotonin and norepinephrine.

Pharmacokinetics

Onset: 15–30 minutes (IM)
Peak Effects: 60 minutes (IM)
Duration: 4–8 hours (IM)
Half-Life: 2–5 hours (IM)

Indications

Acute psychosis and Tourette's syndrome.

Contraindications

Ziprasidone should not be used in patients with hypersensitivity to the medication. Ziprasidone does not appear to prolong the QT/QTc interval to the same degree as seen with the butyrophenones. However, it should be used with caution in patients with a prolonged QT/QTc or history of long QT syndrome.

Precautions

Use with caution in patients with history of seizures, stroke, Alzheimer's disease, or with known cardiovascular disease.

Side Effects

Side effects associated with ziprasidone include myalgias, somnolence, dizziness, tremor, dyskinesia, extrapyramidal effects (dystonia), tachycardia, postural hypotension, nausea, and dry mouth.

Interactions

Carbazepine (Tegretol) may decrease ziprasidone levels. Interactions may occur with antiarrhythmics, antidepressants, and ethanol.

Dosage

Ten mg every 2 hours or 20 mg every 4 hours IM up to a maximum dose of 40 mg. It can be given orally as well.

Rx Olanzapine (Zyprexa, Zyprexa Zydis)

Class Antipsychotic

Description

Olanzapine is a rapidly acting oral antipsychotic agent chemically related to clozapine. Zyprexa Zydis is a rapidly dissolving wafer that can be administered orally or placed in a drink.

Mechanism of Action

Olanzapine inhibits synaptic uptake of serotonin and norepinephrine, producing antipsychotic and anticholinergic effects.

Pharmacokinetics

Onset: < 30 minutes
Peak Effects: 6 hours
Duration: Varies
Half-Life: 21–54 hours

Indications

Acute psychosis and Alzheimer's disease.

Contraindications

Olanzapine should not be used in patients with hypersensitivity to the medication.

Precautions

Use with caution in patients with a history of cardiovascular disease or conditions that may predispose a patient to hypotension. Do not push orally disintegrating tablet through the blister-pack foil. Peel the foil back and remove the tablet.

Side Effects

Side effects associated with olanzapine include myalgias, somnolence, dizziness, tremor, tachycardia, postural hypotension, nausea, and dry mouth.

Interactions

Olanzapine may enhance the hypotensive effects of antihypertensives.

Dosage

Five to 15 mg PO (via rapidly dissolving tablet). May be placed in a drink. *Never place the tablet in the patient's mouth. Allow the patient to place it.* An IM dosage form (available in both a short- and long-acting preparation is available). Typical IM doses range from 2.5 to 30 mg.

℞ Diazepam (Valium)

Class Sedative, anticonvulsant, and antianxiety agent

Description

Diazepam is a benzodiazepine that is frequently used as a sedative, hypnotic, and anticonvulsant.

Mechanism of Action

Benzodiazepines bind to specific sites on gamma-aminobutyric acid (GABA) Type A receptors within the brain. GABA is the major inhibitory neurotransmitter of the central nervous system. Benzodiazepines have no direct effect on the GABA receptors, but do potentiate the effects of GABA within the brain. Increased GABA levels cause sedation. Through this mechanism, the benzodiazepines display their hypnotic, anxiolytic, and anticonvulsant effects. A broad range of side effects including compromised sedation, ataxia, amnesia, alcohol and barbiturate potentiation, tolerance development, and abuse potential, however, limits their usefulness.

Diazepam, one of the most frequently prescribed medications in the United States, is used in the management of anxiety and stress. It is effective in treating the tremors and anxiety associated with alcohol withdrawal. It is also an effective skeletal muscle relaxant, which makes it an effective adjunct in orthopedic injuries. It is a good premedication for minor operative procedures and cardioversion because it induces amnesia, which diminishes the patient's recall of such procedures. In emergency medicine, diazepam is principally used for its anticonvulsant properties. It suppresses the spread of seizure activity through the motor cortex of the brain. It does not appear to abolish the abnormal discharge focus, however.

Pharmacokinetics

Onset: 1–5 minutes (IV), 15–30 minutes (IM)

Peak Effects: 10 minutes (IV), 30–45 minutes (IM)

Duration: 15–60 minutes

Half-Life: 20–50 hours

Indications

Diazepam is used in acute anxiety states, as a premedication before cardioversion, as a skeletal muscle relaxant, in major motor seizures, and in status epilepticus.

Contraindications

Diazepam should not be administered to any patient with a history of hypersensitivity to the medication.

Precautions

Because diazepam is a relatively short-acting medication, seizure activity may recur. In such cases, an additional dose may be required. Flumazenil (Romazicon), a benzodiazepine antagonist, should be available to use as an antidote if required. Injectable diazepam can cause local venous irritation. To minimize irritation, it should only be injected into relatively large veins and should not be given faster than 1 mL/min.

Side Effects

Diazepam can cause hypotension, tachycardia, drowsiness, headache, amnesia, hallucinations, respiratory depression, blurred vision, nausea, and vomiting.

Interactions

Diazepam is incompatible with many medications. Whenever diazepam is given intravenously in conjunction with other medications, the IV line should be adequately flushed. The effects of diazepam can be additive when used in conjunction with other CNS depressants and alcohol.

Dosage

In acute anxiety reactions, the standard dosage is 2–5 mg administered intramuscularly or intravenously. To induce amnesia prior to cardioversion, a dosage of 5–15 mg of diazepam is given intravenously. Peak effects are seen in 5–10 minutes. Diazepam should be given intravenously by slow IV push. It can be injected intramuscularly, but absorption via this route is variable. When an IV line cannot be started, parenteral diazepam can be administered rectally with a similar onset of action. In the management of seizures, the usual dose of diazepam is 5–10 mg administered IV. In many instances it may be necessary to give diazepam directly into the vein, because the seizure activity will prevent the insertion of an indwelling catheter. When given directly into a vein, it is essential that a large vein, preferably in the antecubital fossa, be used.

℞ Lorazepam (Ativan)

Class Anticonvulsant, sedative, and hypnotic

Description

Lorazepam is a benzodiazepine that is used as an anticonvulsant, sedative, and hypnotic.

Mechanism of Action

Benzodiazepines bind to specific sites on GABA Type A receptors within the brain. GABA is the major inhibitory neurotransmitter of the central nervous system. Benzodiazepines have no direct effect on the GABA receptors, but do potentiate the effects of GABA within the brain. Increased GABA levels cause sedation. Through this mechanism, the benzodiazepines display their hypnotic, anxiolytic, and anticonvulsant effects. A broad range of side effects including compromised sedation, ataxia, amnesia, alcohol and barbiturate potentiation, tolerance development, and abuse potential, however, limits their usefulness.

Lorazepam is a benzodiazepine with a shorter half-life than that of diazepam. Its onset of action is approximately the same. It is used in the management of anxiety and stress. It is a good premedication for minor operative procedures and cardioversion because it induces amnesia, which diminishes the patient's recall of such procedures. Lorazepam is often used in pediatrics as an anticonvulsant because of its shorter half-life. Like diazepam, lorazepam suppresses the spread of seizure activity through the motor cortex of the brain. It does not appear to abolish the abnormal discharge focus.

Pharmacokinetics

Onset: 1–5 minutes (IV), 15–30 minutes (IM)
Peak Effects: 15–20 minutes (IV), 2 hours (IM)
Duration: 6–8 hours
Half-Life: 10–20 hours

Indications

Lorazepam is used in major motor seizures, in status epilepticus, as a premedication before cardioversion, and for acute anxiety states.

Contraindications

Lorazepam should not be administered to any patient with a history of hypersensitivity to the medication.

Precautions

Lorazepam should be diluted with normal saline or D_5W prior to intravenous administration. Because lorazepam is a relatively short-acting medication, seizure activity may recur. In such cases, an additional dose may be required. Flumazenil (Romazicon), a benzodiazepine antagonist, should be available to use as antidote if required.

Side Effects

Lorazepam can cause hypotension, drowsiness, headache, amnesia, respiratory depression, blurred vision, nausea, and vomiting.

Interactions

The effects of lorazepam can be additive when used in conjunction with other CNS depressants and alcohol.

Dosage

The usual dose of lorazepam is 0.5–2.0 mg when given intravenously. The dose can be increased to 1.0–4.0 mg when given intramuscularly.

℞ Midazolam (Versed)

Class Sedative and hypnotic

Description

Midazolam is a benzodiazepine with strong hypnotic and amnestic properties.

Mechanism of Action

Benzodiazepines bind to specific sites on GABA Type A receptors within the brain. GABA is the major inhibitory neurotransmitter of the central nervous system. Benzodiazepines have no direct effect on the GABA receptors, but do potentiate the effects of GABA within the brain. Increased GABA levels cause sedation. Through this mechanism, the benzodiazepines display their hypnotic, anxiolytic, and anti-convulsant effects. A broad range of side effects including compromised sedation, ataxia, amnesia, alcohol and barbiturate potentiation, tolerance development, and abuse potential, however, limits their usefulness.

Midazolam is a potent but short-acting benzodiazepine used widely in medicine as a sedative and hypnotic. It is three to four times more potent than diazepam.

Its onset of action is approximately 3–5 minutes when administered intravenously and 15 minutes when administered intramuscularly. Midazolam has impressive amnestic properties. Like other benzodiazepines, it has no effect on pain.

Pharmacokinetics

Onset: 3–5 minutes (IV), 15 minutes (IM)
Peak Effects: 20–60 minutes
Duration: < 2 hours (IV), 1–6 hours (IM)
Half-Life: 1–4 hours

Indications

Midazolam is used as a premedication before cardioversion and other painful procedures. It is also an effective anticonvulsant.

Contraindications

Midazolam should not be administered to any patient with a history of hypersensitivity to the medication. It should not be used in patients who have narrow-angle glaucoma. Midazolam should not be administered to patients in shock, with depressed vital signs, or who are in alcoholic coma.

Precautions

Emergency resuscitative equipment must be available prior to the administration of midazolam. Vital signs must be continuously monitored during and after medication administration. Midazolam has more potential than the other benzodiazepines to cause respiratory depression and respiratory arrest. Flumazenil (Romazicon), a benzodiazepine antagonist, should be available to use as an antidote if required.

Side Effects

Midazolam can cause laryngospasm, bronchospasm, dyspnea, respiratory depression and arrest, drowsiness, amnesia, altered mental status, bradycardia, tachycardia, premature ventricular contractions, and retching.

Interactions

The effects of midazolam can be accentuated by CNS depressants such as narcotics and alcohol.

Dosage

When used for sedation, midazolam must be administered cautiously, because the amount of medication required to achieve sedation varies from individual to individual. Typically, 1–2.5 mg are administered by slow IV injection. Usually, it is best to dilute midazolam with normal saline or D_5W prior to IV administration. Midazolam can be administered intramuscularly at a dose of 0.07–0.08 mg/kg (average adult dose of 5 mg). Recently, many centers have been administering midazolam intranasally or by mouth to sedate children prior to suturing of lacerations.

Hydroxyzine (Vistaril, Atarax)

Class Antianxiety agent and sedative

Description

Hydroxyzine is an antianxiety and sedative agent with sedative properties. It is a versatile medication used frequently in emergency medicine.

Mechanism of Action

Hydroxyzine is chemically unrelated to the phenothiazines. Because of its antihistamine properties, hydroxyzine has been shown to exert a calming effect during acute psychotic states. It is an effective antiemetic and muscle relaxant. When administered concurrently with many analgesics, it tends to potentiate their effects.

Pharmacokinetics

Onset: 15–30 minutes

Peak Effects: 1–2 hours

Duration: 4–6 hours

Half-Life: 20 hours

Indications

Hydroxyzine is used to potentiate the effects of narcotics and synthetic narcotics, for nausea and vomiting, and for anxiety reactions.

Contraindications

Hydroxyzine should not be administered to any patient with a history of hypersensitivity to the medication.

Precautions

Hydroxyzine is given by intramuscular injection only. When administered concomitantly with analgesics, the potentiating effects of hydroxyzine should be kept in mind, and the total analgesic dose should be adjusted accordingly.

Side Effects

Hydroxyzine can cause sedation, dizziness, headache, dry mouth, and seizures.

Interactions

The sedative effects of hydroxyzine can be potentiated by CNS depressants such as narcotics, other antihistamines, sedatives, hypnotics, and alcohol.

Dosage

The standard dosage of hydroxyzine in the management of an acute anxiety reaction is 50–100 mg administered intramuscularly. The standard antiemetic dose is 25–50 mg. Hydroxyzine should be administered by intramuscular injection. Localized burning is a common complaint following an injection of hydroxyzine.

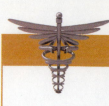

Early on a Saturday morning paramedics are dispatched to a local residence to aid a 40-year-old male patient who is acting violently toward his family members. On arrival paramedics are met by the patient's wife and son, who state they were having breakfast when the patient suddenly "snapped." They state that he keeps talking about how everyone is out to get him and that he seems to think that everyone is part of a conspiracy to "frame" him. His wife and son have tried unsuccessfully to calm him down, but he is getting more aggressive toward them with each attempt to talk to him. Just prior to the arrival of the ambulance, he punched his son and told him "they" would have to kill him before he would leave his house. The police are on the way to back the paramedics up. When the police arrive a few minutes later, paramedics approach the patient. He is standing in the kitchen yelling at everyone to get out before he "kills" them.

Physical Examination

Paramedics are unable to physically assess the patient at this time. A visual survey reveals the following:

CNS:	The patient is conscious, able to speak, and appears in good physical health
Resp:	His respirations are 28 per minute; no obvious signs of trauma
CVS:	His skin is flushed in color
ABD:	Unable to assess
Muscl/Skel:	No injuries noticed

Vital Signs

Paramedics are unable to assess the man's vital signs.

Past Hx:	Over the past couple of weeks, the patient has had several episodes in which he would start raving about being persecuted by everyone around him. Usually they would only last for several minutes and then he would return to normal without any memory of what had just occurred. This time it has been over 30 minutes. This is the worst episode yet and is the first time he has been physically violent toward his family.

Treatment

The paramedics realize that there are several factors to recognize here. First, the patient is 40 years old and appears to be in good physical health. An attempt to physically restrain him could be dangerous for both the patient and the ambulance crew. Second, there is a history of violence, although paramedics are unsure of the extent of that violence. Medical direction was contacted and gave an order for 5 mg of haloperidol (Haldol) and 2 mg of lorazepam (Ativan) mixed together in the same syringe and then given IM. Advice from the medical director was for the paramedics and police to restrain the patient long enough to give the Haldol-Ativan mixture and then release the patient and give the medication time to work. The patient was then to be brought to the hospital, with vital signs monitored en route.

A paramedic explained the situation to the police officers, and with a coordinated effort they were able to restrain the patient and give the medications. Ten minutes later the patient had calmed down significantly and was placed on the stretcher and restrained with straps as a precaution. An uneventful trip to the hospital followed. At the hospital he was admitted to the psychiatric service, where he was treated and then released several days later on medications to help prevent further outbursts.

CHAPTER REVIEW

Summary

It is important to consider and rule out physical causes for bizarre behavior before determining that a patient's disorder is of psychiatric origin. Diabetes, head injury, and alcohol intoxication can cause bizarre behavior easily mistaken for psychosis. The psychotic patient is best handled in an emergency department by personnel skilled in psychiatric intervention. However, some patients may require pharmacological intervention before transport is possible.

Key Words

environmental causes Change in behavior due to conditions in the patient's environment.

excited delirum Condition characterized by a sudden onset of bizarre and/or aggressive behavior, paranoia, panic, agitation, increased physical strength, and hyperthermia. Hyperthermia is often the primary cause of death in these cases.

interpersonal cause Change in behavior due to conditions related to other human beings.

intrapsychic causes Change in behavior due to conditions within one's self.

organic cause Change in behavior due to a structural or metabolic disease process.

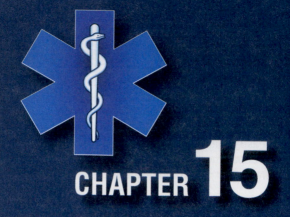

CHAPTER 15

MEDICATIONS USED IN THE TREATMENT OF GASTROINTESTINAL EMERGENCIES

OBJECTIVES

After completing this chapter, the reader should be able to:

- Define the term *antiemetic*.
- Describe and list the indications, contraindications, and dosages for promethazine, dimenhydrinate, prochlorperazine, metoclopramide, ondansetron, and dolasetron.

INTRODUCTION

Nausea and vomiting are common complaints in EMS. They can accompany other conditions or can occur without known cause. Medications used to treat nausea and vomiting are called *antiemetics*. In the past, medications in the phenothiazine class (e.g., promethazine) were commonly used. While effective, they had some untoward effects. Now, with the availability the serotonin antagonists (e.g., ondansetron), nausea and vomiting is much easier to treat and fewer side effects are encountered.

GASTROINTESTINAL MEDICATIONS

Although many medications are available for use in the treatment of gastrointestinal problems, such as peptic ulcers, constipation, diarrhea, emesis, and indigestion, only emesis is treated in prehospital care. These gastrointestinal medications used in prehospital care are *antiemetics*. They are effective in treating nausea and vomiting. Many of these medications are used concomitantly with narcotics, both to potentiate their effects and to reduce the likelihood of the side effects commonly associated with narcotic usage. Antiemetics commonly used in emergency medicine include promethazine (Phenergan), dimenhydrinate (Gravol, Dramamine), prochlorperazine (Compazine), metoclopramide (Reglan), odansetron (Zofran), dolasetron (Anzemet), and trimethobenzamide (Tigan).

The major antiemetics include antihistamines, phenothiazines, and serotonin receptor agonists. Antihistamine antiemetics are absorbed well from the gastrointestinal (GI) tract when administered orally.

Emesis is a complex process that involves various parts of the brain as well as receptors and other structures in the stomach and inner ear. The two involved parts of the brain are the vomiting center and the chemoreceptor trigger zone (CTZ)—both in the medulla. The vomiting center stimulates vomiting directly, while the CTZ does so indirectly.

The vomiting center is stimulated by activation of histamine receptors (specifically H_1 receptors) and acetylcholine (ACH) receptors via the pathway between it and the inner ear. Sensory input from the ears and nose (unpleasant or disturbing sights and smells) and from other parts of the brain in response to an anxiety or fear can stimulate the CTZ which, in turn, stimulates the vomiting center.

Antiemetics

Antiemetics are used in conjunction with chemotherapy, which may cause violent nausea and vomiting. Anitemetics are also indicated in the prophylactic treatment of motion sickness.

Multiple transmitters are involved in the vomiting reflex. They include serotonin, dopamine, acetylcholine, and histamine. Medications that interfere with any of these transmitters can decrease or prevent nausea and vomiting. This functional class includes several pharmacological subclasses: serotonin antagonists, dopamine antagonists, anticholinergics, and cannabinoids.

Serotonin Antagonists

The prototype serotonin antagonist is ondanestron (Zofran). It blocks the serotonin receptors in the CTZ, the stomach, and the small intestine. It is very effective in the treatment of nausea and vomiting associated with chemotherapy, and unlike the dopamine antagonists, it does not cause extrapyramidal effects like dystonia and ataxia. Its most common side effects are headache and diarrhea. Ondansetron is used in some prehospital services.

Dopamine Antagonists

Both phenothiazines and butyrophenones effectively block dopamine receptors in the CTZ. The phenothiazines include prochlorperazine (Compazine), while butyrophenones include haloperidol (Haldol) and droperidol (Inapsine). Agents from both classes cause side effects of extrapyramidal effects and sedation. Another dopamine antagonist, metoclopramide (Reglan) is neither a phenothiazine nor butyrophenone. It is unique in that it blocks both serotonin and dopamine receptors in the CTZ. It also has cholinomimetic effects.

Antihistamines

Antihistamines arrest the effects of histamine release by blocking its receptors. The different classes of antihistamines have the same actions, and they differ in the degree of sedation they cause and in their ability to block other nonhistamine receptors. Several antihistamines have significant anticholinergic properties making them an ideal choice to reduce motion sickness. Promethazine (Phenergan) and dimenhydrinate (Gravol, Dramamine) are occasionally used. These agents' primary side effects includes sedation, constipation, and the effects of muscarinic blockade such as dry mouth. Because they can thicken bronchial secretions, antihistamines should not be used in patients with asthma.

Cannabinoids

The cannabinoids are derivatives of tetrahydrocannabinol (THC) and are effective antiemetics used to treat chemotherapy-induced nausea and vomiting. THC (the active ingredient in marijuana) presents with side efects that include euphoria similar to that effected by marijuana. Although those effects may be desirable for some patients, they may be intensely unpleasant for others. Cannabinoids are not used in the prehospital treatment of nausea and vomiting; however, paramedics may treat patients who are on these medications.

℞ Ondansetron (Zofran)

Class Antiemetic

Description

Serotonin antagonist.

Mechanism of Action

Blocks the serotonin receptors in the CTZ, the stomach, and the small intestine.

Pharmacokinetics

Onset: 10–30 minutes
Peak Effects: 1.5 hours
Duration: 8 hours
Half-Life: 3 hours

Indications

Nausea and vomiting.

Contraindications

Known hypersensitivity to the medication.

Precautions

Patients taking other serotonin blockers.

Side Effects

Headache, lightheadedness, dizziness, tiredness, or constipation.

Interactions

Rifampin (reduces effects of ondansetron).

Dosage

4–8 mg.

Route

IV, PO.

Dolasetron (Anzemet)

Class Antiemetic

Description

Serotonin antagonist.

Mechanism of Action

Blocks the serotonin receptors in the CTZ, the stomach, and the small intestines.

Pharmacokinetics

Onset: 5–10 minutes
Peak Effects: 30–40 minutes
Duration: 8 hours
Half-Life: 7.3 hours

Indications

Nausea and vomiting.

Contraindications

Known hypersensitivity to the medication.

Precautions

Dolasetron can cause prolongation of the QT interval in the ECG. Patients taking other serotonin blockers.

Side Effects

Headache, lightheadedness, dizziness, and diarrhea.

Interactions

None.

Dosage

100 mg over 30 seconds.

Route

IV, PO

Class Antihistamine and antiemetic

Description

Promethazine is a phenothiazine derivative with potent antihistamine (H_1) properties and anticholinergic properties.

Mechanism of Action

Promethazine possesses sedative, antihistamine, antiemetic, and anticholinergic properties. It competitively blocks histamine receptors. The duration of action of promethazine is 4–6 hours. It is an effective and frequently used antiemetic. Promethazine, unlike hydroxyzine, can be given intravenously. It is often administered with analgesics, particularly narcotics, to potentiate their effect.

Pharmacokinetics

Onset: 5 minutes (intravenously [IV], 20 minutes intramuscularly [IM])
Peak Effects: Varies
Duration: 4–6 hours
Half-Life: 10–14 hours

Indications

Promethazine is used for nausea and vomiting, motion sickness, and sedation and to potentiate the effects of analgesics.

Contraindications

Promethazine is contraindicated in patients in comatose states and in those who have received a large amount of depressants. Also, it should not be administered to any patient with a history of hypersensitivity to the medication.

Precautions

Promethazine may impair mental and physical abilities. Care must be taken to avoid accidental intra-arterial injection, as gangrene can result. It should never be administered subcutaneously. Extrapyramidal symptoms (EPS) have been reported following promethazine use. Diphenhydramine (Benadryl) should be available.

Side Effects

Promethazine can cause drowsiness, sedation, blurred vision, tachycardia, bradycardia, and dizziness. Promethazine has been associated with tissue damage (gangrene) when it leaks from the vascular space (extravasates). It now carries a "Black Box" warning by the FDA and is rarely used in EMS and emergency medicine.

Interactions

The depressant effect on the central nervous system (CNS) of narcotics, sedatives or hypnotics, and alcohol is potentiated by promethazine. An increased incidence of EPS has been reported when promethazine is administered to patients taking monamine oxidase inhibitors (MAOIs).

Dosage

The standard dosage of promethazine in the management of nausea and vomiting is 12.5–25 mg administered either intravenously (IV) or intramuscularly (IM). The standard dosage in adjunctive use with analgesics is 25 mg. Promethazine should be given by IV or deep IM injection only. It is rarely used in emergency medicine.

℞ Dimenhydrinate (Gravol, Dramamine)

Class Antiemetic

Description

Dimenhydrinate belongs to the antihistamine class of medications, although it is not commonly used for this action. Its site and action are not precisely known.

Mechanism of Action

The mechanism of action of dimenhydrinate is not precisely known. There is evidence that it acts to depress hyperstimulated labyrinthine functions or associated neural pathways. It is an effective and frequently used antiemetic in Canada. It is often used with analgesics, particularly narcotics. Dimenhydrinate is a combination of two drugs, diphenhydramine and 8-chlorotheophylline. The chlorotheophylline is a salt of theophylline and the belief was that the stimulant properties of the theophylline would offset the sedative properties of the diphenhydramine. The antiemetic properties of the drug are related to the diphenhydramine.

Pharmacokinetics

Onset: Immediate (IV), 20–30 minutes (IM)
Peak Effects: Varies
Duration: 3–6 hours
Half-Life: Unknown

Indications

Dimenhydrinate is used for the prevention or relief of nausea and vomiting, motion sickness, and medication-induced nausea and vomiting (particularly narcotics).

Contraindications

There are no significant contraindications in the emergency setting.

Precautions

Dimenhydrinate should be used with caution in patients with seizure disorders and asthma. Those who are administered the medication should be cautioned against operating motor vehicles or dangerous machinery because of drowsiness associated with the medication.

Side Effects

Dimenhydrinate can cause drowsiness, dizziness, blurred vision, dry mouth, dry nose and bronchi, and tinnitus.

Interactions

The CNS-depressant effect of narcotics, sedatives or hypnotics, and alcohol is potentiated by dimenhydrinate.

Dosage

The standard dose of dimenhydrinate in the management of nausea and vomiting is 12.5–50 mg (diluted with 10 mL normal saline IV over 2 minutes) or 50–100 mg IM or by mouth. This dose can be repeated every 4 hours as needed.

℞ Prochlorperazine (Compazine)

Class Antiemetic

Description

Prochlorperazine is a phenothiazine derivative. It is highly effective in the treatment of severe nausea and vomiting.

Mechanism of Action

Prochlorperazine is an effective and frequently used antiemetic. It does not prevent vertigo and motion sickness, as do many of the other phenothiazines. Prochlorperazine blocks dopaminergic receptors in the brain. It also has weak anticholinergic properties.

Pharmacokinetics

Onset: 10–20 minutes
Peak Effects: Varies
Duration: 4–12 hours
Half-Life: 24–48 hours

Indications

Prochlorperazine is used in severe nausea and vomiting and acute psychosis.

Contraindications

Prochlorperazine should not be used in patients with a history of hypersensitivity to the medication or the phenothiazine class of medications. It should not be administered to comatose patients or those who have received large amounts of CNS depressants.

Precautions

Prochlorperazine may impair mental and physical abilities. It should never be administered subcutaneously because of local tissue irritation. The incidence of EPS appears to be higher with prochlorperazine than with many of the other phenothiazines. Diphenhydramine (Benadryl) should be available.

Side Effects

Prochlorperazine can cause drowsiness, sedation, blurred vision, tachycardia, bradycardia, dizziness, and hypotension.

Interactions

The CNS-depressant effect of narcotics, sedatives or hypnotics, and alcohol is potentiated by prochlorperazine.

Dosage

The standard dose of prochlorperazine is 5–10 mg administered intramuscularly or intravenously. The intravenous route is preferred with severe nausea and vomiting because the onset of action is much more rapid. Often, 10 mg of prochlorperazine is placed into 1 L of normal saline or lactated Ringer's solution and administered. It can be given orally or rectally.

℞ Metoclopramide (Reglan)

Class Antiemetic

Description

Metoclopramide is a medication used in the treatment of gastroesophageal reflux and nausea and vomiting.

Mechanism of Action

Metoclopramide is an effective antiemetic. It stimulates motility of the upper gastrointestinal tract and promotes emptying of the stomach. It increases the tone of the valve between the esophagus and the stomach (lower esophageal sphincter), which reduces reflux of stomach contents into the distal esophagus. Metoclopramide's antiemetic effects appear to result from its blockade of central and peripheral dopamine receptors.

Pharmacokinetics

Onset: 1–3 minutes (IV), 10–15 minutes (IM)

Peak Effects: 1–2 hours

Duration: 1–3 hours

Half-Life: 2.5–6.0 hours

Indications

Metoclopramide is used in severe nausea and vomiting and gastroesophageal reflux.

Contraindications

Metoclopramide should not be used in patients with possible gastrointestinal hemorrhage, bowel obstruction, or perforation. It is also contraindicated in patients with a history of hypersensitivity to the medication.

Precautions

Metoclopramide may impair mental and physical abilities. Mental depression has occurred in patients with and without a prior history of depression following metoclopramide therapy. EPS can occur following metoclopramide administration. Diphenhydramine (Benadryl) should be available.

Side Effects

Metoclopramide can cause drowsiness, fatigue, sedation, dizziness, mental depression, hypertension, hypotension, tachycardia, bradycardia, and diarrhea.

Interactions

The effects of metoclopramide on gastric motility can be antagonized by anticholinergic medications such as atropine. The CNS-depressant effect of narcotics, sedatives or hypnotics, and alcohol can be potentiated by metoclopramide. Hypertension can result when metoclopramide is administered to patients receiving MAOIs (as a part of the serotonin syndrome).

Dosage

The standard dose of metoclopramide is 10–20 mg administered intramuscularly. Metoclopramide can be administered intravenously for severe or intractable nausea and vomiting. The standard intravenous dose is 10 mg administered by slow IV push over 1–2 minutes. Alternatively, 10 mg of metoclopramide can be diluted in 50 mL of normal saline and administered over 15 minutes. The intravenous route is preferred in severe nausea and vomiting because the onset of action is much more rapid.

CHAPTER REVIEW

Summary

Medications are rarely required in the prehospital management of gastrointestinal emergencies. However, many emergency medical services (EMS) systems utilize antiemetics for severe or intractable nausea and vomiting. Prehospital administration of antiemetics decreases the potential for dehydration, improves patient comfort, and reduces exposure of EMS personnel to body fluids. The antiemetics are often used to potentiate the effects of the narcotics. Paramedics are encouraged to be familiar with the antiemetics used in their system.

OBJECTIVES

After completing this chapter, the reader should be able to:

- Discuss the history of pain management in prehospital care.
- Explain the characteristics of the ideal analgesic agent for prehospital care.
- Define the terms *analgesic* and *narcotic*.
- Describe the analgesics available for use in prehospital care.
- Describe and list the indications, contraindications, and dosages for the following medications used in pain management: morphine sulfate, meperidine, fentanyl citrate, nitrous oxide, nalbuphine, butorphanol tartrate, ibuprofen, acetaminophen, and ketorolac.
- Discuss the role of sedatives in prehospital care and give examples of each.
- Describe and list the indications, contraindications, and dosages for the following medications used as neuromuscular-blocking agents: succinylcholine, pancuronium, vecuronium, atricurium, and rocuronium.
- Discuss the role of induction agents in rapid-sequence induction and detail the pharmacology of diazepam, midazolam, ketamine, propofol, and etomidate.
- List the steps in performing rapid-sequence induction (RSI) intubation.
- List the steps in performing pharmacologically-assisted intubation (PAI).

INTRODUCTION

The primary reason people summon an ambulance or present at a hospital emergency department is because of pain. While the patient may not understand the actual cause of the pain, it is the patient's primary concern. The treatment of pain is a primary role of medicine and has roots in ancient medical practice. Pain is an unpleasant sensory and emotional experience associated with actual or perceived tissue or cellular damage. It is among these primitive biological reflexes. The process of alleviating pain is termed *analgesia*. This can be accomplished by medications, physical treatments, and psychological and emotional care. In the emergency setting, medications and physical modalities (e.g., ice, splinting, elevation, immobilization) are the most commonly used although empathy and emotional support play an important role. The provision of analgesia in the prehospital setting is an important aspect of emergency care.

In addition to analgesia, *sedation* has become an important part of emergency care. Sedation is the depression of patients' awareness of their environment and a reduction in their responsiveness to external stimulation. Sedation is generally defined as minimal, moderate, or deep. Levels beyond deep sedation actually fall into the realm of general anesthesia. *Minimal sedation* is primarily designed to relieve anxiety (anxiolysis). Certain medications (anxiolytics) can provide relief for anxiety and allay apprehension without significantly affecting the patient's mental status. *Moderate sedation*, on the other hand, is an actual depression in the patient's level of consciousness, but it does leave the patient able to respond to verbal or tactile stimuli. Generally speaking, with moderate sedation, protective airway reflexes and respiratory and cardiovascular functions are maintained. *Deep sedation* results in depression in the patient's level of consciousness to the point where he or she cannot be aroused. However, the patient can respond to repeated or painful stimuli. With deep sedation the patient may not be able to maintain his or her airway or ventilation. Cardiovascular function is preserved.

In this chapter we will discuss medications used in emergency care for analgesia and sedation. In addition, we will discuss the use of drugs called neuromuscular blockers that cause muscle paralysis allowing airway management and mechanical ventilation.

ANALGESICS

Medications that have proved to be effective in alleviating pain are referred to as **analgesics.** Although they may be administered in many different types of emergencies, they are usually reserved for the treatment of emergencies involving the cardiovascular system and in trauma.

Analgesics used in prehospital care include the following:

- Morphine sulfate
- Hydromorphone (Dilaudid)
- Meperidine (Demerol)
- Fentanyl citrate (Sublimaze)
- Nitrous oxide (Nitronox, Entonox)
- Nalbuphine (Nubain)
- Butorphanol tartrate (Stadol)
- Ketorolac (Toradol)
- Acetaminophen (Tylenol)
- Ibuprofen (Motrin, Advil)

Morphine is derived from the opium plant. It has impressive analgesic effects. Drugs that chemically resemble morphine or that have similar effects are called opiates. The opiates hydromorphone, fentanyl, and meperidine, although similar to morphine in their analgesic effects, are different chemically and are synthetically derived. Opiates interact with opiate receptors located throughout the body. The major opiate receptors are detailed in Table 16–1.

Nalbuphine (Nubain) and butorphanol (Stadol) are synthetic analgesics (opiate-like) with agonist and antagonist properties. This combination reportedly decreases the potential for abuse. Like the opiates, they act to a limited degree on opiate receptors. However, medications in this class have proven less effective than once thought and are rarely used.

TABLE 16–1

Opiate Receptors

Receptors	Location	Effects
Mu (μ)	Brain Spinal Cord GI Tract	μ_1: Supraspinal analgesia Physical dependence μ_2: Respiratory depression Euphoria Miosis Reduced GI motility Physical dependence μ_3: Unknown
Delta (δ)	Brain	Analgesia Antidepressant effects Physical dependence
Kappa (κ)	Brain Spinal Cord	Spinal analgesia Sedation Miosis Dysphoria
Nociceptin	Brain Spinal Cord	Anxiety Depression

TABLE 16–2

Opiate Conversion Chart (Note—These conversion rates are an estimate and should not be considered exact).

Medication	Route	Equianalgesic Dose (mg)
Morphine	IM	10
Hydromorphone	IM	1
Meperidine	IM	75
Fentanyl	IV	0.1 (1 mg = 100 mg morphine)
Nalbuphine	IM	12
Butorphanol	IM	1.5–2.5

Another class of analgesics is the nonsteroidal anti-inflammatory drugs (NSAIDs). Aspirin (discussed in Chapter 7) is the prototypical NSAID. NSAIDs inhibit the enzyme known as cyclooxygenase (COX). As COX levels increase, various mediators of pain and inflammation (e.g., prostaglandins, thromboxane) are increased (causing pain and inflammation). The inhibition of these substances helps to relieve pain and inflammation. Ibuprofen is a common analgesic with anti-inflammatory properties. Acetaminophen is a common analgesic with limited anti-inflammatory properties. Both ibuprofen and acetaminophen are effective in treating fever.

Ketorolac (Toradol) is the first injectable nonsteroidal anti-inflammatory agent. It is often used in emergency medicine as an analgesic because it does not affect the patient's mental status.

Analgesic agents vary in their potency, side effects, and ability to treat pain. Table 16–2 illustrates a relative comparison in potency between agents.

Class **Narcotic** analgesic (Schedule II medication)

Description

Morphine is a central nervous system (CNS) depressant and a potent analgesic. It is commonly used in EMS and emergency medicine. It is a Schedule II controlled substance.

Mechanism of Action

Morphine sulfate is a CNS depressant that acts predominantly on μ opiate receptors in the brain providing both analgesia and sedation. It increases peripheral venous capacitance and decreases venous return. Morphine also decreases myocardial oxygen demand. This action is due to both the decreased systemic vascular resistance and the sedative effects of the medication. Patient apprehension and fear can significantly increase myocardial oxygen demand and in some cases can conceivably increase the size of myocardial infarction.

Pharmacokinetics

Onset: Immediate (IV), 15–30 minutes (IM)
Peak Effects: 20 minutes (IV), 30–60 minutes (IM)
Duration: 2–7 hours
Half-Life: 1–7 hours

Indications

Morphine sulfate is used for severe pain.

Contraindications

Because of the hemodynamic effects described earlier, morphine should not be used in patients who are volume depleted or severely hypotensive. Morphine should not be administered to any patient with a history of hypersensitivity to the medication or to patients with undiagnosed head injury or abdominal pain.

Precautions

Morphine is a narcotic derivative of opium. It has a high tendency for addiction and abuse and is thus covered under the Controlled Substances Act of 1970. It is classified as a Schedule II medication. Consequently, special considerations are involved in the handling of the medication. Morphine causes respiratory depression in higher doses. This is especially true in patients who already have some form of respiratory impairment. The narcotic antagonist naloxone (Narcan) should be readily available whenever the medication is administered.

Side Effects

Morphine can cause nausea, vomiting, abdominal cramps, blurred vision, constricted pupils, altered mental status, headache, and respiratory depression.

Interactions

The CNS depression associated with morphine can be enhanced when administered with antihistamines, antiemetics, sedatives, hypnotics, barbiturates, and alcohol.

Dosage

There are many different approaches to the administration of morphine. An initial dose in the range of 2–10 mg administered intravenously is standard. This dose can be augmented with additional doses of 2 mg every few minutes and can be continued until the pain is relieved or until signs of respiratory depression occur.

Intramuscular injection usually requires 5–15 mg, based on the patient's weight, to attain desired effects. However, morphine is routinely given intravenously in emergency medicine and is often administered with an antiemetic agent such as ondansetron (Zofran). This may help prevent the nausea and vomiting that often accompany morphine administration.

℞ Hydromorphone (Dilaudid)

Class Narcotic analgesic (Schedule II medication)

Description

Hydromorphone (Dilaudid) is a central nervous system (CNS) depressant and a potent analgesic. It is a Schedule II controlled substance.

Mechanism of Action

Hydromorphone is a CNS depressant that acts predominantly on μ opiate receptors in the brain providing both analgesia and sedation.

Pharmacokinetics

Onset: 15–30 minutes (IV/IO)
Peak Effects: 30–90 minutes (IV/IO)
Duration: 4–5 hours
Half-Life: 2.6 hours

Indications

Hydromorphone is used for severe pain.

Contraindications

Hydromorphone should not be administered to any patient with a history of hypersensitivity to the medication or to patients with undiagnosed head injury or abdominal pain.

Precautions

Hydromorphone is a potent opiate. It has a high tendency for addiction and abuse and is thus covered under the Controlled Substances Act of 1970. It is classified as a Schedule II medication. Consequently, special considerations are involved in the handling of the medication. Hydromorphone causes respiratory depression in higher doses. This is especially true in patients who already have some form of respiratory impairment. The narcotic antagonist naloxone (Narcan) should be readily available whenever the medication is administered.

Side Effects

Hydromorphone can cause nausea, vomiting, abdominal cramps, blurred vision, constricted pupils, altered mental status, headache, and respiratory depression.

Interactions

The CNS depression associated with hydromorphone can be enhanced when administered with antihistamines, antiemetics, sedatives, hypnotics, barbiturates, and alcohol.

Dosage

1–2 mg IV. This dose can be augmented with additional doses as needed until the pain is relieved or until signs of respiratory depression occur.

Intramuscular injection usually requires 2–4 mg, based on the patient's weight, to attain desired effects. Hydromorphone is routinely given intravenously in emergency medicine and is often administered with an antiemetic agent such as ondansetron (Zofran). This may help prevent the nausea and vomiting that often accompany morphine administration.

℞ Meperidine (Demerol)

Class Narcotic analgesic (Schedule II medication)

Description

Meperidine is a CNS depressant and a potent analgesic. It is used extensively in medicine in the treatment of moderate to severe pain. It is less potent than morphine sulfate; 60–80 mg of meperidine are roughly equivalent in action to 10 mg of morphine. It is a Schedule II controlled substance.

Mechanism of Action

Meperidine is a CNS depressant that acts on μ and κ opiate receptors in the brain. It has more affinity for the κ receptors than morphine, thus causing more dysphoria. Because of this and other undesired side effects, it is rarely used in emergency medicine.

Pharmacokinetics

Onset: 5 minutes (IV), 10 minutes (IM)
Peak Effects: 1 hour
Duration: 2 hours (IV), 2–4 hours (IM)
Half-Life: 3–5 hours

Indication

Meperidine is used for moderate to severe pain.

Contraindications

Meperidine should not be administered to patients with known hypersensitivity to the medication. In addition, it should not be administered to patients with undiagnosed abdominal pain or head injury, or to patients who are receiving, or who have recently received, monoamine oxidase inhibitors (e.g., Nardil, Parnate, and Eutron). Therapeutic doses of meperidine have occasionally caused severe, and sometimes fatal, reactions in patients receiving these agents.

Precautions

Meperidine can cause respiratory depression. Naloxone (Narcan) should always be available to reverse the effects of the medication if respiratory depression ensues. Like morphine, meperidine should be kept in a secure, locked box. Use with caution in elderly patients and those with hepatic or renal failure.

Side Effects

Meperidine can cause nausea, vomiting, abdominal cramps, blurred vision, constricted pupils, altered mental status, hallucinations, headache, and respiratory depression.

Interactions

Meperidine should not be administered to patients who are receiving, or who have recently received, monoamine oxidase inhibitors (e.g., Nardil, Parnate, and Eutron). These agents are used for certain types of depression and behavioral disorders. Therapeutic doses of meperidine have occasionally caused severe, and sometimes fatal, reactions in patients receiving these agents.

Dosage

The usual dose used in the treatment of severe pain is 25–50 mg administered intravenously. When administered intramuscularly, 50–100 mg is a standard dose. Meperidine is often administered with an antiemetic agent such as ondansetron (Zofran). These agents help prevent the nausea and vomiting that often accompany meperidine administration. Meperidine can be administered either intravenously or intramuscularly.

℞ Fentanyl Citrate (Sublimaze)

Class Narcotic analgesic (Schedule II medication)

Description

Fentanyl, although chemically unrelated to morphine, produces pharmacological effects and a degree of analgesia similar to those of morphine. On a weight basis, however, fentanyl is 50 to 100 times more potent than morphine, but its duration of action is shorter than that of meperidine or morphine. A parenteral dose of 100 mcg of fentanyl is approximately equivalent in analgesic activity to 10 mg of morphine or 75 mg of meperidine. Fentanyl acts primarily on the μ opiate receptors in the brain.

Mechanism of Action

The principal actions of therapeutic value are analgesic and sedative. Fentanyl is a narcotic analgesic with a rapid onset and a short duration of action. Alterations in respiratory rate and alveolar ventilation, associated with narcotic analgesics, may last longer than the analgesic effect. Large doses may produce apnea. Fentanyl appears to have less emetic activity than other narcotic analgesics.

Pharmacokinetics

Onset: Immediate
Peak Effects: 3–5 minutes (IV)
Duration: 30–60 minutes
Half-Life: 6–8 hours

Indications

Fentanyl is used for maintenance of analgesia, as an adjunct in rapid-sequence induction intubation, and for severe pain.

Contraindications

Contraindications include severe hemorrhage, shock, and known hypersensitivity.

Precautions

Vital signs should be monitored routinely. Fentanyl may produce bradycardia, which may be treated with atropine. However, fentanyl should be used with caution in patients with cardiac bradyarrhythmias.

Fentanyl should be administered with caution to patients with liver and kidney dysfunction because of the importance of these organs in the metabolism and excretion of medications. As with other CNS depressants, patients who have received fentanyl should have appropriate surveillance. Resuscitation equipment and a narcotic agonist such as naloxone should be readily available to manage apnea.

Side Effects

As with other narcotic analgesics, the most common serious reactions reported to occur with fentanyl are respiratory depression, apnea, muscle rigidity, and brady-cardia. If these side effects remain untreated, respiratory arrest, circulatory depression, or cardiac arrest could occur.

Interactions

Other medications with a depressant effect on the CNS (e.g., barbiturates, tran-quilizers, narcotics, and general anesthetics) have an additive or potentiating effect with fentanyl. When patients have received such medications, the dose of fentanyl required is less than usual. Likewise, following the administration of fentanyl, the dose of other CNS-depressant medications should be reduced. Severe and unpre-dictable potentiation by monoamine oxidase inhibitors (MAOIs) has been reported with narcotic analgesics. Because the safety of fentanyl in this regard has not been established, its use in patients who have received MAOIs within 14 days is not recommended.

Dosage

Adult dosages are IV, 25–100 mcg (0.025–0.1 mg); direct IV, slowly over at least 1 minute, preferably over 2–3 minutes (not necessary to dilute—may be diluted to facilitate administration); and 100 mcg/2 mL diluted in 3 mL of normal saline for a concentration of 20 mcg/mL. Rapid IV administration can result in chest wall rigidity. This condition is rare and more common in infants and neonates.

Fentanyl can be administered intranasally via a mucosal atomization device (MAD). This allows the provision of effective analgesia without having to start an IV. Absorption of the drug through the nasal mucosa is predictable and safe. This route is particularly useful in children.

Pediatric dosages are 1.7–3.3 mcg/kg for children 2–12 years of age; the dosage should be reduced in very young, elderly, and high-risk patients.

℞ Nitrous Oxide (Nitronox, Entonox)

Class Analgesic and anesthetic gas

Description

Nitronox is a blended mixture of 50 percent nitrous and 50 percent oxygen that has potent analgesic effects.

Mechanism of Action

Nitrous oxide is a CNS depressant with analgesic properties. In the prehospital setting it is delivered in a fixed mixture of 50 percent nitrous oxide and 50 percent oxygen. When inhaled, it has potent analgesic effects. These quickly dissipate, however, within 2–5 minutes after cessation of administration. The Nitronox unit consists of one oxygen and one nitrous oxide cylinder. The gases are fed into a blender that combines them at the appropriate concentration. The mixture is then delivered to a modified demand valve for administration to the patient. Nitronox must be self-administered. It is effective in treating many varieties of pain encountered in the prehospital setting, including pain from many types of trauma. The high concentration of oxygen delivered along with the nitrous oxide will increase the oxygen tension in the blood, thus reducing hypoxia.

Pharmacokinetics

Onset: 2–5 minutes
Peak Effects: 2–5 minutes
Duration: 2–5 minutes
Half-Life: Unknown

Indications

Nitrous oxide is used for pain of musculoskeletal origin, particularly fractures; burns; suspected ischemic chest pain; and states of severe anxiety, including hyperventilation.

Contraindications

Nitronox should not be used in any patient who cannot comprehend verbal instructions or who is intoxicated with alcohol or other medications. It should not be administered to any patient with a head injury who exhibits an altered mental status. Nitronox should not be administered to any patient with chronic obstructive pulmonary disease (COPD) because the high concentration of oxygen (50 percent) might result in respiratory depression. Nitrous oxide tends to diffuse into closed spaces more readily than either carbon dioxide or oxygen. Many COPD patients have air-containing blebs in their lungs, and nitrous oxide can concentrate in these blebs, causing them to swell. Swollen blebs may rupture, causing a pneumothorax. Nitronox should not be administered to patients with a thoracic injury suspicious of pneumothorax, because the gas may accumulate in the pneumothorax, increasing its size. Also, patients with severe abdominal pain and distension suggestive of bowel obstruction should not receive Nitronox. Nitrous oxide can concentrate in pockets of an obstructed bowel, possibly leading to rupture.

Precautions

Nitronox should only be used in areas that are well ventilated. When the gas is used in the patient compartment of an ambulance, a scavenging system should be in place. Nitrous oxide exists in a liquid state inside the gas cylinder. Heat present in the air, in the cylinder wall, or in the various regulators and lines causes the liquid to vaporize. This vaporization process makes the cylinder tank and lines cool to touch. Following prolonged use, frost may develop on the cylinder, regulator, or lines. In very cold environments, generally less than 21°F (6°C), the liquid may be slow to vaporize, and administration may be impossible.

Side Effects

A nitrous oxide–oxygen mixture can cause dizziness, light-headedness, altered mental status, hallucinations, nausea, and vomiting.

Interactions

Nitrous oxide can potentiate the effects of other CNS depressants such as narcotics, sedatives, hypnotics, and alcohol.

Dosage

Nitronox should only be self-administered. Continuous administration may take place until the pain is significantly relieved or until the patient drops the mask. The patient care record should document the duration of medication administration.

℞ Nalbuphine (Nubain)

Class Synthetic analgesic

Description

Nalbuphine is a synthetic analgesic agent with potency equivalent to morphine on a milligram-to-milligram basis.

Mechanism of Action

Like the narcotics, nalbuphine is a centrally acting analgesic (agonist/antagonist) that binds to the opiate receptors in the central nervous system. Its onset of action is considerably faster than that of morphine, occurring within 2–3 minutes after intravenous administration. Its duration of effect is reported to be 3–6 hours. Although nalbuphine causes some respiratory depression in doses up to 10 mg, these effects do not seem to get worse in doses that exceed 10 mg. Naloxone (Narcan) is an effective antagonist and should be available when nalbuphine is administered.

In addition to its effects on opiate receptors, nalbuphine has antagonistic effects similar to those of naloxone. This feature minimizes the abuse potential of the medication and appears to lessen the chances of significant respiratory depression. At this time, nalbuphine is not regulated under the Controlled Substances Act of 1970. Current studies show that it has a minimal tendency for physical dependence and abuse (although some states have specific regulations regarding the drug). However, recent studies have shown nalbuphine to be somewhat unpredictable in terms of analgesia with many authorities discouraging its use in the prehospital setting.

Pharmacokinetics

Onset: 2–3 minutes (IV), 15 minutes (IM)
Peak Effects: 30 minutes
Duration: 3–6 hours
Half-Life: 5 hours

Indication

Nalbuphine is used for moderate to severe pain.

Contraindications

Nalbuphine should not be administered to patients with head injury or undiagnosed abdominal pain.

Precautions

The primary precaution in using nalbuphine is in patients with impaired respiratory function. Small doses of nalbuphine may cause significant respiratory depression. Naloxone should be readily available. Nalbuphine also has narcotic antagonistic properties. Thus, it should be administered with caution to patients dependent on narcotics, because it may cause withdrawal effects. The dosage of nalbuphine should be reduced in older patients because the effects are less predictable in this age group. Small repeated boluses are often safer than a single large dose.

Side Effects

Nalbuphine can cause headache, altered mental status, hypotension, bradycardia, blurred vision, rash, respiratory depression, nausea, and vomiting.

Interactions

Nalbuphine can potentiate the CNS depression associated with narcotics, sedatives, hypnotics, and alcohol. Because of its antagonistic properties, nalbuphine can cause withdrawal symptoms in patients addicted to narcotics. Nalbuphine can interfere with certain types of anesthesia because of its antagonistic properties.

Dosage

The general regimen for nalbuphine administration is 5 mg intravenously initially. This dose may be augmented with additional 2 mg doses if necessary. Nalbuphine can be administered intravenously or intramuscularly.

℞ Butorphanol Tartrate (Stadol)

Class Synthetic analgesic (Class IV medication)

Description

Butorphanol is a synthetic analgesic with analgesic and antagonistic properties. It is quite potent; the analgesic effects of 2 mg of butorphanol are roughly equivalent to 10 mg of morphine.

Mechanism of Action

Butorphanol is a centrally acting analgesic that binds to the opiate receptors in the central nervous system, causing CNS depression and analgesia. Like nalbuphine, it has some antagonistic (naloxone-like) properties. Although butorphanol can cause respiratory depression, this effect usually plateaus following administration of approximately 4 mg. Currently, butorphanol is not restricted under the 1970 act although some states have restrictions on the drug.

Pharmacokinetics

Onset: 10–15 minutes (IM), 2–3 minutes (IV)
Peak Effects: 0.5–1.0 hour (IM), 4–5 minutes (IV)
Duration: 3–4 hours
Half-Life: 3–4 hours

Indication

Butorphanol is used for moderate to severe pain.

Contraindications

Butorphanol should not be administered to any patient with a history of hypersensitivity to the medication. Also, it should not be given to patients dependent on narcotics because it may cause some reversal of the narcotic effects. It should not be administered to patients with head injury or undiagnosed abdominal pain.

Precautions

If butorphanol causes marked respiratory depression, then Narcan can be administered to reverse its effects. When administering any potent analgesic, it is possible to mask other signs and symptoms. All analgesics should be administered only after a thorough physical examination. Butorphanol should not be administered to any patient with head injury because it may cause an increase in cerebrospinal pressure. The dosage of butorphanol should be reduced in older patients because the effects are less predictable in this age group. Small repeated boluses are often safer than a single large dose.

Side Effects

Butorphanol can cause headache, altered mental status, hypotension, bradycardia, blurred vision, rash, respiratory depression, nausea, and vomiting.

Interactions

Like nalbuphine, butorphanol has some narcotic antagonistic properties. Caution should be used when administering butorphanol to patients already dependent on narcotics because it may precipitate withdrawal.

Dosage

The standard dose of butorphanol is 1 mg administered intravenously every 3 to 4 hours. When given intramuscularly, the standard dose is 2 mg. Butorphanol should only be administered intravenously or intramuscularly.

℞ Ketorolac (Toradol)

Class Nonsteroidal anti-inflammatory agent

Description

Ketorolac is the first injectable nonsteroidal anti-inflammatory medication to become available in the United States. It is useful in treating mild to moderate pain.

Mechanism of Action

Ketorolac is a nonsteroidal anti-inflammatory medication (NSAID). It has analgesic, anti-inflammatory, and antipyretic effects. Unlike narcotics, which act on the central nervous system, ketorolac is considered a peripherally acting analgesic. Consequently, it does not have the sedative properties of the narcotics. Ketorolac has been used concomitantly with morphine and meperidine without adverse effects. In dental studies, ketorolac was found to be quite effective as an analgesic.

Pharmacokinetics

Onset: 30 minutes
Peak Effects: 45–60 minutes
Duration: Varies
Half-Life: 4–6 hours

Indication

Ketorolac is used for mild to moderate pain.

Contraindications

Ketorolac should not be used in patients with a known hypersensitivity to the medication. It should not be administered to patients who report allergies to aspirin or NSAIDs, or to patients currently taking aspirin or NSAIDs.

Precautions

Gastrointestinal (GI) irritation and hemorrhage can result from therapy with NSAIDs. Long-term usage increases the incidence of serious GI side effects. Ketorolac is cleared through the kidneys. Long-term usage can result in renal impairment. Use with caution in patients with renal insufficiency.

Side Effects

Ketorolac can cause edema, hypertension, rash, itching, nausea, heartburn, constipation, diarrhea, gastrointestinal hemorrhage, drowsiness, and dizziness.

Interactions

Ketorolac, when administered with other NSAIDs (including aspirin), can worsen the side effects associated with the use of medications in this class. Intramuscular ketorolac has been found to reduce the diuretic response to furosemide (Lasix).

Dosage

The typical dose of ketorolac is 30–60 mg administered intramuscularly. Half the original dose can be repeated every 6 hours. The typical intravenous dose is 30 mg. The dosage should be halved in elderly patients.

℞ Ibuprofen (Motrin, Advil)

Class Nonsteroidal anti-inflammatory agent

Description

Ibuprofen (Motrin, Advil) is among the most used pain and anti-inflammatory medication in the world. It is useful in treating mild to moderate pain. It is also effective in the treatment of fever.

Mechanism of Action

Ibuprofen is a nonsteroidal anti-inflammatory medication (NSAID). It has analgesic, anti-inflammatory, and antipyretic effects. Unlike narcotics, which act on the central nervous system, ibuprofen is considered a peripherally acting analgesic. Consequently, it does not have the sedative properties of the narcotics.

Pharmacokinetics

Onset: 30–60 minutes
Peak Effects: 1–2 hours
Duration: 6–8 hours
Half-Life: 2–4 hours

Indication

Ibuprofen is used for mild to moderate pain.

Contraindications

Ibuprofen should not be used in patients with a known hypersensitivity to the medication. It should not be administered to patients who report allergies to aspirin or NSAIDs, or to patients currently taking aspirin or other NSAIDs.

Precautions

Gastrointestinal (GI) irritation and hemorrhage can result from therapy with NSAIDs. Long-term usage increases the incidence of serious GI side effects. Ibuprofen is cleared through the kidneys. Long-term usage can result in renal impairment.

Side Effects

Ibuprofen can cause edema, hypertension, rash, itching, nausea, heartburn, constipation, diarrhea, drowsiness, and dizziness.

Interactions

Ibuprofen, when administered with other NSAIDs (including aspirin), can worsen the side effects associated with the use of medications in this class.

Dosage

The typical dose of ibuprofen 200–800 mg orally. Typical dosing schemes range from 200 to 400 mg every 6 hours or 200–800 milligrams every 8 hours.

℞ Acetaminophen, Paracetamol (Tylenol)

Class Aniline analgesic and antipyretic

Description

Acetaminophen (Tylenol). It is useful in treating mild to moderate pain.

Mechanism of Action

Acetaminophen is the most widely used analgesic in the United States. Like aspirin, it appears to inhibit the enzyme cyclooxygenase. While it has analgesic and antipyretic properties similar to the NSAIDs, it has little anti-inflammatory properties. It does not have the platelet aggregation inhibition properties of aspirin.

Pharmacokinetics

Onset: 15–30 minutes
Peak Effects: 30–120 minutes
Duration: 3–4 hours
Half-Life: 1–3 hours

Indication

Acetaminophen is used for mild to moderate pain and the treatment of fever.

Contraindications

Acetaminophen is contraindicated in those with a known hypersensitivity to the drug. It should be avoided in patients with liver disease.

Precautions

Acetaminophen is metabolized by the liver and overdoses can be toxic for the liver. In fact, it is the most common cause of acute liver failure.

Side Effects

Minimal within recommended dosage range.

Interactions

Chronic alcohol can increase the hepatotoxicity of acetaminophen.

Dosage

325–650 mg PO every 4–6 hours (up to 1 gram PO is occasionally used as an antipyretic).

℞ Sedatives

Sedatives are medications used to treat anxiety, ease agitation, and promote sleep. They modulate central nervous system neurotransmitters and can affect the patient's level of consciousness. There are three major classes of sedatives:

- *Benzodiazepines.* Examples of benzodiazepines include diazepam, miazolam, lorazepam, and others.
- *Barbiturates.* Examples of barbiturates include amobarbital, thiopental sodium, and phenobarbital.
- *Other agents.* There are various types of sedatives used in emergency medicine that fall into unique classes. These include propofol, ketamine, and etomidate.

Sedatives can depress CNS control systems needed to maintain heart and lung function. Most sedatives also have addictive potential and should be used with caution and stored appropriately.

℞ Diazepam (Valium)

Class Anticonvulsant and sedative (Schedule IV medication)

Description

Diazepam is a benzodiazepine that is frequently used as an anticonvulsant, sedative, and hypnotic.

Mechanism of Action

Benzodiazepines bind to specific sites on gamma-aminobutyric acid (GABA) Type A receptors within the brain. GABA is the major inhibitory neurotransmitter of the central nervous system. Benzodiazepines have no direct effect on the GABA receptors, but do potentiate the effects of GABA within the brain. Increased GABA levels cause sedation. Through this mechanism, the benzodiazepines display their hypnotic, anxiolytic, and anticonvulsant effects. Their usefulness, however, is limited by a broad range of side effects including sedation, ataxia, amnesia, alcohol and barbiturate potentiation, tolerance development, and abuse potential.

In emergency medicine, diazepam is principally used for its anticonvulsant properties and as a sedative. It suppresses the spread of seizure activity through the motor cortex of the brain. It does not appear to abolish the abnormal discharge focus, however. Diazepam, one of the most frequently prescribed medications in the United States, is used in the management of anxiety and stress. It is effective in treating the tremors and anxiety associated with alcohol withdrawal. It is also an effective skeletal muscle relaxant, which makes it an effective adjunct in orthopedic injuries. It is a good premedication for minor operative procedures and cardioversion because it induces amnesia, which dimishes the patient's recall of such procedures.

Pharmacokinetics

Onset: 1–5 minutes (IV), 15–30 minutes (IM)

Peak Effects: 15 minutes (IV), 30–45 minutes (IM)

Duration: 15–60 minutes

Half-Life: 20–50 hours

Indications

Diazepam is used in major motor seizures, status epilepticus, as a sedative prior to painful procedures, as a skeletal muscle relaxant, and in acute anxiety states.

Contraindications

Diazepam should not be administered to any patient with a history of hypersensitivity to the medication.

Precautions

Because diazepam is a relatively short-acting medication, seizure activity may recur. In such cases, an additional dose may be required. Flumazenil (Romazicon), a benzodiazepine antagonist, should be available to use as an antidote if required. Injectable diazepam can cause local venous irritation. To minimize irritation, it should only be injected into relatively large veins and should not be given faster than 1 mL/min.

Side Effects

Diazepam can cause hypotension, drowsiness, headache, amnesia, respiratory depression, blurred vision, nausea, and vomiting.

Interactions

Diazepam is incompatible with many medications. Whenever diazepam is given intravenously in conjunction with other medications, the IV line should be adequately flushed. The effects of diazepam can be cumulative when used in conjunction with other CNS depressants and alcohol.

Dosage

In the management of seizures, the usual dose of diazepam is 5–10 mg IV. In many instances it may be necessary to give diazepam directly into the vein, because the seizure activity will prevent the insertion of an indwelling catheter. When given directly into a vein, it is essential that a large vein, preferably in the antecubital fossa, be used. In acute anxiety reactions, the standard dosage is 2–5 mg administered intramuscularly.

To induce amnesia prior to painful procedures, a dosage of 5–15 mg of diazepam is given intravenously. Peak effects are seen in 5–10 minutes. Diazepam should be given intravenously by slow IV push. It can be injected intramuscularly, but absorption via this route is variable. When an IV line cannot be started, parenteral diazepam can be administered rectally with a similar onset of action.

℞ Midazolam (Versed)

Class Sedative and hypnotic (Schedule IV medication)

Description

Midazolam is a benzodiazepine with strong hypnotic and amnestic properties.

Mechanism of Action

Benzodiazepines bind to specific sites on GABA Type A receptors within the brain. GABA is the major inhibitory neurotransmitter of the central nervous system. Benzodiazepines have no direct effect on the GABA receptors, but do potentiate the effects of GABA within the brain. Increased GABA levels cause sedation. Through this mechanism, the benzodiazepines display their hypnotic, anxiolytic, and anticonvulsant effects. Their usefulness, however, is limited by a broad range of side effects including sedation, ataxia, amnesia, alcohol and barbiturate potentiation, tolerance development, and abuse potential.

Midazolam is a potent but short-acting benzodiazepine used widely in medicine as a sedative and hypnotic. It is three to four times more potent than diazepam. Its onset of action is approximately 1.5 minutes when administered intravenously and 15 minutes when administered intramuscularly. Midazolam has impressive amnestic properties. Like the other benzodiazepines, it has no effect on pain.

Pharmacokinetics

Onset: 1.5 minutes (IV), 15 minutes (IM)

Peak Effects: 20–60 minutes

Duration: < 2 hours (IV), 1–6 hours (IM)

Half-Life: 1–4 hours

Indication

Midazolam is used as a premedication before painful procedures and as a sedative.

Contraindications

Midazolam should not be administered to any patient with a history of hypersensitivity to the medication. It should not be used in patients who have narrow-angle glaucoma. Midazolam should not be administered to patients in shock with depressed vital signs or who are in alcoholic coma.

Precautions

Emergency resuscitative equipment must be available prior to the administration of midazolam. Vital signs must be continuously monitored during and after medication administration. Midazolam has more potential than the other benzodiazepines to cause respiratory depression and respiratory arrest. Flumazenil (Romazicon), a benzodiazepine antagonist, should be available to use as an antidote if required.

Side Effects

Midazolam can cause laryngospasm, bronchospasm, dyspnea, respiratory depression and arrest, drowsiness, amnesia, altered mental status, bradycardia, tachycardia, premature ventricular contractions, and retching.

Interactions

The effects of midazolam can be accentuated by CNS depressants such as narcotics and alcohol.

Dosage

When used for sedation, midazolam must be administered cautiously, because the amount of medication required to achieve sedation varies from individual to individual. Typically, 1–2.5 mg are administered by slow IV injection. Usually, it is best to dilute midazolam with normal saline or D_5W prior to IV administration. Midazolam can be administered intramuscularly at a dose of 0.07–0.08 mg/kg (average adult dose of 5 mg). Recently, many centers have been administering midazolam intranasally or by mouth to sedate children prior to suturing of lacerations.

℞ Ketamine (Ketalar)

Class Anesthetic agents and analgesic agent

Description

Ketamine is a phencyclidine derivative that is unique among sedative, hypnotic, and analgesic agents. It s a dissociative agent for rapid sequence induction/intubation and for sedation. Ketamine has strong amnestic properties.

Mechanism of Action

Ketamine is thought to cause a dissociation between the cortical and limbic system, resulting in a seemingly awake patient who is dissociated from the environment. It has powerful analgesic and sedative properties.

Pharmacokinetics

Onset: < 1 minute (IV), < 5 minutes (IM)
Peak Effects: Varies
Duration: 10–15 minutes (IV), 20–30 minutes (IM)
Half-Life: 1–2 hours

Indication

Ketamine is used as a sedative and induction agent for RSI (particularly in children).

Contraindications

Ketamine is contraindicated in those with a significant elevation in blood pressure and in those who have a hypersensitivity to the medication.

Precautions

Ketamine can cause hallucinations following waking (emergence hallucinations) that can be quite severe. The incidence of hallucinations is higher in adults than in children. Much of this can be avoided by keeping the environment quiet when the patient emerges from anesthesia. Ketamine is usually used with a low dose of a benzodiazepine such as lorazepam, diazepam, or midazolam. Resuscitation equipment must be immediately available. All monitors (ECG, SpO_2, $ETCO_2$) must be in place prior to administration. Monitor vital signs closely.

Side Effects

Side effects associated with ketamine include increased hallucinations, increased skeletal muscle tone, nausea, and vomiting. Protective airway reflexes may actually be enhanced with ketamine. Ketamine can cause excessive bronchial secretions.

Interactions

Recovery time may be prolonged if narcotics and barbiturates are also used.

Dosage

The usual dose is 0.5–1.0 mg/kg IV given over 30–60 seconds. For the IM route, 2–4 mg/kg may be used.

℞ Etomidate (Amidate)

Class Sedative and hypnotic

Description

Etomidate is an ultra-short-acting, nonbarbiturate, nonbenzodiazepine hypnotic. It does not have any analgesic properties. It is used as an induction agent for RSI. Of the sedatives used in RSI, etomidate has the best safety profile.

Mechanism of Action

Etomidate produces a rapid induction of anesthesia with minimal respiratory and cardiovascular effects. Unlike other types of sedative/hypnotics, etomidate does not cause histamine release.

Pharmacokinetics

Onset: 10–20 seconds

Peak Effects: < 1 minute

Duration: 3–5 minutes

Half-Life: 30–70 minutes

Indication

Etomidate is used as an induction agent for rapid-sequence induction/intubation.

Contraindication

Etomidate is contraindicated in patients with a hypersensitivity to the medication.

Precautions

Etomidate should be used with caution in patients with marked hypotension, severe asthma, or severe cardiovascular disease.

Side Effects

Side effects associated with etomidate include myoclonic skeletal muscle movement, apnea, hyperventilation or hypoventilation, laryngospasm, hypertension or hypotension, tachycardia or bradycardia, nausea, and vomiting. Injection site pain is common. Several studies have shown some adrenal suppression following the administration of etomidate but these are not geneally thought to be clinically problematic.

Interaction

Verapamil may cause prolonged respiratory depression and apnea.

Dosage

Give 0.1–0.3 mg/kg IV over 15–30 seconds.

℞ Propofol (Diprivan)

Class Sedative and hypnotic

Description

Propofol (Diprivan) is an ultra-short-acting, nonbarbiturate, nonbenzodiazepine hypnotic used as an induction agent in sedation and anesthesia.

Mechanism of Action

Propofol produces a rapid induction of anesthesia. The mechanism of action is unclear.

Pharmacokinetics

Onset: 9–36 seconds
Peak Effects: 3–5 minutes
Duration: 6–10 minutes
Half-Life: 5–12 hours

Indications

Propofol is used as an induction agent for sedation and intubation as well as for maintenance of sedation.

Contraindications

Propofol is contraindicated in patients with a hypersensitivity to the medication. Propofol is in an emulsion made from soybean an egg products. It shoud not be used in patients with increased cranial pressure.

Precautions

Propofol is a potent sedative. Patients should be constantly monitored and equipment facilities for maintenance of a patent airway, artificial ventilation, oxygen administration, and other resuscitative facilities should be readily available at all times.

Side Effects

Pain on induction is common. Be prepared for respiratory depression. Other common side effects include hypotension, bradycardia, transient apnea during induction, nausea and vomiting during recovery phase, and headache during recovery phase.

Interaction

No pharmacological incompatibility has been encountered.

Dosage

2 mg/kg IV for induction followed by 25–75 mcg/kg/minute infusion as needed. Procedural sedation usually requires a lesser dose (0.5–1.0 mg/kg)

NEUROMUSCULAR BLOCKERS

Establishment and protection of the airway has the highest priority in emergency care. On certain occasions patients who are still responsive may have trouble maintaining their airway and may require endotracheal intubation. This situation most commonly occurs in patients with medication overdoses, in patients with status epilepticus, and in trauma patients with closed-head injuries. Often, however, intubation is difficult because of the presence of gag reflexes, clenched teeth, or general combativeness. In these cases endotracheal intubation can be carried out after administration of a neuromuscular-blocking agent.

Neuromuscular-blocking agents are medications that cause muscle relaxation, thus facilitating endotracheal intubation (see Table 16–3). All skeletal muscles, including the muscles of respiration, respond to these medications. Following administration, the patient will become apneic and require mechanical ventilation. Neuromuscular-blocking agents have no effect on the patient's level of consciousness or pain sensation. Neuromuscular-blocking medications are classified as *depolarizing* and *nondepolarizing* based on their mechanism of action. The most commonly used depolarizing medication is succinylcholine, and vecuronium and pancuronium are the most frequently used nondepolarizing agents.

TABLE 16–3

Common Neuromuscular Blockers Used in Rapid-Sequence Induction (RSI)

Generic	Trade	Class	Adult Dose	Pediatric Dose	Onset	Duration
Succinylcholine	Anectine	Depolarizing	1.0–1.5 mg/kg	1.0–2.0 mg/kg	30–60 seconds (IV) 2–3 minutes (IM)	2–3 minutes (IV) 10–30 minutes (IM)
Pancuronium	Pavulon	Nondepolarizing	0.04–0.1 mg/kg	0.04–0.1 mg/kg	35–45 seconds	30–60 minutes
Vecuronium	Norcuron	Nondepolarizing	0.08–0.10 mg/kg	≥ 1 year: adult dose	< 1 minute	25–40 minutes
Atracurium	Tracurium	Nondepolarizing	0.4–0.5 mg/kg	1 month–2 years: 0.3–0.4 mg/kg	1–2 minutes	60–70 minutes
Rocuronium	Zemuron	Nondepolarizing	0.6 mg/kg	> 2 years: adult dose 0.6 mg/kg	30–60 seconds	30–60 minutes

1. *Succinylcholine (Anectine).* Succinylcholine is a depolarizing neuromuscular blocker commonly used in emergency medicine. It acts in approximately 60–90 seconds and lasts approximately 3–5 minutes. Succinylcholine causes muscle fasciculations progressing to total paralysis, including paralysis of the diaphragm.

2. *Pancuronium (Pavulon).* Pancuronium is a long-acting, nondepolarizing neuromuscular-blocking agent. It acts in 30–45 seconds and lasts 30–60 minutes.

3. *Vecuronium (Norcuron).* Vecuronium is a nondepolarizing neuromuscular-blocking agent with a rapid onset and short duration of action. It has fewer cardiovascular side effects than succinylcholine and does not cause fasciculations.

4. *Atracurium (Tracurium).* Atracurium is a nondepolarizing neuromuscular-blocking agent with a rapid onset and short to intermediate duration of action.

5. *Rocuronium (Zemuron).* Rocuronium is a nondepolarizing neuromuscular-blocking agent with a rapid to intermediate onset, depending on dose, and an intermediate duration of action. At equivalent doses, rocuronium has approximately the same clinically effective duration of action as vecuronium.

Depolarizing Blocking Agents

Succinylcholine is the only therapeutic depolarizing blocking agent. Although it is similar to nondepolarizing blockers in its therapeutic effect, its mechanism of action differs. Because succinylcholine is absorbed poorly from the gastrointestinal tract, the preferred administration route is IV. Succincylcholine is primarily metabolized in the blood by the enzyme pseudocholinesterase. The remainder is metabolized in the liver and excreted via the kidneys.

Pharmacodynamics

Succinylcholine has a biphasic effect. In phase I blockade, it acts like acetylcholine and depolarizes the synaptic membrane of the muscle. However, succinylcholine is resistant to acetylcholinesterase (in the neuromuscular junction), so the depolarization persists, resulting in brief periods of excitation, manifested by muscle fasciculations (uncoordinated contractions of muscle fibers), followed by muscle paralysis and flaccidity. Phase II is normally not seen except in high medication concentrations. Succinylcholine is the medication of choice for short-term muscle relaxation, such as during intubation. The primary adverse medication reactions to succinylcholine are the same as those to nondepolarizing blockers: prolonged apnea and cardiovascular alterations. Patients commonly experience muscle pain from the fasciculations that occur in phase I.

℞ Succinylcholine (Anectine)

Class Depolarizing neuromuscular blocker

Description

Succinylcholine is a short-acting, depolarizing skeletal muscle relaxant used to facilitate endotracheal intubation.

Mechanism of Action

Succinylcholine is a short-acting, depolarizing skeletal muscle relaxant. Like acetylcholine, it combines with cholinergic receptors in the motor nerves to cause depolarization. Neuromuscular transmission is thus inhibited, which renders the muscles unable to be stimulated by acetylcholine. Following IV injection, complete paralysis is obtained within 30–60 seconds and persists for approximately 2–3 minutes. Effects then start to fade, and a return to normal is seen within 6 minutes. Muscle relaxation begins in the eyelids and jaw. It then progresses to the limbs, the abdomen, and finally the diaphragm and intercostals. It has no effect on consciousness.

Pharmacokinetics

Onset: 30–60 seconds (IV), 2–3 minutes (IM)
Peak Effects: 1–3 minutes
Duration: 2–3 minutes (IV), 10–30 minutes (IM)
Half-Life: 5–10 minutes

Indication

Succinylcholine is used to achieve temporary paralysis when endotracheal intubation is indicated and muscle tone or seizure activity prevents it.

Contraindications

Succinylcholine is contraindicated in patients with a history of hypersensitivity to the medication. It should not be used with penetrating eye injuries or in patients with a history of narrow-angle glaucoma. Succinylcholine should not be administered by persons inexperienced with its use.

Precautions

Succinylcholine should not be administered unless personnel skilled in endotracheal intubation are present and ready to perform the procedure. Oxygen therapy equipment should be readily available, as should all emergency resuscitative medications and equipment. Fractures have been reported in children following the use of depolarizing neuromuscular blockers due to strong and sustained muscle fasciculations. Cardiac arrest and ventricular arrhythmias have been reported when succinylcholine was administered to patients with severe burns and severe crush injuries.

Side Effects

Succinylcholine can cause wheezing, respiratory depression, apnea, aspiration, arrhythmias, bradycardia, sinus arrest, hypertension, hypotension, hyperkalemia, increased intraocular pressure, and increased intracranial pressure. Malignant hyperthermia has been reported.

Interactions

Certain medications can enhance the neuromuscular-blocking action of succinylcholine: lidocaine, procainamide, β-blockers, magnesium sulfate, and other neuromuscular blockers.

Dosage

The dosage for succinylcholine is 1–1.5 mg/kg administered intravenously. The preferred route for succinylcholine administration is intravenously. It can be administered intramuscularly if required, however.

Nondepolarizing Blocking Agents

The nondepolarizing blocking agents, also called competitive or stabilizing agents, are derived curare alkaloids and their synthetic analogues. We discuss four such agents: pancuronium bromide, vecuronium bromide, atracurium, and rocuronium bromide. These medications produce intermediate to prolonged muscle relaxation, such as that required for intubation and ventilation during surgery. Because nondepolarizing blockers are poorly absorbed from the gastrointestinal tract, they are administered parenterally, with the IV route preferred. A variable but large proportion of the nondepolarizing agents is excreted unchanged in the urine. Some of the medications, such as pancuronium and vecuronium, are metabolized partially in the liver.

Pharmacodynamics

The nondepolarizing blockers compete with acetylcholine at the cholinergic sites of the skeletal muscle membrane. This action blocks acetylcholine's neurotransmitter action, preventing the muscle membrane from depolarizing. The effect can be counteracted clinically by anticholinesterase medications, such as neostigmine or pyridostigmine, which inhibit the action of acetylcholinesterase, the enzyme that destroys acetylcholine.

The initial muscle weakness produced by the medications quickly changes to flaccid paralysis that affects the muscles in a specific sequence. The first muscles to exhibit flaccid paralysis are those innervated by the motor portions of the cranial nerves and small, rapidly moving muscles in the eyes, face, and neck. Next, the limb, abdomen, and trunk muscles become flaccid. Finally, the intercostal muscles and diaphragm are paralyzed. Recovery from the paralysis usually occurs in the reverse order.

Because these medications do not cross the blood–brain barrier, no alterations in consciousness or pain perception occur. Thus patients are aware of what is happening to them and may experience extreme anxiety and pain, but they cannot communicate their feelings.

Nondepolarizing blockers are used for intermediate or prolonged muscle relaxation. They facilitate endotracheal intubation and are used during surgery to decrease the amount of anesthetic required and to facilitate manipulations. They are also used to paralyze patients who need ventilatory support but who fight the endotracheal tube and ventilator.

Pancuronium selectively blocks the vagus nerve and may result in tachycardia, cardiac arrhythmias, and hypertension.

℞ Pancuronium Bromide (Pavulon)

Class Nondepolarizing neuromuscular blocker

Description

Pancuronium bromide is a derivative of curare and is used to provide muscle relaxation to facilitate endotracheal intubation.

Mechanism of Action

Pancuronium competes with acetylcholine for cholinergic receptor sites on the postjunctional membrane. This results in paralysis of muscle fibers served by the occupied neuromuscular junction. It does not cause an initial depolarization wave, as does succinylcholine. The onset of action of pancuronium is 30–45 seconds, and the effect may persist for up to 60 minutes. Effects may begin to subside after 35–45 minutes.

Pharmacokinetics

Onset: 30–45 seconds
Peak Effects: 3–5 minutes
Duration: 30–60 minutes
Half-Life: 2 hours

Indication

Pancuronium is used to achieve temporary paralysis when endotracheal intubation is indicated and muscle tone, seizures, or laryngospasm prevents it.

Contraindications

Pancuronium is contraindicated in patients with a history of hypersensitivity to the medication. It should not be administered by persons inexperienced with its use.

Precautions

Pancuronium should not be administered unless personnel skilled in endotracheal intubation are present and ready to perform the procedure. Oxygen therapy equipment should be readily available, as should all emergency resuscitative medications and equipment. Hypotension can occur. Thus, the vital signs must be constantly monitored. Pancuronium can increase intracranial pressure. In patients with head injuries, vecuronium is often preferred.

Side Effects

Pancuronium can cause wheezing, respiratory depression, apnea, aspiration, arrhythmias, bradycardia, sinus arrest, hypertension, hypotension, increased intraocular pressure, and increased intracranial pressure.

Interactions

Certain medications can enhance the neuromuscular-blocking action of pancuronium: lidocaine, procainamide, β-blockers, magnesium sulfate, certain antibiotics (aminoglycosides), and other neuromuscular blockers.

Dosage

The adult and pediatric dosage for pancuronium is 0.04 to 0.1 mg/kg administered intravenously. Repeat doses of 0.01–0.02 mg/kg administered intravenously may be required every 20–40 minutes.

℞ Vecuronium (Norcuron)

Class Nondepolarizing neuromuscular blocker

Description

Vecuronium is a derivative of pancuronium and is used to provide muscle relaxation to facilitate endotracheal intubation.

Mechanism of Action

Vecuronium has a similar mechanism of action as pancuronium. However, it is approximately one-third more potent, with a shorter duration of effect. Vecuronium competes with acetylcholine for cholinergic receptor sites on the postjunctional membrane. This competition results in paralysis of muscle fibers served by the occupied neuromuscular junction. It does not cause an initial depolarization wave, as does succinylcholine. The onset of action of vecuronium is < 1 minute, with good to excellent intubation conditions within 2.5–3 minutes.

Pharmacokinetics

Onset: < 1 minute
Peak Effects: 3–5 minutes
Duration: 25–40 minutes
Half-Life: 30–80 minutes

Indication

Vecuronium is used to achieve temporary paralysis when endotracheal intubation is indicated and muscle tone or seizure activity prevents it.

Contraindications

Vecuronium is contraindicated in patients with a history of hypersensitivity to the medication.

Precautions

Vecuronium should not be administered unless personnel skilled in endotracheal intubation are present and ready to perform the procedure. Oxygen therapy equipment should be readily available, as should all emergency resuscitative medications and equipment.

Side Effects

Vecuronium can cause wheezing, respiratory depression, apnea, aspiration, arrhythmias, bradycardia, sinus arrest, and hypertension.

Interactions

Certain medications can enhance the neuromuscular-blocking action of vecuronium: lidocaine, procainamide, β-blockers, magnesium sulfate, and other neuromuscular blockers.

Dosage

Adult dose. Vecuronium is 0.08–0.10 mg/kg administered intravenously. Neuromuscular blockade should last 25–30 minutes.

℞ Atracurium (Tracurium)

Class Nondepolarizing neuromuscular blocker

Description

Atracurium is used to provide muscle relaxation to facilitate endotracheal intubation.

Mechanism of Action

Atracurium has a similar mechanism of action as vecuronium. Atracurium competes with acetylcholine for cholinergic receptor sites on the postjunctional membrane. This competition results in paralysis of muscle fibers served by the occupied neuromuscular junction. It does not cause an initial depolarization wave, as does succinylcholine. The onset of action of atracurium is 2 minutes, with good to excellent intubation conditions within 2.5–3 minutes.

Pharmacokinetics

Onset: 2 minutes
Peak Effects: 3–5 minutes
Duration: 60–70 minutes
Half-Life: 20 minutes

Indication

Atracurium is used to achieve temporary paralysis when endotracheal intubation is indicated and muscle tone or seizure activity prevents it.

Contraindications

Atracurium is contraindicated in patients with a history of hypersensitivity to the medication.

Precautions

Atracurium should not be administered unless personnel skilled in endotracheal intubation are present and ready to perform the procedure. Oxygen therapy equipment should be readily available, as should all emergency resuscitative medications and equipment. Use with caution in asthmatics.

Side Effects

Atracurium can cause wheezing, respiratory depression, apnea, aspiration, arrhythmias, bradycardia, sinus arrest, hypertension, hypotension, increased intraocular pressure, and increased intracranial pressure.

Interactions

Certain medications can enhance the neuromuscular-blocking action of atracurium: lidocaine, procainamide, β-blockers, magnesium sulfate, and other neuromuscular blockers.

Dosage

Adult dose. Atracurium is 0.4–0.5 mg/kg administered intravenously. Neuromuscular blockade should last 60–70 minutes.

℞ Rocuronium Bromide (Zemuron)

Class Nondepolarizing neuromuscular blocker

Description

Rocuronium is a nondepolarizing neuromuscular-blocking agent with a rapid to intermediate onset, depending on dose, and intermediate duration of action.

Mechanism of Action

Rocuronium acts by binding competitively to cholinergic receptors at the motor end plate to antagonize the action of acetylcholine, an effect that is reversible in the presence of acetylcholinesterase inhibitors, such as neostigmine and edrophonium.

Pharmacokinetics

Onset: 30–60 seconds
Peak Effects: 1–3 minutes
Duration: 30–60 minutes
Half-Life: 14–18 minutes

Indications

Rocuronium is indicated as an adjunct to general anesthesia to facilitate both rapid-sequence (initiated at 60–90 seconds postadministration) and routine endotracheal intubation and to provide skeletal muscle relaxation during surgery or mechanical ventilation.

Contraindications

Rocuronium is contraindicated in patients with a history of hypersensitivity to the medication.

Precautions

Rocuronium should be administered in carefully adjusted dosages by or under the supervision of experienced clinicians who are familiar with its actions and the possible complications of its use. Rocuronium is associated with a slight elevation of heart rate and blood pressure; tachycardia may occur in children.

Side Effects

Bronchospasm is a rare side effect of rocuronium.

Interactions

Intensity and duration of paralysis may be prolonged by pretreatment with succinylcholine, general anesthesia (inhalation), lidocaine, quinidine, procainamide, beta-adrenergic-blocking agents, potassium-losing diuretics, or magnesium.

Dosage

Rapid-sequence tracheal intubation dosage for adults and children is 600 mcg (0.6 mg/kg). Maintenance dose is 100–200 mcg (0.1–0.2 mg/kg) continuous infusion.

INDUCTION AGENTS

Neuromuscular-blocking agents have no effect on consciousness. Thus, when performing rapid-sequence induction (RSI) on all but unconscious patients, it is necessary to first administer a sedative/hypnotic induction agent. Administering a neuromuscular blocker to a conscious patient can be terrifying because they will be unable to move or breathe, yet will remain conscious and alert throughout the procedure.

The classic anesthetic induction agent is the barbiturate thiopental sodium. In emergency medicine and in the prehospital setting, the benzodiazepines diazepam (Valium) and midazolam (Versed) are sometimes used although other agents (e.g., etomidate [Amidate] and ketamine [Ketalar]) are frequently used. Ketamine is a dissociative agent that does not affect breathing or airway reflexes. It is used primarily in children because of its tendency to cause hallucinations in older patients. Etomidate is an ultra-fast-acting nonbarbiturate, nonbenzodiazepine sedative/hypnotic popular in EMS.

RAPID-SEQUENCE INDUCTION

The procedure for RSI is as follows: Place the patient in a supine position. Preoxygenate with 100 percent oxygen for 5 minutes (spontaneous respirations) or ventilate with a bag-valve-mask device and 100 percent oxygen for at least five tidal volumes prior to intubation to facilitate nitrogen washout (allows 3–5 minutes of apnea without serious hypoxemia).

1. Establish IV normal saline with large-bore catheter (two IVs if time and personnel permit).
2. Monitor ECG, SpO_2, waveform capnography, and vital signs as closely as possible throughout procedure.
3. Perform a thorough neurological exam.
4. Prepare for rapid administration of fentanyl, midazolam, lidocaine, atropine, and succinylcholine.
5. Assemble and prepare equipment (suction, endotracheal tube, endotracheal tube stylet, syringe, lubricant, and cricothyrotomy and PTTV kits).

6. Administer atropine 1.0 mg IV push if
   - Bradycardia is present (fentanyl may induce bradyarrhythmias)
   - Cervical-spine injury
   - Patient is under age 16 (pediatric dose 0.02 mg/kg IV push)

7. Prepare paralytic agents.

8. Consider fentanyl as a preinduction agent.

9. Administer induction agent (e.g., etomidate, midazolam, ketamine, propofol).

10. As patient becomes sedated, check adequacy of sedation and administer 1.5 mg/kg succinylcholine or 0.01 mg/kg vecuronium IV push and stop ventilating if doing so.

11. Apnea and jaw relaxation are indications that the patient is sufficiently relaxed to proceed with endotracheal intubation. If patient is not adequately relaxed, then administer atropine and a second dose of succinylcholine 1.5 mg/kg.

12. Position head, visualize larynx, and intubate.

13. Observe lung inflations, check endotracheal tube for fogging, and auscultate the chest for adequate ventilation. Ventilate with 100 percent oxygen at 16–20 per minute. (Use ETCO$_2$ to determine effective ventilatory rate.)

14. Inflate cuff on endotracheal tube.

15. Reassess patient's vital signs.

16. The effects of the succinylcholine will wear off in 3–5 minutes (vecuronium will wear off in 25–30 minutes).

17. Medical control or standing orders may request the administration of pancuronium or vecuronium if continued paralysis is warranted.

18. The maintenance dose of pancuronium is 0.01 mg/kg; the maintenance dose of vecuronium is 0.01 mg/kg.

19. Assess patient for adequacy of sedation. It may be necessary to administer more fentanyl, midazolam, or propofol for long transports.

PHARMACOLOGICALLY-ASSISTED INTUBATION

An alternative to rapid-sequence induction is the use of many of the same medications, without the use of paralytics. This procedure is referred to as pharmacologically-assisted intubation (PAI). The advantage to this procedure is that paralytics are not used, and a reversal of some of the respiratory depressant effects (from the narcotic fentanyl) is possible with the administration of Narcan. A disadvantage to this procedure occurs in the patient with trismus or a clenched jaw. In spite of the administration of the PAI medications, it may be impossible to pass the endotracheal tube. In this case a surgical airway may be warranted.

The procedure for PAI is as follows: Place the patient in a supine position. Preoxygenate with 100 percent oxygen for 5 minutes (spontaneous respirations) or ventilate with a bag-valve-mask device and 100 percent oxygen for at least five tidal volumes prior to intubation to facilitate nitrogen washout (allows 3–5 minutes of apnea without serious hypoxemia).

1. Establish IV normal saline with large-bore catheter. Monitor ECG, SpO$_2$, ETCO$_2$ and vital signs as closely as possible throughout procedure.

2. Prepare for rapid administration of fentanyl, midazolam, and atropine. Assemble and prepare equipment (suction, endotracheal tube, endotracheal tube stylet, syringe, lubricant, and cricothyrotomy and PTTV kits).

3. Administer atropine 1.0 mg IV push if
   - Bradycardia is present (fentanyl may induce bradyarrhythmias)
   - Spine injury
   - Patients under age 16 (pediatric dose 0.02 mg/kg IV push)

4. Administer fentanyl 1.0 mcg/kg IV push or for the adult patient 100 mcg initially, redosing with 50 mcg or 0.5 mcg/kg increments as necessary to a maximum of 4 mcg/kg.

5. Administer midazolam 0.09–0.3 mg/kg slow IV push or for the adult patient 2.5–5 mg if the patient is responsive to voice or pain and blood pressure is over 100 systolic. Redose with up to three 1 mg boluses if necessary, the blood pressure is over 100 systolic, and the patient becomes responsive to voice or pain.

6. As patient becomes relaxed, approximately 1–2 minutes after administration of midazolam, apply cricoid pressure.

7. Check adequacy of sedation and administer additional fentanyl and midazolam if required.

8. Position head, visualize larynx, apply lidocaine spray, and intubate. Observe lung inflations, check endotracheal tube for fogging, and auscultate the chest for adequate ventilation. Ventilate with 100 percent oxygen at 16–20 per minute. Monitor ECG, vital signs, and SpO_2 every 3–5 minutes.

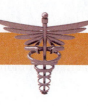

CASE PRESENTATION

At 1430 hours paramedics are called to a football field to help a 16-year-old male who has injured his leg playing football. En route the dispatcher tells the paramedics that the 16-year-old male is conscious and breathing and has a possible fracture of his left leg. On arrival paramedics are directed to the center of the field, where a group of players and coaches are standing. They find their patient lying on the ground with an obviously deformed left ankle. He is wearing football equipment, and first-aid providers have already removed the patient's shoes, socks, and helmet. The patient states that he was running with the ball when he stepped in a small hole in the field. He felt a "pop" in his ankle and then extreme pain. He states he attempted to get up but was unable to because of the pain.

Physical Examination

CNS:	The patient is conscious, alert, and oriented × 4; in extreme pain
Resp:	Respirations are 24; trachea is midline; no signs of trauma; lung sounds are clear bilaterally
CVS:	Carotid and radial pulses are present and strong; skin is pink and warm
ABD:	Soft and nontender
Extremities:	Arms and right leg intact with good pulses, sensation, and strength; left leg is deformed at the ankle, with the left foot rotated externally; distal pulse is palpable in left foot, although it is cooler to touch than the right foot

Vital Signs

Pulse:	96/min, regular, strong
Resp:	24/min, shallow
BP:	122/80 mmHg
SpO$_2$:	99 percent
ECG:	Regular sinus rhythm
Hx:	The patient is not taking any medications, has no known allergies, and states he is a healthy person.

Treatment

Paramedics examine the patient thoroughly and determine that because of the mechanism of the injury the patient does not need to be spinal immobilized. His left ankle is severely angulated, with obvious external rotation. His left foot is cool to touch but has a strong pulse and is pink in color. During attempts to splint the ankle the patient screams in pain, and therefore paramedics decide to give an analgesic prior to completion of the splinting to make it more bearable for the patient. An IV is initiated using an 18-gauge catheter in the right forearm. The IV of normal saline is run TKVO. Paramedics give the patient 5 mg of morphine IV over 2 minutes as per standing order. The paramedics immobilize the ankle in a pillow splint. The patient is moved to the ambulance. The patient is still in considerable pain, and another 5.0 mg of morphine is administered. The patient's vital signs, especially respirations and blood pressure, are closely monitored. En route to the hospital the patient starts to complain about feeling nauseated and is therefore given 25 mg of dimenhydrinate (Gravol) IV. The rest of the trip to the hospital is uneventful. On arrival at the hospital, the patient is assessed and treated for a severe dislocation fracture of his left ankle.

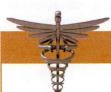

CASE PRESENTATION

At 1900 hours on a fall evening, paramedics are called to the high school football stadium to aid a football player who has injured his shoulder. On arrival they are directed to the sidelines, where the coaches are attending to a player. The player is not wearing shoulder pads and is slouched to his right side.

Physical Examination

CNS:	The patient is conscious, alert, and oriented × 4; in moderate pain
Resp:	Respirations are 24; trachea is midline
CVS:	Carotid and radial pulses are present; skin is warm and dry
ABD:	Soft and nontender
Extremities:	Dislocation of right shoulder

(continued)

Case Presentation (continued)

Vital Signs

Pulse:	88/min, regular
Resp:	18/min, shallow
BP:	118/72 mmHg
SpO$_2$:	96 percent
Hx:	The patient is not taking any medications, has no known allergies, and states he is a healthy person. The coaches tell the paramedics that the football player is the team quarterback. He was sacked on a play and landed heavily on his shoulder.

Treatment

On assessment paramedics find that the shoulder is dislocated anteriorly. They give the patient nitrous oxide to self-administer. After several minutes of breathing the nitrous oxide, the patient states that the pain is not as intense. Paramedics sling and swathe the arm and shoulder and move the patient to the ambulance. Once in the unit, they administer 2 mg of hydromorphone IM in the left deltoid. The combination of nitrous oxide and hydromorphone give the patient almost total pain relief. The transport to the hospital is uneventful.

CHAPTER REVIEW

Summary

Paramedics can reliably manage most patients who complain of pain. With their expanded understanding of pain medications, oversight by medical direction, and use of critical thinking skills, paramedics are ready to relieve the pain many patients suffer.

Key Words

analgesic   A medication used in the relief of pain.

narcotic   A substance that works on the central nervous system to decrease or relieve the sensation of pain. Narcotic pain killers (analgesics) are made from opium or made artificially.

CHAPTER 17

WEAPONS OF MASS DESTRUCTION

OBJECTIVES

After completing this chapter, the reader should be able to:

- Define the terms *weapons of mass destruction (WMD)* and *CBRNE agent*.
- Understand the importance of using personal protective equipment during WMD incidents.
- Describe the common CBRNE agents and their prehospital treatments: nerve agents, vesicants, blood agents, choking agents, viruses, toxins, bacteria, and radiological agents.

INTRODUCTION

Our world changed on September 11, 2001. The reality of the terrorist attacks against the United States on that day was graphically brought into our living rooms through our television sets. Many witnessed the attacks firsthand. However, these attacks were not the first terrorist attacks to use weapons of mass destruction against civilian targets.

Terrorists have clearly indicated their ability and desire to utilize nontraditional weapons in their attacks. In 1984, the Bhagwan Shree Rajneesh cult contaminated salad bars in restaurants in The Dalles, Oregon, with salmonella bacteria, sickening 751 people. Their goal was to cause widespread illness during local elections so the cult would dominate the county commission and sheriff's offices. In 1995, members of the Aum Shinrikyo religious cult launched a sarin nerve gas attack on the Tokyo subway that killed 13 people and sent over 5,500 people to hospitals. Of these patients, 1,038 were suffering effects from the sarin while the others were the "worried well" who had to be distinguished from those who were ill. Letters containing anthrax were sent to news media and government offices in 2001 shortly after the September 11 attacks. These letters killed five people and infected 17 others. Terrorists have even embraced a heretofore rare form of terrorism called *homicide bombing*. In homicide bombings, terrorists hide high-power explosives on their bodies or in their cars and detonate these when they are most apt to injure a large number of people—usually civilians. In Iraq, placing the bombs on chlorine tanker trucks added a toxic chemical hazard to the damage from the explosion. As terrorists resort to nontraditional weapons, the task of protecting a nation and a people becomes more and more difficult.

Emergency Medical Services (EMS) personnel, by the nature of their work, are on the front line of defense and will play a major role in any future terrorist attacks. Because of this, EMS personnel must be familiar with what has come to be known as *weapons of mass destruction (WMD)*. These include *chemical, biological, radiological, nuclear, and explosive (CBRNE) agents* that can be introduced through various mechanisms. CBRNE agents, depending on the particular agent involved, can enter the body through the skin or be ingested, inhaled, or introduced via a vector or weapon. As a general rule, personal protective equipment (PPE) can be used to prevent entry of these agents. Many of these agents are known, and antidotes and treatments are available.

In this chapter, we address the issue of WMD from a prehospital pharmacological standpoint. The field of WMD is diverse and complicated and it is not possible to discuss it comprehensively within the scope of this book. Instead, we concentrate on common pharmacological agents EMS personnel may be called on to administer (or take) in the event of a terrorist attack.

PERSONAL PROTECTIVE EQUIPMENT

Your personal safety and that of your team should always be your main priority when responding to a possible WMD incident. Because of the nature of CBRNE agents, it is essential that EMS personnel use personal protective equipment (PPE) to minimize the risk of exposure and subsequent illness or death. PPE may involve specialized suits, gloves, boots, and respiratory protection. It is essential that you understand the suspected CBRNE agent that you are dealing with in order to take the appropriate precautions. Always refer to local guidelines and recommendations regarding the use and level of PPE. It is paramount that all personnel who might be called on to respond to a WMD incident be trained in the appropriate protective measures and response. Remember, you cannot help others if you become a victim!

CHEMICAL AGENTS

Chemical agents used in WMD affect people in different ways. Nerve agents affect the autonomic and voluntary nervous systems, causing increased parasympathetic symptoms and ultimately flaccid paralysis. Vesicants cause damage to the skin, eyes, and mucous membranes. Blood agents profoundly and adversely affect the cellular use of oxygen, resulting in cellular hypoxia and rapid death. Choking agents cause pulmonary destruction, ultimately leading to pulmonary edema, hypoxia, and death. Chemical agents may appear as vapors, aerosols, or liquids and may be delivered by conventional or nonconventional weapons.

Nerve Agents

Nerve agents are potent chemicals that profoundly affect the nervous system. They are organophosphorus compounds that are much stronger than—but similar to—many commercial insecticides used in agriculture. They include tabun, sarin, soman, and VX.

Nerve agents may present as a liquid, vapor, or both and are capable of being absorbed through the skin or inhaled and absorbed through the respiratory tract. These agents are compounds that have a very high affinity for the enzyme acetylcholinesterase. Acetylcholinesterase is responsible for breaking down the neurotransmitter acetylcholine in the autonomic nervous system and in the neuromuscular junction. When the nerve agent bonds to the enzyme, acetylcholinesterase no longer has the ability to metabolize acetylcholine, leading to unrelenting stimulation of the target receptor site.

This causes the patient to exhibit symptoms of parasympathetic stimulation. These result from the direct effects on the parasympathetic nervous system (miosis, increased intestinal contractions) and from stimulation of glands innervated by the parasympathetic nervous system (increased salivation, increased acid secretion in the stomach, runny nose, tearing, and sweating). Likewise, the skeletal muscles will be affected. Initially, there will be some twitching, which will lead to muscle fasciculations. This may lead to seizures or complete motor paralysis. Exposure leads to a series of signs and symptoms where the amount and route of exposure can cause varying symptoms:

- *Mild symptoms* of nerve agent poisoning include miosis, rhinorrhea, shortness of breath, chest tightness, gastrointestinal upset, sweating, and muscle fasciculations.
- *Moderate symptoms* include wheezing, profuse airway secretions, respiratory distress, muscle weakness, vomiting, and diarrhea.
- *Severe symptoms* include unconsciousness, seizures, flaccid paralysis, cyanosis, and apnea.

The mnemonic *SLUDGEM* can be used to remember these: *S*alivation, *L*acrimation, *U*rination, *D*efecation, *G*astrointestinal upset, *E*mesis, *M*iosis.

The severity of exposure can be determined by the speed of the onset of symptoms; the sooner the onset of symptoms, the more severe the exposure. It is important to remember that, with exposure to liquid nerve agents, the onset of symptoms may be delayed for up to 18 hours. Delay of symptoms is also seen with ingestion of these agents such as might occur when insecticides are used during a suicide attempt.

Treatment of nerve agent poisoning involves the administration of specific **antidotes**. The antidotes are atropine sulfate and pralidoxime (2-PAM). These are often supplied in a kit referred to as a Mark I kit (Figure 17–1). The Mark I kit contains 2 mg of atropine and 600 mg of 2-PAM in spring-driven autoinjectors. Atropine helps to block the effects of acetylcholine at the neuromuscular junction and in the synapses of the autonomic nervous system by binding to acetylcholine receptors. This is a temporary benefit and repeat doses of atropine may be needed if signs or symptoms of nerve agent poisoning recur. It is important to remember that larger than usual doses of atropine are usually required for nerve agent poisoning. 2-PAM serves to reactivate

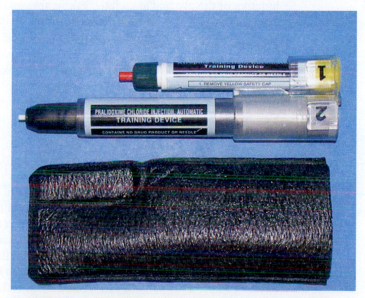

● **FIGURE 17–1** Mark I autoinjector.

the acetylcholinesterase by competitively binding with the nerve agent and releasing the nerve agent from the acetylcholinesterase molecule, thus allowing acetylcholinesterase to again function. If the patient is symptomatic with moderate symptoms, they should be administered one or two Mark I kits and receive additional doses every 5 minutes until secretions begin to dry and ventilatory status improves. For severe exposures, start with two to three Mark I kits and consider the addition of diazepam for seizure prophylaxis. Pediatric patients will require less medication because of their size. Atropine should be dosed at 0.5 mg intramuscularly (IM) for children younger than 2 years of age. Children 2 to 10 years of age should receive 1 mg IM, and children older than 10 years of age should receive 2 mg IM. 2-PAM is given at 15 mg/kg intravenously (IV) to children weighing less than 44 lb (20 kg). Those weighing more than 44 lb (kg) can receive the 600 mg IM adult dose. Newer, military versions of the Mark I kit also contain diazepam.

Vesicants

Vesicants, also called blistering agents, have been the mainstays of chemical warfare until international treaties banned their use. They are still used by certain rogue nations and pose a threat as WMDs.

Vesicants are normally a dark brown oily liquid and are very persistent agents meaning that they remain in the environment for a long time and are difficult to remove. They burn and blister the skin or any other part of the body they contact. It is essential that responding personnel wear appropriate respiratory protection when irritant gases are suspected. The three common vesicants are discussed next.

Mustard

Mustard agents are strong alkylating agents that, in addition to causing extensive genetic damage, are capable of exerting effects in a variety of tissues. The most common hazard from mustard is that of liquid contact with the skin, although vapor may be absorbed readily through the respiratory tract and eyes. Mustard produces a garlic-like odor that quickly becomes unnoticeable because exposure to the agent causes the olfactory nerves to become insensitive.

There are no immediate signs of mustard exposure; however, some 4 to 8 hours later, redness of the skin may appear. In addition there may be reddening of the conjunctiva of the eye and associated eye itching and pain. The eyes will often feel gritty. The patient may also exhibit upper respiratory symptoms such as sinus pain, cough, and scratchy throat. Eventually, small fluid-filled blisters (vesicles) will appear; however, no mustard is present in the blister fluid. Mustard eventually causes cellular death.

The mechanism of action of mustard is unknown and consequently there is no specific antidote for mustard poisoning. The only initial action is to decontaminate the victim as soon as possible. Decontamination of the mustard agent victim after 5 minutes will not prevent the development of toxic effects, but will protect others from cross-contamination.

Lewisite

The hazards from lewisite are similar to those of the other vesicant agents; however, the vapor causes immediate burning and pain in the eyes and exposed mucous membranes. The skin will exhibit a grayish color reflective of tissue destruction within minutes after contact with lewisite. Later, severe damage of the skin, eyes, and airway may appear. Edema of the lungs is more marked than that caused by mustard and frequently is accompanied by pleural fluid. When inhaled in high concentration, it may be fatal in as short a time as 10 minutes. Lewisite causes leakage from systemic capillaries resulting in hypovolemia and, ultimately, hypotension.

EMS personnel must be ready to provide airway assistance. Decontamination should be performed as soon as possible. Skin lesions from vesicant agents should be treated as you would treat a thermal burn with Silvadene or Neosporin. Artificial tears and topical ophthalmic antibiotics may help with eye involvement. Airway involvement may lead to laryngeal edema; EMS personnel should have a low threshold for intubating the patient and providing mechanical ventilation. There is an antidote for lewisite called British Anti-lewisite (BAL). If administered early after exposure, it may decrease some of the internal damage, but will not help skin, eye, or airway damage.

Phosgene Oxime

Phosgene is a chemical that can be encountered in certain manufacturing processes. Phosgene oxime and lewisite are similar in their effects. Like lewisite, phosgene causes immediate effects. The vapor causes immediate burning and pain in the eyes and exposed mucous membranes. The skin will exhibit a grayish color reflective of tissue destruction within minutes after contact with phosgene oxime. Later, severe damage of the skin, eyes, and airway may appear.

Decontamination should be performed as soon as possible. There is no antidote for phosgene oxime. Calamine lotion may be applied to the skin. Artificial tears and topical ophthalmic antibiotics may help with eye involvement. Airway involvement may lead to laryngeal edema; EMS personnel should have a low threshold for intubating the patient and providing mechanical ventilation. Consider administering analgesics.

Blood Agents

Blood agents are chemicals that interfere with the cellular metabolism of oxygen. Their usual route of entry is by inhalation. The most common blood agent is cyanide.

Cyanide is a product of many chemical processes and occurs naturally in some foods. It is also produced by combustion when certain items are burned. The two general forms of cyanide are hydrogen cyanide and cyanogen chloride. Cyanide can enter the body through the respiratory tract, by ingestion, or through the skin. It is rapidly distributed by the blood. Once in the body, the toxin directly poisons the respiratory mechanism of the cells. This leads to cellular hypoxia and, ultimately, death.

Cyanide inactivates an enzyme called *cytochrome a_3*. This enzyme is an important part of cellular respiration and deactivation of the enzyme leads to cellular hypoxia. The administration of supplemental oxygen cannot overcome this problem.

Following exposure, the victim will begin to demonstrate symptoms in 15 to 30 seconds. Initially, the respiratory rate will increase. Later, dizziness, weakness, anxiety, and nausea will occur. Ultimately, the patient will lose consciousness and stop breathing. This progression of events is quite rapid. In fact, many victims of cyanide poisoning die before help reaches them. Occasionally, rescuers have reported the smell of bitter almonds in cyanide victims.

Treatment includes maintenance of the airway and respirations and administration of an antidote. All cyanide exposure victims should receive high-flow, high-concentration oxygen and mechanical ventilation, if required. Antidote therapy should be provided as soon as possible. The preferred antidote is hydroxocobalamin (CyanoKit) (Figure 17–2). However, if hydroxocobalamin is unavailable, the older cyanide kit (Lilly, Pasadena) can be used (Figure 17–3). This kit contains amyl nitrite, sodium nitrite, and sodium thiosulfate. The nitrite causes the iron in hemoglobin to change to a form called methemoglobin. Methemoglobin has a high affinity for cyanide and can actually remove cyanide off the *cytochrome a_3* enzyme and out of the cells. Once removed, it must be detoxified with sodium thiosulfate, where it is excreted by the kidneys. Methemoglobin will gradually return to normal hemoglobin through natural biochemical processes.

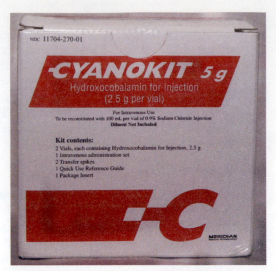

● **FIGURE 17–2** CyanoKit. © Bryan E. Bledsoe

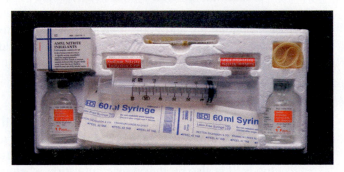

● **FIGURE 17–3** Cyanide antidote kit. © Jeff Forster

Amyl nitrite is supplied in ampules for inhalation. It can be immediately administered by inhalation or with a bag-valve-mask unit while IV access is obtained. Once IV access is obtained, sodium nitrite can be administered intravenously. Half the original dose can be repeated in 30 minutes as needed. Finally, following nitrite therapy, sodium thiosulfate can be administered intravenously to detoxify and remove the cyanide. The antidotes are much less effective when given individually as compared to giving them in the sequence described.

Choking Agents

Choking agents primarily affect the respiratory system. They include ammonia, chlorine, and phosgene (a different agent than phosgene oxime). There is usually associated eye irritation. Ammonia and chlorine can cause pulmonary edema with high-level exposures—usually taking 2 to 24 hours to develop. These agents physically damage the membranes of the lungs, causing fluid to enter the interstitial space and ultimately leading to pulmonary edema. The patient eventually becomes hypoxic. The first symptom is usually shortness of breath, which becomes progressively worse.

It is important to remove the victim from the source and administer high-flow, high-concentration oxygen. Mechanical ventilation should be provided as needed. There are no specific antidotes. It is important to remember that pulmonary edema caused by these agents is not cardiac in origin and diuretics may be of limited use. Supplemental oxygen and inhaled bronchodilators are useful. Riot control agents can cause many of the same effects as choking agents and sometimes it is hard to distinguish between the two.

BIOLOGICAL AGENTS

Biological agents include those derived from viruses, bacteria, fungi, and other organisms. In some cases, the biological agent itself is responsible for infection. In others, toxins produced by the bacteria are responsible. Fungi attack mainly plants and therefore are really a threat only to the agricultural system. The following are common biological agents that can be used as WMDs.

Viruses

Viruses are a group of submicroscopic infective agents that are regarded either as extremely simple microorganisms or as extremely complex molecules. They typically contain a protein coat surrounding an RNA or DNA core of genetic material but no semipermeable membrane. They are capable of growth and multiplication only in living cells.

Smallpox

Smallpox is caused by the variola virus. It was declared eradicated from the earth by the World Health Organization in 1980. Two research labs were allowed to keep strains of the variola virus: the Centers for Disease Control and Prevention in Atlanta, Georgia, and the Vector Center in Koltsovo, Russia. Following the fall of the Soviet Union it became uncertain whether all vials of the virus at Vector were accounted for. In addition, concerns have been raised that clandestine stockpiles of the virus might remain even though all stocks were supposed to have been destroyed by 1999. Its lethality and ease of transmission make smallpox an attractive WMD agent.

The incubation period for smallpox is approximately 12 days. Signs and symptoms of infection include malaise, fever, chills (rigors), vomiting, headache, and backache. Some patients will develop a delirium. Approximately 2 to 3 days after the onset of symptoms, a rash develops on the face, hands, and forearms, and then spreads to the trunk. The lesions then form red spots and ultimately pustules. The pustules will later scab over.

A vaccine for smallpox is available and vaccination against smallpox was once routine. However, once the disease was eradicated, vaccine administration stopped. The vaccine lasted from 3 to 10 years and booster doses are administered as needed. Specific therapy for those infected is vaccinia immune globulin, which is most effective when administered within 24 hours of exposure.

Ebola

Ebola virus is one of the deadliest viruses known and causes hemorrhagic fever. It causes death in 50 to 90 percent of all infected patients. It is transmitted through direct contact with the blood, urine, stool, semen, or organs of infected persons. Inhalation transmission has been reported. The incubation period is 2 to 21 days. Hemorrhagic fever usually begins with a sudden onset of fever, weakness, muscle pain, headache, and sore throat. Later, the patient will develop nausea, vomiting, diarrhea, and rash. Organ failure (renal and hepatic) usually begins secondary to internal and external bleeding. The hemorrhagic symptoms usually begin on the fifth day. Ebola is a prime candidate for an agent in a WMD. No vaccines are available, nor is antiviral therapy available. Treatment consists of isolation and supportive care.

Marburg

The Marburg virus is closely related to the Ebola virus. It was first identified following an outbreak of hemorrhagic fever in Germany after importation of African green monkeys. The symptoms are similar to Ebola. The mortality rate is approximately 25 percent. Marburg can be aerosolized, thus making it an attractive weapon. No vaccine or treatment is available.

Toxins

Toxins are poisonous substances that are produced by a living organism and are usually very unstable, notably toxic when introduced into the tissues, and typically capable of inducing antibody formation.

Botulism

Botulinum toxin, one of the most lethal compounds known to man, is produced by the bacteria *Clostridium botulinum*. Members of the *Clostridium* species are spore formers. **Spores** are special reproductive cells produced by certain bacteria. Botulism most commonly results from improperly canned or undercooked foods that contain the bacteria. The bacteria themselves are harmless, but the toxin they produce is extremely toxic. Botulism is not contagious. Without prophylaxis or treatment, victims stand little chance of survival.

There are seven or more types of botulinum toxin. The toxin affects the neuromuscular junction much like a neuromuscular blocker. The first symptoms develop within 1 to 12 hours of exposure and include drooping of the eyelids, dry mouth, difficulty swallowing, difficulty talking, blurred vision, and double vision. The paralysis then moves downward from the face to the throat, chest, abdomen, and extremities. Ultimately, the muscles of respiration will be fully paralyzed and asphyxia death results.

Treatment consists of ventilatory assistance and the administration of an antitoxin. The antitoxin (trivalent botulinum antitoxin) should be administered as soon as possible once botulism is suspected. If treatment is not promptly administered, the paralysis will set in and may take several months for function to return. A vaccine is now available for many of the botulinum types.

Ricin

Ricin is a toxin derived from the processing of castor beans (*Ricinus communis*) and inhibit protein synthesis. It is easy to produce, and stable. Ricin can be ingested, injected, or inhaled. Symptoms begin approximately 3 hours after inhaling ricin and include coughing, chest tightness, fever, dyspnea, nausea, and muscle aches. Symptoms following ingestion include nausea, vomiting, internal bleeding, liver failure, and ultimately, multiple organ failure. If injected, ricin causes death of muscles and lymph nodes near the injection site. This can lead to organ failure and death.

No vaccine or antitoxin is available for ricin. Treatment is supportive and fluid replacement is paramount. If ingested, lavage with activated charcoal may be beneficial.

Bacteria

Bacteria are living organisms made up of nuclear material, cytoplasm, and a cell membrane.

Tularemia

Tularemia, also known as *rabbit fever* or *deer fly fever*, is caused by the bacterium *Francisella tularensis*. The bacteria are highly infective; in fact, a single bacterium has the potential to infect a human. It is contracted through open wounds and inhalation resulting in two forms: ulceroglandular tularemia and inhalational tularemia. A biological warfare attack with tularemia would most likely be delivered by aerosol. A vaccine is available and tularemia is treated with doxycycline, ciprofloxacin, gentamicin, or streptomycin.

Ulceroglandular tularemia is usually contracted under natural conditions through inoculation by contact with the skin or mucous membranes of an infected animal or from the bites of infected deer flies, mosquitoes, and ticks. This results in the formation of an ulcer at the site of inoculation. Later, lymph nodes proximal to the ulcer become swollen and tender. The patient will usually develop fever and malaise.

Inhalational tularemia is less common, and is a result of inhaling contaminated dust. It is characterized by the sudden onset of chills, fever, headache, muscle aches, fatigue, cough, and loss of body fluids. The incubation period is 1 to 21 days with 3 days being average. The illness can last up to 3 weeks. The mortality rate is approximately 30 percent.

Anthrax

Anthrax is caused by the bacterium *Bacillus anthracis*. Although rare in humans, this organism is often seen in veterinary practice. This bacterium produces specialized reproductive cells known as spores. Bacterial spores have thick walls and are able to withstand varying temperatures, humidity, and other unfavorable conditions. In fact, anthrax spores can survive in sunlight for several days and steam heat up to 318°F. They can remain viable in soil or water for years waiting to infect a host organism where they will begin to reproduce. The anthrax bacteria (or its spores) can enter the body through breaks in the skin, inhalation, or ingestion. The incubation period for anthrax is typically 1 to 6 days (although longer incubation periods have been documented). Anthrax cannot be spread from person to person. A vaccine for anthrax is available.

Depending on the route of exposure, anthrax can affect the skin, lungs, or gastrointestinal tract. When anthrax is limited to the skin, it is referred to as *cutaneous anthrax*. This form is usually contracted from tissues of infected animals (sheep, goats, cattle). Cutaneous anthrax can be treated with antibiotics including penicillin, doxycycline, and ciprofloxacin (Cipro). Treatment usually lasts for at least 60 days because spores can take that long to germinate.

Inhaling the anthrax spores into the lungs leads to *inhalational anthrax*, which is more common in cattle. This results in fever and fatigue (flu-like symptoms) within 1 to 7 days after exposure. This is often followed by a slight improvement. Then, there is an abrupt onset of respiratory distress (cough and dyspnea), tachycardia, shock, and eventually death. The fatality rate for untreated inhalational anthrax is greater than 90 percent. Antibiotics (often a combination of antibiotics) are the treatment of choice. Persons possibly exposed to anthrax should be immediately started on antibiotic therapy and remain on it until tests have excluded or confirmed infection.

A new medication, Raxibacumab, is a human monoclonal antibody drug for inhalational anthrax. While antibiotics can kill the anthrax bacteria, they are not effective against the deadly toxins that the bacteria produce. Raxibacumab targets anthrax toxins after they are released by the bacteria. In an inhalation anthrax attack, people may not know they are infected with anthrax until the toxins are already circulating in their blood. At this point, it may be too late for antibiotics alone to be effective. Raxibacumab has been added to the United States Strategic National Stockpile.

Intestinal anthrax has been reported and causes abdominal distress, vomiting, and in some cases, bloody diarrhea. It can be caused by ingesting contaminated meat, and it takes a large spore load to infect a person. Intestinal anthrax can lead to septicemia and death.

Plague

Plague, also referred to as the *Black Death*, killed millions of people in the pre-antibiotic era and still poses a threat as a WMD. Plague is caused by *Yersinia pestis* bacteria, which is not a spore former. The two types of plague infection are bubonic plague and pneumonic plague.

Bubonic plague is the most common and is transmitted from rodents to humans by the bite of an infected flea. The infection spreads through the lymphatic system, causing swollen lymph nodes in the groin (known as *buboes*). The infection can invade the bloodstream, causing septicemia.

Pneumonic plague can result from septicemia or inhalation of the organism. The bacteria spread rapidly in the lungs, causing a hemorrhagic pneumonia. This feature makes plague an attractive agent for biological warfare. Untreated pneumonic plague is usually fatal. The incubation period is 2 to 10 days. The patient with plague is highly infectious. The illness usually lasts 1 to 2 days. Symptoms include malaise, high fever, tender lymph nodes, skin lesions, chills, headaches, bloody sputum, pneumonia, circulatory failure, and death.

Persons exposed to plague should be treated with doxycycline or ciprofloxacin. No vaccine is available. Pneumonic plague can be treated successfully if antibiotics are started within 24 hours of the onset of symptoms. Antibiotics used in pneumonic plague include streptomycin, gentamicin, doxycycline, chloramphenicol, and ciprofloxacin.

Brucellosis

Brucellosis, also known as undulant fever, is caused by bacteria in the *Brucella* species (*Brucella suis, Brucella melitensis, Brucella abortus*). The *Brucella* species is not a spore former. The infection is spread via inhalation. The incubation period is 5 to 21 days, but can occasionally take up to 2 months. Brucellosis tends to cause incapacitation rather than death in most cases. Initially the patient will develop flu-like symptoms (fever, chills, headache, loss of appetite, mental depression, extreme fatigue, aching joints, sweating, nausea, and vomiting). Brucellosis is treated with the antibiotics doxycycline and rifampin. Treatment is usually for a minimum of 6 weeks. The relapse rate is high.

Patients infected with smallpox, plague, and Ebola are contagious. The key to exposure prevention is the use of appropriate PPE, which is used in EMS every day to control the spread of bloodborne pathogens.

RADIOLOGICAL AGENTS

Radiological agents are substances that emit ionizing radiation, which is harmful to all living creatures. They may be solids, liquids, or gases. These agents can be delivered through the use of nuclear weapons, conventional explosives that disperse a radioactive material ("dirty" bombs), or the manual dispersal of radioactive material. Exposure can occur in three ways. Persons can become contaminated, irradiated, or have radioactive material incorporated into the body.

Contamination occurs when radioactive materials get onto the body or clothing of the victim. Removal is accomplished through thorough decontamination and clothing removal. Follow your local procedures for radiation decontamination. Do not shower in an attempt to remove the contamination, as that will spread the contamination.

Irradiation occurs when a person is near a radioactive source and the energy from that source damages the person's cells. Nuclear radiation cannot be felt, seen, or otherwise detected by any of our senses. However, it damages the cells of the human body as it passes through them. Radiation passage changes the structure of molecules and essential elements of the cell by transferring its energy to the cell. Damaged cells then go on to repair themselves, die, or to produce altered or damaged cells. It is possible for someone to be irradiated without being contaminated by the material and these patients do not pose a risk to anyone else.

If a radioactive material is inhaled, ingested, or penetrates the skin (fragments from a dirty bomb), then the patient will be exposed to the radiation internally from that material. Internal exposure is much more significant than external exposure as the body's tissues receive a higher level of irradiation.

Protection from radiological agents is simple and easy to follow, and is based on the following points.

Time. Reducing the time spent in the area of radiation will reduce the radioactive dose received.

Distance. The effects of radiation decrease as you move away from the radiation source. This is an inverse square relationship where if you double the distance you are from the source, you will receive one-quarter of the radiation.

Shielding. Protective barriers and clothing between you and the radioactive material will decrease the amount of radiation reaching your body. It is important to choose a material that is appropriate for the type of radiation present.

There are four main types of radiation: alpha, beta, gamma, and neutrons.

Alpha particles are large, heavy subatomic particles that produce dense ionization along their path. They can be stopped by as little as a few centimetres of air, a sheet of paper, or the outer layers of our skin. Because of this limited penetrating capability, alpha sources that are outside the body do not present a radiation hazard. However, when the particles are inside the body, they become an internal radiation hazard and can do significant damage.

Beta particles are small, light subatomic particles and can penetrate much deeper into tissue than alpha particles. Beta radiation of sufficient energy will penetrate the outer layers of skin and reach the deeper tissues. However, it does not normally penetrate to the internal organs. Beta particles can generally be stopped by as little as a sheet of plywood or plastic.

Gamma radiation is electromagnetic waves of energy that travel long distances in air and are very penetrating. When gamma rays pass through matter they may be scattered and/or absorbed. They have substantial penetrating power but quickly lose their energy as they interact with atoms along their path. Interactions with body cells may damage skin or internal tissues. Lead, concrete, and other heavy materials are needed to shield against gamma radiation.

Neutron radiation may be produced by a variety of nuclear reactions. It is normally encountered only around a nuclear reactor or after the detonation of a nuclear weapon. Neutrons are uncharged particles and can penetrate through the skin and internal organs. Neutron radiation can be stopped by concrete, water, or a paraffin barrier.

Symptoms of radiation poisoning can vary, but include nausea, vomiting, severe burns, fatigue, and then death. Persons exposed to radiation should be decontaminated as soon as possible following accepted procedures. Patients with internal radiation exposure (ingestion or inhalation) cannot be decontaminated.

CHAPTER REVIEW

Summary

EMTs and paramedics must be familiar with common WMDs. In dealing with a possible WMD attack, it is important to remain calm, put on personal protective equipment, and stay upwind and uphill until the scene has been deemed safe to approach. Always use the Incident Command System or Incident Management System as appropriate. When the agent is identified, apply treatment per local protocol. EMS personnel may be in particular demand when antidote administration is required. Therefore, EMS personnel must be familiar with the common WMD antidotes and treatments. Regardless, your personal safety and that of your crew should always be your first priority.

Key Words

antidote   A remedy for counteracting a poison.

contamination   Occurs when radioactive materials get onto the body or clothing of the victim.

irradiation   Occurs when a person is near a radioactive source and the energy from that source damages the person's cells.

spore   An oval body, formed within certain species of bacteria. It is regarded as a resting phase during the life cycle of the cell and is extremely resistant to environmental factors.

vesicant   A blistering drug or agent.

CENTRAL NERVOUS SYSTEM STIMULANTS

A
Amp
Bam
Batu (methcathinone)
Beans (MDMA)
Bennies
Bennie (Benzidrine)
Black and white
Black beauties
Black birds
Blue angels
Blue beauties
Bombido (injectable amphetamine)
Bombita (Spanish-speaking community)
Candy
Cartwheels
Cat (methcathinone)
Chalk
Chicken powder
Chocolate
Chris
Christine
Christmas eve
Christmas trees
Christy (smokable meth)
Coast to coast
Coke (cocaine)
Copilot
Crack (cocaine)
Crank
Crink
Cris
Crisscross
Crissroads

Croak (meth and crack)
Crystal (methamphetamine)
Dexies
Disco pellets
Dominoes
Double cross
Eye openers
Fire (meth and crack)
Flake (cocaine)
Footballs
Glass
Go-fast
Gold dust (cocaine)
Granulated orange
Green and clears
Greenies
Hanyak
Head drugs
Hearts
Hiropon (smokable methamphetamine or methcathinone)
Ice
Inbetweens
Jam
Jelly baby
Jolly baby
Jugs
Kaksonjae
LA (long-acting amphetamines)
LA glass (smokable LA)
LA turnarounds
Leapers
Lid poppers
Lid proppers

Little bomb
Max (dissolved gamma hydroxy buterate mixed with amphetamine)
Meth
Mexican crack
Minibennie
Nugget
Oranges
Peaches
Pep pills
Pink and green
Pinks
Quartz
Rippers
Rock (cocaine)
Rosa (Spanish-speaking community)
Roses
Shabu (methcathinone)
Snap
Snow (cocaine)
Speed
Speedball (heroin plus cocaine)
Toot
Truck drivers
Turnarounds
Uppers
Ups
Wake-ups
Whiffledust
Whites
X
XTC
Yellow jackets

PHENCYCLIDINE (PCP)

A Beam me up Scotty (PCP and crack)
Ace
Ad
Amoeba
Angel dust
Animal tranquilizer
Aurora
Black acid (PCP and LSD)
Bush
Bust bee
Cheap cocaine
Cosmos
Criptal
Devil's dust
Dipper
DOA
Domex (PCP and ecstasy)
Dummy mist
El Diablito (for combination of PCP, marijuana, cocaine, and heroin in Spanish-speaking community)
Frios (marijuana laced with PCP in Spanish-speaking community)
Goon
Green
Guerrilla
Hog
Jet
K
Kools (marijuana laced with PCP)
Lemon 714
Lovely
Magic dust
Mauve
Mist
Monkey tranquilizers
Mumm dust
Niebla (Spanish-speaking community)
Octane (PCP laced with gasoline)
Ozone
Peace pill
Purple
Rocket fuel
Shermans
Sherms
Special LA coke
Superacid
Supercoke
Supergrass
Superjoint
Trangs
Tranq
Wack

HEROIN

Black tar
Brown
Chinese white
H
H and stuff
Horse
Junk
Mexican mud
Scat
Shit
Skag
Smack
Snow
Stuff
Tango and Cash

OTHER ANALGESICS

Black (opium)
Blue velvet (paregoric plus amphetamine)
Dollies (methadone)
M (morphine)
Microdots (morphine)
PG or PO (paregoric)
Pinks and grays (propoxyphene hydrochloride)
Poppy (opium)
Tar (opium)
Terp (terpin hydrate or cough syrup with codeine)

CENTRAL NERVOUS SYSTEM DEPRESSANTS

Blue birds
Blue devil
Blue heaven
Blues
Bullets
Dolls
Double trouble
Downs
Goofballs
Green and whites (chlordiazepoxide)
Greenies
Ludes
Nembies
Peanuts
Peter (chloral hydrate)
Rainbows
Red Devils

Roaches (chlordiaepoxide)
Seccy
Seggy

T-birds
Toolies
Tranqs

Wallbangers
Yellow jackets
Yellows

HALLUCINOGENS

Acid (LSD)
Blue dots (LSD)
Cactus (mescaline)
Crystal

Cube (LSD)
D (LSD)
Mesc (mescaline)
Mexico mushroom (psilocybin)

Owsleys (LSD)
Pearly gates (morning glory seeds)

CANNABINOLS

Acapulco gold
Bhang
Brick
Charas
Colombian
Gage
Ganja
Grass
Hash
Hay
Hemp

J
Jane
Jive
Joint
Key or Kee
Lid
Locoweed
Mary Jane
Mexican
MJ
Muggles

Pot
Reefer
Roach
Rope
Sativa
Stick
Sweet Lucy
Tea
Texas tea
Weed
Yesca

SOLVENTS AND INHALANTS

Air blast
Ames
Amies
Aroma of men
Bang
Boopers
Bullet
Buzz bomb
Climax

Honey oil
Huff
Huffing
Jac aroma
Kicks
Laughing gas (nitrous oxide)
Locker room (isobutyl nitrate)
Medusa
Moon gas

Oz
Pearls (amyl nitrite)
Poppers (isobutyl or amyl nitrate)
Poppers (isobutyl or amyl nitrite)
Rush
Snappers
Sniffers
Whiteout

INHALANTS

Air blast
Ames
Amies
Amys
Aroma of men
Bang
Boppers

Bullet
Buzz bomb
Climax
Honey oil
Huff
Laughing gas (nitrous oxide)
Locker room (isobutyl nitrate)

Medusa
Moon gas
Oz
Pearls (amyl nitrite)
Poor man's pot
Poppers (isobutyl or amyl nitrate)
Whiteout

STREET DRUG LINGO

Abe's cape: $5 bill

Agonies: withdrawal symptoms

All star: user of many types of drugs

Amped out: fatigue after using methamphetamine

Baby habit: occasional user of drugs

Bad go: bad reaction to a drug

Bagging: using inhalants

Batt: hypodermic needle

Bedbugs: fellow addicts

Bender: drug party

Bone: $50 piece of crack

Boulder: $20 worth of crack

Cooker: one who manufactures methamphetamine

Deck: 1 to 15 g of heroin

Demo: sample size of crack

Deuce: $2 worth of drug

Eight ball: 1/8 ounce of any type of drug

Gluey: one who sniffs or inhales glue

Huffer: one who uses inhalants

Hype: an addict, most frequently refers to IV drug users

Lid: 1 ounce of marijuana

Meth head: regular meth user

Meth monster: one who gets a violent reaction to methamphetamine

Rolling: getting high on Ecstasy

Snot: residue left after smoking amphetamines

Snotball: rubber cement rolled into balls and burned so the fumes can be inhaled

Speed freak: regular meth user

Spike: hypodermic needle

Plasma Protein Fraction (Plasmanate)

Class	Protein colloid
Action	Plasma volume expander
Indication	Hypovolemic states (especially burn shock)
Contraindication	None when used in the management of life-threatening situations
Precautions	Hypertension
	Short shelf life
Side Effect	Edema
Dosage	Dosage should be titrated according to patient's hemodynamic response; follow accepted resuscitation formulas in the management of burn shock
	Adult: 250–500 mL (12.5–25 g protein) not to exceed 10 mL/min
Route	IV infusion
Pediatric Dosage	10–30 mL/kg at 5–10 mL/min

Dextran

Class	Imitation protein (sugar) colloid
Action	Plasma volume expander
Indication	Hypovolemic shock
Contraindication	Patients with known hypersensitivity to the drug
	Congestive heart failure
	Renal failure
	Bleeding disorders
Precautions	Severe anaphylactic reactions have been known to occur
	Monitor for circulatory overload
	Can impede accurate blood typing because dextran molecule coats the erythrocytes; draw tube of blood for blood typing before administering dextran
Side Effects	Nausea
	Vomiting
	Rash
	Itching

Dosage	Dosage should be titrated according to patient's hemodynamic response
	500 mL over 15–30 minutes
Route	IV infusion
Pediatric Dosage	Same as adult

 ## Hetastarch (Hespan)

Class	Artificial colloid
Action	Plasma volume expander
Indication	Hypovolemic states
	Septic shock
Contraindication	Few in life-threatening conditions
Precautions	Monitor for circulatory overload
	Large volumes of hetastarch may alter the coagulation mechanism
Side Effects	Nausea
	Vomiting
Dosage	Dosage should be titrated according to patient's hemodynamic response
	500–1000 mL, not to exceed 20 mL/kg/hr; total dose not to exceed 1500 mL in 24 hours
Route	IV infusion
Pediatric Dosage	Safety in children has not been established

 ## Polygeline (Haemaccel)

Class	Artificial colloid
Action	Plasma volume expander
Indication	Hypovolemic states
Contraindication	Patients with known hypersensitivity to the drug
Precautions	Allergic reactions (rare)
Side Effects	Urticaria
	Tachycardia
	Bradycardia
	Dyspnea
Dosage	Dosage should be titrated according to patient's hemodynamic response
Route	IV
Pediatric Dosage	Dosage should be titrated according to the patient's hemodynamic response

 ## Lactated Ringer's Solution

Class	Isotonic crystalloid
Action	Approximates the electrolyte concentration of the blood
Indication	Hypovolemic shock

Contraindications	Congestive heart failure
	Renal failure
Precaution	Monitor for circulatory overload
Side Effects	Rare
Dosage	*Hypovolemic shock (systolic less than 90 mmHg):* Infuse "wide open" until a systolic of 100 mmHg is attained; once a systolic of 100 mmHg has been attained, infusion should be slowed to 100 mL/hr
	Other: As indicated by the patient's condition and situation being treated
Route	IV infusion
Pediatric Dosage	20 mL/kg repeated as required based on hemodynamic response

5 Percent Dextrose in Water (D$_5$W)

Class	Sugar solution
Action	Glucose nutrient solution
Indications	IV access for emergency drugs
	For dilution of concentrated drugs for IV infusion
Contraindication	Should not be used as a fluid replacement for hypovolemic states.
	Avoid in head injury and stroke
Precautions	Monitor for circulatory overload
	Draw tube of blood before administering to diabetics
Side Effects	Rare
Dosage	Generally administered TKO
Route	IV infusion
Pediatric Dosage	Same as adult

10 Percent Dextrose in Water (D$_{10}$W)

Class	Hypertonic sugar solution
Action	Replaces blood glucose
Indications	Hypoglycemia
	Neonatal resuscitation
	Rarely used as an IV infusion; rather, as a bolus dose as needed
Contraindication	Should not be used as fluid replacement for hypovolemic states
	Avoid in head injury and stroke
Precautions	Monitor for circulatory overload
	Draw tube of blood before administering D$_{10}$W to diabetics
Side Effects	Rare
Dosage	Dependent on patient's condition and condition being treated
Route	IV infusion
Pediatric Dosage	< 3 months of age, 2–6 mL/kg IV/IO

0.9 Percent Sodium Chloride (Normal Saline)

Class	Isotonic electrolyte
Action	Fluid and sodium replacement
Indications	Heat-related problems (heat exhaustion and heat stroke)
	Freshwater drowning
	Hypovolemia
	Diabetic ketoacidosis
Contraindication	Congestive heart failure
Precaution	Electrolyte depletion (K^+, Mg^{2+}, Ca^{2+}, among others) can occur following administration of large amounts of normal saline
Side Effect	Thirst
Dosage	Dependent on patient's condition and situation being treated; in freshwater drowning and heat emergencies, the administration is usually rapid
Route	IV infusion
Pediatric Dosage	Dose is dependent on patient's size and condition

0.45 Percent Sodium Chloride (One-Half Normal Saline)

Class	Hypotonic electrolyte
Action	Slow rehydration
Indications	Patients with diminished renal or cardiovascular function for which rapid rehydration is not indicated
Contraindications	Cases in which rapid rehydration is indicated
Precaution	Electrolyte depletion can occur following administration of large amounts of one-half normal saline
Side Effects	Rare
Dosage	Dependent on patient's condition and situation being treated
Route	IV infusion
Pediatric Dosage	Dose is based on patient's size and condition

5 Percent Dextrose in 0.9 Percent Sodium Chloride (D₅NS)

Class	Hypertonic sugar and electrolyte solution
Action	Provides electrolyte and sugar replacement
Indications	Heat-related disorders
	Freshwater drowning
	Hypovolemia
	Peritonitis
Contraindications	Should not be administered to patients with impaired renal or cardiovascular function
	Avoid in head injury and stroke
Precaution	Draw tube of blood before administering to diabetics

Side Effects	Rare
Dosage	Dependent on patient's condition and situation being treated
Route	IV infusion
Pediatric Dosage	Dose is dependent on patient's size and condition

5 Percent Dextrose in 0.45 Percent Sodium Chloride (D₅1/2NS)

Class	Slightly hypertonic sugar and electrolyte solution
Action	Provides electrolyte and sugar replacement
Indications	Heat exhaustion
	Diabetic disorders
	For use as a TKO solution in patients with impaired renal or cardiovascular function
Contraindications	Situations in which rapid fluid replacement is indicated
	Avoid in head injury and stroke
Precaution	Draw tube of blood before administering to diabetics
Side Effects	Rare
Dosage	Dependent on patient's condition and situation being treated
Route	IV infusion
Pediatric Dosage	Dose is dependent on patient's size and condition

5 Percent Dextrose in Lactated Ringer's Solution (D₅LR)

Class	Hypertonic sugar and electrolyte solution
Action	Provides electrolyte and sugar replacement
Indications	Hypovolemic shock
	Hemorrhagic shock
	Certain cases of acidosis
Contraindications	Should not be administered to patients with decreased renal or cardiovascular function
	Avoid in head injury and stroke
Precautions	Monitor for signs of circulatory overload
	Draw tube of blood before administering to diabetics
Side Effects	Rare
Dosage	Dependent on patient's condition and situation being treated
Route	IV infusion
Pediatric Dosage	Dose is dependent on patient's size and condition

Pediatric Fluid Resuscitation

Bolus #1	20 mL normal saline or lactated Ringer's solution
Bolus #2	20 mL normal saline or lactated Ringer's solution
Bolus #3	10 mL/kg of colloid or blood

INTRODUCTION

This appendix provides a quick reference to the most commonly used emergency medications. The dosages and indications have been taken from the most recent Advanced Cardiac Life Support (ACLS) standards of the American Heart Association. Medications not covered in ACLS are taken from the American Medical Association's *Drug Evaluation*. It is important to remember that specific medications, dosages, indications, and routes may vary by area. It is essential that paramedics be familiar with these variations and follow the guidelines established by the medical director of the system in which they work.

 ### Abciximab (ReoPro)

Class	Glycoprotein IIB/IIIA inhibitor
Action	Inhibits platelet aggregation by blocking glycoprotein IIA/IIIB receptors
Indication	Adjunct to percutaneous coronary intervention (PCI)
Contraindications	Internal bleeding (within 6 weeks), GI/GU bleeding, stroke (within 2 years), bleeding disorders, recent major surgery (within 6 weeks), known hypersensitivity to the medication.
Precautions	Abciximab should be used with caution in patients who have an increased risk of bleeding. Allergic reactions have been reported with abciximab.
Side Effects	Increased risk of bleeding, nausea, vomiting, abdominal pain, anemia, pain, sweating.
Dosage	*UA/NSTEMI with planned PCI in < 24 hours*: 0.25 mg/kg IV bolus administered 10–60 minutes prior to PCI, followed by a continuous infusion 0f 0.125 mcg/kg/minute for 12 hours (maximum dose is 10 mcg/min).
Route	IV
Pediatric Dosage	Not routinely used

 ### Acetaminophen, Paracetamol (Tylenol)

Class	Nonnarcotic analgesic, antipyretic
Action	Inhibits cyclooxygenase
Indications	Mild to moderate pain, fever
Contraindications	Known hypersensitivity to the medication.

Precautions	Use with caution in children < 3 years and patients with known liver disease
Side Effects	Minimal within recommended dosage range
Dosage	325–650 mg every 4–6 hours (up to 1 gram is occasionally used as an antipyretic)
Route	PO
Pediatric Dosage	10–15 mg/kg every 4–6 hours

Adenosine (Adenocard)

Class	Antiarrhythmic
Action	Slows atrioventricular conduction
Indication	Regular tachyarrhythmias (narrow- and wide-complex)
Contraindications	*Torsades de pointes* (polymorphic ventricular tachycardia), atrial fibrillation, second- or third-degree heart block, known hypersensitivity to the medication
Precautions	Arrhythmias, including blocks, are common at the time of cardioversion
	Use with caution in patients with asthma
Side Effects	Facial flushing
	Headache
	Shortness of breath
	Dizziness
	Nausea
Dosage	6 mg given as a rapid intravenous (IV) bolus over a 1- to 2-second period; if, after 1–2 minutes, cardioversion does not occur, administer a 12 mg dose over 1–2 seconds
Route	IV; should be administered directly into a vein or into the medication administration port closest to the patient and followed by flushing of the line with IV fluid
Pediatric Dosage	*< 50 kg:* 0.05–0.1 mg/kg IV; Maximum dose: 0.3 mg/kg/dose up to 12 mg
	> 50 kg: Same as adult dose

Albuterol (Proventil)

Class	Sympathomimetic (β_2 selective)
Action	Bronchodilation
Indications	Asthma
	Reversible bronchospasm associated with chronic obstructive pulmonary disease
Contraindications	Known hypersensitivity to the medication
	Symptomatic tachycardia
Precautions	Blood pressure, pulse, and electrocardiogram (ECG) results should be monitored
	Use caution in patients with known heart disease

Side Effects	Palpitations
	Anxiety
	Headache
	Dizziness
	Sweating
Dosage	*Metered-dose inhaler:* One to two sprays (90 mcg per spray)
	Small-volume nebulizer: 0.5 mL (2.5–5.0 mg) in 2.5 mL normal saline over 5–15 minutes
	Rotohaler: One 200 mcg Rotocap should be placed in the inhaler and breathed by the patient
Route	Inhalation
Pediatric Dosage	< 1 year: 0.05–0.15 mg/kg/dose every 4–6 hours
	1–5 years: 1.25–2.5 mg/dose every 4–6 hours
	5–12 years: 2.5 mg/dose every 4–6 hours
	> 12 years: 2.5–5.0 mg/dose every 6 hours

 ## Alteplase, Recombinant Tissue Plasminogen Activator (rtPA) (Activase)

Class	Fibrinolytic
Action	Dissolves blood clots
Indication	Acute coronary syndrome
Contraindications	1. Any prior intracranial hemorrhage
	2. Known structural cerebral vascular lesion (e.g., AVM)
	3. Known malignant intracranial neoplasm (primary or metastatic)
	4. Ischemic stroke within 3 months EXCEPT acute ischemic stroke within 3 hours
	5. Suspected aortic dissection
	6. Active bleeding or bleeding diathesis (excluding menses)
	7. Significant closed head trauma or facial trauma within 3 months

It is relatively contraindicated (i.e., the risks must be weighed against the potential benefits) in the following cases:

1. History of chronic, severe, poorly controlled hypertension
2. Severe uncontrolled hypertension on presentation (SBP > 180 mm Hg or DBP > 110 mm Hg). This could be an absolute contraindication in low-risk patients with myocardial infarction.
3. History of prior ischemic stroke > 3 months, dementia, or known intracranial pathology not covered in contraindications
4. Traumatic or prolonged (< 10 minutes) CPR or major surgery (< 3 weeks)
5. Recent (within 2 to 4 weeks) internal bleeding
6. Noncompressible vascular punctures
7. For streptokinase/anistreplase: prior exposure (> 5 days ago) or prior allergic reaction to these agents

Anaphylaxis can occur with alteplase therapy but is very rare. Emergency resuscitative medications and equipment should be immediately available. Reperfusion arrhythmias are common once the occluded artery opens. Antiarrhythmic medications should be immediately available.

Side Effects	Bleeding
	Allergic reactions
	Anaphylaxis
	Fever
	Nausea and vomiting
Dosage	Loading dose of 15 mg is administered as an IV bolus over 1 to 2 minutes. This is followed by an infusion of 0.75 mg/kg (up to 50 mg) IV over the first 30 minutes then 0.5 mg/kg (up to 35 mg) IV over 60 minutes. The infusion must be carefully administered via a controlled IV pump.
Route	IV (slow)
Pediatric Dosage	Not recommended

Aminophylline

Class	Xanthine bronchodilator
Actions	Smooth muscle relaxant
	Causes bronchodilation
	Has mild diuretic properties
	Increases heart rate
Indications	Bronchial asthma
	Reversible bronchospasm associated with chronic bronchitis and emphysema
	Congestive heart failure
	Pulmonary edema
Contraindications	Patients with history of hypersensitivity to the medication
	Hypotension
	Patients with peptic ulcer disease
Precautions	Monitor for arrhythmias
	Monitor blood pressure
	Do not administer to patients on chronic theophylline preparations until the theophylline blood level has been determined
Side Effects	Convulsions
	Tremor
	Anxiety
	Dizziness
	Vomiting
	Palpitations
	PVCs
	Tachycardia

Dosages	*Method 1:* 250–500 mg in 90 or 80 mL of D_5W infused over 20–30 minutes (approximately 5–10 mg/kg/hr)
	Method 2: 250–500 mg (5–7 mg/kg) in 20 mL of D_5W infused over 20–30 minutes
Route	Slow IV infusion
Pediatric Dosage	6 mg/kg loading dose to be infused over 20–30 minutes; maximum dose not to exceed 12 mg/kg over 24 hours

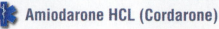

Amiodarone HCL (Cordarone)

Class	Antiarrhythmic (Class III)
Action	Prolongs action potential and refractory period
	Slows the sinus rate; increases PR and QT intervals
	Decreases peripheral vascular resistance (α and β adrenergic blockade)
Indications	Life-threatening cardiac arrhythmias such as ventricular tachycardia and ventricular fibrillation
Contraindications	Severe sinus node dysfunction
	Sinus bradycardia
	Second- and third-degree atrioventricular block
	Hemodynamically significant bradycardia
Precaution	Heart failure
Side Effects	Hypotension
	Nausea
	Anorexia
	Malaise, fatigue
	Tremors
	Pulmonary toxicity
	Ventricular ectopic beats
Dosage	*Ventricular fibrillation or pulseless ventricular tachycardia (adults):* 300 mg. May be repeated at 150 mg for recurrent or refractory arrhythmias.
	Narrow-complex tachycardias: Amiodarone should be dosed at 150 mg IV/IO over 10 minute and repeated as necessary. This can be followed by a 1 mg/min infusion over 6 hours, followed by a 0.5 mg/min infusion as needed. The total 24-hour dose should not exceed 2.2 gm.
Route	IV
Pediatric Dosage	5 mg/kg IV or IO over 30 minutes. May repeat twice up to 15 mg/kg. Maximum single dose 300 mg

Amyl Nitrite

Class	Nitrate
Actions	Causes coronary vasodilation
	Removes cyanide ion via complex mechanism
Indication	Cyanide poisoning (bitter almond smell to breath)

Contraindications	None when used in the management of cyanide poisoning
Precaution	Has tendency for abuse
Side Effects	Headache
	Hypotension
	Reflex tachycardia
	Nausea
Dosage	Inhalant should be broken and inhaled; repeated as needed until patient is delivered to emergency department; effects diminish after 20 minutes
Route	Inhalation
Pediatric Dosage	Inhalant should be broken and inhaled; repeated until patient is delivered to emergency department

Anistreplase (Eminase)

Class	Fibrinolytic
Action	Dissolves blood clots
Indication	Acute coronary syndrome
Contraindications	1. Any prior intracranial hemorrhage

2. Known structural cerebral vascular lesion (e.g., AVM)
3. Known malignant intracranial neoplasm (primary or metastatic)
4. Ischemic stroke within 3 months EXCEPT acute ischemic stroke within 3 hours
5. Suspected aortic dissection
6. Active bleeding or bleeding diathesis (excluding menses)
7. Significant closed head trauma or facial trauma within 3 months

It is relatively contraindicated (i.e., the risks must be weighed against the potential benefits) in the following cases:

1. History of chronic, severe, poorly controlled hypertension
2. Severe uncontrolled hypertension on presentation (SBP > 180 mm Hg or DBP > 110 mm Hg). This could be an absolute contraindication in low-risk patients with myocardial infarction.
3. History of prior ischemic stroke > 3 months, dementia, or known intracranial pathology not covered in contraindications
4. Traumatic or prolonged (> 10 minutes) CPR or major surgery (< 3 weeks)
5. Recent (within 2 to 4 weeks) internal bleeding
6. Noncompressible vascular punctures
7. For streptokinase/anistreplase: prior exposure (> 5 days ago) or prior allergic reaction to these agents

Precautions	May be ineffective if administered within 12 months of prior streptokinase or anistreplase therapy
	Antiarrhythmic and resuscitative medications should be available

Side Effects	Bleeding
	Allergic reactions
	Anaphylaxis
	Fever
	Nausea and vomiting
Dosage	30 units slow intravenously over 4–5 minutes as part of Eminase protocol
Route	IV (slow)
Pediatric Dosage	Not recommended

✡ Aspirin

Class	Platelet inhibitor and anti-inflammatory
Action	Inhibits platelet aggregation
Indications	New chest pain suggestive of acute myocardial infarction
	Signs and symptoms suggestive of recent stroke (cerebrovascular accident)
Contraindication	Patients with known hypersensitivity to the medication
Precautions	Gastrointestinal bleeding and upset stomach
Side Effects	Heartburn
	Nausea and vomiting
	Wheezing
Dosage	160 or 325 mg by mouth chewed
Route	Oral
Pediatric Dosage	10–15 mg/kg/dose every 4–6 hours

✡ Atracurium (Tracrium)

Class	Nondepolarizing neuromuscular blocker
Action	Paralyzes skeletal muscles including respiratory muscles
Indication	To achieve paralysis for endotracheal intubation (rapid-sequence induction)
Contraindication	Patients with known hypersensitivity to the medication
Precautions	Should not be administered unless persons skilled in endotracheal intubation are present
	Endotracheal intubation equipment must be available
	Oxygen equipment and emergency resuscitative medications must be available
	Paralysis occurs in 2 minutes and lasts 35–70 minutes
Side Effects	Prolonged paralysis
	Hypotension
	Bradycardia
Dosage	0.4–0.5 mg/kg IV
Route	IV
Pediatric Dosage	< 2 years: 0.3–0.4 mg/kg; > 2 years: 0.4–0.5 mg

Atropine

Class	Parasympatholytic (anticholinergic)
Actions	Blocks acetylcholine receptors
	Increases heart rate
	Decreases gastrointestinal secretions
Indications	Hemodynamically significant bradycardia
	Organophosphate poisoning
Contraindication	None when used in emergency situations
Precautions	Dose of 3 mg should not be exceeded except in cases of organophosphate poisonings
	Tachycardia
	Hypertension
Side Effects	Palpitations
	Tachycardia
	Headache
	Dizziness
	Anxiety
	Dry mouth
	Pupillary dilation
	Blurred vision
	Urinary retention (especially in older men)
Dosage	*Bradycardia:* 0.5 mg every 3–5 minutes to maximum of 3.0 mg
	Organophosphate poisoning: 2–5 mg or more
Routes	Intravenous (IV)
	Endotracheal (endotracheal dose 2 to 2.5 times the IV dose)
Pediatric Dosage	*Bradycardia:* 0.02 mg/kg (minimum dose of 0.1 mg)
	Maximum single dose: child, 0.5 mg

Bumetanide (Bumex)

Class	Potent diuretic
Actions	Inhibits reabsorption of sodium chloride
	Promotes prompt diuresis
	Slight vasodilation
Indications	Congestive heart failure
	Pulmonary edema
Contraindications	Dehydration
	Pregnancy
Precautions	Should be protected from light
	Dehydration
Side Effects	Few in emergency usage
Dosage	0.5–1.0 mg
Routes	IV, IM
Pediatric Dosage	≥ 6 months: 0.015–0.1 mg/kg/dose

✹ Butorphanol (Stadol)

Class	Synthetic analgesic
Actions	Central nervous system depressant
	Decreases sensitivity to pain
Indication	Moderate to severe pain
Contraindications	Patients with a history of hypersensitivity to the medication
	Head injury
	Use with caution in patients with impaired respiratory function
Precautions	Respiratory depression (naloxone should be available)
	Patients dependent on narcotics
Side Effects	Symptoms of withdrawal when administered to persons dependent on narcotics
	Nausea
	Altered levels of consciousness
Dosage	*Intravenous:* 1 mg
	Intramuscular: 2 mg
Routes	IV, IM
Pediatric Dosage	Rarely used

✹ Calcium Chloride

Class	Electrolyte
Action	Increases cardiac contractility
Indications	Acute hyperkalemia (elevated potassium level)
	Acute hypocalcemia (decreased calcium level)
	Calcium channel blocker (e.g., nifedipine, verapamil) overdose
	Abdominal muscle spasm associated with spider bite and Portuguese man-of-war stings
	Antidote for magnesium sulfate
Contraindication	Patients receiving digitalis
Precautions	IV line should be flushed between calcium chloride and sodium bicarbonate administration
	Extravasation may cause tissue necrosis
Side Effects	Arrhythmias (bradycardia and asystole)
	Hypotension
Dosage	2–4 mg/kg of a 10 percent solution; may be repeated at 10-minute intervals
Route	IV
Pediatric Dosage	5–7 mg/kg of a 10 percent solution

✹ Captopril (Capoten)

Class	Angiotensin-converting enzyme (ACE) inhibitor
Actions	Peripheral smooth muscle relaxant thus lowering blood pressure (both systolic and diastolic)

Indications	Hypertension
	Congestive heart failure
Contraindications	Pregnancy, angioedema (swelling of the tongue and mouth) and known hypersensitivity to the medication
Precautions	Hypotension
Side Effects	Cough
	Headache
	Dizziness
	Syncope
Dosage	12.5–25 mg
Route	Sublingually
Pediatric Dosage	Not indicated in prehospital setting

Chlorpromazine (Thorazine, Largactil)

Class	Major tranquilizer (Phenothiazine)
Actions	Blocks dopamine receptors in brain associated with mood and behavior
	Has antiemetic properties
Indications	Acute psychotic episodes
	Mild alcohol withdrawal
	Intractable hiccoughs
	Nausea and vomiting
Contraindications	Comatose states
	Presence of sedatives
	Presence of hallucinogens or phencyclidine-like compounds
Precautions	Orthostatic hypotension
	May cause extrapyramidal reactions (Parkinsonian), especially in children
Side Effects	Physical and mental impairment
	Drowsiness
Dosage	25–100 mg
Route	IM
Pediatric Dosage	0.5 mg/kg

Clevidipine (Cleviprex)

Class	Calcium channel blocker
Actions	Causes vascular smooth muscle relaxation reducing peripheral vascular resistance and blood pressure
Indications	Hypertensive emergencies
Contraindications	Patients who are hypotensive or who have known hypersensitivity to the drug
Precautions	Can cause significant drop in blood pressure. Do not give with beta blockers.

Side Effects	Nausea
	Vomiting
	Dizziness
	Headache
Dosage	Initial dose of 1–2 mg/hr titrated to achieve desired BP. Dose may be doubled as often as every 90 seconds. The rate of clevidipine titration may become less rapid as BP nears the goal, with dose increases every 5–10 minutes at a rate of 1–2 mg/hr. Dosage should not exceed 32 mg/hr based on available studies.
Route	IV
Pediatric Dosage	Not indicated

✴ Clopidogrel (Plavix)

Class	Platelet aggregate inhibitor
Actions	Inhibits platelet aggregation by binding to ADP receptors on the surface of platelets
Indications	Acute coronary syndrome
	Stroke
	Peripheral vascular disease
Contraindications	Bleeding disorders
	Peptic ulcer
	Known hypersensitivity to the medication
Precautions	Do not use with nonsteroidal anti-inflammatory drugs (NSAIDs)
Side Effects	Bleeding
	Fever
	Allergic reactions
	Myalgias
	Rash
Dosage	*Acute coronary syndrome:* Non-ST-segment elevation ACS (UA/NSTEMI): 300 mg loading dose followed by 75 mg once daily, in combination with aspirin (75–325 mg once daily)
	STEMI: 75 mg once daily, in combination with aspirin (75–325 mg once daily), with or without a loading dose and with or without thrombolytics
	Recent MI, recent stroke, or established peripheral arterial disease: 75 mg once daily
Route	PO
Pediatric Dosage	Not indicated

✴ Dexamethasone (Decadron, Hexadrol)

Class	Steroid
Actions	Possibly decreases cerebral edema
	Anti-inflammatory
	Suppresses immune response (especially in allergic reactions)

Indications	Anaphylaxis (after epinephrine and diphenhydramine)
	Asthma
	Chronic obstructive pulmonary disease
Contraindications	None in the emergency setting
Precautions	Should be protected from heat
	Onset of action may be 2–6 hours and thus should not be considered to be of use in the critical first hour following an anaphylactic reaction
Side Effects	Gastrointestinal bleeding
	Prolonged wound healing
Dosage	4–24 mg
Routes	IV, IM
Pediatric Dosage	0.2–0.5 mg/kg

Dextrose (50 Percent)

Class	Carbohydrate
Action	Elevates blood glucose level rapidly
Indication	Hypoglycemia
Contraindications	None in the emergency setting
Precaution	A blood sample should be drawn before administering 50 percent dextrose
Side Effect	Local venous irritation
Dosage	25 g (50 mL)
Route	IV
Pediatric Dosage	0.5 g/kg slow IV; should be diluted 1:1 with sterile water to form a 25 percent solution

Diazepam (Valium)

Class	Tranquilizer (benzodiazepine)
Actions	Anticonvulsant
	Skeletal muscle relaxant
	Sedative
Indications	Major motor seizures
	Status epilepticus
	Premedication before cardioversion
	Skeletal muscle relaxant
	Acute anxiety states
Contraindication	Patients with a history of hypersensitivity to the medication
Precautions	Can cause local venous irritation
	Has short duration of effect
	Do not mix with other medications because of possible precipitation problems
	Flumazenil (Romazicon) should be available

Side Effects	Drowsiness
	Hypotension
	Respiratory depression and apnea
Dosage	*Status epilepticus:* 5–10 mg intravenously (IV)
	Acute anxiety: 2–5 mg intramuscularly (IM) or IV
	Premedication before cardioversion: 5–15 mg IV
Routes	IV (care must be taken not to administer faster than 1 mL/min), IM, rectal
Pediatric Dosage	*Status epilepticus:* 0.1–0.2 mg/kg

Digoxin (Lanoxin)

Class	Cardiac glycoside, antiarrhythmic, inotrope
Actions	Increases cardiac contractile force
	Increases cardiac output
	Reduces edema associated with congestive heart failure
	Slows atrioventricular conduction
Indications	Congestive heart failure
	Rapid atrial arrhythmias, especially atrial flutter and atrial fibrillation
Contraindications	Any patient with signs or symptoms of digitalis toxicity
	Ventricular fibrillation
Precautions	Monitor for signs of digitalis toxicity
	Patients who have recently suffered a myocardial infarction have greater sensitivity to the effects of digitalis
	Calcium should not be administered to patients receiving digitalis
Side Effects	Nausea and vomiting
	Arrhythmias
	Yellow vision
Dosage	0.25–0.50 mg
Route	IV
Pediatric Dosage	Rarely used in prehospital setting

Diltiazem (Cardizem)

Class	Calcium channel blocker
Actions	Slows conduction through the atrioventricular mode
	Causes vasodilation
	Decreases rate of ventricular response
	Decreases myocardial oxygen demand
Indications	Stable, narrow-complex tachycardias if rhythm remains uncontrolled or unconverted by adenosine or vagal maneuvers or if SVT is recurrent
	Control ventricular rate in patients with atrial fibrillation or atrial flutter

Contraindications	Hypotension
	Wide-complex tachycardia
	Conduction system disturbances
Precautions	Should not be used in patients receiving intravenous β-blockers
	Hypotension
	Must be kept refrigerated
Side Effects	Nausea and vomiting
	Hypotension
	Dizziness
Dosage	15–20 mg IV bolus (0.25 mg/kg) over 2 minutes. Additional bolus doses of 20–25 mg (0.35 mg/kg) can be administered in 15 minutes as needed. A maintenance infusion of 5–15 mg/hr can be administered for rate control (titrated to the desired rate).
Routes	IV, IV drip
Pediatric Dosage	Rarely used

Dimenhydrinate (Gravol, Dramamine)

Class	Antihistamine
Action	Antiemetic
Indications	Nausea and vomiting
	Motion sickness
	To potentiate the effects of analgesics
Contraindications	Comatose states
	Patients who have received a large amount of depressants (including alcohol)
Precautions	Use with caution in patients with seizure disorders
	Asthma
Side Effects	May impair mental and physical ability
	Drowsiness
Dosage	*Slow intravenous:* 12.5–25.0 mg
	Intramuscular or oral: 50–100 mg
Routes	IV, IM, oral
Pediatric Dosage	Pediatric data unavailable

Diphenhydramine (Benadryl)

Class	Antihistamine
Actions	Blocks histamine receptors
	Has some sedative effects
Indications	Anaphylaxis
	Allergic reactions
	Dystonic reactions due to phenothiazines

Contraindications	Asthma
	Nursing mothers
Precautions	Hypotension
Side Effects	Sedation
	Dries bronchial secretions
	Blurred vision
	Headache
	Palpitations
Dosage	25–50 mg
Routes	Slow IV push, deep IM
Pediatric Dosage	2–5 mg/kg

Dobutamine (Dobutrex)

Class	Sympathomimetic
Actions	Increases cardiac contractility
	Little chronotropic activity
Indication	Short-term management of congestive heart failure
Contraindication	Should only be used in patients with an adequate heart rate
Precautions	Ventricular irritability
	Use with caution following myocardial infarction
	Can be deactivated by alkaline solutions
Side Effects	Headache
	Hypertension
	Palpitations
Dosage	2.5–20 mcg/kg/min
	Method: 250 mg should be placed in 500 mL of D_5W, which gives a concentration of 0.5 mg/mL
Route	IV drip
Pediatric Dosage	2–20 mcg/kg/min

Dolasetron (Anzemet)

Class	Antiemetic
Actions	Blocks the serotonin receptors in the CTZ, the stomach, and the small intestines
Indications	Nausea, vomiting
Contraindications	Known hypersensitivity to the medicine
Precautions	Use with caution in patients taking serotonin blockers
Side Effects	Headache, lightheadedness, dizziness
Dosage	100 mg IV over 30 seconds
Route	IV, PO
Pediatric Dosage	Rarely used in prehospital setting

✳ Dopamine (Intropin)

Class	Sympathomimetic
Actions	Increases cardiac contractility
	Causes peripheral vasoconstriction
Indications	Hemodynamically significant hypotension (systolic blood pressure of 70–100 mmHg) not resulting from hypovolemia
	Symptomatic bradycardia refractory to atropine
Contraindications	Hypovolemic shock in which complete fluid resuscitation has not occurred
	Pheochromocytoma
Precautions	Presence of severe tachyarrhythmias
	Presence of ventricular fibrillation
	Ventricular irritability
	Beneficial effects lost when dose exceeds 20 mcg/kg/min
Side Effects	Ventricular tachyarrhythmias
	Hypertension
	Palpitations
Dosage	*Initial dose:* 2–5 mcg/kg/min; increase as needed
	Method: 800 mg should be placed in 500 mL of D_5W, giving a concentration of 1600 mg/mL
Route	IV drip only
Pediatric Dosage	2–20 mcg/kg/min

✳ Droperidol (Inapsine)

Class	Butyrophenone antipsychotic/antiemetic
Actions	Antagonizes the effects of medications that act on the chemoreceptor trigger zone (CTZ)
	Reduces anxiety and produces sedation
Indication	Acute psychosis
	Nausea/vomiting
Contraindication	Patients with known hypersensitivity to the medication
Precautions	"Black box" warning regarding QT interval prolongation
	Use with caution in the elderly, debilitated, or poor-risk patients
	Monitor vital signs and ECG
Side Effects	Drowsiness
	EPS symptoms (dystonia)
	Dizziness
	Restlessness
	Hypotension
	Tachycardia
Dosage	2.5–10.0 mg IV
Route	IV
Pediatric Dosage	0.088–0.165 mg/kg IV (children > 2 years)

Edrophonium (Tensilon)

Class	Anticholinesterase
Actions	Inhibits action of enzyme cholinesterase, thus potentiating acetylcholine
	Increases parasympathetic tone
Indications	PSVT refractory to vagal maneuvers; considered a second-line agent to verapamil or adenosine
Contraindication	Patients with a history of hypersensitivity to the medication
Precautions	Respirations must be constantly monitored
	Bradycardia
	Hypotension
	Avoid exposure to dextrose solutions
Side Effects	Dizziness
	Syncope
Dosage	5 mg
Route	IV
Pediatric Dosage	0.1–0.2 mg/kg

Enalaprilat (Vasotec)

Class	Angiotensin-converting enzyme (ACE) inhibitor
Actions	Peripheral smooth muscle relaxant thus lowering blood pressure (both systolic and diastolic)
Indications	Hypertension
	Congestive heart failure
Contraindications	Pregnancy, angioedema (swelling of the tongue and mouth) and known hypersensitivity to the medication.
Precautions	Hypotension
Side Effects	Cough, headache, dizziness, syncope
Dosage	1.25–5.0 mg (typically 1.25 mg)
Route	IV
Pediatric Dosage	Not indicated in prehospital setting

Enoxaparin (Lovenox)

Class	Anticoagulant (low molecular-weight heparin)
Action	Acts as effective anticoagulant
Indications	Unstable angina
	Non-Q-wave myocardial infarction
	Pulmonary embolism
	Deep venous thrombosis
Contraindication	Patients with a known hypersensitivity to the medication or heparin
Precaution	Do not use in patients with major bleeding or at increased risk of bleeding

Side Effects	Confusion
	Dizziness
	Edema
	Bleeding complications
Dosage	*Adult dose (STEMI):* 30 mg IV plus a 1 mg/kg SQ dose followed by 1 mg/kg SQ SC every 12 hours (maximum 100 mg for the first two doses only).
	Adult dose (unstable angina (UA)/non-ST segment elevation myocardial infarction (NSTEMI)): 1 mg/kg administered SQ every 12 hours in conjunction with oral aspirin therapy (100–325 mg once daily)
Routes	SC, IV
Pediatric Dosage	1 mg/kg SQ

✴ Epinephrine 1:1 000

Class	Sympathomimetic
Action	Bronchodilation
Indications	Bronchial asthma
	Exacerbation of chronic obstructive pulmonary disease
	Allergic reactions
	Pediatric cardiac arrest (after initial epinephrine dosage)
Contraindications	Patients with underlying cardiovascular disease
	Hypertension
	Pregnancy
	Patients with tachyarrhythmias
Precautions	Should be protected from light
	Blood pressure, pulse, and electrocardiogram (ECG) results must be constantly monitored
Side Effects	Palpitations and tachycardia
	Anxiousness
	Headache
	Tremor
Dosage	0.3–0.5 mg
Route	IM
Pediatric Dosage	0.01 mg/kg up to 0.3 mg

✴ Epinephrine 1:10 000

Class	Sympathomimetic
Actions	Increases heart rate and automaticity
	Increases cardiac contractile force
	Increases myocardial electrical activity
	Increases systemic vascular resistance
	Increases blood pressure
	Causes bronchodilation

Indications	Cardiac arrest
	Anaphylactic shock
	Severe reactive airway disease
Contraindications	Epinephrine 1:10 000 is for intravenous (IV) or endotracheal use; it should not be used in patients who do not require extensive resuscitative efforts
Precautions	Should be protected from light
	Can be deactivated by alkaline solutions
Side Effects	Palpitations
	Anxiety
	Tremulousness
	Nausea and vomiting
Dosage	*Cardiac arrest:* 1 mg repeated every 3–5 minutes; higher doses may be ordered by medical control
	Severe anaphylaxis: 0.05–0.1 mg (5–10 percent of the epinephrine dose used routinely in cardiac arrest) IV/IO. An epinephrine drip may be required.
Routes	IV, IV drip, endotracheal (endotracheal dose 2–2.5 times IV dose)
Pediatric Dosage	0.01 mg/kg initially; with subsequent doses every 3–5 minutes as needed

Eptifibatide (Integrillin)

Class	Glycoprotein IIB/IIIA inhibitor
Action	Inhibits platelet aggregation by blocking glycoprotein IIA/IIIB receptors
Indication	ACS patients undergoing percutaneous coronary intervention (PCI) as well as those who will be managed medically
Contraindications	Known hypersensitivity to the drug, active internal bleeding or history of bleeding within previous 30 days, severe uncontrolled hypertension (systolic BP $>$ 200 mm Hg and/or diastolic BP $>$ 110 mm Hg), major surgical procedure within 6 weeks, history of hemorrhagic stroke or other stroke within 30 days, concurrent use of other glycoprotein IIb/IIIa receptor antagonists, platelet count $<$ 100,000/mm^3, severe renal insufficiency or dependency on renal dialysis.
Precautions	Eptifibatide should be used with caution in patients who have an increased risk of bleeding
Side Effects	Increased risk of bleeding, hypotension
Dosage	*Acute Coronary Syndrome:* 180 mcg/kg as a bolus dose, followed by 2 mcg/kg/min until hospital discharge or surgical intervention (up to 72 hours)
	Percutaneous Coronary Intervention: 180 mcg/kg as a bolus dose, immediately before PCI, followed by 2 mcg/kg/min infusion followed by a second bolus of 180 mcg/kg is given 10 min after first bolus; infusion should continue for 18–24 or hospital discharge (minimum of 12 hours)

Route	IV
Pediatric Dosage	Not routinely used

✦ Esmolol (Brevibloc)

Class	Beta-blocker (β_1 selective)
Actions	Decreases heart rate
	Decreases atrioventricular conduction
Indications	Stable, narrow-complex tachycardias
	Rate control in atrial fibrillation or atrial flutter
	Certain forms of polymorphic VT
Contraindications	Sinus bradycardia
	Heart block greater than first degree
	Cardiogenic shock
	Overt congestive heart failure
	Patients with bronchospastic disease (asthma)
Precautions	Hypotension is common and is usually dose related
	Patients with congestive heart failure may have worsening of their symptoms
	May worsen bronchospastic disease
Side Effects	Dizziness
	Diaphoresis
	Hypotension
	Nausea
Dosage	*Preparation:* Place two 2.5 g ampules in 500 mL of D_5W, yielding a concentration of 10 mg/mL
	Loading dose: 500 mcg/kg/min for 1 minute, then reduce to maintenance dose
	Maintenance dose: 50 mcg/kg/min; if ineffective after 4 minutes, repeat loading dose and increase maintenance dose to 100 mcg/kg/min; may repeat as needed until a total maintenance dose of 300 mcg/kg/min has been achieved
Route	IV infusion only
Pediatric Dosage	100–500 mcg/kg/min loading dose over 1 minute, followed 25–50 mcg/kg/minute maintenance infusion

✦ Etomidate (Amidate)

Class	Sedative/hypnotic
Action	Creates an ultra-short-acting sedative/hypnotic effect
Indication	Induction agent for rapid-sequence induction
Contraindication	Known hypersensitivity to the medication
Precautions	Marked hypotension
	Severe asthma
	Severe cardiovascular disease
	Adrenal suppression

Side Effects	Myoclonic skeletal muscle movement
	Apnea
	Laryngospasm
Dosage	0.1–0.3 mg/kg IV over 15–30 seconds
Route	IV
Pediatric Dosage	*> 10 years:* same as adult dose;
	< 10 years: not indicated

 ## Fentanyl Citrate (Sublimaze)

Class	Narcotic
Actions	Central nervous system depressant
	Decreases sensitivity to pain
Indications	Severe pain
	Adjunct to rapid-sequence induction
	Maintenance of analgesia
Contraindications	Shock
	Severe hemorrhage
	Patients with history of hypersensitivity to the medication
Precautions	Respiratory depression (naloxone should be available)
	Hypotension
	Nausea
Side Effects	Dizziness
	Altered level of consciousness
	Bradycardia
Dosage	25–100 mcg
Route	IV, IN
Pediatric Dosage	2–12 years: 1–2 mcg/kg/dose

Flumazenil (Romazicon)

Class	Benzodiazepine antagonist
Action	Reverses the effects of benzodiazepines
Indication	To reverse central nervous system respiratory depression associated with benzodiazepines
Contraindications	Flumazenil should not be used as a diagnostic agent for benzodiazepine overdose in the same manner naloxone is used for narcotic overdose
	Known hypersensitivity to the medication
Precautions	Administer with caution to patients dependent on benzodiazepines because it may induce life-threatening benzodiazepine withdrawal
	Should not be used as part of a "coma cocktail"
Side Effects	Fatigue
	Headache

	Nervousness
	Dizziness
Dosage	0.2 mg IV over 30 seconds, repeated as needed to a maximum dose of 1.0 mg
Route	IV
Pediatric Dosage	0.01 mg/kg (max dose = 0.2 mg)

 ## Fosphenytoin (Cerebyx)

Class	Anticonvulsant
Actions	Converts to phenytoin
	Suppresses seizure activity
Indications	Major motor seizures
	Antiarrhythmic
Contraindication	Hypersensitivity to the medication or to the phenytoin (hydantoin) class of medications
Precautions	Patients with impaired renal function
	Alcoholism
	Hypotension
	Heart block
Side Effects	Dizziness
	Somnolence
	Hypotension
	Heart block
Dosage	15–20 mg phenytoin equivalent/kg IV, IM
Route	IV, IM
Pediatric Dosage	15–20 mg phenytoin equivalent/kg IV/IM

Furosemide (Lasix)

Class	Potent diuretic
Actions	Inhibits reabsorption of sodium chloride
	Promotes prompt diuresis
	Vasodilation
Indications	Congestive heart failure
	Pulmonary edema
Contraindications	Pregnancy
	Dehydration
Precautions	Should be protected from light
	Dehydration
Side Effects	Few in emergency usage
Dosage	40–80 mg
Route	IV
Pediatric Dosage	0.5–2.0 mg/kg/dose

Glucagon

Class	Hormone (antihypoglycemic agent)
Actions	Causes breakdown of glycogen to glucose
	Inhibits glycogen synthesis
	Elevates blood glucose level
	Increases cardiac contractile force
	Increases heart rate
Indications	Hypoglycemia
	Beta-blocker overdose
Contraindication	Hypersensitivity to the medication
Precautions	Effective only if there are sufficient stores of glycogen within the liver
	Use with caution in patients with cardiovascular or renal disease
	Draw blood for glucose test before administration
Side Effects	Few in emergency situations
Dosage	*Intravenous:* 0.25–0.5 unit
	Intramuscular: 1.0 mg
Routes	IV, IM
Pediatric Dosage	0.03 mg/kg

Haloperidol (Haldol)

Class	Major tranquilizer (butyrophenone)
Actions	Blocks dopamine receptors in brain responsible for mood and behavior
	Has antiemetic properties
Indication	Acute psychotic episodes
Contraindications	Should not be administered in the presence of other sedatives
	Should not be used in the management of dysphoria caused by Talwin
Precaution	Orthostatic hypotension
Side Effects	Physical and mental impairment
	Parkinson-like reactions have been known to occur, especially in children
Dosage	2–5 mg
Route	IM
Pediatric Dosage	Rarely used

Heparin

Class	Anticoagulant (unfractionated)
Actions	Direct inhibitor of thrombin
Indications	Acute Coronary Syndrome (ACS)
	Pulmonary embolism

Contraindications	Known hypersensitivity to the drug and/or beef or pork products
Precautions	Do not use in patients with active major bleeding or thrombocytopenia. Use with caution in the elderly or any patient with increased risk of bleeding
Side Effects	Confusion, edema, dizziness, bleeding complications
Dosage	*Adult dose (acute STEMI and unstable angina):* 60 U/kg IV (maximum 4,000 units) followed by 12 U/kg/hr (maximum 1,000 U/hr). This is often given with alteplase (rtPA) *Adult dose (NSTEMI and unstable angina):* 60–70 U/kg IV (maximum, 5000 U) as initial bolus followed by a 12–15-U/kg/h infusion
Route	IV
Pediatric Dosage	50 units/kg followed by IV infusion

 ## Hydralazine (Apresoline)

Class	Antihypertensive (potent vasodilator)
Actions	Relaxes vascular smooth muscle
	Decreases arterial pressure (diastolic greater than systolic)
	Increases cardiac output
Indications	Hypertensive emergency in which a prompt reduction in blood pressure is required
	Hypertension accompanying pregnancy
Contraindications	Patients with a known history of coronary artery disease
	Rheumatic heart disease involving the mitral valve
	History of hypersensitivity to the medication
Precautions	May induce angina
	May cause electrocardiogram (ECG) changes and cardiac ischemia
	Blood pressure, pulse rate, and ECG results should be constantly monitored
Side Effects	Headache
	Nausea
	Vomiting
	Tachycardia
	Palpitations
	Diarrhea
Dosage	20–40 mg given by slow IV bolus; may be repeated, if required
Route	IV
Pediatric Dosage	Safety in children has not been established

Hydrocortisone (Solu-Cortef)

Class	Steroid
Actions	Anti-inflammatory
	Suppresses immune response (especially in allergic and anaphylactic reactions)
Indications	Severe anaphylaxis
	Asthma and chronic obstructive pulmonary disease
	Urticaria (hives)
Contraindications	None in the emergency setting
Precautions	Must be reconstituted and used promptly
	Onset of action may be 2–6 hours, and thus the medication should not be expected to be of use in the critical first hour following an acute anaphylactic reaction
Side Effects	Gastrointestinal bleeding
	Prolonged wound healing
	Suppression of natural steroids
Dosage	100–250 mg
Routes	IV, IM
Pediatric Dosage	30 mg/kg

Hydromorphone (Dilaudid)

Class	Narcotic
Actions	Central nervous system depressant
	Decreases sensitivity to pain
Indications	Severe pain
Contraindications	Shock
	Severe hemorrhage
	Patients with history of hypersensitivity to the medication
Precautions	Respiratory depression (naloxone should be available)
	Hypotension
	Nausea
Side Effects	Dizziness
	Altered level of consciousness
	Bradycardia
Dosage	1–4 mg
Route	IV, IM, PO
Pediatric Dosage	0.015 mg/kg/dose IV

Hydroxocobalamin (CyanoKit)

Class	Cyanide antidote
Actions	Chelates cyanide ion from cytochrome oxidase
Indications	Presumed or confirmed cyanide poisoning
Contraindications	None when used in the setting of cyanide poisoning

Precautions	Allergic reactions and transient hypertension reported
Side Effects	Red skin and urine, elevated blood pressure, flushing
Dosage	5 g IV infusion over 15 minutes. A second dose of 5 g may be administered as needed by IV infusion for a total dose of 10 g
Route	IV
Pediatric Dosage	Not studied, although there are some reported cases of successful usage

Hydroxyzine (Vistaril)

Class	Antihistamine
Actions	Antiemetic
	Antihistamine
	Antianxiety
	Potentiates analgesic effects of narcotics and related agents
Indications	To potentiate the effects of narcotics and synthetic narcotics
	Nausea and vomiting
	Anxiety reactions
Contraindication	Patients with a history of hypersensitivity to the medication
Precautions	Orthostatic hypotension
	Analgesic dosages should be reduced when used with hydroxyzine
	Urinary retention
Side Effect	Drowsiness
Dosage	50–100 mg
Route	Deep IM
Pediatric Dosage	1 mg/kg

Ibuprofen (Motrin, Advil)

Class	NSAID
Action	Anti-inflammatory, prostaglandin inhibitor
Indications	Mild to moderate pain
	Fever
Contraindication	Patients with known hypersensitivity to the medication, patients taking other NSAIDs
Precautions	Gastrointestinal bleeding and upset stomach
Side Effects	Heartburn
	Nausea and vomiting
	Wheezing
Dosage	200–800 mg/dose
Route	PO
Pediatric Dosage	5–10 mg/kg/dose every 4–6 hours

Inamrinone (Inocor)

Class	Cardiac inotrope
Actions	Increases cardiac contractility
	Vasodilator
Indication	Short-term management of severe congestive heart failure
Contraindication	Patients with history of hypersensitivity to the medication
Precautions	May increase myocardial ischemia
	Blood pressure, pulse, and electrocardiogram (ECG) results should be constantly monitored
	Inamrinone should only be diluted with normal saline or one-half normal saline; no dextrose solutions should be used
	Furosemide (Lasix) should not be administered into an IV line delivering inamrinone
Side Effects	Reduction in platelets
	Nausea and vomiting
	Cardiac arrhythmias
Dosage	0.75 mg/kg bolus given slowly over 2–5-minute interval followed by maintenance infusion of 2–15 mg/kg/min
Route	IV bolus and infusion as described earlier
Pediatric Dosage	Safety in children has not been established

Insulin (Humilin, Novolin, Iletin)

Class	Hormone (hypoglycemic agent)
Actions	Causes uptake of glucose by the cells
	Decreases blood glucose level
	Promotes glucose storage
Indications	Elevated blood glucose
	Diabetic ketoacidosis
Contraindications	Avoid overcompensation of blood glucose level; if possible, administration should wait until the patient is in the emergency department
Precautions	Administration of excessive dose may induce hypoglycemia
	Glucose should be available
Side Effects	Few in emergency situations
Dosage	10–25 units regular insulin IV followed by an infusion at 0.1 units/kg/hr
Routes	IV, SQ
Pediatric Dosage	Dosage is based on blood glucose level

Ipecac

Class	Emetic
Actions	Irritates the enteric tract
	Acts on vomiting center in the brain
Indication	Poisoning in conscious patient

Contraindications	Vomiting should not be induced in any patient with impaired consciousness
	Poisonings involving strong acids, bases, or petroleum distillates
	Antiemetic poisonings, especially of the phenothiazine type
Precautions	Monitor and ensure a patent airway
	The risk of aspiration is increased when using ipecac
Side Effects	Rare
Dosage	30 mL (1 oz) followed by 15 mL/kg of warm water
Route	Oral
Pediatric Dosage	*< 1 year of age:* 10 mL
	1–12 years of age: 15 mL
	> 12 years of age: 30 mL

 Ipratropium (Atrovent)

Class	Anticholinergic
Actions	Causes bronchodilation
	Dries respiratory tract secretions
Indications	Bronchial asthma
	Reversible bronchospasm associated with chronic bronchitis and emphysema
Contraindications	Should not be used in patients with history of hypersensitivity to the medication
	Should not be used as primary acute treatment of bronchospasm
Precaution	Monitor vital signs
Side Effects	Palpitations
	Dizziness
	Anxiety
	Headache
	Nervousness
Dosage	500 mcg placed in small-volume nebulizer (typically administered with a β-agonist)
Route	Inhaled
Pediatric Dosage	350–500 mcg/dose

 Isoetharine (Bronkosol)

Class	Sympathomimetic (β2 selective)
Actions	Bronchodilation
	Increases heart rate
Indications	Asthma
	Reversible bronchospasm associated with chronic bronchitis and emphysema
Contraindication	Patients with history of hypersensitivity to the medication

Precautions	Blood pressure, pulse, and electrocardiogram (ECG) results must be constantly monitored
Side Effects	Palpitations
	Tachycardia
	Anxiety
	Tremors
	Headache
Dosage	*Hand nebulizer:* Four inhalations
	Small-volume nebulizer: 0.5 mL (1:3 with saline)
Route	Inhalation only
Pediatric Dosage	0.25–0.5 mL diluted with 4 mL normal saline

Isoproterenol (Isuprel)

Class	Sympathomimetic
Actions	Increases heart rate
	Increases cardiac contractile force
	Causes bronchodilation
Indications	Bradycardias refractory to atropine (when transcutaneous pacing is unavailable)
	Severe status asthmaticus
Contraindication	Should not be used to increase blood pressure in cardiogenic shock
Precautions	Can cause ventricular irritability
	Can be deactivated by alkaline solutions
	Should be used with caution for recent myocardial infarction
	External pacing, if available, should be used instead of isoproterenol
Side Effects	Tachyarrhythmias
	Tremors
	Palpitations
	Headache
Dosage	1 mg should be placed in 500 mL of D_5W and then slowly infused at 2–10 µg/min and titrated until the desired rate is obtained or until PVCs occur
Route	IV drip only
Pediatric Dosage	0.1 mcg/kg/min

Ketamine (Ketalar)

Class	Sedative/hypnotic and analgesic
Action	Causes dissociative state
Indication	Induction agent for rapid-sequence induction
Contraindications	Patients with hypersensitivity to the medication
	Significantly elevated blood pressure

Precautions	Hallucinations can occur with emergency, particularly on emergence
	Emergency airway and resuscitative equipment and medications must be available
Side Effects	Hallucinations
	Increased skeletal muscle tone
Dosage	1.0–4.5 mg/kg IV
	3.0–8.0 mg/kg IM
Routes	IV, IM
Pediatric Dosage	0.5–3.0 mg/kg IV, IM

Ketorolac (Toradol)

Class	Nonsteroidal anti-inflammatory agent
Actions	Anti-inflammatory
	Analgesic (peripherally acting)
Indication	Mild to moderate pain
Contraindications	Patients with a history of hypersensitivity to the medication
	Patients allergic to aspirin
Precautions	Gastrointestinal irritation or hemorrhage can occur
Side Effects	Edema
	Rash
	Heartburn
Dosage	*Intravenous:* 15–30 mg
	Intramuscular: 30–60 mg
Routes	IV, IM
Pediatric Dosage	0.5 mg/kg/dose (max dose = 30 mg)

Labetalol (Trandate, Normodyne)

Class	Sympathetic blocker
Actions	Selectively blocks α_1-receptors and nonselectively blocks β-receptors
Indication	Hypertensive emergency
Contraindications	Bronchial asthma
	Congestive heart failure
	Heart block
	Bradycardia
	Cardiogenic shock
Precautions	Blood pressure, pulse, and electrocardiogram (ECG) results must be constantly monitored
	Atropine should be available

Side Effects	Bradycardia
	Heart block
	Congestive heart failure
	Bronchospasm
	Postural hypotension
Dosage	20 mg by slow IV infusion over 2 minutes; doses of 40 mg can be repeated in 10 minutes until desired supine blood pressure is obtained or until 300 mg of the medication has been given
	200 mg placed in 500 mL D$_5$W to deliver 2 mg/min
Route	IV infusion or slow IV bolus as described earlier
Pediatric Dosage	Safety in children has not been established

 ## Levalbuterol (Xopenex)

Class	Sympathetic agonist (β_2 selective)
Action	Bronchodilation
Indications	Asthma
	Reversible bronchospasm associated with chronic obstructive pulmonary disease
Contraindications	Known hypersensitivity to the medication
	Symptomatic tachycardia
Precaution	Blood pressure, pulse, and electrocardiogram (ECG) results should be monitored
Side Effects	Palpitations
	Anxiety
	Headache
	Dizziness
Dosage	0.63 mg in 3.0 mL normal saline every 6–8 hours
Route	Inhalation
Pediatric Dosage	0.31 mg in 3.0 mL normal saline 3 times a day

 ## Lidocaine (Xylocaine)

Class	Antiarrhythmic (Class IB)
Actions	Suppresses ventricular ectopic activity
	Increases ventricular fibrillation threshold
	Reduces velocity of electrical impulse through conductive system
Indications	Ventricular tachycardia/fibrillation refractory to amiodarone
Contraindications	High-degree heart blocks
	PVCs in conjunction with bradycardia
Precautions	Dosage should not exceed 300 mg/hr
	Monitor for central nervous system toxicity
	Dosage should be reduced by 50 percent in patients older than 70 years of age or who have liver disease
	In cardiac arrest, use only bolus therapy

Side Effects	Anxiety
	Drowsiness
	Dizziness
	Confusion
	Nausea and vomiting
	Convulsions
	Widening of QRS complex
Dosage	*Bolus:* Initial bolus of 1.0–1.5 mg/kg; additional boluses of 0.5–0.75 mg/kg can be repeated at 5- to 10-minute intervals until the arrhythmia has been suppressed or until 3.0 mg/kg of the medication has been administered; reduce dosage by 50 percent in patients older than 70 years of age
	Drip: After the arrhythmia has been suppressed, a 2–4 mg/min infusion may be started to maintain adequate blood levels
Routes	IV bolus, IV infusion
Pediatric Dosage	1 mg/kg

Lorazepam (Ativan)

Class	Tranquilizer (benzodiazepine)
Actions	Anticonvulsant
	Sedative
Indications	Major motor seizures
	Status epilepticus
	Premedication before cardioversion
	Acute anxiety states
Contraindication	Patients with a history of hypersensitivity to the medication
Precautions	Has short duration of effect
	Do not mix with other medications because of possible precipitation problems
	Flumazenil (Romazicon) should be available
	Dilute with normal saline of D_5W prior to IV administration
Side Effects	Drowsiness
	Hypotension
	Respiratory depression and apnea
Dosage	0.5–2.0 mg IV; may be increased to 1.0–4.0 mg IV
Routes	IV, IM, rectal
Pediatric Dosage	0.05–0.10 mg/kg (maximum dose 4 mg)

Magnesium Sulfate

Class	Anticonvulsant and antiarrhythmic
Actions	Central nervous system depressant
	Anticonvulsant
	Antiarrhythmic

Indications	*Obstetrical:* Eclampsia (toxemia of pregnancy)
	Cardiovascular: Torsade de pointes (irregular, polymorphic ventricular tachycardia)
Contraindications	Shock
	Heart block
Precautions	Caution should be used in patients receiving digitalis
	Hypotension
	Calcium chloride should be readily available as an antidote if respiratory depression ensues
	Use with caution in patients with renal failure
Side Effects	Flushing
	Respiratory depression
	Drowsiness
Dosage	1–4 g
Routes	IV, IM
Pediatric Dosage	Not indicated

 Mannitol (Osmotrol)

Class	Osmotic diuretic
Actions	Decreases cellular edema
	Increases urinary output
Indications	Acute cerebral edema
	Blood transfusion reactions
Contraindications	Pulmonary edema
	Patients who are dehydrated
	Hypersensitivity to the medication
Precautions	Rapid administration can cause circulatory overload
	Crystallization of the medication can occur at lower temperatures
	An in-line filter should be used
Side Effects	Pulmonary congestion
	Sodium depletion
	Transient volume overload
Dosage	1.5–2.0 g/kg
Routes	IV slow bolus or infusion
Pediatric Dosage	0.25–0.5 g/kg IV over 60 minutes

 Meperidine (Demerol)

Class	Narcotic
Actions	Central nervous system depressant
	Decreases sensitivity to pain
Indication	Moderate to severe pain

Contraindications	Patients receiving monoamine oxidase inhibitors
	Undiagnosed abdominal pain
	Patients with history of hypersensitivity to the medication
Precautions	Respiratory depression (naloxone should be available)
	Hypotension
	Nausea
Side Effects	Dizziness
	Altered level of consciousness
Dosage	*Intravenous:* 25–50 mg
	Intramuscular: 50–100 mg
Routes	IV, IM
Pediatric Dosage	1 mg/kg

 ## Metaproterenol (Alupent)

Class	Sympathomimetic (β_2 selective)
Actions	Bronchodilation
	Increases heart rate
Indications	Bronchial asthma
	Reversible bronchospasm associated with chronic bronchitis and emphysema
Contraindications	Patients with cardiac arrhythmias or significant tachycardia
Precautions	Blood pressure, pulse, and electrocardiogram (ECG) results must be constantly monitored; occasional nausea and vomiting reported
Side Effects	Palpitations
	Anxiety
	Headache
	Nausea and vomiting
	Dizziness
	Tremor
Dosage	*Metered-dose inhaler:* Two to three inhalations; can be repeated in 3–4 hours if required
	Small-volume nebulizer: 0.2–0.3 mL diluted in 2–3 mL normal saline administered over 5–15 minutes
Route	Inhalation only
Pediatric Dosage	0.05–0.3 mL in 4 mL normal saline

 ## Methylprednisone (Solu-Medrol)

Class	Steroid
Actions	Anti-inflammatory
	Suppresses immune response (especially in allergic reactions)
Indications	Severe anaphylaxis
	Asthma and chronic obstructive pulmonary disease

Contraindications	None in the emergency setting
Precautions	Must be reconstituted and used promptly
	Onset of action may be 2–6 hours, and thus the medication should not be expected to be of use in the critical first hour following an anaphylactic reaction
Side Effects	Gastrointestinal bleeding
	Prolonged wound healing
	Suppression of natural steroids
Dosage	*General usage:* 125–250 mg
Routes	IV, IM
Pediatric Dosage	30 mg/kg

 ## Metoclopramide (Reglan)

Class	Phenothiazine antiemetic
Actions	Antiemetic
	Reduces gastroesophageal reflux
Indications	Nausea and vomiting
	Gastroesophageal reflux
Contraindications	Gastrointestinal hemorrhage
	Bowel obstruction or perforation
	Patients with a history of hypersensitivity to the medication
Precaution	Extrapyramidal (dystonic) symptoms have been reported
Side Effects	May impair mental and physical ability
	Drowsiness
Dosage	*Intramuscular:* 10–20 mg
	Intravenous: 10 mg by slow IV push over 1–2 minutes
Routes	IV, IM
Pediatric Dosage	Rarely used

 ## Metoprolol (Lopressor)

Class	Sympathetic blocker (β_2 selective), Antiarrhythmic (Class II)
Action	Selectively blocks β_2-adrenergic receptors (cardioprotective)
Indication	Suspected or definite acute myocardial infarction in patients who are hemodynamically stable
	Stable, narrow-complex tachycardias if rhythm remains uncontrolled or unconverted by adenosine or vagal maneuvers or if SVT is recurrent
	Control ventricular rate in patients with atrial fibrillation or atrial flutter
	Certain forms of polymorphic VT (associated with acute ischemia, familial Long QT Syndrome, catecholaminergic)

Contraindications	Heart rate less than 45 beats per minute
	Systolic blood pressure <100 mmHg
	Heart block
	Shock
	History of asthma
Precautions	Blood pressure, pulse, and electrocardiogram (ECG) results must be constantly monitored
	Atropine and transcutaneous pacing should be available
Side Effects	Bradycardia
	Heart block
	Congestive heart failure
	Depression
	Bronchospasm
Dosage	Initial bolus of 5 mg slow IV injection
	May repeat 5 mg bolus in 5 minutes if vital signs are stable
	May repeat 5 mg bolus in 10 minutes if vital signs are stable
Route	Slow IV bolus
Pediatric Dosage	Safety in children has not been established

Midazolam (Versed)

Class	Tranquilizer (benzodiazepine)
Actions	Hypnotic
	Sedative
Indications	Premedication before cardioversion
	Acute anxiety states
Contraindications	Patients with a history of hypersensitivity to the medication
	Narrow-angle glaucoma
	Shock
Precautions	Emergency resuscitative equipment must be available
	Flumazenil (Romazicon) should be available
	Dilute with normal saline of D_5W prior to intravenous administration
	Respiratory depression more common with midazolam than with other benzodiazepines
Side Effects	Drowsiness
	Hypotension
	Amnesia
	Respiratory depression and apnea
Dosage	1.0–2.5 mg administered IV
Routes	IV, oral, intranasal
Pediatric Dosage	0.03 mg/kg

Milrinone (Primacor)

Class	Cardiac inotrope
Actions	Increases cardiac contractility
	Vasodilator
Indication	Short-term management of severe congestive heart failure
Contraindication	Patients with history of hypersensitivity to the medication
Precautions	May increase myocardial ischemia
	Blood pressure, pulse, and electrocardiogram (ECG) results should be constantly monitored
	Milrinone should only be diluted with normal saline or one-half normal saline
	Furosemide (Lasix) should not be administered into an IV line delivering milrinone
Side Effects	Reduction in platelets
	Nausea and vomiting
	Cardiac arrhythmias
Dosage	50 mcg/kg IV/IO over a 10-minute interval followed by maintenance infusion of 0.375 mcg/kg/min
Route	IV bolus and infusion
Pediatric Dosage	Limited data

Morphine

Class	Narcotic
Actions	Central nervous system depressant
	Causes peripheral vasodilation
	Decreases sensitivity to pain
Indications	Severe pain
Contraindications	Head injury
	Volume depletion
	Undiagnosed abdominal pain
	History of hypersensitivity to the medication
Precautions	Respiratory depression (naloxone should be available)
	Hypotension
	Nausea
Side Effects	Dizziness
	Altered level of consciousness
Dosage	*Intravenous:* 2–5 mg followed by 2 mg every few minutes until the pain is relieved or until respiratory depression ensues
	Intramuscular: 5–15 mg based on patient's weight
Routes	IV, IM
Pediatric Dosage	0.1–0.2 mg/kg IV

Nalbuphine (Nubain)

Class	Synthetic analgesic
Actions	Central nervous system depressant
	Decreases sensitivity to pain
Indication	Moderate to severe pain
Contraindication	Patients with a history of hypersensitivity to the medication
Precautions	Use with caution in patients with impaired respiratory function
	Respiratory depression (naloxone should be available)
	Patients dependent on narcotics may experience symptoms of withdrawal
	Nausea
Side Effects	Dizziness
	Altered mental status
Dosage	5–10 mg
Routes	IV, IM
Pediatric Dosage	Rarely used

Naloxone (Narcan)

Class	Narcotic antagonist
Action	Reverses effects of narcotics
Indications	Narcotic overdoses including the following: morphine, hydromorphone, fentanyl, Demerol, paregoric, methadone, heroin, hydrocodone, oxycodone
	Synthetic analgesic overdoses including the following: Nubain, Stadol, Talwin, Darvon
	To rule out narcotics in coma of unknown origin
Contraindication	Patients with a history of hypersensitivity to the medication
Precautions	May cause withdrawal effects in patients dependent on narcotics
	Short acting; should be augmented every 5 minutes
	Should never be used as part of a "coma cocktail"
Side Effects	Rare
Dosage	1–2 mg
Routes	IV, IM, endotracheal (endotracheal dose 2–2.5 times IV dose)
Pediatric Dosage	*< 5 years old:* 0.1 mg/kg
	> 5 years old: 2.0 mg

Nesiritide (Natrecor)

Class	Natriuretic polypeptide
Actions	Vasodilation
	Sodium excretion
	Diuresis

Indication	Acutely decompensated congestive heart failure (CHF)
Contraindications	CHF secondary to valvular heart disease
	Patients with known hypersensitivity to the medication
Precautions	Use with caution in patients receiving ACE inhibitors
	Physiological monitors should be applied
Side Effects	Headaches
	Back pain
	Catheter/injection site pain
	Fever
	Leg cramps
Dosage	Initial bolus of 2.0 mcg/kg over 60 seconds followed by continuous infusion of 0.01 mcg/kg/min
Route	IV
Pediatric Dosage	Not indicated

 ## Nifedipine (Procardia)

Class	Calcium channel blocker
Actions	Relaxes smooth muscle, causing arteriolar vasodilation
	Decreases peripheral vascular resistance
Indications	Chronic hypertension
	Angina pectoris
Contraindications	Known hypersensitivity to the medication
	Hypotension
Precautions	Blood pressure should be constantly monitored
	May worsen congestive heart failure
	Nifedipine should not be administered to patients receiving intravenous β-blockers
Side Effects	Dizziness
	Flushing
	Nausea
	Headache
	Weakness
Dosage	10 mg sublingually; puncture the capsule several times with a needle and place it under the patient's tongue and have him or her withdraw the liquid medication
Routes	Oral, sublingual
Pediatric Dosage	0.25–0.5 mg/kg

 ## Nicardipine (Cardene)

Class	Calcium channel blocker
Actions	Relaxes smooth muscle, causing arteriolar vasodilation
	Decreases peripheral vascular resistance
Indications	Hypertensive emergency

Contraindications	Known hypersensitivity to the medication
	Hypotension
Precautions	Blood pressure should be constantly monitored
	May worsen congestive heart failure
	Nicardipine should not be administered to patients receiving intravenous β-blockers
Side Effects	Dizziness
	Flushing
	Nausea
	Vomiting
	Headache
	Weakness
Dosage	5 mg/hour via infusion pump. Increase by 2.5 mg/hour every 5–15 minutes as needed to a maximum of 15 mg/hour
Routes	Oral, sublingual
Pediatric Dosage	0.5–3.0 mcg/kg/min

Nitroglycerin (Nitrostat)

Class	Antianginal
Actions	Smooth muscle relaxant
	Reduces cardiac work
	Dilates coronary arteries
	Dilates systemic arteries
Indications	Angina pectoris
	Chest pain associated with myocardial infarction
Contraindications	Children younger than 12 years of age
	Hypotension
Precautions	Constantly monitor blood pressure
	Syncope
	Medication must be protected from light
	Expires quickly once bottle is opened
Side Effects	Headache
	Dizziness
	Hypotension
Dosage	One tablet repeated at 3- to 5-minute intervals up to three times
Route	Sublingual
Pediatric Dosage	Not indicated

✳ Nitroglycerin Paste (Nitro-Bid)

Class	Antianginal
Actions	Smooth muscle relaxant
	Decreases cardiac work
	Dilates coronary arteries
	Dilates systemic arteries
Indications	Angina pectoris
	Chest pain associated with myocardial infarction
Contraindications	Children younger than 12 years of age
	Hypotension
Precautions	Constantly monitor blood pressure
	Syncope
	Medication must be protected from light
	Expires quickly once bottle is opened
Side Effects	Dizziness
	Hypotension
Dosage	1/2 to 1 inch
Route	Topical
Pediatric Dosage	Not indicated

✳ Nitroglycerin Spray (Nitrolingual Spray)

Class	Antianginal
Actions	Smooth muscle relaxant
	Decreases cardiac work
	Dilates coronary arteries
	Dilates systemic arteries
Indications	Angina pectoris
	Chest pain associated with myocardial infarction
Contraindication	Hypotension
Precautions	Constantly monitor vital signs
	Syncope can occur
Side Effects	Dizziness
	Hypotension
	Headache
Dosage	One spray administered under the tongue; may be repeated in 3–5 minutes; no more than three sprays in 15-minute period; spray should not be inhaled
Route	Sprayed under tongue on mucous membrane
Pediatric Dosage	Not indicated

✳ Nitrous Oxide (Nitronox, Entonox)

Class	Gas
Action	Central nervous system depressant

Indications	Pain of musculoskeletal origin, particularly fractures
	Burns
	Suspected ischemic chest pain
	States of severe anxiety including hyperventilation
Contraindications	Patients who cannot comprehend verbal instructions
	Patients intoxicated with alcohol or medications
	Head-injury patients who exhibit an altered mental status
	Chronic obstructive pulmonary disease; increased oxygen concentration may cause respiratory depression
	Thoracic injury suspicious of pneumothorax
	Abdominal pain and distension suggestive of bowel obstruction
Precautions	Use only in well-ventilated area
	Gas-scavenging system is recommended
	May not operate properly at low temperatures
Side Effects	Headache
	Dizziness
	Giddiness
	Nausea
	Vomiting
Dosage	Self-administered only using fixed 50 percent nitrous oxide and 50 percent oxygen blender
Route	Inhalation only
Pediatric Dosage	Self-administered only

Norepinephrine (Levophed)

Class	Sympathomimetic
Action	Causes peripheral vasoconstriction
Indications	Hypotension (systolic blood pressure < 70 mmHg) not due to hypovolemia
Contraindication	Hypotensive states due to hypovolemia
Precautions	Can be deactivated by alkaline solutions
	Constant monitoring of blood pressure is essential
	Extravasation can cause tissue necrosis
Side Effects	Anxiety
	Palpitations
	Headache
	Hypertension
Dosage	0.5–30 mcg/min
	Method: 8 mg should be placed in 500 mL of D_5W, giving a concentration of 16 mcg/mL
Route	IV drip only
Pediatric Dosage	0.01–0.5 mcg/kg/min (rarely used)

Olanzapine (Zyprexia, Zyprexia Zydis)

Class	Atypical antipsychotic
Action	Sedative
	Antipsychotic
Indication	Acute psychosis
Contraindication	Patients with known hypersensitivity to the medication
Precaution	Patients with cardiovascular disease
Side Effects	Myalgias
	Somnolence
	Dizziness
	Postural hypotension
Dosage	5–15 mg PO
Route	PO (rapidly dissolving)
Pediatric Dosage	Not indicated

Ondansetron (Zofran)

Class	Antiemetic
Actions	Blocks the serotonin receptors in the CTZ, the stomach, and the small intestines
Indications	Nausea, vomiting
Contraindications	Known hypersensitivity to the medicine
Precautions	Use with caution in patients taking serotonin blockers
Side Effects	Headache, lightheadedness, dizziness
Dosage	4–8 mg
Route	IV, IM, PO
Pediatric Dosage	0.15 mg/kg IV

Oxygen

Class	Gas
Action	Necessary for cellular metabolism
Indication	Hypoxia
Contraindications	Non-hypoxic patients
Precautions	Avoid hyperoxia
	Use cautiously in patients with chronic obstructive pulmonary disease (COPD)
	Humidify when providing high-flow rates
Side Effect	Drying of mucous membranes
Dosage	*Cardiac arrest:* 100 percent
	Other critical patients: 100 percent
	Other: Administer only enough to correct hypoxia
Route	Inhalation
Pediatric Dosage	24–100 percent as required

Oxytocin (Pitocin)

Class	Hormone (oxytocic)
Actions	Causes uterine contraction
	Causes lactation
	Slows postpartum vaginal bleeding
Indication	Postpartum vaginal bleeding
Contraindications	Any condition other than postpartum bleeding
	Cesarean section
Precautions	Essential to ensure that the placenta has delivered and that there is not another fetus before administering oxytocin
	Overdosage can cause uterine rupture
	Hypertension
Side Effects	Anaphylaxis
	Cardiac arrhythmias
Dosage	*Intravenous:* 10–20 units in 500 mL of D_5W administered according to uterine response
	Intramuscular: 3–10 units
Routes	IV drip, IM
Pediatric Dosage	Not indicated

Pancuronium Bromide (Pavulon)

Class	Neuromuscular-blocking agent (nondepolarizing)
Actions	Skeletal muscle relaxant
	Paralyzes skeletal muscles including respiratory muscles
Indication	To achieve paralysis to facilitate endotracheal intubation
Contraindication	Patients with known hypersensitivity to the medication
Precautions	Should not be administered unless persons skilled in endotracheal intubation are present
	Endotracheal intubation equipment must be available
	Oxygen equipment and emergency resuscitative medications must be available
	Paralysis occurs within 3–5 minutes and lasts for approximately 60 minutes
Side Effects	Prolonged paralysis
	Hypotension
	Bradycardia
Dosage	0.04–0.1 mg/kg; repeat doses of 0.01–0.02 mg/kg intravenously as required every 20–40 minutes
Route	IV
Pediatric Dosage	0.1 mg/kg

Phenobarbitol (Luminal)

Class	Barbiturate
Actions	Suppresses spread of seizure activity through the motor cortex
	Central nervous system depressant
Indications	Major motor seizures
	Status epilepticus
	Acute anxiety states
Contraindication	History of hypersensitivity to the medication
Precautions	Respiratory depression
	Hypotension
	Can cause hyperactivity in children
	Extravasation may cause tissue necrosis
Side Effects	Drowsiness
	Children may become hyperactive
Dosage	100–250 mg
Routes	IV slowly, IM
Pediatric Dosage	10 mg/kg

Phenytoin (Dilantin)

Class	Anticonvulsant and antiarrhythmic
Actions	Inhibits spread of seizure activity through motor cortex
	Antiarrhythmic
Indications	Major motor seizures
	Status epilepticus
	Arrhythmias due to digitalis toxicity
Contraindications	Any arrhythmia except those due to digitalis toxicity
	High-grade heart blocks
	Patients with history of hypersensitivity to the medication
Precautions	Should not be administered with glucose solutions
	Hypotension
	Electrocardiogram (ECG) monitoring during administration is essential
Side Effects	Local venous irritation
	Itching
	Central nervous system (CNS) depression
Dosage	*Status epilepticus:* 150–250 mg (10–15 mg/kg) not to exceed 50 mg/min
	Digitalis toxicity: 100 mg over 5 minutes until the arrhythmia is suppressed or until a maximum dose of 1000 mg has been administered or symptoms of CNS depression occur
Route	IV (dilute with saline)
Pediatric Dosage	*Status epilepticus:* 8–10 mg/kg IV
	Digitalis toxicity: 3–5 mg/kg IV over 100 minutes

Physotigmine (Antilirium)

Class	Cholinesterase inhibitor
Actions	Inhibits cholinesterase
	Potentiates acetylcholine
Indications	Tricyclic antidepressant overdoses (Elavil, Tofranil, Triavil, Norpramin)
	Atropine (belladonna) overdoses
Contraindications	Asthma and chronic obstructive pulmonary disease
	Gangrene
	Diabetes
	Cardiovascular disease
Precautions	Monitor for bronchospasm and laryngospasm
	Seizures
Side Effects	Excessive salivation
	Bradycardia
	Emesis
Dosage	0.5–2.0 mg
Route	IV
Pediatric Dosage	0.5–1.0 mg over 5 minutes

Pralidoxime (2-Pam, Protopam)

Class	Cholinesterase reactivator
Actions	Reactivates cholinesterase in cases of organophosphate poisoning
	Deactivates certain organophosphates by direct chemical reaction
Indications	Severe organophosphate poisoning as characterized by muscle twitching, respiratory depression, and paralysis
Contraindications	Poisonings due to inorganic phosphates
	Poisonings other than organophosphates
Precautions	Always ensure safety and protection of rescue personnel
	Laryngospasm, tachycardia, and muscle rigidity have occurred following rapid administration
	Should only follow atropinization
Side Effects	Excitement
	Manic behavior
Dosage	1–2 g in 250–500 mL of normal saline infused over 30 minutes
Route	IV drip
Pediatric Dosage	20–40 mg/kg by the same method

Procainamide (Pronestyl)

Class	Antiarrhythmic (Class IA)
Actions	Slows conduction through myocardium
	Elevates ventricular fibrillation threshold
	Suppresses ventricular ectopic activity
Indications	Ventricular tachycardia with pulse
	Pre-excited atrial fibrillation
Contraindications	High-degree heart blocks
	PVCs in conjunction with bradycardia
Precautions	Dosage should not exceed 17 mg/kg
	Monitor for central nervous system toxicity
Side Effects	Anxiety
	Nausea
	Convulsions
	Widening of QRS complex
Dosage	*Initial:* 20 mg/min until arrhythmia is abolished, hypotension ensues, QRS complex is widened by 50 percent of original width, or total of 17 mg/kg has been given
	Maintenance: 1–4 mg/min
Routes	Slow IV bolus, IV drip
Pediatric Dosage	Rarely used

Prochlorperazine (Compazine)

Class	Phenothiazine antiemetic
Action	Antiemetic
Indications	Nausea and vomiting
	Migraine headache
Contraindications	Comatose states
	Patients who have received a large amount of depressants (including alcohol)
	Patients with a history of hypersensitivity to the medication
Precautions	Extrapyramidal (dystonic) symptoms have been reported
Side Effects	May impair mental and physical ability
	Drowsiness
Dosage	5–10 mg slow IV or IM
Routes	IV, IM
Pediatric Dosage	Not recommended

Promethazine (Phenergan)

Class	Phenothiazine antihistamine (H_1 antagonist)
Actions	Mild anticholinergic activity
	Antiemetic
	Potentiates actions of analgesics

Indications	Nausea and vomiting
	Motion sickness
	To potentiate the effects of analgesics
	Sedation
Contraindications	Comatose states
	Patients who have received a large amount of depressants (including alcohol)
Precautions	Avoid accidental intraarterial injection
	Extravasation can cause tissue damage ("Black Box" warning)
Side Effects	May impair mental and physical ability
	Drowsiness
Dosage	12.5–25.0 mg
Routes	IV, IM
Pediatric Dosage	0.5 mg/kg

 ## Propofol (Diprovan)

Class	Sedative/hypnotic
Actions	Unclear but appear to inhibit GABA activity in the brain
Indications	Induction and maintenance of sedation
Contraindications	Known hypersensitivity to the drug or egg or soybean products
Precautions	Propofol is a potent sedative to be used only with adequate monitoring and adequate resuscitation equipment available
Side Effects	Pain on induction
	Hypotension
	Apnea
	Headache
	Nausea and vomiting
Dosage	25–75 mcg/kg as needed
Route	IV, PO
Pediatric Dosage	1 mg/kg IV

Propranolol (Inderal)

Class	Sympathetic blocker
Action	Nonselectively blocks β-adrenergic receptors
Indications	Stable, narrow-complex tachycardia
	Rate control in atrial fibrillation or flutter
	Certain forms of polymorphic ventricular tachycardia
Contraindications	Asthma and chronic obstructive pulmonary disease
	Patients dependent on sympathetic agonists
	Congestive heart failure

Precautions	Should not be given concurrently with verapamil
	Atropine and transcutaneous pacing should be readily available
Side Effects	Bradycardia
	Heart blocks
	Congestive heart failure
	Bronchospasm
Dosage	1–3 mg diluted in 10–30 mL of D_5W given slowly IV
Route	Slow IV bolus
Pediatric Dosage	0.01 mg/kg

 ## Racemic Epinephrine (MicroNEFRIN)

Class	Sympathomimetic
Actions	Bronchodilation
	Increases heart rate
	Increases cardiac contractile force
Indication	Croup (laryngotracheobronchitis)
Contraindications	Epiglottitis
	Hypersensitivity to the medication
Precautions	Vital signs should be constantly monitored
	Should be used only once in the prehospital setting
Side Effects	Palpitations
	Anxiety
	Headache
Dosage	0.25–0.75 mL of a 2.25 percent solution in 2.0 mL normal saline
Route	Inhalation only (small-volume nebulizer)
Pediatric Dosage	0.25–0.75 mL of a 2.25 percent solution in 2.0 mL normal saline

 ## Retaplase (Retavase)

Class	Fibrinolytic
Action	Increases plasmin by increasing the conversion of plasminogen
Indication	Acute myocardial infarction
Contraindications	Reteplase is absolutely contraindicated in the following cases:

1. Any prior intracranial hemorrhage
2. Known structural cerebral vascular lesion (e.g., AVM)
3. Known malignant intracranial neoplasm (primary or metastatic)
4. Ischemic stroke within 3 months EXCEPT acute ischemic stroke within 3 hours

5. Suspected aortic dissection

6. Active bleeding or bleeding diathesis (excluding menses)

7. Significant closed head trauma or facial trauma within 3 months

It is relatively contraindicated (i.e., the risks must be weighed against the potential benefits) in the following cases:

1. History of chronic, severe, poorly controlled hypertension

2. Severe uncontrolled hypertension on presentation (SBP > 180 mm Hg or DBP > 110 mm Hg). This could be an absolute contraindication in low-risk patients with myocardial infarction.

3. History of prior ischemic stroke > 3 months, dementia, or known intracranial pathology not covered in contraindications

4. Traumatic or prolonged (> 10 minutes) CPR or major surgery (> 3 weeks)

5. Recent (within 2 to 4 weeks) internal bleeding

6. Noncompressible vascular punctures

7. For streptokinase/anistreplase: prior exposure (> 5 days ago) or prior allergic reaction to these agents

8. Pregnancy

Precautions	Emergency resuscitative medications and equipment should be immediately available
	Antiarrhythmic medications should be readily available
Side Effects	Bleeding
	Allergic reactions
	Fever
	Nausea and vomiting
Dosage	10 units IV over 2 minutes. Repeat 10 units IV (over 2 minutes) in 30 minutes (20 units total)
Route	IV
Pediatric Dosage	Not indicated

Rocuronium Bromide (Zemuron)

Class	Nondepolarizing neuromuscular blocker
Action	Prevents neuromuscular transmission by blocking the effect of acetylcholine
	Skeletal muscle paralysis
Indication	Induction of skeletal muscle paralysis
Contraindication	Hypersensitivity to the medication
Precautions	Underlying cardiovascular disease
	Dehydration or electrolyte abnormalities

Side Effect	Bronchospasm
Dosage	*Initial dose rapid-sequence induction:* 600 mcg/kg
	Maintenance dose: 100–200 mcg/kg continuous infusion
Route	IV, IV drip
Pediatric Dosage	*Initial dose:* 600 mcg/kg
	Maintenance dose: 75–125 μg/kg continuous infusion

✠ Salbutamol (Ventolin)

Class	Sympathomimetic (β_2 selective)
Action	Bronchodilation
Indications	Asthma
	Reversible bronchospasm associated with chronic obstructive pulmonary disease
Contraindications	Known hypersensitivity to the medication
	Symptomatic tachycardia
Precautions	Blood pressure, pulse, and electrocardiogram (ECG) results should be monitored
	Use caution in patients with known heart disease
Side Effects	Palpitations
	Anxiety
	Headache
	Dizziness
	Sweating
Dosage	*Metered-dose inhaler:* One to two sprays (90 mcg per spray)
	Small-volume nebulizer: 0.5 mL (2.5 mg) in 2.5 mL normal saline over 5–15 minutes
	Rotohaler: One 200 mcg Rotocap should be placed in the inhaler and breathed by the patient
Route	Inhalation
Pediatric Dosage	0.15 mg/kg (0.03 mL/kg) in 2.5 mL normal saline by small-volume nebulizer

✠ Sodium Bicarbonate

Class	Alkalinizing agent
Actions	Combines with excessive acids to form a weak volatile acid
	Increases pH
Indications	Tricyclic antidepressant overdose
	Severe acidosis refractory to hyperventilation
Contraindication	Alkalotic states
Precautions	Correct dosage is essential to avoid overcompensation of pH
	Can deactivate catecholamines
	Can precipitate with calcium
	Delivers large sodium load

Side Effect	Alkalosis
Dosage	1 mEq/kg initially followed by 0.5 mEq/kg every 10 minutes as indicated by blood gas studies
Route	IV
Pediatric Dosage	1 mEq/kg initially followed by 0.5 mEq/kg every 10 minutes

Sodium Nitrite

Class	Nitrate/cyanide antidote
Action	Converts hemoglobin to methemoglobin for treatment of cyanide poisoning
Indication	Cyanide poisoning
Contraindication	Should not be administered to asymptomatic individuals
Precaution	Hypotension common with rapid IV administration
Side Effects	Exessive methemoglobinemia
	Hypotension
Dosage	300 mg IV; half-original dose repeated as needed (every 30 minutes) or if initial dose is ineffective
Route	IV
Pediatric Dosage	10 mg/kg IV; half-original dose repeated as needed (every 30 minutes) or if initial dose is ineffective

Sodium Nitroprusside (Nipride, Nitropress)

Class	Potent vasodilator
Actions	Peripheral arterial and venous vasodilator
	Decreases blood pressure
	Increases cardiac output in congestive heart failure
Indication	Hypertensive emergency
Contraindications	None when used in the management of life-threatening emergencies
Precautions	Bottle must be wrapped in foil to protect from light
	Should not be administered to children or pregnant women in the prehospital setting
	Reduce the dosage in elderly patients
	Blood pressure, pulse, and electrocardiogram (ECG) results must be diligently monitored
Side Effects	Nausea
	Retching
	Vomiting
	Palpitations
	Diaphoresis
	Tachycardia
	Dizziness
	Side effects often diminish as dosage is reduced

Dosage	0.5 mg/kg/min
Route	IV infusion only
Pediatric Dosage	Not indicated in prehospital setting

Sodium Thiosulfate

Class	Cyanide antidote
Action	Converts cyanide to thiocyanate where it can be eliminated by the body
Indication	Cyanide poisoning
Contraindication	None in the setting of cyanide poisoning
Precautions	None in the setting of cyanide poisoning
Side Effects	Nausea
	Vomiting
	Arthralgias
	Psychosis
Dosage	12.5 g IV; half-original dose repeated as needed
Route	IV
Pediatric Dosage	400 mg/kg IV; half-original dose repeated as needed

Sotalol HCL (Betapace, Sotacor)

Class	Antiarrhythmic (Class II) and β-adrenergicblocking agent (nonselective)
Actions	Blocks stimulation of β_1 (myocardial) and β_2 (pulmonary, vascular, and uterine) adrenergic receptor sites
	Suppression of arrhythmias
Indication	Hemodynamically-stable monomorphic ventricular tachycardia
Contraindications	Uncompensated congestive heart failure
	Pulmonary edema
	Cardiogenic shock
	Bradycardia or heart block
Precautions	Renal impairment
	Hepatic impairment
Side Effects	Fatigue
	Weakness
	Anxiety
	Dizziness
	Drowsiness
	Insomnia
	Memory loss
	Mental depression
	Mental status changes
	Nervousness
	Nightmares

Dosage	1.5 mg/kg IV over 5 minutes (slower infusion preferred)
Route	IV, PO
Pediatric Dosage	Not indicated

✠ Streptokinase (Strepase)

Class	Fibrinolytic
Action	Dissolves blood clots
Indication	Acute myocardial infarction
Contraindications	Persons with internal bleeding
	Suspected aortic dissection
	Traumatic cardiopulmonary resuscitation
	Severe persistent hypertension
	Recent head trauma or known intracranial tumor
	History of stroke in the past 6 months
	Pregnancy
Precautions	May be ineffective if administered within 12 months of prior streptokinase or anistreplase therapy
	Antiarrhythmic and resuscitative medications should be available
Side Effects	Bleeding
	Allergic reactions
	Anaphylaxis
	Fever
	Nausea and vomiting
Dosage	1.5 million units over 1 hour
Route	IV drip
Pediatric Dosage	Not recommended

✠ Succinylcholine (Anectine)

Class	Neuromuscular blocking agent (depolarizing)
Actions	Skeletal muscle relaxant
	Paralyzes skeletal muscles, including respiratory muscles
Indication	To achieve paralysis to facilitate endotracheal intubation
Contraindication	Patients with known hypersensitivity to the medication
Precautions	Should not be administered unless persons skilled in endotracheal intubation are present
	Endotracheal intubation equipment must be available
	Oxygen equipment and emergency resuscitative medications must be available
	Paralysis occurs within 1 minute and lasts for approximately 8 minutes
Side Effects	Prolonged paralysis
	Hypotension
	Bradycardia

Dosage	1–1.5 mg/kg (40–100 mg in an adult)
Route	IV
Pediatric Dosage	1 mg/kg

 ## Terbutaline (Brethine)

Class	Sympathomimetic
Actions	Bronchodilator
	Increases heart rate
Indications	Bronchial asthma
	Reversible bronchospasm associated with chronic obstructive pulmonary disease
	Preterm labor
Contraindication	Patients with known hypersensitivity to the medication
Precautions	Blood pressure, pulse, and electrocardiogram (ECG) results must be constantly monitored
Side Effects	Palpitations
	Tachycardia
	Premature ventricular contractions
	Anxiety
	Tremors
	Headache
Dosage	*Metered-dose inhaler:* Two inhalations, 1 minute apart
	Subcutaneous injection: 0.25 mg; may be repeated in 15–30 minutes
Routes	Inhalation, Subcutaneous injection, IV drip (in preterm labor)
Pediatric Dosage	0.01 mg/kg subcutaneously

Thiamine (Vitamin B$_1$)

Class	Vitamin
Action	Allows normal breakdown of glucose
Indications	Coma of unknown origin
	Alcoholism
	Delirium tremens
Contraindications	None in the emergency setting
Precautions	Rare anaphylactic reactions have been reported
	Should not be used as part of a "coma cocktail"
Side Effects	Rare, if any
Dosage	100 mg
Routes	IV, IM
Pediatric Dosage	Rarely indicated

Tirofiban (Aggrastat)

Class	Glycoprotein IIB/IIIA inhibitor
Action	Inhibits platelet aggregation by blocking glycoprotein IIA/IIIB receptors
Indication	Acute coronary syndrome
Contraindications	Internal bleeding (within 6 weeks), GI/GU bleeding, stroke (within 2 years), bleeding disorders, recent major surgery (within 6 weeks), known hypersensitivity to the medication.
Precautions	Tirofiban should be used with caution in patients who have an increased risk of bleeding. Allergic reactions have been reported with abciximab
Side Effects	Increased risk of bleeding, nausea, vomiting, abdominal pain, anemia, pain, sweating
Dosage	0.4 mcg/kg/min for 30 minutes and then continued at 0.1 mcg/kg/min
Route	IV
Pediatric Dosage	Not indicated

Trimethobenzamide (Tigan)

Class	Antiemetic
Action	Antiemetic with fewer sedative effects than other common antiemetic medications
Indications	Nausea and vomiting
Contraindications	Children (injectable form only)
	Patients with a history of hypersensitivity to the medication
Precaution	Extrapyramidal (dystonic) symptoms have been reported
Side Effects	May impair mental and physical ability
	Drowsiness
Dosage	200 mg IM
Route	IM
Pediatric Dosage	Parenteral administration not recommended

Vasopressin

Class	Hormone, vasoconstrictor
Actions	Antidiuretic hormone
	Potent vasoconstrictor
Indication	Cardiac arrest
Contraindication	None when used in the emergency setting
Precautions	Few in emergency setting
Side Effects	Blanching of skin
	Hypertension
	Bradycardia
Dosage	40 units IV (single dose only)
Route	IV
Pediatric Dosage	Not indicated

✦ Vecuronium (Norcuron)

Class	Neuromuscular-blocking agent (nondepolarizing)
Action	Skeletal muscle relaxant
	Paralyzes skeletal muscles including respiratory muscles
Indication	To achieve paralysis to facilitate endotracheal intubation
Contraindication	Patients with known hypersensitivity to the medication
Precautions	Should not be administered unless persons skilled in endotracheal intubation are present
	Endotracheal intubation equipment must be available
	Oxygen equipment and emergency resuscitative medications must be available
	Paralysis occurs within 1 minute and lasts for approximately 30 minutes
Side Effects	Prolonged paralysis
	Hypotension
	Bradycardia
Dosage	0.08–0.1 mg/kg
Route	IV
Pediatric Dosage	0.1 mg/kg

✦ Verapamil (Isoptin, Calan)

Class	Calcium channel blocker
Actions	Slows conduction through the atrioventricular node
	Inhibits reentry during paroxysmol supraventricular tachycardia (PSVT)
	Decreases rate of ventricular response
	Decreases myocardial oxygen demand
Indications	Narrow-complex tachycardias including:
	Stable, narrow-complex tachycardias if rhythm remains uncontrolled or unconverted by adenosine or vagal maneuvers or if SVT is recurrent
	Control ventricular rate in patients with atrial fibrillation or atrial flutter
Contraindications	Heart block
	Conduction system disturbances
Precautions	Should not be used in patients receiving intravenous β-blockers
	Hypotension
Side Effects	Nausea
	Vomiting
	Hypotension
	Dizziness
Dosage	2.5–5 mg; a repeat dose of 5–10 mg can be administered after 15–30 minutes if PSVT does not convert; maximum dose is 30 mg in 30 minutes

Route	Intravenous
Pediatric Dosage	*0–1 year:* 0.1–0.2 mg/kg (maximum of 2.0 mg) administered slowly
	1–15 years: 0.1–0.3 mg/kg (maximum of 5.0 mg) administered slowly

Ziprasidone (Geodon)

Class	Atypical antipsychotic
Actions	Sedative
	Antipsychotic
Indication	Acute psychosis
Contraindications	Patients with known hypersensitivity to the medication
	Patients with prolonged QT syndrome
Precautions	History of seizures
	Stroke
	Alzheimer's disease
Side Effects	Myalgias
	Somnolence
	Dizziness
	Postural hypotension
Dosage	10–20 mg IM
Route	IM
Pediatric Dosage	Not indicated

The following information pertains to immediate prehospital emergencies. Some of these classifications cover a broad range of drugs. The information provided is very general and is intended only for use as a quick reference.

Classification/Type

Type(s)	Therapeutic classification
Actions	The major mechanism or mechanisms of action and how the drug exerts its therapeutic effects
Indications	Condition or conditions for which the drugs are commonly prescribed
Adverse Effects	Any effect other than those that were therapeutically intended; usually undesirable, specific, and predictable; often a result of too much of the drug; may include any combination of those listed
Interactions	Presence of another drug or drugs may alter the effects of either drug or promote entirely different effects
How Supplied	Most common forms of the drug
Note	Miscellaneous relevant or nice-to-know information
Common Examples	A few examples (listed by trade name) of drugs in this class; when given, generic names are indicated by boldface type

Antianginals

Type(s)	Nitrates and nitrites (primarily) (*see also* Beta-Blockers and Calcium Channel Blockers)
Actions	Nitrates and nitrites (coronary vasodilators) Vasodilation Decreases myocardial work and reduces MVO_2 by Reducing preload and afterload Improving coronary perfusion (including collateral) May relieve coronary vasospasm
Indications	Angina, acute myocardial infarction, congestive heart failure, and after myocardial infarction Coronary artery spasm and SVTs To increase exercise tolerance

Adverse Effects	*Cardiovascular system:* Hypotension, bradycardia, paradoxical angina, flushing, feeling of warmth, syncope, reflex tachycardia, palpitation, and possible reperfusion arrhythmias (via relief of coronary vasospasm)
	Central nervous system: Transient or persistent headache, dizziness, weakness, and anxiety
	Other: N/V, may cause slight SL burning sensation
Interactions	Hypotensives, ETOH: May potentiate hypotension
How Supplied	Tablet, ointment or paste, aerosol, and transdermal patch
Note	These patients usually have coronary artery disease
	Tablets may lose potency within a few months
	Aerosols maintain potency for up to 3 years
	Tolerance and dependence may develop after prolonged use
	Paramedics should avoid (prolonged) contact with nitro paste (e.g., during chest compression) because it will be absorbed through their skin
	Canister should *not* be shaken; if it is, that dose is sprayed out and the next dose is administered to the patient

Common Examples	Cardilate	Nitrol
	Coronex	Nitrolingual spray
	Isordil	Nitrong
	Nitrobid	Nitrostablin
	Nitrogard	Nitrostat

 ## Antiarrhythmics

Type(s)	Various (classes I–IV)
Actions	Various, depends on specific antiarrhythmic:
	(−) chronotropy
	(+) or (−) inotropy
	(−) dromotropy
	Depresses automaticity
	Reduces MVO_2
	Suppresses PVCs
	Suppresses reentry activity
	Vagolytic
	May elevate the threshold for VF
Indications	To maintain NSR (or a controlled or stable abnormal rhythm)
	To prevent chronic rhythm disturbances
Adverse Effects	*Cardiovascular system:* Arrhythmia, conduction disturbances, hypotension, myocardial depression, may induce or exacerbate congestive heart failure or pulmonary edema, and may precipitate angina
	Central nervous system: Headache, central nervous system depression, altered level of consciousness
	Other: N/V
Interactions	Other antiarrhythmics: May potentiate or depress effects

How Supplied	Tablet and capsule	
Note	Usually prescribed after some type of cardiac insult	
Common Examples	Antiarrythmics may be classified by their predominant electrophysiological effects (e.g., Vaughn-Williams-Singh Classification).	

Class I	Class II	Class III
Biquin	*Primarily β-Blockers*	Bretylate
Dilantin	Betaloc	Bretylol
Mexitil	Biocadren	Cordarone (amiodarone)
Norpace	Corgard	
Procan	Inderal	
Pronestyl	Lopressor	
Prosedyl	Sotacor	
Quinate	Tenormin	
Quinidex	Visken	
Quinine		
Rhythmodan		
Tonocard		
Xylocaine		

Class IV	
Calcium channel blockers	*Cardiac glycosides*
Adalat	Cedilanid
Cardizem	Crystodigin
Isoptin	Digitaline
	Lanoxin
	Norvasc
	Novodigozin

 Anticoagulants

Type(s)	Warfarin or Coumadin derivatives
Actions	Decreases the ability of blood to clot:

     Prevents further extension of the clot

     Prolongs blood-clotting time

     May prevent clotting

Indications	Prophylaxis or treatment of blood clotting:

     Venous thrombosis, pulmonary embolism

     Adjunct in the treatment of coronary occlusion and transient ischemic accidents

     Home dialysis

     Recurrent problems with blood clots

     Treatment of embolization in A-fib

     Postfibrinolytic therapy

Adverse Effects	Hemorrhage (from any organ or tissue)
	Excessive bleeding from minor cuts, menstruation, or nosebleed
	Melena, petechiae
	N/V/D
Interactions	Salicylates, some antibiotics: May prolong clotting time and increase risk of hemorrhage
How Supplied	Tablet
Note	Also known as "blood thinners"
	Patients on home dialysis may take heparin intravenously
	Antiplatelet (e.g., aspirin Persantine) effects are similar to anticoagulant effects
Common Examples	Coumadin Minihep
	Hepalean Sintrom
	Heparin Warfilone

 ## Anticonvulsants

Type(s)	Benzodiazepines, barbiturates, hydantoins, and succinimides
Actions	Prevents and suppresses the spread of seizure activity in the motor cortex
	Elevates seizure threshold
	Skeletal muscle relaxation
Indications	Epilepsy
	Chronic seizures
	Generalized tonic-clonic seizures
	"Absence spells" seizures
	Simple partial, complex partial, or myoclonic seizures
Adverse Effects	*Cardiovascular system:* Hypotension and arrhythmia
	Central nervous system: Respiratory depression, apnea, excessive central nervous system depression, ataxia, dizziness, drowsiness, fatigue, weakness, confusion, behavioral disturbances, sedation, coma, amnesia, irritability, nervousness, headache, tremor, and paradoxical seizure (from overdose)
	Other: N/V/D, anorexia, abdominal pain, indigestion, constipation, visual disturbances, and nystagmus
Interactions	Central nervous system depressants: Potentiate effects
How Supplied	Tablet, capsule, and syrup
Note	Many patients are on combination therapy
Common Examples	Celontin Milontin
	Depakene Mogadon
	Dilantin Mysoline
	Epival Rivotril
	Mebaral Tegretol
	Mebroin Zarontin
	Mesantoin

Antidepressants: Monoamine Oxidase Inhibitors

Type(s)	Monoamine oxidase inhibitors (psychotropics)
Actions	Affects mood and behavior:
	Blocks impulse transmission at the synapse
	Inhibits catecholamine breakdown
Indications	Moderate-severe depression (usually refractory to tricyclic antidepressants)
	Atypical depression and phobic disorders (drug of choice)
	Prevention of panic attacks
	Depressive disorders (atypical, neurotic, or reactive)
Adverse Effects	*Cardiovascular system:* Tachycardia, PVCs, VT, hypotension, and sweating
	Central nervous system: Respiratory depression, central nervous system depression, dizziness, headache, irritability, anxiety, paresthesia, tremor, seizure, coma, ataxia, fever, and insomnia
	Other: N/V, urine retention, constipation, stiff neck, and dry mouth
Interactions	Antihypertensives: May potentiate effects
	Sympathomimetics or tyramine-rich foods and drinks: May potentiate effects (may induce hypertensive crisis)
	Central nervous system depressants: May potentiate effects
How Supplied	Tablet
Note	Overdose effects may persist for days
Common Examples	Marplan Parnate
	Nardil

Antidepressants: Tricyclic Antidepressants

Type(s)	Tricyclic antidepressants (psychotropics)
Actions	Mechanism of action is not exactly clear:
	Antidepressant effects
	Mild sedative effects
	Cholinergic blockade
	May inhibit catecholamine breakdown
	Peripheral α blockade
	Impairs cardiac depolarization and conduction
	$(-)$ inotropy
Indications	Severe endogenous depression (drug of choice)
	Prevention of panic attacks
	Pain control (some benefit for patients with fibromyalgia)
Adverse Effects	*Cardiovascular system:* Orthostatic hypotension, bradycardia, (wide complex) tachycardia, arrhythmia, PVCs, conduction defects (widened QRS complex, prolonged PR and QT intervals, ST and T wave abnormalities, and atrioventricular blocks) may precipitate congestive heart failure

Central nervous system: Initially confusion, anxiety, sweating, ataxia, and vomiting are seen; may precipitate mania and psychosis. Later central nervous system depression, delirium, hallucinations, coma, muscle rigidity, seizure, respiratory depression, and apnea may be present

Other: Anticholinergic effects (fever, hot flushed skin, dry mucous membranes, pupil dilation, urine retention) and anti-α effects (hypotension, sedation, cardiac depression)

Interactions	Sympathomimetics: May potentiate effects
	Central nervous system depressants: May potentiate effects
How Supplied	Tablet and capsule
Note	Ingestion of 1–2 g is potentially lethal and hard to treat
	Physostigmine (Antilirium), a cholinergic, may reverse some cholinergic symptoms
	Clinically related to phenothiazines
	Overdose effects may persist for days

Common Examples

Adapin	Norpramin
Anafranil	Pamelor
Asendin	Pertofrane
Aventyl	Sinequan
Desyrel	Surmontil
Elavil	Tofranil
Etrafon	Triadapin
Limbitrol	Triptil
Ludiomil	Vivactil

 ## Antidiabetics: Insulins

Type(s)	Insulin (pancreatic hormone)
Actions	Facilitates glucose transmembrane transport and stimulates carbohydrate metabolism
	Facilitates glucose storage (as glycogen), primarily in the liver, muscle, and kidney

	Time (hour)		
Insulin type	**Onset**	**Peak**	**Duration**
Short acting			
Regular (Toronto)	0.5–1	2.5–5	5–8
Similente	1–1.5	5–10	12–16
Intermediate acting			
NPH	1.5–2	4–12	24–48
Lente	2–2.5	7–15	22–48
Long acting			
PZI	4–7	10–30	36+
Ultralente	4–7	8–30	28–36+

Indications	Diabetes that cannot be controlled by diet alone
	Diabetics who cannot produce or excrete adequate amounts of insulin: usually type I (insulin-dependent diabetes mellitus), or juvenile diabetics
	In place of oral hypoglycemic therapy in patients with complications
Adverse Effects	*Other:* Hypoglycemia, hypokalemia, and electrolyte depletion
Interactions	ETOH, β-blockers, monoamine oxidase inhibitors, anabolic steroids, salicylates: May potentiate hypoglycemic effects
	Corticosteroids, thiazides, catecholamines: May diminish hypoglycemic effects
How Supplied	Multidose vial and penfill (subcutaneous or intramuscular injection); some are combination products
Note	Epinephrine may reverse hypoglycemic effects
	May be on combination of different insulin preparations
	Extracted from beef or pork pancreas or produced from genetic engineering
	Insulin preparations differ primarily in onset, peak, and duration of action, which may vary slightly among manufacturers
	Insulin is a protein and is destroyed in the gastrointestinal tract. It must be given parenterally. The abdomen, thigh, and arm are common sites.
Common Examples	Humilin Novolin
	Iletin Velosulin

 ## Antidiabetics: Oral Hypoglycemics

Type(s)	Oral hypoglycemics (sulfonylureas)
Actions	Stimulates pancreatic beta cells to produce and secrete insulin
Indications	To control hyperglycemia in patients whose diabetes cannot be controlled by diet alone and when insulin therapy is inappropriate; usually type II (non-insulin-dependent diabetes mellitus or adult) diabetics
Adverse Effects	Severe and prolonged hypoglycemia (especially when accompanied by acute ETOH overdose); possible associated hypoglycemic seizure
Interactions	ETOH, anabolic steroids, monoamine oxidase inhibitors, oral anticoagulants, salicylates, sulfonamides, β-blockers: May potentiate hypoglycemic effects
	Corticosteroids, glucagon, thiazides, catecholamines: May diminish hypoglycemic effects
How Supplied	Tablet
Note	Provides an alternative to intravenous insulin
	Oral hypoglycemics differ primarily in onset, peak, and duration of action

Hypoglycemia may persist despite intravenous dextrose or may recur (because oral hypoglycemics are longer lasting than dextrose)

Common Examples

Diabeta	Euglucon
Diabinese	Mobenol
Dimelor	Orinase

Antihypertensives

Type(s)
Various (vasodilators, sympatholytics, β-blockers, diuretics, and combination products)

Actions
Vasodilation (decreased blood pressure)
ACE inhibitors (reduced vasoconstriction)
Sympatholytics (reduced vessel tone)
α-Blockade (reduced SVR)
Diuresis (decreased volume)

Indications
Hypertension, congestive heart failure
Sodium retention, edema, ascites

Adverse Effects
Cardiovascular system: Orthostatic to profound hypotension, syncope, flushing, rebound hypertension, reflex tachycardia, arrhythmia, angina, and PVCs

Central nervous system: Drowsiness, dizziness, confusion, sedation, and headache

Other: Fluid and Na^+ retention, congestive heart failure, electrolyte imbalance, N/V/D, abdominal pain, and muscle cramps

Interactions
Monoamine oxidase inhibitors: May potentiate hypotensive effects

How Supplied
Tablet and capsule

Note
Some are combination products

Common Examples

Aldomet	Loniten
Capoten	Minipress
Catapres	Serparsil
Combipres	Viskazide

Antipsychotics

Type(s)
Primarily phenothiazines (major tranquilizers) (psychotropics)

Actions
Phenothiazines alter behavior in such a way as to enable the patient to cope with illness and function in daily activities without excessive sedation
Some also have antiemetic or anticholinergic effects

Indications	Acute and chronic control of behavioral disorders resulting from mental illness:
	Schizophrenia, recurrent mania
	Psychotic disorders
	Anxiety disorders
	Prevention of N/V
Adverse Effects	*Cardiovascular system:* Hypotension, bradycardia, arrhythmia, and atrioventricular blocks
	Central nervous system: Respiratory depression, central nervous system depression, sedation, drowsiness, confusion, dizziness, weakness, tremor, seizure, and coma
	Other: Extrapyramidal effects (primarily muscle spasms) and anticholinergic effects (dry mouth, nasal congestion, blurred vision, salivation)
Interactions	Opiates, barbiturates, ETOH, and other central nervous system depressants: May potentiate effects
	"Epi": May be ineffective in reversing hypotension (may in fact potentiate the hypotension)
How Supplied	Tablet, solution, suspension, syrup, and suppository
Note	Diphenhydramine (Benadryl) or benztropine (Cogentin) may counteract some
	Tranquilizers induce calmness and sedation without excessively depressing level of consciousness

Common Examples			
	Haldol	Peridol	Sparine
	Haloperidol	Permitil	Stelazine
	Mellaril	Quide	Trilafon
	Nozinan	Serentil	

Anxiolytics (Antianxiety)

Type(s)	Primarily benzodiazepines (minor tranquilizers) and carbamates
Actions	Central nervous system depressant, sedation
	Skeletal muscle relaxation
Indications	Excessive anxiety and tension (acute or chronic):
	Stresses of everyday life
	Emotional and physical disorders
	Tension from insomnia
	Anticonvulsant
	Muscle spasms
	Adjunctive management of acute ETOH or opiate withdrawal

Adverse Effects	*Cardiovascular system:* Hypotension and tachycardia
	Central nervous system: Respiratory depression, apnea, excessive central nervous system depression or sedation, coma, drowsiness, dizziness, vertigo, confusion, ataxia, slurred speech, headache, amnesia, fatigue, weakness, occasional paradoxical irritability, excitability, aggression, hallucinations, and delirium
	Other: N/V, pupil dilation
Interactions	Central nervous system depressants, including ETOH: Potentiate effects
How Supplied	Tablet, capsule, and caplet
Note	This is probably the most widely prescribed class of drugs in the world
	There is potential for tolerance, abuse, and addiction
	A withdrawal syndrome may result from abrupt cessation after chronic use

Common Examples	Atarax	Multipax
	Ativan (lorazepam)	Serax
	Donnatal	Stelzine
	Lectopam	Tranxene
	Librium (chlordiazepoxide)	Valium (diazepam) Vivol (diazepam)
	Loftran	Xanax
	Mellaril	

Beta-Blockers

Type(s)	Sympathetic blocker
Actions	Some selectively block β_1 (cardioselective) or β_2 (bronchoselective) receptors; some are nonselective
Indications	Mild to moderate hypertension
	Prevention of recurrent angina
	Prevention of recurring tachyarrhythmias
	Migraines
Adverse Effects	*Cardiovascular system:* May precipitate or aggravate chronic obstructive pulmonary disease, asthma, bronchospasm, increased airway resistance, hypotension, bradycardia, atrioventricular block, and congestive heart failure
	Central nervous system: Fatigue, headache, hallucinations, seizure, and coma
	Other: N/V, may induce hypoglycemia

Interactions	Sympathomimetics: Block β effects (patient may be unable to mount a tachycardic response to hypovolemia)
	Calcium blockers: Potentiate bradycardia and myocardial depression
	Cardiac glycosides: Potentiate bradycardia
	Epinephrine: Severe vasoconstriction
	Diuretics: May potentiate antihypertensive effects
How Supplied	Tablet
Note	Acute withdrawal may precipitate angina (due to increased sensitivity to catecholamines)
	Often used in combination therapy
	Selective β-blockers are usually dose dependent (tend to lose β selectivity in higher doses)
Common Examples	Betaloc Lopressor
	Blocardren Sotacor
	Corgard Tenormin
	Inderal Visken

Bronchodilators: Sympathomimetics

Type(s)	Sympathomimetics
Actions	Most are β selective (some are not)
	Bronchodilation (via β_2 stimulation)
	Some β effects
	Little or no α stimulation
Indications	Prevention or treatment of bronchospasm caused by reversible obstructive airway disease (chronic obstructive pulmonary disease, asthma, bronchitis, and emphysema)
Adverse Effects	*Cardiovascular system:* Excessive cardiac stimulation, tachycardia, palpitation, and hypertension; may precipitate angina, acute myocardial infarction, PVCs, and arrhythmia; possible hypotension, sweating
	Central nervous system: Excessive central nervous system stimulation (anxiety to seizure), headache, dizziness, drowsiness, weakness, fatigue, and paresthesia
	Other: N/V, heartburn, bad taste, muscle cramps, and dry nose and throat; may cause severe paradoxical bronchospasm from repeated excessive use
Interactions	β-blocker: May block effects
	Monoamine oxidase inhibitors, tricyclic antidepressants: May potentiate effects
How Supplied	Aerosol, tablet, suppository, and nebulizer solution
Note	Aerosolized drugs may not reach the smaller airways, especially in the presence of bronchospasm and thick mucous plugs (the nebulizer solution will be much more effective)
	Aerosol sympathomimetics have the potential for patient tolerance and abuse

These patients may also be on steroids and antibiotics

Some are combination products

Overdose effects may be reversed by a β-blocker such as propranolol (Inderal)

Some are catecholamines, and some are not; they differ primarily in their onset and duration

There is also a long-acting salbutamol called Serevent; it is not to be used for the compromised patient due to its longer onset of action

Common Examples	Alupent	Bronkometer
	Berotec	Bronkosol
	Brethaire	Serevent
	Brethine	Vaponefrin
	Bricanyl	Ventolin
	Bronkaid	

 ## Bronchodilators: Theophyllines

Type(s)	Theophyllines
Actions	Bronchodilation and vasodilation
	Respiratory stimulation
	Diuresis
	(+) chronotropy, (+) inotropy
Indications	Prevention and treatment of bronchospasm caused by reversible obstructive airway disease (chronic obstructive pulmonary disease, asthma, bronchitis, emphysema) and related bronchospastic disorders
Adverse Effects	*Cardiovascular system:* Hypotension, angina, tachycardia, palpitation, arrhythmia, PVCs, and flushing
	Central nervous system: Headache, nervousness, irritability, anxiety, excitement, dizziness, mild delirium, insomnia, fever, tremor, seizure, coma, and increased respiratory rate
	Other: N/V/D, anorexia, abdominal cramps, hematemesis, diuresis, dehydration, and visual or auditory disturbances
Interactions	β-blockers: May oppose effects
	Barbiturates, phenytoin: May decrease theophylline blood levels
How Supplied	Tablet, aerosol, elixir, syrup, and suppository
Note	Children are very sensitive: Toxic-to-therapeutic ratio is small
	Some are combination products
Common Examples	Choledyl	Somophyllin
	Phyllocontin	Tedral
	Quibron	Theo-Dur

Calcium Channel Blockers

Type(s)	Antiarrhythmic, antihypertensive, and antianginal
Actions	Blocks entry of calcium into the cell (especially cardiac and vascular smooth muscle):

(−) chronotropy

(−) inotropy

(−) dromotropy

Vasodilation (including coronary)

Bronchodilation

Inhibits coronary artery spasm

Indications	Nifedipine, verapamil, and diltiazem: Angina from coronary artery spasm and chronic stable angina (effort associated)
	Verapamil: PSVT, A-fib, A-flutter
Adverse Effects	**Verapamil and Nifedipine:**

Cardiovascular system: Conduction disturbances, arrhythmia, hypotension, bradycardia, congestive heart failure, flushing, and peripheral edema

Central nervous system: Headache, fatigue, drowsiness, dizziness, nervousness, central nervous system depression, confusion, and insomnia

Other: N/V/D/ and rash

Diltiazem

Interactions	Digoxin: May increase digoxin blood levels
	β-blockers: May potentiate some effects
How Supplied	Tablet and capsule (oral and sublingual)
Note	Often used in combination therapy
	Verapamil's most potent activity is electrophysiological, and nifedipine's most potent activity is hemodynamic; diltiazem acts like a less potent combination of the two
Common Examples	Adalat Isoptin
	Cardizem

 Cardiotonics: Cardiac Glycosides

Type(s)	Digitalis ("Dig") preparations
Actions	Promotes movement of calcium into the cell:

(+) inotrope

(−) chronotrope

(−) dromotrope

Improves atrial conduction

Indications	Congestive heart failure, after myocardial infarction
	A-fib, A-flutter
	SVTs

Adverse Effects	*Cardiovascular system:* May exacerbate congestive heart failure and almost any arrhythmia or conduction defect (usually conduction disturbances, PACs, PVCs, SVTs); hypotension
	Central nervous system: Fatigue, weakness, agitation, hallucinations, behavioral changes, headache, dizziness, vertigo, confusion, anxiety, paresthesia, and insomnia
	Other: N/V/D/, anorexia, malaise, visual disturbances, and hypokalemia
Interactions	Diuretics, Ca^{2+}, quinidine, amiodarone, Ca^{2+} blockers, catecholamines: May precipitate digitalis toxicity
How Supplied	Tablet and capsule
Note	Toxicity is more frequent in patients with hypokalemia, hypocalcemia, or hypomagnesemia
	About 7 to 40 percent of patients on digitalis develop some symptoms of toxicity
	Digitalized patients may develop more serious and resistant arrhythmias following cardioversion; use of very low energy levels and prophylactic lidocaine or phenytoin may prevent this
	Digitalis glycosides vary in potency, onset, and duration of action; they are generally long acting
Common Examples	Cedilanid Lanoxin
	Crystodigin Novodigoxin
	Digitaline

Diuretics

Type(s)	Various (primarily thiazides, loop, and combination products with antihypertensives, β-blockers, and aldosterone antagonists)
Actions	Diuresis
	Promotes sodium (Na^+) excretion
	Vasodilation
Indications	Hypertension
	Chronic fluid overload (congestive heart failure, pulmonary, peripheral edema)
	Liver cirrhosis with ascites and edema
	Decreased renal function (impairment)
	Edema (drug induced or from renal origin)
Adverse Effects	*Cardiovascular system:* Hypovolemia, hypotension, tachycardia, and arrhythmia
	Central nervous system: Drowsiness, confusion, delirium, dizziness, weakness, seizure, and coma
	Other: Dehydration, electrolyte imbalance (most commonly K^+), hyperosmolality, dry mouth or thirst, cramps, N/V/D, and visual or auditory disturbances; may inhibit insulin release (hyperglycemia)

Interactions	Antihypertensives: Increased antihypertensive effects
How Supplied	Tablet, capsule, and suppository
Note	Also known as "water pills"
	These patients are often on potassium (K$^+$) supplements
	Electrocardiogram may show prominent P waves, diminished T waves, and presence of U waves
Common Examples	Aldactazide Dyazide
	Aldactone Lasix
	Duretic Moduret

Narcotic: Analgesics

Type(s)	Narcotic (opiate) (natural, semisynthetic, synthetic)
Actions	Analgesia (increases pain threshold)
	Decreases anxiety, apprehension, fear
	Central nervous system depressant, sedation
	Cardiovascular (decreased anxiety reduces catecholamine release; vasodilation reduces preload)
Indications	Pain relief
	Cough suppression
	Sedation for anxiety, apprehension, and fear
	Antidiarrheal
Adverse Effects	*Cardiovascular system:* Hypotension, bradycardia, flushing, sweating, and pulmonary edema (noncardiogenic)
	Central nervous system: Respiratory depression, apnea, central nervous system depression, euphoria, drowsiness, dizziness, weakness, excessive sedation, apathy, paradoxical central nervous system, stimulation, nervousness, anxiety, headache, seizure, coma, hallucinations, delusions, and mood change
	Other: N/V, urine retention, may constrict or dilate pupils, and may suppress cough or corneal reflex
Interactions	Central nervous system depressants, tricyclic antidepressants, and monoamine oxidase inhibitors: Potentiate effects
How Supplied	Tablet, capsule, caplet, elixir, suppository, and intravenous
Note	Narcotics have the potential for patient tolerance, abuse, and addiction
	A withdrawal syndrome may result from abrupt cessation after chronic use
Common Examples	Ancasal Morphine
	Atasol Numorphan
	Codeine Oxycocet
	Darvon Oxycodan
	Demerol (meperidine) Percocet
	Percodan

Dilaudid
(hydromorphone)
Empracet
Exdol

Talwin
Tylenol with codeine
(Nos. 1, 2, 3, and 4)

Sedatives and Hypnotics

Type(s)	Primarily barbiturates, benzodiazepines; also piperidines, carbamates
Actions	Sedatives induce central nervous system depression and sedation, and "calm the nerves" Hypnotics induce and maintain sleep
Indications	Some are for daytime use, some are for nighttime use Anxiety, tension, stress, apprehension, irritability, excitement, and insomnia Chronic behavioral disorders Psychotherapy Seizure disorders
Adverse Effects	*Cardiovascular system:* Hypotension and pulmonary edema *Central nervous system:* Central nervous system or respiratory depression, drowsiness, dizziness, weakness, confusion, delirium, headache, ataxia, slurred speech, hypnosis (paradoxical excitement in the elderly), possible paresthesia, seizure, coma, nightmares, and hangover *Other:* Extrapyramidal reactions, anticholinergic effects, Parkinson-like reactions (especially in children), N/V/D, rash, and withdrawal syndrome
Interactions	ETOH, other central nervous system depressants: Excessive central nervous system and respiratory depression Monoamine oxidase inhibitors: Inhibit barbiturate metabolism
How Supplied	Tablet, capsule, and suppository
Note	Some have potential for tolerance, abuse, and addiction from chronic use Some are combination products Duration of action varies with each drug; some may be extremely long acting

Common Examples

Amytal	Nembutal
Butisol	Nodular
Dalmane	Placidyl
Day-Barb	Plexonal
Doriden	Restoril
Halcion	Seconal
Mandrax	Tranxene
Mogadon	Tuinal

COMMON EXAMPLES OF HOME MEDICATIONS

Narcotic: Analgesics

Ancasal	Morphine
Atasol	Numorphan
Codeine	Oxycocet
Darvon	Oxycodan
Demerol	Percocet
Dilaudid	Percodan
Empracet	Talwin
Exdol	Tylenol with Codeine (Nos. 1, 2, 3, and 4)

Antianginals

Cardilate	Nitrol
Coronex	Nitrolingual Spray
Isordil	Nitrong
Nitrobid	Nitrostablin
Nitrogard	Nitrostat

Anxiolytics (Antianxiety)

Atarax	Multipax
Ativan	Serax
Donnatal	Stelzine
Lectopam	Tranxene
Librium	Valium
Loftran	Vivol
Mellaril	Xanax

Anticoagulants

Coumadin	Minihep
Hepalean	Sintrom
Heparin	Warfilone

Anticonvulsants

Celontin	Milontin
Depakene	Mogadon
Dilantin	Mysoline
Epival	Rivotril
Mebaral	Tegretol
Mebroin	Zarontin
Mesantoin	

Antidepressants: Monamine Oxidase Inhibitors

Marplan	Parnate
Nardil	

Antidepressants: Tricyclic Antidepressants

Adapin	Norpramin
Anafranil	Pamelor
Asendin	Pertofrane
Aventyl	Sinequan
Desyrel	Surmontil
Elavil	Tofranil
Etrafon	Triadapin
Limbitrol	Triptil
Ludiomil	Vivactil

Antidiabetics: Insulins

Humilin	Novolin
Iletin	Velosulin

Antidiabetics: Oral Hypoglycemics

Diabeta	Euglucon
Diabinese	Mobenol
Dimelor	Orinase

Antlarrhythmics

Antiarrhythmics may be classified by their predominant electrophysiological effects (e.g., Vaughn-Williams-Singh Classification).

Class I	Class II	Class III
Biquin	*Primarily β-blockers*	Bretylate
Dilantin	Betaloc	Bretylol
Mexitil	Biocadren	Cordarone
Norpace	Corgard	
Procan	Inderal	
Pronestyl	Lopressor	
Prosedyl	Sotacor	
Quinate	Tenormin	
Quinidex	Visken	
Quinine		
Rhythmodan		
Tonocard		
Xylocaine		

(continued)

Class IV

Ca^{2+} channel blockers	Cardiac glycoside
Adalat	Cedilanid
Cardizem	Crystodigin
Isoptin	Digitaline
	Lanoxin
	Novodigozin

Antihypertensives

Aldomet	Loniten
Capoten	Minipress
Catapres	Serparsil
Combipres	Viskazide

Antipsychotics

Haldol	Peridol	Sparine
Haloperidol	Permitil	Stelazine
Mellaril	Quide	Trilafon
Nozinan	Serentil	

Beta-Blockers

Betaloc	Lopressor
Blocardren	Sotacor
Corgard	Tenormin
Inderal	Visken

Bronchodilators: Sympathomimetics

Alupent	Bronkaid
Berotec	Bronkometer
Brethaire	Bronkosol
Brethine	Vaponefrin
Bricanyl	Ventolin

Bronchodilators: Theophyllines

Choledyl	Somophyllin
Phyllocontin	Tedral
Quibron	Theo-Dur

Calcium Channel Blockers

Adalat   Isoptin

Cardizem

Cardiotonics: Cardiac Glycosides

Cedilanid   Lanoxin

Crystodigin   Novodigoxin

Diuretics

Aldactazide   Dyazide

Aldactone   Lasix

Duretic   Moduret

Digitaline

Sedatives and Hypnotics

Amytal   Nembutal

Butisol   Nodular

Dalmane   Placidyl

Day-Barb   Plexonal

Doriden   Restoril

Halcion   Seconal

Mandrax   Tranxene

Mogadon   Tuinal

Subcutaneous Medication Administration

Intramuscular Injection

Intravenous Setup

Procedure for Intravenous Cannulation

External Jugular Vein Cannulation

Intravenous Bolus

Intravenous Infusion Administration

Endotracheal Tube Administration

Intraosseous Infusion

Nebulized Inhalation

Bag-Valve Nebulized Medication Administration

Self-Administered Nitrous Oxide

Epinephrine Autoinjectors (Epi-Pen)

Umbilical Vein Catheterization

SUBCUTANEOUS MEDICATION ADMINISTRATION

Subcutaneous injection is a method of administering medications directly into subcutaneous or fatty tissue, where they are absorbed into the general circulation (see Procedure E–1). Medication injected subcutaneously is typically absorbed more slowly than through the intravenous routes but faster than through the oral route. The subcutaneous injection of epinephrine may be lifesaving in severe cases of asthma or allergic reactions. Glucagon can also be administered subcutaneously for the treatment of insulin shock. The medication must be administered into the subcutaneous tissue and not into the more superficial dermis or deeper muscle, connective tissue, or blood vessels.

The procedure for subcutaneous administration is as follows:

1. Confirm medication order by protocol or direct on-line medical control.
2. Observe Standard Precautions (gloves and glasses).
3. Prepare the necessary equipment):
   - 1-cc syringe
   - One needle (preferably 1 to 1½ inches in length, 16 to 22 gauge) to withdraw medication
   - One needle (preferably ½ to ⅝ inch in length, 25 gauge) for medication administration
   - Antiseptic swab

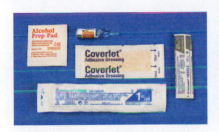

E–1a Prepare the equipment.

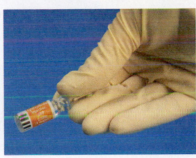

E–1b Check the medication.

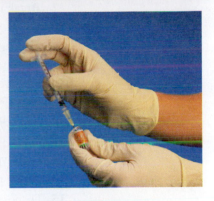

E–1c Draw up the medication.

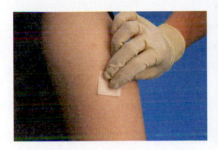

E–1d Prep the site.

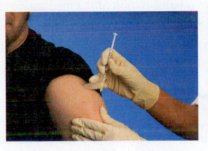

E–1e Insert the needle at a 45° angle.

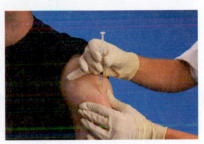

E–1f Remove the needle and cover the puncture site.

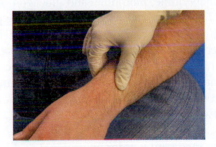

E–1g Monitor the patient.

- 2 × 2 gauze pad
- Medication
- Sharps container

4. Explain to the patient what you are going to do and reconfirm that the patient is not allergic to the medication. Be sure to advise the patient of any complications that might result from the administration.

5. Examine the ampule of medication, including name and expiration date. Hold it up to the light and inspect for discoloration or particles in the solution. Do not administer if discolored or if particles are present.

6. "Shake down" the ampule. This will force the liquid to the lower portion of the ampule so that it can be broken without spillage of the medication.

7. Break the ampule using a 2×2 gauze pad to prevent injury.

8. Draw the medication into the syringe. Invert the syringe and expel any air present.

9. Choose a suitable site. The easiest and most accessible site is the subcutaneous tissue over the deltoid muscle in the arm.

10. Prepare the site by cleansing it with an antiseptic swab using a firm circular motion from the vein outward.

11. Pinch up the skin and insert the needle into the tissue at a 45-degree angle.

12. Inject the medication into the subcutaneous tissue slowly.

13. Remove the syringe. Do not recap the needle.

14. Apply pressure to the site with sterile gauze pad.

15. Dispose of the syringe and medication container in appropriate sharps container.

16. Apply pressure to the administration site and cover with an adhesive strip.

17. Confirm administration of the medication.

18. Closely monitor the patient for the desired therapeutic effect and possible side effects.

19. Document time of procedure and patient effects.

INTRAMUSCULAR INJECTION

Intramuscular (IM) injection is a method of administering medications directly into muscle, where it is absorbed into the general circulation. Prehospital administration of IM medications is relatively uncommon but is useful when other administration routes fail. Several prehospital medications can be administered IM, the most common being diazepam, meperidine, morphine, and glucagon. Absorption by the IM route is slower than by the IV route; because it requires adequate perfusion, it may be ineffective in the hypotensive patient. IM injections may be contraindicated in patients with coagulopathies (a defect in the clotting mechanism of the body) or those who take anticoagulants.

Several sites are used for intramuscular injections (see Figure E–1). Epinephrine 1:1000 for anaphylaxis is the emergency medication most commonly administered IM.

The procedure for intramuscular medication administration is as follows (see Procedure E–2):

1. Confirm medication order by protocol or direct on-line medical control.

2. Observe Standard Precautions (gloves and glasses).

3. Prepare the necessary equipment:
   • Syringe of sufficient size to contain the medication
   • One needle (preferably 1 to 1½ inches in length, 16 to 22 gauge) to withdraw medication
   • One needle (preferably ¾ to 1 inch in length, 21 to 25 gauge) for medication administration
   • Antiseptic swab
   • 2×2 gauze pad
   • Medication
   • Sharps container

4. Explain to the patient what you are going to do and reconfirm that the patient is not allergic to the medication. Be sure to advise the patient of any complications that might result from the administration.

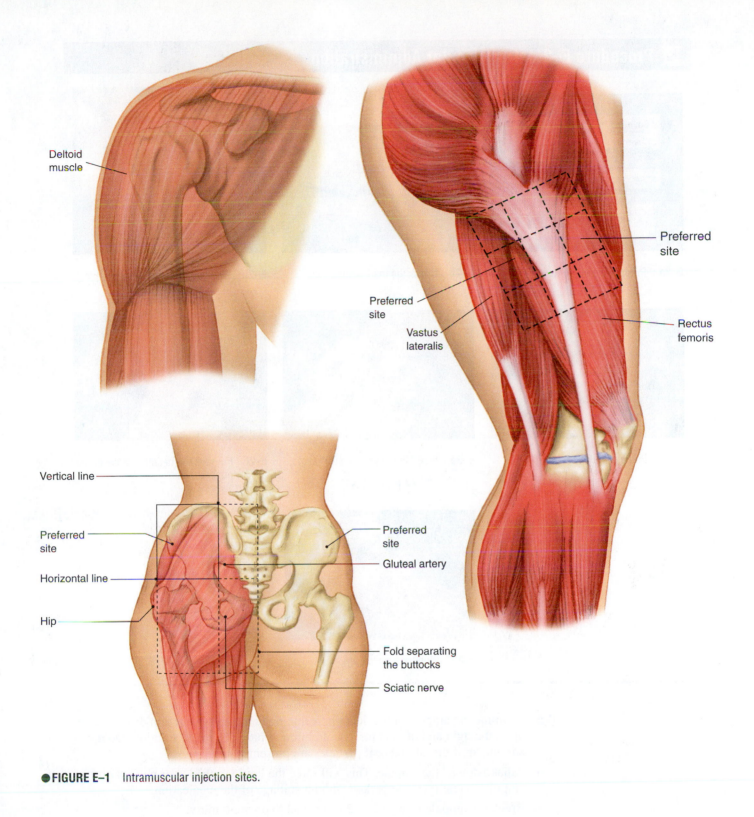

Deltoid
muscle

Preferred
site

Preferred
site

Vastus
lateralis

Rectus
femoris

Vertical line

Preferred
site

Horizontal line

Hip

Preferred
site

Gluteal artery

Fold separating
the buttocks

Sciatic nerve

●FIGURE E–1   Intramuscular injection sites.

℞ Procedure E-2 Intramuscular Administration

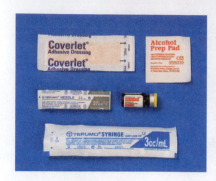

E-2a Prepare the equipment.

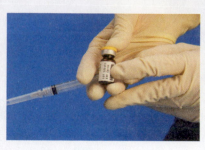

E-2b Check the medication.

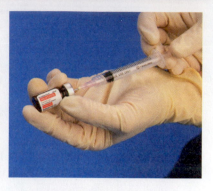

E-2c Draw up the medication.

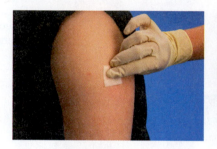

E-2d Prepare the site.

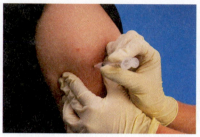

E-2e Insert the needle at a 90° angle.

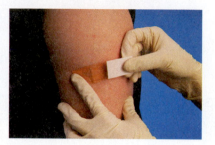

E-2f Remove the needle and cover the puncture site.

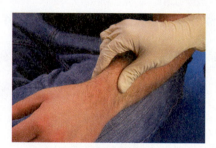

E-2g Monitor the patient.

5. Examine the ampule of medication, including name and expiration date. Hold it up to the light and inspect for discoloration or particles in the solution. Do not administer if discolored or if particles are present.

6. "Shake down" the ampule. This will force the liquid to the lower portion of the ampule so that it can be broken without spillage of the medication.

7. Break the ampule using a 2 × 2 gauze pad to prevent injury.

8. Draw the medication into the syringe. Invert the syringe and expel any air present.

9. Choose a suitable site. The most accessible sites are the deltoid muscle in the arm, the vastus lateralis in the leg and the gluteous muscle in the buttocks (see Figure E-1).

10. Prepare the site by cleansing it with an antiseptic swab using a firm circular motion from the vein outward.

11. Insert the needle with a rapid motion into the tissue at a 90-degree angle (see Procedure E–2e).

12. Aspirate the syringe to ensure that you are not in a blood vessel. If you get any blood return, you should withdraw the needle and reattempt administration at another site.

13. Inject the medication slowly.

14. Remove the syringe. Do not recap the needle.

15. Dispose of the syringe and medication container in appropriate sharps container.

16. Apply pressure to the administration site and cover with an adhesive strip.

17. Confirm administration of the medication.

18. Closely monitor the patient for the desired therapeutic effect and possible undesired side effects.

19. Document time of procedure and patient effects.

INTRAVENOUS SETUP

1. Prepare the necessary equipment and observe Standard Precautions (gloves, glasses, or goggles):
   - Appropriate IV fluid
   - Appropriate administration set

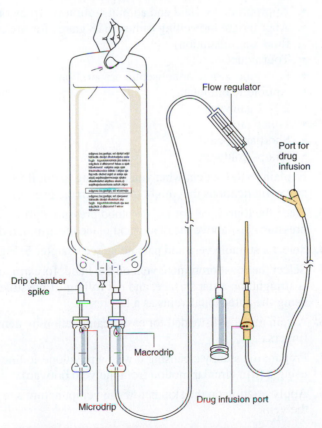

● **FIGURE E–2** Macrodrip and microdrip administration sets.

- Appropriate indwelling catheter
- Extension IV tubing if necessary

2. Remove the envelope from the IV fluid.

3. Inspect the fluid, making sure that it is not discolored and does not contain any particulate matter; check that it contains the correct amount of fluid. Do not administer if discolored, if particles are present, or if less than the indicated quantity of fluid is present.

4. Open and inspect the IV tubing.

5. Attach the extension tubing.

6. Close the clamp on the tubing.

7. Remove the sterile cover from the IV fluid and the administration set.

8. Insert the administration set into the IV fluid.

9. Squeeze the drip chamber to fill it with fluid.

10. Bleed all of the air out of the IV tubing.

11. Hang the bag on an IV pole (or have a bystander hold it) at the appropriate height.

PROCEDURE FOR INTRAVENOUS CANNULATION

The procedure is as follows (see Procedure E–3):

1. Prepare the necessary equipment and observe Standard Precautions (gloves and goggles):
   - Appropriate IV fluid and administration set (previously set up)
   - Appropriate indwelling catheter (18 gauge for lifelines and 12 to 16 gauge for fluid administration)
   - Tourniquet
   - Povidone-iodine or antiseptic preparation
   - Antibiotic ointment
   - 2 × 2 gauze pad
   - 1-inch tape
   - Short arm board
   - Sharps container

2. Explain to the patient what you are going to do. Be sure to advise the patient of any complications that might result from the procedure.

3. Place the tourniquet (or inflate blood pressure cuff to 20 mmHg below systolic pressure) just above the elbow and place the arm in a dependent position.

4. Select a suitable vein and palpate it (see Chapter 5, Figures 5–6 and 5–7).

5. Select the most prominent vein on the hand, forearm, or antecubital space that is straight, on a flat surface, and not rolling. If possible, avoid veins over joints, using the antecubital veins as a last resort.

6. A vein may be distended for easier cannulation by gently tapping on it with the fingers.

7. Prepare the site by cleansing it with a povidone-iodine or antiseptic preparation using a firm circular motion from the vein outward.

8. Apply traction on the skin below the venipuncture site and stabilize the vein.

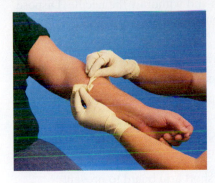

E–3a Place the constricting band.

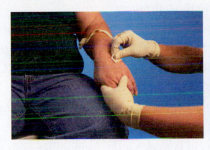

E–3b Cleanse the venipuncture site.

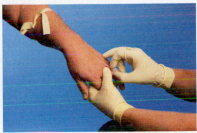

E–3c Insert the intravenous cannula into the vein.

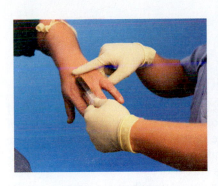

E–3d Withdraw any blood samples needed.

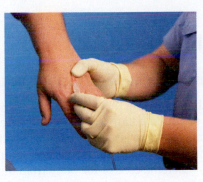

E–3e Connect the IV tubing.

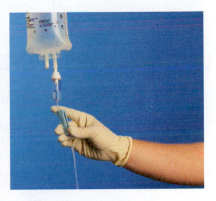

E–3f Turn on the IV and check the flow.

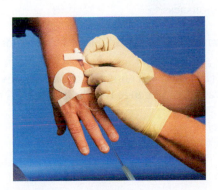

E–3g Secure the site.

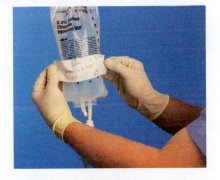

E–3h Label the intravenous solution bag.

9. Tell the patient there will be a quick, painful stick.

10. With the bevel of the needle upward, puncture the skin using a 30- to 45-degree angle. Enter the vein directly from above or from the side.

11. When the vein is entered, you should feel a "pop" and see flashback into the catheter (see Chapter 5, Figures 5–8 through 5–10).

12. Carefully lower the catheter and advance the needle and catheter approximately 2 mm to stabilize the needle in the vein.

13. Slide the catheter off the needle into the vein and withdraw the needle. Dispose of the needle in a puncture-proof (sharps) container.

14. Remove the tourniquet.

15. Connect the IV tubing and slowly open the valve.

16. Confirm that the fluid is flowing freely without any evidence of infiltration.

17. Cover the IV site with an sterile dressing (Op Site).

18. Securely tape the IV catheter.

19. Make a loop with the infusion tubing and tape the loop to the arm.

20. Adjust the flow rate.

21. If the vein is over a joint, immobilize with a short arm board to prevent dislodgment of the catheter.

22. Document the successful completion of the IV.

23. Monitor the patient for the desired effects and any undesired ones as well.

EXTERNAL JUGULAR VEIN CANNULATION

Intravenous Access in the External Jugular Vein

The external jugular vein is a large peripheral vein in the neck, between the angle of the jaw and the middle third of the clavicle. It connects into the central circulation of the subclavian vein. Because it lies so close to the central circulation, cannulation here offers many of the same benefits afforded central venous access. Fluids and medications rapidly reach the core of the body from this site.

Consider the external jugular vein only after you have exhausted other means of peripheral access or when a patient requires immediate fluid administration. This is an extremely painful site to access, so you typically will reserve its use for patients with a decreased or total loss of consciousness.

1. Prepare the necessary equipment and observe Standard Precautions (gloves, glasses, or goggles):
   - Appropriate intravenous (IV) fluid and administration set (previously set up)
   - Appropriate indwelling catheter (18 gauge for lifelines and 14 to 16 gauge for fluid administration)
   - Povidone-iodine or antiseptic preparation
   - Antibiotic ointment
   - 2 × 2 gauze pad
   - 1-inch tape
   - Sharps container

2. Explain to the patient what you are going to do (if the patient is conscious). Be sure to advise the patient of any complications that might result from the procedure.

3. Position the patient supine with feet elevated (when possible).

4. Turn the head in the direction away from the side to be cannulated.

5. Select a suitable vein and palpate it.

6. Prepare the site by cleansing it with a povidone-iodine or antiseptic preparation.

7. Apply traction on the vein just below the clavicle.

8. Attach a 10 mL syringe to an IV catheter. Align the catheter and point the tip of the catheter toward the feet.

9. Tell the patient there will be a quick, painful stick.

10. With the bevel of the needle upward, puncture the skin using a 30-degree angle. The needle tip should enter midway between the angle of the jaw and the clavicle and should be aimed toward the shoulder on the same side as the vein. Apply suction to the syringe. As the vein is entered, note a flashback of blood.

11. Carefully lower the catheter and advance the needle and catheter approximately 2 mm to stabilize the needle in the vein.

12. Slide the catheter off the needle into the vein and then remove the needle. Dispose of the needle into a puncture-proof (sharps) container.

13. Connect the IV tubing and slowly open the valve.

14. Confirm that the fluid is flowing freely without any evidence of infiltration.

15. Cover the IV site with an sterile dressing (Op Site).

16. Securely tape the IV catheter.

17. Make a loop with the infusion tubing and tape the loop to the neck.

18. Adjust the flow rate.

19. Document the successful completion of the IV.

20. Monitor the patient for the desired effects and any undesired ones as well.

INTRAVENOUS BOLUS

Intravenous bolus, or IV push, is a method of administering medications directly into the bloodstream (see Procedure E–4). This method provides a rapid route for medications. Because this is a rapid method of medication administration, it is the most commonly used route for life-threatening emergencies. These emergencies include the following:

- Ventricular arrhythmias
- Supraventricular tachycardia
- Symptomatic bradycardia
- Hypoglycemia
- Metabolic acidosis
- Seizures
- Acute pulmonary edema
- Cardiopulmonary arrest
- Narcotic overdose
- Pain control

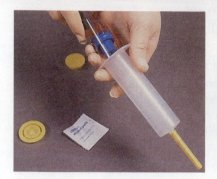

E–4a Prepare the equipment.

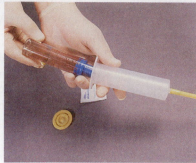

E–4b Prepare the medication.

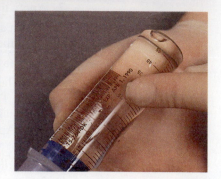

E–4c Check the label.

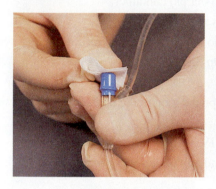

E–4d Select and clean an administration port.

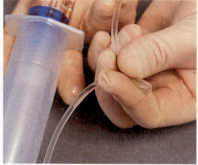

E–4e Pinch the line.

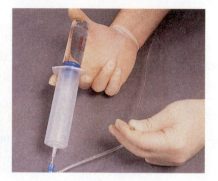

E–4f Administer the medication.

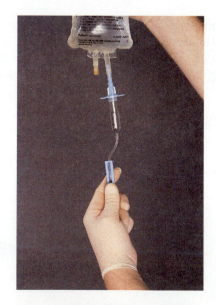

E–4g Adjust the IV flow rate.

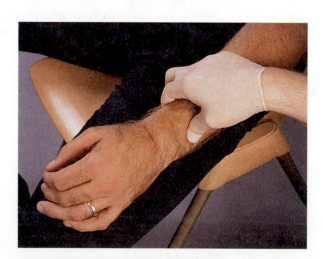

E–4h Monitor the patient.

1. Confirm medication order by protocol or direct on-line medical control.
2. Observe Standard Precautions (gloves and glasses).
3. Prepare the necessary equipment
   - Syringe of sufficient size to contain the medication (or prefilled syringe)
   - Needle (preferably 1 inch long, 18 gauge)
   - Antiseptic or povidone-iodine preparation
   - 2 × 2 gauze pad
   - Medication
   - Sharps container
4. Explain to the patient what you are going to do and reconfirm that the patient is not allergic to the medication. Be sure to advise the patient of any complications that might result from the administration.
5. Examine the ampule of medication, including name and expiration date. Hold it up to the light and inspect for discoloration or particles in the solution. Do not administer if discolored or if particles are present.
6. "Shake down" the ampule. This will force the liquid to the lower portion of the ampule so that it can be broken without spillage of the medication.
7. Break the ampule using a 2 × 2 gauze pad to prevent injury.
8. Draw the medication into the syringe. Invert the syringe and expel any air.
9. Locate the medication port on the IV administration set and cleanse it with an antiseptic swab.
10. Insert the needle into the medication port.
11. Pinch the IV line off above the medication port.
12. Administer the medication in a slow, deliberate fashion.
13. Remove the needle and wipe the medication port with an antiseptic swab.
14. Release the pinched line and confirm free flow of IV fluid. Set IV flow rate.
15. Confirm administration of the medication.
16. Closely monitor the patient for the desired therapeutic effects as well as any undesired side effects.

INTRAVENOUS INFUSION ADMINISTRATION

Intravenous piggyback or IV drip infusion provides a route for continuous medication administration (see Procedure E–5). It offers the advantage of being easily titrated to increase or decrease the rate of flow or to discontinue the infusion based on the patient's response.

1. Confirm medication order by protocol or direct on-line medical control.
2. Observe Standard Precautions (gloves and glasses).
3. Prepare the necessary equipment:
   - Medication
   - Syringe to transfer the medication from the ampule to the diluent
   - Antiseptic preparation or other antibacterial scrub
   - Two 18-gauge, 1-inch needles
   - Label for the bag
   - Sharps container

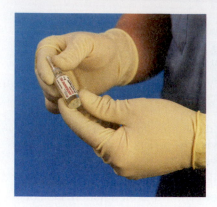

E–5a Select the medication.

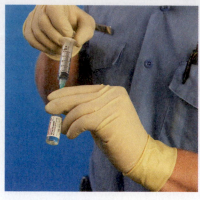

E–5b Draw up the medication.

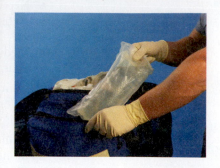

E–5c Select the IV fluid for dilution.

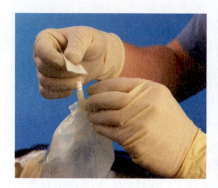

E–5d Clean the medication addition port.

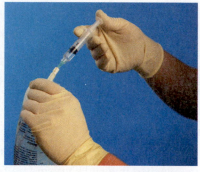

E–5e Inject the medication into the fluid.

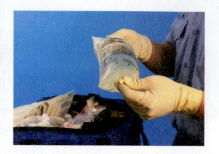

E–5f Mix the solution.

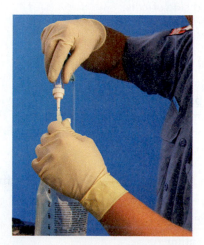

E–5g Insert an administration set and connect to main IV line with needle.

4. Explain to the patient what you are going to do and reconfirm that the patient is not allergic to the medication. Be sure to advise the patient of any complications that might result from the administration.

5. Examine the medication, including name and expiration date.

6. Assemble the equipment and attach the needle to the syringe if not preattached.

7. Calculate and draw up desired volume of medication into syringe.

8. Draw the medication into the syringe using aseptic technique. Invert and expel any air.

9. Cleanse the medication port on the IV bag into which the medication will be added.

10. Invert the bag and add the medication through the medication addition port.

11. Remove the needle and dispose of in sharps container and cleanse the medication addition port.

12. Invert the bag several times and place an administration set into it.

13. Bleed the air out of the administration set and attach a 1-inch, 18-gauge needle.

14. Cleanse the medication port on the administration set of the already established IV line and insert the needle.

15. Tape the needle securely.

16. Set the primary IV rate to TKO.

17. Adjust the flow rate of the piggyback infusion to the desired dose.

18. Label the bag.

19. Confirm establishment of the infusion.

20. Closely monitor the patient for the desired therapeutic effects as well as any undesired side effects.

ENDOTRACHEAL TUBE ADMINISTRATION

Endotracheal bolus is a procedure that allows the delivery of a medication directly to the tracheobronchial tree and lung tissue via an endotracheal tube. While the administration of medications through the endotracheal tube has theoretical application, current literature has not shown this method of medication administration to be effective and therefore other routes of administration, such as intraosseous infusion, should be used.

The number of medications administered via an endotracheal tube (ETT) is limited, and it is generally used during cardiac arrest when intravenous access is not available. The three medications most commonly administered via an ETT are atropine, epinephrine, and lidocaine. Although Narcan can be given via the ETT, other routes are available and may be preferable. There is some debate as to the exact amount of medication to be administered. However, the dose of medication should be at least equal to the IV dose and should be delivered in a volume of 5 to 10 mL.

The procedure is as follows:

1. Confirm medication order by protocol or direct on-line medical control.

2. Observe Standard Precautions (gloves and face shield).

3. Prepare the necessary equipment
   - Prefilled syringe and needle or 18- or 19-gauge needle with syringe
   - Sterile saline or water for dilution
   - Sharps container

4. Examine the ampule of medication, including name and expiration date. Hold it up to the light and inspect for discoloration or particles in the solution. Do not administer if discolored or if particles are present.

5. Pre-oxygenate the patient in anticipation of medication administration.

6. Remove the bag-valve-mask unit and inject the medication down the tube.

7. Replace the bag-valve-mask unit and resume ventilation.

8. Monitor the patient for the desired therapeutic effect and any possible undesired side effects.

9. Dispose of needle in sharps container.

INTRAOSSEOUS INFUSION

Intraosseous (IO) infusion is a puncture into the medullary cavity of a bone that provides the paramedic with a rapid access route for fluids and medications. The IO site is for temporary use only. Once the patient's condition has stabilized, another form of intravenous therapy should be initiated. Prolonged use of IO infusion has led to infection more often than traditional IV lines. IOs are indicated in the following cases:

- Hemodynamic instability
- Altered level of consciousness
- Respiratory compromise
- Cardiac arrest
- Critical burns
- Status seizures

Contraindications

- Recent fracture or absent pulses to limbs considered for access
- Skin infection or cellulitis at insertion site
- Excessive tissue or absence of adequate anatomical landmarks
- Certain orthopedic procedures (at or near site)
- Recent IO placement at insertion site (within 24 hours)

Complications

- Extravasation
- Dislodgement
- Compartment syndrome
- Target bone fracture
- Pain
- Fluid overload or reduced flow
- Cellulitis and osteomyelitis
- Growth plate injury

The procedure is as follows:

1. Confirm medication order by protocol or direct on-line medical control.
2. Observe Standard Precautions (gloves and glasses).

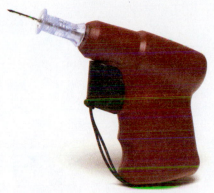

● FIGURE E–3 Intraosseous needle or
16- to 18-gauge spinal
needle. Courtesy of VidaCare

3. Prepare the necessary equipment:
   - Medication
   - Intravenous fluid and tubing
   - 10 mL syringe
   - Injectable saline
   - Intraosseous needle and needle driver (see Figure E–3)
   - Povidone-iodine preparation
   - Antibiotic ointment
   - Several rolls of Kling

4. Prepare equipment using appropriate needle set and charge the IV line.

5. Locate insertion sites using appropriate land-marking techniques.

   Proximal Tibia

   - Palpate the patella, then 2 finger widths distally, then 1 finger width medially
   - OR 1–3 cm below the tibial tuberosity (the protrusion that extends out from below the kneecap)

   Distal Tibia

   - Anteromedial tibial plane: 2 finger widths (2–3cm) above the medial malleolus (instep ankle protrusion) Remember "BIG TOE GO EASY IO" The big toe is on the medial aspect of the foot which can help us remember the alternate site.

   Humeral Head

   - Proximal aspect or humeral head. As you near the shoulder you will note a protrusion. This is the base of the greater tubercle insertion site.

6. Using aseptic technique, prepare the insertion site.

7. Select the appropriate needle set, and attach the needle hub to the EZ-IO driver.

8. Stabilize the site and insert the needle into the skin over the target site at a 90° angle to the bone. Verify that the 5 mm "No Go" line is visible on the needle/stylet. If the line is not visible, select the next larger size needle.

9. Lightly hold the driver. DO NOT PUSH, but gently guide the driver. Avoid rocking or pulsating the trigger.

10. Evidence that insertion is complete:
    - Sudden lack of resistance
    - Catheter flange touches skin

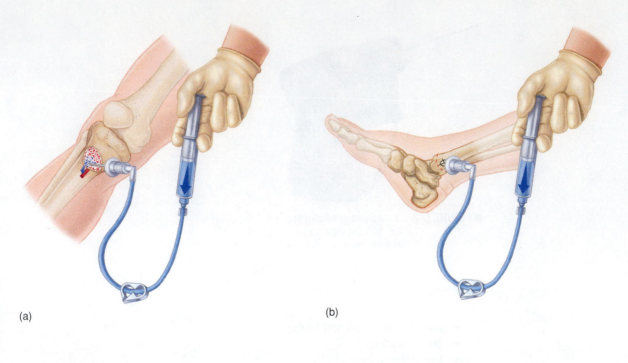

(a)

(b)

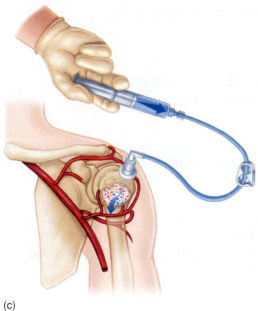

(c)

● **FIGURE E–4** Intraosseous infusion.

11. Remove the EZ-IO driver from the needle set while stabilizing the catheter hub.

12. Remove the stylet from the catheter by holding the hub and gently unscrewing counter clockwise. The cartridge shuttle is designed as a sharps container; dispose properly.

13. Attach primed EZ-Connect and secure.

14. Confirm placement by:
   • Noting blood in catheter hub prior to EZ-Connect placement.
   • Catheter is firmly seated and does not move.
   • Blood or marrow can be aspirated from the catheter (not always present).

15. Attempt saline flush with the appropriate amount of normal saline: 10 mL for adults, 5 mL for pediatrics.

16. If there is no flow, slightly adjust the needle back out and attempt to flush again. If no flow, attempt placement in an alternate site. Leave the needle and IV loop in place—DO NOT remove the IO needle.

17. If fluid administration is required, attach an IV set to the EZ-Connect and administer fluids as per MCPs.
    - 150–300 mmHg of pressure must be maintained for continuous fluid infusion. This can be obtained with the use of a pressure infuser or by administering fluid boluses with a syringe. To ensure accuracy of administration, fluid should be administered using a 60 mL syringe. Be cautious of fluid overload.

18. Secure the catheter hub and the EZ-Connect to prevent dislodgement.

19. Apply wrist band with applicable information recorded.

20. Monitor site and patient condition.

21. Catheter should be removed within 24 hours of insertion.

NEBULIZED INHALATION

Nebulized inhalation of medications is a method of delivering medications via the tracheobronchial tree using a nebulizer. Nebulized inhalation mixes oxygen with a medication, which results in a vapor that the patient can inhale. Nebulized medication administration is used in the prehospital setting for asthma and chronic obstructive pulmonary disease (COPD). Commonly used medications include albuterol (Proventil), salbutamol (Ventolin), ipatropium (Atrovent) and metaproterenol (Alupent).

1. Confirm medication order by protocol or direct on-line medical control.

2. Observe Standard Precautions (gloves and face shield).

3. Prepare the necessary equipment:
   - Side-stream nebulizer
   - Oxygen tubing
   - Medication
   - Normal saline for dilution of the bronchodilator

4. Explain procedure to the patient.

5. Take the patient's vital signs and connect the patient to a cardiac monitor.

6. Assemble the nebulizer and place the bronchodilator and saline solution in the reservoir of the side-stream nebulizer.

7. Connect the device and administer oxygen at 6 to 12 lpm and start treatment.

8. Have the patient inhale normally through the mouthpiece or through the mask.

9. Have the patient take a deep breath every three to five inhalations.

10. Continue treatment until the solution is depleted.

11. Administer supplemental oxygen following treatment.

12. Reassess the patient's vital signs and monitor the electrocardiogram results.

BAG-VALVE NEBULIZED MEDICATION ADMINISTRATION

Nebulized medication administration may be required in patients with serious airway compromise due to a severe asthma attack. In these situations, the intubated patient may receive nebulized ventolin via the bag-valve device. Commonly used medications include albuterol (Proventil), salbutamol (Ventolin), ipatropium (Atrovent) and metaproterenol (Alupent).

1. Confirm medication order by protocol or direct on-line medical control.
2. Observe Standard Precautions (gloves and face shield).
3. Prepare the necessary equipment
   - Side-stream nebulizer
   - Oxygen tubing
   - Bag-valve-mask device
   - Intubation equipment
   - Medication
   - Normal saline for dilution of the bronchodilator
4. Take the patient's vital signs and connect the patient to a cardiac monitor and O_2 saturation monitor.
5. Assemble the nebulizer and place the bronchodilator and saline solution in the reservoir of the side-stream nebulizer.
6. Connect the nebulizer to the bag-valve device and administer oxygen at 6 to 12 lpm and start treatment.
7. Ventilate the patient 12 to 20 times per minute.
8. Continue treatment until the solution is depleted.
9. Continue to assist ventilations following treatment.
10. Reassess the patient's vital signs, and monitor the electrocardiogram results.
11. Repeat treatment as necessary per protocol.

SELF-ADMINISTERED NITROUS OXIDE

A 50:50 nitrous and oxygen mixture allows the patient to regulate his or her pain control by self-administering the gas. This mixture has a rapid effect on the central nervous system and depresses cortical function with no direct effects on the respiratory system. It has an extremely short half-life. Nitrous oxide is indicated in the following situations:

- Musculoskeletal trauma
- Thermal burns
- Childbirth

Nitrous oxide is contraindicated in the following situations:

- Altered mental status
- Alcohol intoxication
- Head injury
- Abdominal or chest trauma
- Shock
- Pneumothorax
- Pulmonary disease (chronic obstructive pulmonary disease or asthma)
- Inability to comprehend or respond to verbal commands
- Inability to self-administer
- Abdominal distension suggestive of bowel obstruction

1. Confirm medication order by protocol or direct on-line medical control.
2. Observe Standard Precautions (gloves and face shield/glasses).
3. Prepare the necessary equipment
   - Medication tank(s)
   - Face mask
4. Invert the nitrous tank several times to create vaporization and mix the gases.
5. Open the pressure valves on the oxygen and nitrous tanks.
6. Explain to the patient what you are going to do and reconfirm that the patient is not allergic to the medication. Be sure to advise the patient of any complications that might result from the administration.
7. Instruct the patient on the use of the device.
8. Place the patient in a sitting position (if possible) and instruct and assist the patient in creating a tight face mask seal.
9. Coach the patient to inhale and exhale normally.
10. If the patient feels uncomfortable for any reason during the procedure, the patient should remove the mask and breathe normally.
11. No one should apply or hold the face mask to the patient except the patient.
12. Monitor the patient for changes in level of consciousness and other vital signs.

EPINEPHRINE AUTOINJECTORS (EPI-PEN)

Patients who experience severe allergic reactions often carry epinephrine autoinjectors. These injectors deliver an intramuscular dose of 0.3 mg of epinephrine for adults or 0.15 mg for children. These injectors are indicated for severe allergic reactions due to insect stings or bites, foods, medications, or other allergens.

1. Confirm medication order by protocol or direct on-line medical control.
2. Observe Standard Precautions (gloves and face shield/glasses).
3. Prepare the necessary equipment:
   - Epinephrine autoinjector
   - Personal protective equipment
4. Explain to the patient what you are going to do and reconfirm that the patient is not allergic to the medication. Be sure to advise the patient of any complications that might result from the administration.
5. Assess need for epinephrine administration.
6. Examine the autoinjector for name, dose, and expiration date.
7. Remove safety cap from autoinjector.
8. Place autoinjector on outer thigh.
9. Press hard until you hear the injector function.
10. Hold autoinjector in place for several seconds.
11. Take the patient's vital signs, connect the patient to a cardiac monitor, and watch for a change in the patient's condition.

UMBILICAL VEIN CATHETERIZATION

Umbilical vein catheterization (UVC) is a method of gaining access by placing a special catheter or tubing into the umbilical vein of the neonatal umbilicus. This procedure allows the paramedic to administer fluids or medications when percutaneous cannulation into a small vein is impossible. Indications include a neonatal patient, less than 1 week of age, in need of intravenous (IV) access but without accessible peripheral veins.

This procedure is complex and requires extensive initial training and regular updates to retain the necessary skills to perform the procedure. The immediate need for the procedure must outweigh the transport decision as this procedure cannot be accomplished in a moving ambulance. Distance to hospital may dictate that rapid transport is preferred over this procedure.

The procedure is as follows:

1. Confirm medication order by protocol or direct on-line medical control.
2. Observe Standard Precautions (gloves and face shield/glasses).
3. Prepare the necessary equipment:
   - Appropriate IV fluid and administration set (previously set up)
   - Appropriate indwelling catheter
   - Povidone-iodine or antiseptic preparations
   - Antibiotic ointment
   - 2 × 2 gauze pad
   - 1-inch tape
   - Sharps container
4. Explain to the patient's parents what you are going to do. Be sure to advise the patient's parents of any complications that might result from the procedure.
5. Restrain the infant, if necessary.
6. Clean and drape the area. The umbilicus should be cleansed, using povidone-iodine solution.
7. Place a loose tie of umbilical tape around the base of the umbilicus.
8. Locate the two umbilical arteries and one umbilical vein. The vein has a thin wall and larger lumen compared with the thick walls and smaller lumen of the umbilical arteries. Trim the cord approximately 1 cm to provide a fresh opening.
9. Using a sterile hemostat, insert the tip of the hemostat into the lumen of the vein. Gently open the hemostat to dilate the vessel.
10. Introduce and advance a heparinized–saline flushed umbilical catheter approximately 2 to 4 inches. This will place the catheter into the inferior vena cava of the infant. You should note blood return after inserting the catheter. Do not force the catheter because severe hemorrhage or liver injury may occur.
11. Hook up the catheter to a three-way stopcock. Flush the catheter with 1 mL heparin solution.
12. Secure the catheter, using the piece of umbilical tape, by tying the tape around the umbilicus.
13. After securing the catheter, hook the IV tubing to the stopcock to allow for the administration of fluids and/or medications.
14. Monitor the umbilicus for bleeding. A dressing is usually not used in this situation, so that the umbilicus can be viewed.

HERB	SOURCE: MEDICINAL INGREDIENTS	CLASSIFICATION	SUGGESTED USES
Alfalfa (*Medicago sativa*)	**Leaves and flowers:** Vitamins, minerals, proteins, enzymes	Diuretic, tonic	Helpful in stomach ailments including aiding peptic ulcers; improves appetite; relieves urinary and bowel disorders; eliminates retained water
Aloe vera (*Aloe vera*)	**Leaves:** Polysaccharides, amino acids, vitamins, minerals, aloin	Emollient, purgative	Healing and soothing for the stomach; effective laxative; useful for bug bites, skin irritation, burns, minor cuts, and scratches; helps the body to eliminate waste material in adults with bronchial asthma
Bilberry (*Vaccinium myrtillus*)	**Fruit:** Anthocyanosides	Antiseptic, astringent	Improves nighttime vision, helps preserve eyesight, prevents eye damage, regulates bowel action, and stimulates appetite
Cascara sagrada (*Rhamnus purshiana*)	**Dried bark:** Hydroxianthracene derivative (HAD), free anthraquinone	Laxative, tonic	Acts on large intestine and stimulates peristalsis; useful in constipation, dyspepsia, and other digestive complaints; liver tonic *Caution: Contraindicated in lactating or pregnant women*
Cat's claw (*Uncaria tomentosa*)	**Bark:** Proanthocyanidins, alkaloids, phytochemicals	Antiviral, antioxidant	Useful in stimulating the flow of gastric juices and pancreatic secretions; beneficial for irritable bowel syndrome and Crohn's disease; anti-inflammatory, immune system booster
Cayenne (*Capsicum frutescens*)	**Fruit:** Capsaicin, carotenoids, capsicidins heat value 40,000 scovill units per gram	Stimulant, digestive	Used to stimulate appetite and aid digestion; increases production of gastric juices and relieves gas and bowel pains or cramps; irritating to hemorrhoids *Caution: Do not use in gastrointestinal problems*
Chamomile (*Maticaria chamomilla*)	**Flower:** Volatile oil, bisabolols, flavonoids	Anti-inflammatory, antispasmodic, anti-infective, mild sedative, calmative	Calms the nerves and upset stomach; reduces anxiety, soothes ulcers, and reduces mucous membrane inflammations; good antibacterial action; rare cases of allergic reaction in those with severe hypersensitivity to ragweed pollen
Coltsfoot (*Tussilago farfara*)	**Leaves:** Flavonoids, mucilage, tannin	Expectorant, anticatarrhal, antispasmodic, demulcent	Pulmonary coughs and colds; used for asthma, bronchitis, and emphysema
Cranberry (*Vaccinium macrocrarpon*)	**Twig and fruit:** Anthocyanidins	Antioxidant, bacteriostatic effect	Cleanses and stops infections in the urinary tract

(continued)

HERB	SOURCE: MEDICINAL INGREDIENTS	CLASSIFICATION	SUGGESTED USES
Damiana (*Turnera aphrodisiaca*)	**Leaves and flowers:** Volatile oil, flavonoids, hydroquinine, glycoside	Tonic, nervine, aphrodisiac, antidepressant	Recommended as a laxative and as a general tonic; helps relieve anxiety and may enhance sexual performance *Caution: Damiana interferes with iron absorption*
Dandelion (*Taraxacum officinale*)	**Leaves and roots:** Sesquiterpenes, triterpenes, phenolic acids, carotenoids	Used in kidney and liver disorders; a natural diuretic and digestive aid; reduces blood pressure, may help prevent iron deficiency, anemia, chronic rheumatism, gout, and stiff joints	Used in kidney and liver disorders; a natural diuretic and digestive aid; reduces blood pressure and may help prevent iron deficiency, anemia, chronic rheumatism, gout, and stiff joints
Devil's claw (*Harpagophytum procumbens*)	**Root:** Harpogoside, beta-sitosterol	Anti-inflammatory, antirheumatic, analgesic, sedative	For arthritis and rheumatism; helpful to reduce swelling, relieve pain, and improve mobility in the joints *Caution: Contraindicated during pregnancy*
Dong quai (*Angelica sinensis*)	**Root:** Volatile aromatic oil, polysaccharides	Tonic immuno-stimulant, antispasmodic	Used to treat all symptoms of menopause as an alternative to estrogen therapy; regulates the hormonal system; overall tonic for female reproductive system; reduces high blood pressure and premenstrual syndrome *Caution: Contraindicated in pregnancy*
Echinacea (*Echinacea angustifolia* and *E. purpurea*)	**Root:** Echinacosides, polysaccharides, phytosterols	Antibiotic, antifungal immunostimulant	Stimulates and boosts immune function; has cortisone-like activity that helps wound healing; fights bacterial and viral infections *Caution: Contraindicated in pregnancy*
Evening primrose (*Oenothera biennis*)	**Plant:** Gamma-linolenic acid (GLA), mixed tocopherols	Antispasmodic	Used in treatment of multiple sclerosis and premenstrual syndrome; helps prevent heart disease and stroke and maintains healthy skin *Caution: Excess consumption can result in oily skin*
Eyebright (*Euphrasia officinalis*)	**Herb:** Iridoid glycosides, tannins, phenolic acids, volatile oil	Astringent, tonic	Strengthens the eye and assists in aiding the body to dissolve cataracts, heal lesions, and heal conjunctivitis
Fenugreek (*Trigonella foenum-graecum*)	**Seeds:** Flavonoids, saponin, vitamins	Demulcent, expectorant	Helpful in stomach and intestinal problems; good expectorant for coughs and colds
Feverfew (*Tanacetum parthenium*)	**Leaves:** Sesquiterpene lactones (parthenolide)	Anti-inflammatory, emmenagogue	Helps prevent migraine headaches and also useful against swelling and arthritis; stimulates digestion and improves liver function *Caution: Contraindicated in lactating or pregnant women*
Ginger (*Zingiber officinale*)	**Root:** Volatile oil, phenylalkylketones	Diaphoretic, cholagogue, carminative, stimulant	Relieves indigestion and abdominal cramping; benefit in relieving motion sickness, dizziness, nausea, and colds; ginger lowers blood clotting

HERB	SOURCE: MEDICINAL INGREDIENTS	CLASSIFICATION	SUGGESTED USES
Ginkgo biloba (*Ginkgo biloba*)	**Leaves:** Flavoglycosides (quercetin, proanthocyanidins); also contains terpenes	Antiasthmatic, bronchodilator, platelet activating factor (PAF) inhibitor	Increases blood flow to the brain; decreases memory loss, Alzheimer's disease, cerebral vascular insufficiency, and blood clotting; has the ability to neutralize free radicals and also beneficial for asthma, stress, vertigo, and tinnitus *Caution: Potential drug interaction with warfarin and aspirin; take with food*
Ginseng (*Panax schinseng*)	**Root:** Ginsenosides (triterpene saponins), glycosides	Tonic, stimulant, demulcent, stomachache	Stimulates both physical and mental activity; antifatigue (insomnia, nervousness, poor appetite); enhances immune system, inhibits exhaustion of adrenal gland; antistress *Caution: If you are pregnant or if you have high blood pressure, consult with your physician or health practitioner before using*
Goldenseal (*Hydrastis canadensis*)	**Root:** Alkaloids (hydrastine), fatty acids, volatile oil	Anti-inflammatory, tonic, mild laxative	Strengthens the immune system to help cold and flu symptoms; acts as an anti-inflammatory; helpful in constipation and in stomach disorders such as indigestion *Caution: Contraindicated during pregnancy*
Guggulipids (*Commiphora mukul*)	**Stem:** Essential oil, guggulsterone, oleoresin	Anticholesterenic	Lowers blood cholesterol by 14 to 27 percent and can lower triglycerides by 22 to 23 percent; helps reduce atherosclerotic plaques; improves the heart metabolism and increases liver metabolism of low-density lipoprotein cholesterol *Caution: Contraindicated during pregnancy*
Hawthorn (*Crategus oxyacantha*)	**Berries:** Flavonoids, glycosides, saponins, catechins, tannins, procyanidins	Cardiac tonic, hypotensive, antisclerotic	Alleviates hypertension and high blood pressure and reduces the severity of angina attacks; sedative and antispasmodic effects
Horsetail (*Equisetum arvense*)	**Herb:** Silicic acid, minerals, silica, flavoglucosides, saponins, alkaloids	Astringent, diuretic	Genitourinary complaints, mild diuretic, broken nails, hair loss, skin; stimulates an increase in white blood cells; used for arteriosclerosis and inflamed or enlarged prostate
Licorice (*Glycyrrhiza glabra*)	**Root:** Glycyrrhizin, flavonoids	Demulcent, diuretic, expectorant, laxative	Gastric ulcers, adrenal insufficiency, and hypoglycemia; good for coughs and other bronchial complaints *Caution: Contraindicated for those with high blood pressure or if pregnant*
Milk thistle (*Siybum marianum*)	**Seeds and leaves:** Flavonoids (silymarin)	Hepatoprotective, cholagogue	Promotes flow of bile; tonic for spleen, stomach, kidney, and gallbladder; beneficial for liver disease (jaundice, hepatitis, and cirrhosis)
Oats (*Avena sativa*)	**Stems and seeds:** Proteins, c-glycosyl flavones, avenacosides	Antidepressant, cardiac tonic, nervine	Lessens debility, depression, stress, and menopause symptoms; good for skin disease; tonic for impotence

(continued)

HERB	SOURCE: MEDICINAL INGREDIENTS	CLASSIFICATION	SUGGESTED USES
Parsley (*Petroselinum sativum*)	**Seeds and leaves:** Volatile oil, coumarins, flavonoids	Carminative, diuretic, expectorant, antispasmodic	Relieves gas and is a natural diuretic; good for coughs, asthma, and suppressed or difficult menstruation
Peppermint (*Mentha piperita*)	**Leaves:** Essential oil, flavonoids, carotenes	Diaphoretic, carminative, antispasmodic	Aids in digestion, flatulence, colds, influenza, and migraines
Pumpkin (*Cucurbita pepo*)	**Seeds:** Linoleic acid, cucurbitacins, zinc	Diuretic, demulcent, taeniacide, anthelmintic	Effective in reducing the size and symptoms of an enlarged prostate. Helps to expel tapeworms
Pygeum (*Pygeum africanum*)	**Bark:** Phytosterols (sitosterols), terpenoids, ferulic esters	Anti-inflammatory, diuretic, antiedema	Prostatitis, benign prostatic hypertrophy (BPH), incontinence, painful urination, dysuria, cancer of the prostate, and urinary tract disorders
Rosehips (*Rosa species*)	**Fruit:** Bioflavonoids, vitamins (C, B-complex)	Astringent, diuretic, tonic	Excellent source of vitamin C for nervous and stressful situations; helps prevent infections; blood purifier
Saw palmetto (*Serenoa serrulata*)	**Berries:** Saponins, phytosterols, fatty acids, volatile oil	Tonic, diuretic, sedative, endocrine agent	Benign prostatic hypotrophy, antiallergic and anti-inflammatory; urinary tract disorders, impotence, and infertility in women
Slippery elm (*Ulmus fulva*)	**Inner bark:** Mucilage: galactose, galacturonic acid	Demulcent, emollient, astringent, mucilage	Gastric or duodenal ulcers; inflammation of stomach, colitis, coughs, sore throat, and soothes skin disorders
St. John's wort (*Hypericum perforatum*)	**Herb:** Essential oil, glycosides (hypericin), flavonoids	Sedative, anti-inflammatory, astringent	Antidepressant; stress and irritability; immune support, anti-inflammatory, antiviral, AIDS *Caution: Avoid excessive exposure to sunlight since hypericin may render the skin photosensitive; note: most resembles monoamine oxidase inhibitors*
Valerian (*Valeriana officinalis*)	**Root:** Valerinic acid, sequiterpenes, glycoside, essential oils	Sedative, hypnotic, nervine, hypotensive	Balancing agent for hyperexcitability and exhaustion; calms nervous disorders and acts as both sedative and tranquilizer; helps headaches, high blood pressure, and stomach and menstrual cramps *Caution: Contraindicated in pregnancy; high doses should be avoided over a long period of time*
White willow (*Salix alba*)	**Bark:** Salicin, tannins, flavonoid glycosides (quercetin)	Analgesic, anti-inflammatory, tonic	Soothes headaches and reduces fevers; helps stomach ailments and heartburn; mild analgesic for arthritic and rheumatic conditions
Wild yam (*Dioscorea villosa*)	**Root:** Diosgenins, saponins, glycosides	Anti-inflammatory, cholagogue, mild diaphoretic, spasmolytic	Menopause, menstrual cramps, ovarian pain; various types of rheumatism and intestinal colic

SPECIALTY PRODUCTS

HERB	SOURCE: MEDICINAL INGREDIENTS	CLASSIFICATION	SUGGESTED USES
Bee pollen	**Bee pollen:** Vitamins, minerals, enzymes, amino acids	Supplement	Provides energy and essential nutrients; helpful in stomach ailments, hormonal system, allergies, hay fever, and exhaustion and builds resistance to diseases *Caution: Some people may be allergic to bee pollen; try small amounts of doses daily*
Coenzyme Q10	**CO Q10 Ubiquinone:** Japanese source	Supplement	Vital role in energy production at the cellular level and recommended in the treatment of cardiovascular disease; revitalizes the immune system
Flaxseed	**Seed:** Alpha-linolenic acid (ALA), omega-3 series of essential fatty acids	Purgative, demulcent, emollient	Helps lower cholesterol and blood triglyceride levels and helps prevent clot formation; digestive and urinary disorders
Glucosamine sulfate	**Crab shell:** Glucose, amino and sulfate group, mucopolysaccharides, glycoproteins	Supplement	Stimulates the synthesis of cartilage in the joints; relief from pain and inflammation around joints associated with osteoarthritis
Pycnogenol	**Pine bark extract:** Proanthocyanidins, natural soluble organic acids, glucose, bioflavonoid	Antioxidant	Strengthens blood vessels and useful for allergies; anti-inflammatory and antiaging; neutralizes existing free radicals in the blood

COMMON USES OF HERBAL EXTRACTS

Note: The following information should not be used for the diagnosis, treatment, or prevention of disease in humans. The information contained herein is in no way intended to be a guide to medical practice or a recommendation that herbs be used for medicinal purposes. This information is presented here for its educational value and as information for medical personnel.

CONDITION	COMMON HERBS
Allergy	Nettles, echinacea, goldenseal, bee pollen
Antibacterial	Echinacea, garlic, angelica, barberry
Anticatarrhal	Elder, goldenseal, sandalwood, hyssop
Antidepressant	Lavender, St. John's wort, oats, damiana, rosemary, schizandra
Antifungal	Garlic, propolis, cinnamon, black walnut
Anti-inflammatory	Oak bark, thyme, peppermint, propolis, sage
Antiseptic	Peppermint, thyme, propolis, sage, oak bark, black walnut
Antispasmodic	Valerian, passion flower, peppermint, red clover, catnip, rosemary, motherwort, thyme
Antiviral	St. John's wort, echinacea, garlic, astragalus
Aphrodisiac	Schizandra, ginseng, damiana
Arthritis or rheumatism	Devil's claw, alfalfa, wild yam, white willow, black cohosh, sarsaparilla, glucosamine

(continued)

CONDITION	COMMON HERBS
Asthma	Mullein, coltsfoot, goldenseal, ginkgo biloba, horehound, licorice, elecampane, blessed thistle, wild cherry, blue cohosh
Astringent	Nettles, plantain, red raspberry, oak bark, goldenseal, rhubarb, sage, true unicorn, yellow dock, wild cherry bark, wood betony
Blood purifiers	Red clover, blessed thistle, burdock, sarsaparilla
Bronchial support	Schizandra, mullein, coltsfoot, fenugreek, horehound, hyssop, licorice, elecampane, thyme, myrrh, goldenseal
Cardiovascular	Hawthorn, fo-ti, oats, reishi, motherwort
Cholesterol	Hawthorn, reishi, linden, guggulipids
Circulatory	Ginkgo biloba, garlic, ginger, gotu kola, capsicum, prickly ash, hawthorn, bioflavonoids
Colds or flu	Echinacea, catnip, peppermint, boneset, elder, zinc lozenge
Cough	Wild cherry bark, licorice (daytime usage), slippery elm, coltsfoot, horehound
Diarrhea (*also see* Astringent)	Oak bark, plantain, thyme, chamomile
Digestive aids	Barberry, true unicorn, yellow dock, wild cherry bark, wood betony
Diuretics	Parsley, corn silk, couch grass, dandelion (also natural potassium source), buchu, uva ursi, rosehips, sandalwood
Earache	Mullein oil, garlic, sage (to swab in and around ear)
Eczema	Nettles, chickweed, goldenseal, red clover, burdock
Expectorant	Elecampane, fenugreek, plantain, thyme, horehound, hyssop, licorice, sage, mullein, garlic
Eyes	Eyebright, chamomile (eyewash)
Fever	Sage, thyme, echinacea, white willow, nettles, wild indigo, yarrow
Flatulence	Fennel, peppermint, ginger, sage
Hay fever	Nettles, echinacea (*see* Allergy)
Headache	White willow, peppermint, lavender, passion, flower, wood betony, linden, ginger, rosemary, valerian
High blood pressure	Garlic, hawthorn, yarrow
Immune support	Astragalus, reishi, nettles, shiitake, schizandra, echinacea, propolis, garlic, Pau D'Arco, cat's claw
Impotency	Oats, ginseng, damiana, sarsaparilla
Kidney or bladder	Couch grass, meadowsweet, uva ursi, cranberry
Laxative	Cascara sagrada, rhubarb
Liver	Yellow dock, milk thistle, boneset, fo-ti, blessed thistle, barberry, lipoic acid
Lymphatics	Echinacea, red clover
Male hormonals	Sarsaparilla, ginseng, damiana, oats
Menopause or premenstrual syndrome	Dong quai, evening primrose, licorice, black cohosh
Mental alertness	Ginkgo biloba, rosemary, gotu kola, periwinkle (helpful with senility)
Migraine headaches	Feverfew

CONDITION	COMMON HERBS
Nausea	Peppermint, gingerroot, red raspberry
Nervine	Oats, passion flower, hops, chamomile, valerian, linden, reishi, rosemary, skullcap
Oral (mouthwash or antiseptics)	Myrrh gum, oak bark, goldenseal, chlorophyll
Pain (reduction)	Hops, white willow, valerian (also add immune herbal)
Prostate	Saw palmetto, pygeum, pumpkin seed
Psoriasis	Burdock, red clover, echinacea, chickweed, yellow dock, sarsaparilla
Respiratory	Horehound, mullein, myrrh, astragalus, goldenseal, elecampane
Shingles	Passion flower, echinacea, oats (proper nutritional and stress support)
Sore throat	Sage, slippery elm, wild indigo, red raspberry, echinacea
Stomachache	Fennel, ginger, peppermint, chamomile
Thyroid	Bladderwrack
Tonic	Ginseng, reishi, schizandra, gotu kola, fo-ti, nettles, oat
Ulcers	Marshmallow, licorice, slippery elm (gastric peptic), meadowsweet, red clover

APPENDIX G
PRACTICE PROBLEMS ANSWER KEY—CHAPTER 4

SECTION 1
1. 1 g   = 1000 mg
2. 1 mg   = 1000 mcg
3. 1 mg   = 0.001 g
4. 0.8 mg   = 800 mcg
5. 1.5 L   = 1500 mL
6. 400,000 mg   = 400 g
7. 800 mg   = 0.8 g
8. 500 mL   = 0.5 L
9. 37°C   = 98.6°F
10. 104°F   = 40°C
11. 1/4 gr   = 16.25 mg
12. 2 Tbsp   = 30 mL
13. 180 lb   = 82 kg
14. 7 lb   = 3.2 kg
15. 25 kg   = 55 lb

SECTION 2
1. 10 mL
2. 2 mL
3. 5 mL
4. 2 mL
5. 2.5 mL
6. 4 mL
7. 0.3 mL
8. 4 mL
9. 10 mL
10. 50 mL

SECTION 3
1. 6.8 mL
2. 1.4 mL
3. 8 mL
4. 72 mL
5. 0.2 mL

SECTION 4
1. 3200 mg/mL
2. 9 grams
3. 10 mg/mL
4. 50 mg/mL
5. 16 mcg/mL
6. 8 mg/mL
7. 1600 mg/mL
8. 60 mcg/mL
9. 10 mg/mL
10. 5 mg/mL

SECTION 5
1. 15 gtt/min
2. 15 gtts/min
3. 30 gtts/min
4. 22.5 or 23 gtt/min
5. 30 gtt/min
6. 5 gtt/min
7. 10 gtt/min
8. 18.75 or 19 gtt/min
9. 4.7 or 5 gtt/min
10. 60 gtt/min

SECTION 6
1. 7.5 gtt/min
2. 15 gtt/min
3. 30 gtt/min
4. 28.5 or 29 gtt/min
5. 10 gtt/min
6. 1 gtt
7. 12.75 or 13 gtt/min
8. 37.5 or 38 gtt/min
9. 10 mcg/kg/min
10. 4 mcg/kg/min

SECTION 7
1. 75 gtt/min
2. 50 gtt/min
3. 20 gtt/min
4. 100 gtt/min over first hour then 12.5 gtts/min over next 8 hours
5. 100 gtt/min

Loading dose, defined, 33, 34, 44
Local effects of rectal medication
    administration, 51, 61
Lopressor. *See* metoprolol
Lorazepam
    behavioral emergencies, 345, 354–355
    beta-blocker toxic exposure, 317
    excited delirium, 346
    flumazenil toxic exposure, 315
    ketamine, 388
    quick reference, 455
    rectal route of administration, 60
    sedative, as, 384
    seizures, 286, 288–289, 297
    sublingual route of administration, 57
    TCA toxicity, 326
Lovenox. *See* enoxaparin
LSD (lysergic acid diethylamide, acid), 15t, 345
Luminal. *See* phenobarbital
Lysergic acid diethylamide (LSD, acid), 15t, 345

Macrodrip administration sets, 108
Magnesium (Mg^{2+}), 86
Magnesium sulfate
    antiarrhythmic, 127, 157, 170–172
    atracurium, 397
    mineral sources for medication, 3f, 4
    pancuronium bromide, 394
    preeclampsia and eclampsia, 299,
        300–301, 306
    quick reference, 455–456
    respiratory emergencies, 226, 244–245
    rocuronium bromide, 398
    succinylcholine, 393
    vecuronium, 396
Magnesium supplements
    digoxin/digitalis toxic exposure, 327
    ethylene glycol toxic exposure, 329
    neuroleptic toxic exposure, 314
Maintenance dose, 34, 44
Mannitol
    blood osmolarity, changing, 37
    neurological trauma, 283, 284–285
    quick reference, 456
MAOIs. *See* monoamine oxidase inhibitors
    (MAOIs)
Marburg virus, 409
Mark I kit, 405–406, 405f
Mast cells, 253, 263
Mast-cell membrane stabilizers, 231t
Maxalt. *See* rizatriptan
Mazindol, 15t
MDMA (ecstasy), 15t, 345
Mechanism of action
    chemically combining with other substances, 37
    medication profile, 18
    medications, of, 25, 44
    normal metabolic pathway, altering, 37
    physical properties, changing, 37
    receptor site, binding to, 35–37, 44
Medical asepsis, 54–55, 60, 61
Medical control
    on- and off-line, 12, 24
    protocols and guidelines, 12–13, 24
Medical direction for medication
    administration, 54
Medical director, defined, 12, 24
Medical oversight of prehospital care
    drug names, 17–18
    medical control, 12, 24
    medical control protocols and guidelines,
        12–13, 24

medical director, 12, 24
medication storage, 16–17, 17f, 23
overview of, 11
regulations, standards, and legislation,
    13–16, 15f, 23, 24
Medically clean techniques, 55, 61
Medication dosage calculations
    chapter objectives, 62
    concentration problems, 71–73, 80
    IV drip, calculating, 74–76, 80–81
    IV drip based on patient weight, calculating,
        76–77, 81–82
    metric system, 63–67, 64t, 65t, 78
    milliliters per hour to drops per minute,
        converting to, 77–78, 82–83
    ordered dose, finding, 67–69, 78–79
    practice problems, 78–83, 530
    units per kilogram, finding, 69–70, 79
Medication dose-response curve, 33, 33f
Medication orders, components of, 47–48
Medication profile, components of, 18–21,
    20f, 23, 24
Medication reservoirs, 31, 44, 45
Medications. *See also* administration of
    medications; pharmacokinetics and
    pharmacodynamics; prescription drug
    information
    administration of, steps in, 56
    animal sources for, 3f, 4
    defined, 1, 24
    development, phases of, 9–10
    expedited approval, 10
    forms of
        inhalants, 21
        liquids, 19–21, 20f, 23, 24
        solid medications, 21
        suppositories, 21
    laboratory-produced sources for, 3f, 4, 24, 271
    mineral sources for, 3f, 4
    names of, 17–18
    newly approved, classification of, 8–9
    plant sources for, 3–4, 3f
    preparation of, 53, 61
    research and bringing to market, 6, 6f, 24
    response to, factors altering, 39–40
    sources of information about, 4–5, 5f, 5t
    standards for, 16–17, 23
    storage of, 16, 23
    unlabeled uses, 11, 24
Mental status change, 270. *See also* behavioral
    emergencies, medications for
Meperidine
    controlled drug schedule, 15t
    miosis, 310
    overdose, 333, 334
    pain management, 370, 371t, 374–375
    quick reference, 456–457
Mescaline, 15t
Metabolic acidosis, 194
Metabolic-endocrine emergencies, medications
    for. *See also* insulin
    blood glucose levels, regulation of, 265,
        267, 282
    case presentations, 271–272, 279–280,
        280–281
    chapter objectives, 264
    chapter summary, 281
    dextrose in water, 276–277
    diabetes, types of, 267–268
    diabetes mellitus, described, 265, 266t, 281, 282
    diabetic ketoacidosis, 266t, 268, 269, 281, 282
    glucagon, 274–276, 281, 282

hyperosmolar hyperglycemic nonketotic state,
    266t, 269
hypoglycemia, 266t, 270–271
insulin, 270t, 271–272
key words, 281–282
oral hypoglycemics, 268, 488–489, 499
overview of, 264, 281
thiamine, 277–278
Metabolism, defined, 32, 44
Metaproterenol
    allergic reactions and anaphylaxis, 262
    asthma, 231t
    inhalational route of administration, 58
    quick reference, 457
    respiratory emergencies, 226, 239–240
    sympathomimetic syndrome, 311
Metered-dose inhalers, 58–59, 61
Methadone, 15t, 16, 334
Methanol exposure, 331–332
Methaqualone, 15t
Methemoglobin, 320, 321, 343, 407
Methoxamine, 311
Methylphenidate, 15t
Methylprednisolone
    allergic reactions, 255, 258–259
    asthma, 231t, 232
    quick reference, 457–458
    respiratory emergencies, 226, 245–246
    spinal cord injury, 283
Methyltestosterone, 15t
Methylxanthines, 231t, 232
Metoclopramide, 360, 361, 367–368, 458
Metoprolol
    antiarrhythmic, 155t
    quick reference, 458–459
    selective beta-blocker, 127, 149–151
Metric system
    conversions within and with customary
        system, 64–65, 65t
    multiples, submultiples, and prefixes, 64, 64t
    rules of, 65–67
    units of, 63–64, 65
Mexiletine, 155t
MicroNefrin. *See* racemic epinephrine
Midazolam
    behavioral emergencies, 345, 355–356
    excited delirium, 346
    flumazenil toxic exposure, 315
    induction agent, 398, 399
    intranasal route of administration, 57
    ketamine, 388
    PAI, 399, 400
    quick reference, 459
    sedative, as, 384, 386–387
    seizures, 286, 289–291
Milk thistle, 525
Milrinone, 127, 144–145, 460
Mineral sources for medications, 3f, 4
Minidrip administration sets, 108
Minimal sedation, 370
Minimum effective concentration,
    defined, 38, 39f, 45
Moderate sedation, 370
Monoamine oxidase inhibitors (MAOIs)
    fentanyl, 376
    meperidine, 375
    metoclopramide, 368
    prescription drug information, 486, 499
    promethazine, 365
Moricizine, 155t
Morphine sulfate
    agonist property, 37

Opium plant, 3f, 4
Oraflex. *See* benoxaprofen
Oral hypoglycemics
    prescription drug information, 488–489, 499
    type II diabetes, 268
Oral route of administration
    enteral tract, 51
    rate of absorption, 29t, 30f
    toxic substances, 309
Organic causes of behavioral emergencies,
        345, 359
Organophosphates
    atropine sulfate, 173
    toxic exposure, 334–338
Orogastric/nasogastric tube route of medication
        administration, 51
Orphan Drug Act of 1983, 10–11
Orphan drugs, 10–11
Osmosis, 26, 27, 88, 88f, 113
Osmotrol. *See* mannitol
Ouabain, 174
Over-the-needle catheters, 107
Oxidative stress, 129
Oxycodone
    controlled drug schedule, 15t
    naloxone, 334
Oxygen
    administration, purpose of, 226–227
    anaphylaxis, 255
    asthma, 230–231
    capnography, 229, 250
    carbon monoxide exposure, 318, 319
    cardiovascular medication, 127, 129–131,
        131t, 223, 224
    cylinders, common sizes of, 131t
    devices for, 227–228
    flow rate by device, 131t
    hyperbaric oxygen therapy, 318, 319, 322
    pulse oximetry, 228–229, 250
    quick reference, 466
    respiratory emergencies, 225, 226–229, 250
    ventilatory support, 228–229, 250
Oxygen devices
    nasal cannula, 227
    non-rebreather mask, 227–228
    simple face mask, 227
    Venturi mask, 228
Oxygen free radicals, 129
Oxygen saturation. *See* pulse oximetry
Oxytocin
    animal source for medication, 3f, 4
    postpartum hemorrhage, 299, 302–303, 306
    quick reference, 467

Pacing, overdrive, 314
Pacing, transcutaneous
    beta-blocker toxic exposure, 317
    calcium channel blocker toxic
        exposure, 318
    organophosphate and carbamate toxic
        exposure, 336
PAI (pharmacologically-assisted intubation),
        399–400
Pain management. *See* analgesics; sedation and
        pain management; specific medications
Pancreas, 265
Pancreatin, 4
Pancuronium bromide
    neuromuscular blocker, 390, 391, 391t, 393,
        394–395
    quick reference, 467
    rapid-sequence induction, 399

Paracetamol. *See also* acetaminophen
    pain management, 383–384
    quick reference, 424–425
Paraquat, 130
Parasympathetic nervous system (PNS)
    ACh receptors, 116, 117f, 121–123, 122f,
        123f, 123t
    ANS division, 115, 115f, 116t, 117f
    cholinergic system, 131
    defined, 125
    ganglia, 116, 117f, 120, 121f
    organization of, 120, 121f
    organs, actions on, 132t
    stimulation of, 120–121
Parasympatholytics, 123, 128. *See also*
        anticholinergics
Parasympathomimetics, 123
Paregoric, 334
Parenteral medications. *See also* specific routes
        of administration
    advantages and disadvantages, 51t
    defined, 20–21, 20f, 23, 24
    endotracheal, 52, 58, 61
    inhalational, 53, 56, 58–59, 61
    intradermal, 52, 61
    intramuscular, 52, 57, 59–60, 61
    intranasal, 52, 57, 61
    intraosseous, 52, 58, 61
    intravenous, 52, 57–58, 60, 61
    subcutaneous, 52, 57, 60, 61
    sublingual injection, 52, 61
    topical/transdermal, 52, 56
    umbilical, 53
    use by paramedics, 50
    vaginal, 53
Parnate. *See* tranylcypromine
Paroxetine
    serotonin syndrome, 311
    toxic exposure, 339
Paroxysmal supraventricular tachycardia, 169
Parsley, 526
Partial (focal) seizures, 285
Pasadena Cyanide Antidote Kit, 320, 321–324,
        322f, 407–408, 408f
Passive transport, 26–27, 45
Pathologic state, and response to medications, 40
Patient history, and toxicological emergencies,
        308–309
Patient weight
    IV drip, calculating, 76–77, 81–82
    units per kilogram, finding, 69–70, 79
Pavulon. *See* pancuronium bromide
Paxil. *See* paroxetine
PCP (phencyclidine), 15t, 345, 416
Peak concentration of medication, 35
Pediatric patients
    fluid resuscitation, 423
    medication administration techniques, 59–60
    medication therapy, 40–41, 41f
Pellagra, 277
Penicillin
    anaphylaxis, 253
    cutaneous anthrax, 411
Pentazocine, 15t, 310, 333, 334, 347
Pepcid. *See* famotidine
Peppermint, 526
Pepsin, 4
Percocet. *See* oxycodone
Percodan. *See* oxycodone
Periods, metric system, 66
Peripheral nervous system, 114–115, 115f, 125
Personal protective equipment, 404, 412

Peyote, 15t
PH
    blood, of, 228, 250
    medication, of, 28, 45
Pharmacognosy
    animal sources of medications, 3f, 4
    defined, 2, 24
    laboratory-produced medications,
        3f, 4, 24, 271
    medication information, sources of, 4–5, 5f, 5t
    mineral sources of medications, 3f, 4
    plant sources of medications, 2, 3–4, 3f
Pharmacokinetics and pharmacodynamics
    case study, 43
    chapter objectives, 25
    chapter summary, 43
    key words, 44–45
    pharmacodynamics
        defined, 25, 45
        geriatric patients, 41–42
        mechanisms of action of medications,
            35–37, 44
        medication potency and efficacy, 37–38,
            38f, 44
        medication response, factors altering,
            39–40
        pediatric patients, 40–41, 41f
        pregnancy and lactation, 42–43, 42t
        therapeutic index, 38–39, 45
    pharmacokinetics
        absorption, 27–30, 29f, 29t, 30f, 45
        accumulation, 34, 44
        biotransformation, 32, 33f, 44
        clearance, 34
        defined, 25, 45
        distribution, 30–31, 44, 45
        elimination, 32–33, 44
        medication dosing, 33, 33f, 44
        medication half-life, 34, 44
        medication profile, 18
        onset, peak, and duration of action,
            34–35, 45
        physiology of transport, 26–27, 44, 45
        processes in, 26, 44
    pharmacology, defined, 25–26
Pharmacological class (family) of
    drugs, 18
Pharmacologically-assisted intubation (PAI),
    399–400
Pharmacologists, defined, 1, 24
Pharmacology, defined, 1, 24
Pharmacology, general information about
    case study, 22–23
    chapter objectives, 1
    chapter summary and key words, 23–24
    drugs, defined, 1, 23
    FDA classification of newly approved
        medications, 8–9
    general terminology and abbreviations,
        6–7, 7–8t
    historical considerations, 1–2
    medical oversight, 11–18, 15t, 17f, 23, 24
    medication, unlabeled uses of, 11, 24
    medication profile, components of, 18–21,
        20f, 23, 24
    medication research and bringing a
        medication to market, 6, 6f, 24
    new medication development, 9–11
    pharmacognosy, 2–5, 3f, 5f, 5t, 24
    pharmacological terminology, 21–22
Phencyclidine (PCP), 15t, 345, 416
Phenelzine, 375

Phenergan. *See* promethazine
Phenobarbital
    beta-blocker toxic exposure, 317
    controlled drug schedule, 15t
    neuroleptic toxic exposure, 314
    quick reference, 468
    sedative, 384
    seizures, 286, 293, 294
Phenothiazines
    anticholinergic properties, 312
    neuroleptic toxic exposure, 314
    pralidoxime, 338
Phentermine, 15t
Phentolamine, 136
Phenylephrine
    neuroleptic toxic exposure, 314
    sympathetic agonist, 127, 137–138
    sympathomimetic syndrome, 311
Phenylpropanolamine, 311
Phenytoin
    antiarrhythmic and anticonvulsant, 127, 155t, 157, 168–169
    beta-blocker toxic exposure, 317
    dextrose-containing IV solutions, 292
    digoxin/digitalis toxic exposure, 327
    neuroleptic toxic exposure, 314
    quick reference, 468
    seizures, 286, 291–292
"Phenytoin equivalents," 292
Pheochromocytoma, 140, 223
Phosgene, 408
Phosgene oxime poisoning, 407
Phosphate (HPO_4-), 86
Phosphodiesterase inhibitors, 143–145
Physicians' Desk Reference, 11
Physiological barriers, to medication distribution, 31, 44
Physostigmine
    anticholinergic toxicity, 313
    edrophonium chloride, 169
    quick reference, 469
Piggyback infusion, 52, 61, 513–515
Pindolol, 316
Pitressin. *See* vasopressin
Placebos, 10
Placenta previa, 302, 306
Placental barrier to medication distribution, 31
Plague, 411–412
Plant sources for medications, 2, 3–4, 3f
Plasma, 89, 89f, 113
Plasma protein fraction, 91, 93–94, 419
Plasma reservoirs, 31
Plasmanate. *See* plasma protein fraction
Platelet aggregation inhibitors, 128, 176–185
Platelets (thrombocytes), 89f, 90, 113
Plavix. *See* clopidogrel
Plurals, metric system, 66
Pneumonic plague, 412
Pneumothorax, and nitrous oxide, 199, 378
PNS. *See* parasympathetic nervous system (PNS)
Poison ivy, 252, 252t
Polygeline, 92, 97–98, 420
Postganglionic nerves, 115, 116–118, 117f, 118f
Postpartum hemorrhage, 299, 302–303, 306
Potassium (K^+), 86
Potassium channel blockers, 155t, 156f
Potassium levels
    DKA, 268
    insulin therapy, 273
Potassium supplements, 339
Potency of medications, 37
Potentiation, defined, 22

Powder (medication form), 21
Pralidoxime
    nerve agents, 405–406, 405f
    quick reference, 469
    toxic exposures, 335, 336, 337–338
Prednisone
    allergic reactions, 255
    asthma, 231t
Preeclampsia, 244, 300, 306
Prefilled syringes, 20, 20f, 24
Preganglionic nerves, 115, 117f
Pregnancy, 42, 42t. *See also* obstetrical and gynecological emergencies, medications for
Prescription drug information. *See also* specific medications
    analgesics, 496–497, 498
    antianginals, 482–483, 498
    antiarrhythmics, 483–484, 499–500
    anticoagulants, 484–485, 498
    anticonvulsants, 485, 498
    antidepressants, 486–487, 499
    antidiabetics, 487–489, 499
    antihypertensives, 489, 500
    antipsychotics, 489–490, 500
    anxiolytics, 490–491, 498
    beta-blockers, 491–492, 500
    bronchodilators, 492–493, 500
    calcium channel blockers, 494, 501
    cardiac glycosides, 494–495, 501
    cardiotonics, 494–495, 501
    diuretics, 495–496, 501
    hypnotics, 497, 501
    insulins, 487–488, 499
    MAOIs, 486, 499
    narcotics, 496–497, 498
    oral hypoglycemics, 488–489, 499
    sedatives, 497, 501
    sympathomimetics, 492–493, 500
    theophyllines, 493, 500
    tricyclic antidepressants, 486–487, 499
Preterm labor
    described, 303
    magnesium sulfate, 244, 301
    medications for, 299, 303–304
    terbutaline, 237
Primacor. *See* milrinone
Procainamide
    antiarrhythmic, 127, 155, 155t, 160–161, 161f
    anticholinergic toxicity, 313
    atracurium, 397
    digoxin/digitalis toxic exposure, 327
    neuroleptic toxic exposure, 315
    pancuronium bromide, 394
    quick reference, 470
    rocuronium bromide, 398
    sotalol, 149
    succinylcholine, 393
    vecuronium, 396
Procardia. *See* nifedipine
Prochlorperazine
    antiemetic, 360, 361, 366–367
    neuroleptic malignant syndrome, 311
    quick reference, 470
Prodrug, defined, 32
Promethazine
    allergic reactions and anaphylaxis, 257
    antiemetic, 360, 361, 364–365
    quick reference, 470–471
Pronestyl. *See* procainamide
Propafenone, 155t
Propofol, 384, 389–390, 471
Propranolol

    antiarrhythmic, 155t, 157
    efficacy of, 37, 38, 38f
    neuroleptic toxic exposure, 314
    nonselective beta-blocker, 127, 147–148
    quick reference, 471–472
Proprietary (trade) names of drugs, 17, 18
ProSom. *See* estazolam
Protocols
    medication administration, 54
    medication orders, 57
    treat-and-release, 13
    treatment protocols, 13, 24
Protopam. *See* pralidoxime
Proventil. *See* albuterol
Prozac. *See* fluoxetine
Psychological factors, in response to medications, 40
Pulmonary edema, 240
Pulse oximetry
    carbon monoxide exposure, 319
    defined, 129, 223, 250
    false readings, 228–229
    normal values, 228
    purpose of, 228
Pulseless ventricular tachycardia, 244
Pumpkin, 526
Pure Food and Drug Act of 1906, 13
Purity standards for medications, 16–17
Purple foxglove plant, 2, 3f, 327
Pycnogenol, 527
Pygeum, 526
Pyridoxine, 329

Quinidine
    anticholinergic toxicity, 313
    digoxin/digitalis toxic exposure, 327
    neuroleptic toxic exposure, 315
    rocuronium bromide, 398
    sodium channel blocker, 155t
    sotalol, 149

Rabbit fever, 410
Racemic epinephrine. *See* epinephrine, racemic
Radiological agents
    overview of, 412, 414
    protection from, 413
    types of radiation, 413
Ranitidine, 254, 257
Rapid-sequence induction, 398–399
Ratio and proportion method
    concentration of solution, finding, 73
    dose, calculation of, 68
    solute, amount of, 72
    units per kilogram, finding, 70
    volume to infuse, based on concentration, 72
Raxibacumab, 411
Reactive oxygen species, 129
"Rebound worsening," 236
Receptor sites for medications, 35–37, 44
Recombinant DNA technology, defined, 2, 24
Recombinant tissue plasminogen activator (rtPA) (alteplase), 2, 128, 189–190, 426–427
Rectal route of administration
    defined, 61
    general use, 51–52
    pediatric use, 60
    rate of absorption, 29t
Refractory, defined, 22
Regional blood flow, and distribution of medication, 31
Regional poison centers, 308